17
EDITION

Basic Pharmacology for Nurses

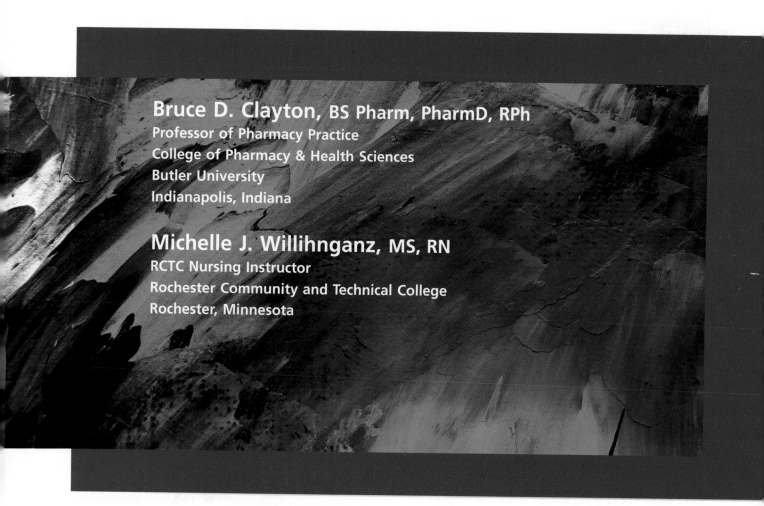

Bruce D. Clayton, BS Pharm, PharmD, RPh
Professor of Pharmacy Practice
College of Pharmacy & Health Sciences
Butler University
Indianapolis, Indiana

Michelle J. Willihnganz, MS, RN
RCTC Nursing Instructor
Rochester Community and Technical College
Rochester, Minnesota

ELSEVIER

ELSEVIER

3251 Riverport Lane
St. Louis, Missouri 63043

BASIC PHARMACOLOGY FOR NURSES, SEVENTEENTH EDITION   ISBN: 978-0-323-31112-0

Notices

Knowledge and best practice in this field are constantly changing. As new research and experience broaden our understanding, changes in research methods, professional practices, or medical treatment may become necessary.

Practitioners and researchers must always rely on their own experience and knowledge in evaluating and using any information, methods, compounds, or experiments described herein. In using such information or methods they should be mindful of their own safety and the safety of others, including parties for whom they have a professional responsibility.

With respect to any drug or pharmaceutical products identified, readers are advised to check the most current information provided (i) on procedures featured or (ii) by the manufacturer of each product to be administered, to verify the recommended dose or formula, the method and duration of administration, and contraindications. It is the responsibility of practitioners, relying on their own experience and knowledge of their patients, to make diagnoses, to determine dosages and the best treatment for each individual patient, and to take all appropriate safety precautions.

To the fullest extent of the law, neither the Publisher nor the authors, contributors, or editors, assume any liability for any injury and/or damage to persons or property as a matter of products liability, negligence or otherwise, or from any use or operation of any methods, products, instructions, or ideas contained in the material herein.

Previous editions copyrighted 2013, 2010, 2007, 2004, 2001, 1997, 1993, 1989, 1985, 1981, 1977, 1973, 1969, 1965, 1961, and 1957.

Library of Congress Cataloging-in-Publication Data

Names: Clayton, Bruce D., 1947- , author. | Willihnganz, Michelle J., author.
Title: Basic pharmacology for nurses / Bruce D. Clayton, Michelle Willihnganz.
Description: 17th edition. | St. Louis, Missouri : Elsevier, [2016] |
    Includes bibliographical references and index.
Identifiers: LCCN 2015046359 | ISBN 9780323311120 (pbk.)
Subjects: | MESH: Pharmaceutical Preparations—administration & dosage |
    Pharmacological Phenomena | Patient Education as Topic | Nurses'
    Instruction
Classification: LCC RM300 | NLM QV 4 | DDC 615/.1—dc23 LC record available at
http://lccn.loc.gov/2015046359

Senior Content Strategist: Nancy O'Brien
Content Development Manager: Jean Sims Fornango
Senior Content Development Specialist: Laura Selkirk
Publishing Services Manager: Julie Eddy
Senior Project Manager: Mary Stueck
Design Direction: Renée Duenow

Printed in Canada

Last digit is the print number: 9 8 7 6 5 4 3 2 1

Working together
to grow libraries in
developing countries

www.elsevier.com • www.bookaid.org

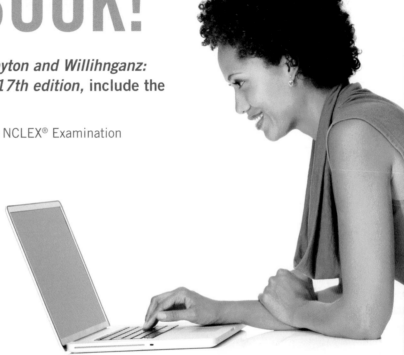

To Francine,
for her unfailing support and encouragement,
and to Sarah, Nathaniel, and Evelyn,
and
Beth, Nicholas, and Clayton,
the lights of our lives!

—BDC

To Kevin, the love of my life;
and to my wonderful daughters who always stand beside me.

—MJW

Reviewers and Ancillary Contributors

REVIEWERS

Frances Ann Bivens, RN, BSN
Coordinator, School of Practical Nursing
McDowell County Career and Technology Center
Welch, West Virginia

Edwin A. Caniete, MBM, LVN
Instructor
Preferred College of Nursing
Van Nuys, California

Fleurdeliza T. Cuyco, BS
Pharmacology Instructor
Preferred College of Nursing
Los Angeles, California

Sally A. Fitzgerald, MSN, RN, CCM
Associate Professor, Nursing
Community College of Beaver County
Monaca, Pennsylvania

Wendy Greenspan, MSN, RN, CCRN, CNE
Assistant Professor, Nursing
Rockland Community College
Suffern, New York

Janis Grimland, RN, BSN
Vocational Nursing Program Coordinator
Hill College
Hillsboro, Texas

Sarah E. (Herron) Johnson, FNP-BC
Family Nurse Practitioner
Wellmont Medical Associates
Abingdon, Virginia

Kimberly Kelly, RN, BSN, MSN
School Director, VN Program Director
The Vocational Nursing Institute, Inc.
Houston, Texas

Kristi S. Miller, RN, OCN, MSN
Associate Chair of Nursing
Asheville Buncombe Technical Community College
Asheville, North Carolina

Nora MacLeod-Glover, BSc (Pharm), PharmD
Associate Professor, Health Systems
University of Toronto
Toronto, Ontario, Canada

Cassandra Porter, RN, MSN
Nursing Instructor
Lake Land College
Mattoon, Illinois

Diana Seekely, RN, BSN
Clinical Coordinator
The Vocational Nursing Institute, Inc.
Houston, Texas

Travis E. Sonnett, PharmD
Clinical Pharmacy Specialist/Adjunct Clinical Professor
Mann-Grandstaff VA Medical Center
College of Pharmacy, Washington State University
Spokane, Washington

Sister Ann Wiesen, RN, BSN, MRA
Director of Practical Nursing
Erwin Technical Center
Tampa, Florida

ANCILLARY CONTRIBUTORS

Laura Bevlock Kanavy, RN, BSN, MSN
Director, Practical Nursing Program
Career Technology Center of Lackawanna County
Scranton, Pennsylvania
Test Bank

Charla K. Hollin, RN
Rich Mountain Community College
Allied Health Division Chair
Mena, Arkansas
TEACH

Mark Matusiak
Instructor
Rockwood Summit High School
St. Louis, Missouri
Open Book Quizzes

Advisory Board

Preface

The seventeenth edition of *Basic Pharmacology for Nurses*, in the tradition of the book's standards first established in 1957, advocates the administration of medication with safety and precision while focusing on medication safety through medication monitoring and patient education. In the practice setting, the nurse not only must demonstrate knowledge of the underlying disease process but also must be able to perform an accurate assessment to identify individualized nursing diagnoses. The nurse must also plan and implement care in a manner that involves the patient as an active participant in decisions affecting care. Therefore a primary concern throughout this book is the integration of patient teaching about drug therapy to enable the patient to reach therapeutic goals and attain an optimum level of health. The nurse must also validate patient understanding to ensure that the individual has the ability to provide safe self-care and monitoring of the prescribed treatment plan. User friendly in content, structure, and layout, the text is concise and easy to read. With its emphasis on the seven Rights of Drug Administration (right drug, right time, right indication, right dosage, right patient, right route, and right documentation), *Basic Pharmacology for Nurses* provides students with the information needed to provide safe, effective nursing care for patients receiving drug therapy.

ORGANIZATION AND SPECIAL FEATURES

CONTENT THREADS

Basic Pharmacology for Nurses, seventeenth edition, shares some features and design elements with other Elsevier books that you may be using. The purpose of these Content Threads is to make it easier for students and instructors to use the variety of books required by a fast-paced and demanding curriculum.

The shared features in *Basic Pharmacology for Nurses*, seventeenth edition, include the following:
- Cover and internal design similarities; the colorful, student-friendly design encourages reading and learning of this core content
- Numbered lists of Objectives that begin each chapter
- Key Terms with pronunciations at the beginning of each chapter; the key terms are in color when they are defined in the chapter
- Bulleted lists of Key Points at the end of each chapter

- Multiple-choice and multiple-response Review Questions for the NCLEX® Examination at the end of each chapter; answers are provided on the Evolve student website.

In addition to content and design threads, these textbooks benefit from the advice and input of the Elsevier Advisory Board.

CONTENTS

Unit I explores pharmacology foundations, principles, lifespan considerations, the nursing process with pharmacology, and patient education. Unit II contains the unique Illustrated Atlas of Medication Administration that provides extensive step-by-step instructions and illustrations that show primary routes of administration and proper administration techniques for all forms of medications.

Units III through X provide an overview of each drug class, followed by narrative discussions of the most common individual drugs. The units and chapters are organized by body system.

CHAPTER ORGANIZATION

- Each drug chapter in Units III through X begins with an overview of a clinical problem and its management.
- The general nursing implications section focuses on how the nursing process is applied to the medical condition being discussed, including clearly identified headings for Assessment, Implementation, and Patient Education. The Patient Education section helps the nurse incorporate patient education designed to promote health into the overall treatment plan.
- Drug monographs are provided for each major drug class. These monographs describe Actions, Uses, and Therapeutic Outcomes for each class.
- A drug class–specific nursing implications section for each drug monograph highlights Premedication Assessment, Product Availability, Dosing Instructions, Common Adverse Effects, Serious Adverse Effects, and Drug Interactions.

SPECIAL FEATURES

Basic Pharmacology for Nurses includes special features designed to foster effective learning and comprehension.

- Chapter opening features include lists of Objectives and Key Terms with pronunciations.
- Clinical Pitfall and Medication Safety Alert boxes highlight critically important clinical considerations to help students practice safety and reduce medication errors.
- Clinical Goldmine boxes put a spotlight on tips and best practices for clinical procedures.
- Lifespan Considerations boxes focus on the implications of drug therapy for children, pregnant and breastfeeding women, and older adults.
- Herbal Interactions boxes discuss well-documented interactions among drugs, herbal therapies, and dietary supplements.
- A handy bulleted list of Key Points at the end of most chapters facilitates review of essential chapter content.

NEW TO THIS EDITION

- This edition includes the latest FDA approvals and withdrawals, including up-to-date clinical drug indications and new drugs.
- Increased emphasis on medication safety stresses imperative information for patient protection.
- Additional information on genetics, pharmacogenomics, and racial/gender factors in drug actions is included to highlight the most up-to-date research.

TEACHING AND LEARNING PACKAGE

FOR STUDENTS

- The Evolve Website provides free student resources, including answers and rationales for in-text Review Questions for the NCLEX® Examination, a math review, links to the FDA's *Catalog of FDA-Approved Drug Products* and *Safety Information and Adverse Event Reporting Program*, a collection of Patient Teaching handouts, and a Spanish/English audio glossary. Helpful features also include a Key Terms Glossary, fully customizable Patient Self-Assessment Forms provided as "completable" PDF documents, a collection of 500 NCLEX®-style Review Questions, and interactive Drug Dosage Calculators.

- The revised Study Guide provides additional learning resources that complement those in the textbook. Questions for each chapter follow the objectives in the book for additional focus on these key concepts. A new section on matching starts each chapter, and a patient scenario is included with the chapters that detail the medications. Each question has a page number identified to help the student find the answer in the textbook. Answers to the Study Guide questions are available from instructors.

FOR INSTRUCTORS

The comprehensive *Evolve Resources with TEACH Instructor Resource* provides a rich array of resources that includes the following:

- Updated TEACH Lesson Plans, based on textbook learning objectives, provide ready-to-use lesson plans that tie together all of the text and ancillary components provided for *Basic Pharmacology for Nurses*.
- The collection of PowerPoint Lecture Slides is specific to the text.
- A Test Bank, delivered in ExamView, now provides an expanded collection of approximately 900 multiple-choice and alternate-format NCLEX®-style questions. Each question includes the Correct Answer, Rationale, Step of the Nursing Process, and NCLEX® Patient Needs Category, as well as corresponding text page numbers.
- Open Book Quizzes that feature at least 5 questions for every chapter.
- A collection of five Audience Response Questions per chapter—discussion-oriented questions with correct answer and rationale—are provided within the TEACH PowerPoint lecture outlines for use with iClicker and other audience response systems.
- The Image Collection contains every reproducible image from the text. Images are suitable for incorporation into classroom lectures, PowerPoint presentations, or distance-learning applications.
- Answer keys are provided for the Study Guide.

Special Features

Basic Pharmacology for Nurses focuses on medication safety through medication monitoring and patient education. Full-color art and design features accompany detailed, understandable discussions of drugs organized by body system.

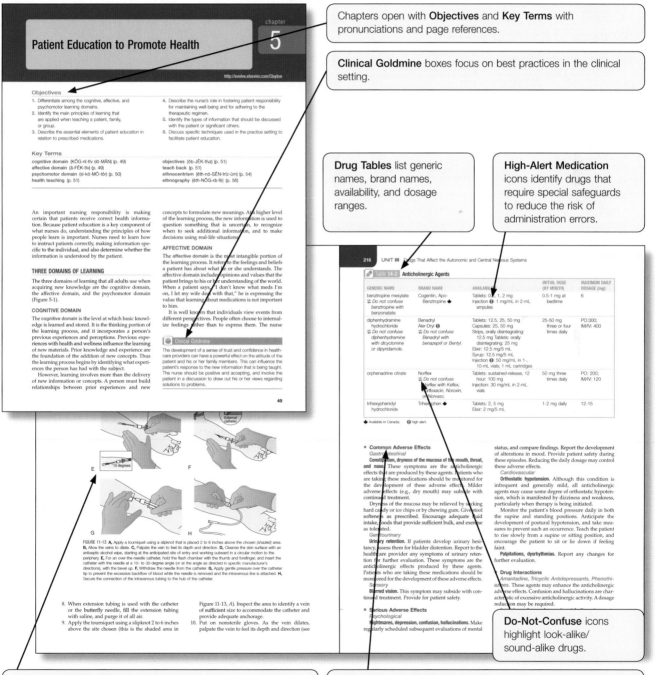

Chapters open with **Objectives** and **Key Terms** with pronunciations and page references.

Clinical Goldmine boxes focus on best practices in the clinical setting.

Drug Tables list generic names, brand names, availability, and dosage ranges.

High-Alert Medication icons identify drugs that require special safeguards to reduce the risk of administration errors.

Do-Not-Confuse icons highlight look-alike/sound-alike drugs.

Step-by-step **full-color art** shows proper medication administration techniques.

Comprehensive **Drug Class** discussions with clearly identified **Nursing Implications** are featured.

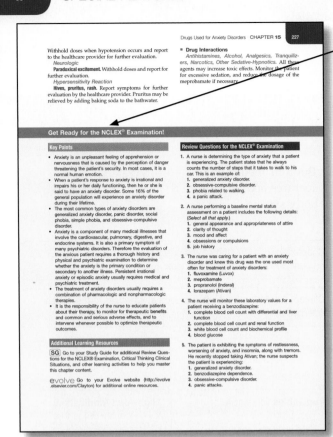

Get Ready for the NCLEX® Examination! sections include Key Points, Additional Learning Resources, and Review Questions for the NCLEX® Examination.

- **Patient Education and Health Promotion** is emphasized in the overall treatment plan.
- **Lifespan Considerations** boxes focus on implications of drug therapy for children, pregnant and breastfeeding women, and older adults.
- **Clinical Pitfall and Medication Safety Alert** boxes highlight critically important clinical considerations.
- **Herbal Interactions** boxes describe possible adverse effects of alternative therapies.

STUDY GUIDE

Includes *Practice Questions for the NCLEX® Examination* for each textbook chapter. Answers to the revised study guide are available from your instructor.

Contents

chapter

Drug Definitions, Standards, and Information Sources

1

http://evolve.elsevier.com/Clayton

Objectives

1. Differentiate between the chemical, generic, and brand names of drugs.
2. Identify the various methods used to classify drugs.
3. Identify sources of drug information available for healthcare providers.
4. Cite sources of credible drug information on the Internet.
5. Discuss the difference between prescription and nonprescription drugs.
6. Describe the process of developing and bringing new drugs to market.
7. Differentiate between the Canadian *chemical* names and the *proper* name of a drug.

Key Terms

pharmacology (făr-mă-KŎL-ŏ-jē) (p. 1)
therapeutic methods (thĕr-ă-PYŪ-tĭk MĔTH-ĕdz) (p. 1)
drugs (p. 1)
chemical name (KĔM-ĭ-kŭl) (p. 1)
generic name (jĕ-NĂR-ĭk) (p. 1)
brand name (p. 2)
prescription drugs (p. 2)
nonprescription drugs (p. 2)

over-the-counter (OTC) drugs (p. 2)
illegal drugs (ĭl-LĒ-gŭl) (p. 2)
schedules (SKĔD-jūlz) (p. 5)
black box warnings (p. 8)
orphan drugs (ŌR-făn) (p. 8)
Food and Drugs Act and Regulations (p. 9)
Controlled Drugs and Substances Act (p. 10)

Pharmacology (from the Greek *pharmakon,* meaning "drugs," and *logos,* meaning "science") deals with the study of drugs and their actions on living organisms. Diseases that cause illness may be treated in several different ways, which are referred to as *therapies.* The various approaches to therapy are called *therapeutic methods.* Examples of therapeutic methods include the following:

- **Drug therapy:** Treatment with drugs
- **Diet therapy:** Treatment with diet (e.g., a low-salt diet for patients with cardiovascular disease)
- **Physiotherapy:** Treatment with natural physical forces (e.g., water, light, heat)
- **Psychological therapy:** The identification of stressors and methods that can be used to reduce or eliminate stress

Most illnesses caused by diseases require a combination of therapeutic methods for successful treatment.

Drugs (from the Dutch *droog,* meaning "dry") are chemical substances that have an effect on living organisms. Therapeutic drugs, which are often called *medicines,* are those drugs that are used for the prevention or treatment of diseases. Up until the early

to mid-twentieth century, dried plants were the most abundant source of medicines; thus the word *drug* was applied to them.

DRUG NAMES, STANDARDS, LEGISLATION, AND DEVELOPMENT IN THE UNITED STATES

DRUG NAMES

All drugs have several names, which may cause confusion. When administering the prescribed drug, the spelling on the drug package must correspond exactly with the spelling of the drug ordered to ensure that the proper medicine is administered.

Each drug has three names: (1) a *chemical* name; (2) a *generic* name; and (3) a *brand* name. The **chemical name** is most meaningful to the chemist. By means of the chemical name, the chemist understands the exact chemical constitution of the drug and the exact placement of its atoms or molecular groupings.

Before a drug becomes official, it is given a **generic name** or common name. The generic name is simpler than the chemical name. It may be used in any country and by any manufacturer. The first letter of the generic name is not capitalized. Students are strongly encouraged to learn and refer to drugs by their generic names because formularies (i.e., lists of medicines available through a pharmacy) are maintained by generic names. When a therapeutically equivalent drug becomes available in generic form, the generic medicine is routinely substituted for the brand-name medicine.

Generic names are provided by the U.S. Adopted Names Council, which is an organization sponsored by the U.S. Pharmacopeial Convention, the American Medical Association, and the American Pharmacists Association. The official name, which is virtually always the generic name in the United States, is the name under which the drug is listed by the U.S. Food and Drug Administration (FDA). The FDA is empowered by federal law to generically name the drugs for human use in the United States.

A trademark or **brand name** is followed by the symbol ®. This symbol indicates that the name is registered and that the use of the name is restricted to the owner of the drug, which is usually the manufacturer. Most drug companies place their products on the market under brand names rather than generic names. The brand names are deliberately made easier to pronounce, spell, and remember. The first letter of the brand name is capitalized.

> **EXAMPLE:** See Figure 1-1.
>
> *Chemical name:* 4-Thia-1-azabicyclo(3.2.0)heptane-2-
> carboxylic acid, 6-([aminophenylacetyl]amino)-3,3-
> dimethyl-7-oxo-, (2S-[2α,-5α,6β(S*)])-
> *Generic name:* ampicillin
> *Brand names:* Principen, Polycillin

Drugs may be classified by a variety of methods according to the *body system* that they affect (e.g., the central nervous system, the cardiovascular system, the gastrointestinal system); their *therapeutic use* or *clinical indications* (e.g., antacids, antibiotics, antihypertensives, diuretics, laxatives); and their *physiologic* or *chemical action* (e.g., anticholinergics, beta-adrenergic blockers, calcium channel blockers, cholinergics).

Drugs may be further classified as prescription or nonprescription. **Prescription drugs** require an order by a health professional who is licensed to prescribe drugs, such as a physician, a nurse practitioner, a physician assistant, a pharmacist, or a dentist. **Nonprescription,** or **over-the-counter (OTC), drugs** are sold without a prescription in a pharmacy or in the health section of department or grocery stores. **Illegal drugs,** sometimes referred to as *recreational drugs,* are drugs or chemical substances used for nontherapeutic purposes. These substances either are obtained illegally or have not received approval for use by the FDA. See Chapter 48 for further information about substance abuse.

SOURCES OF DRUG STANDARDS AND DRUG INFORMATION

Drug products made by different manufacturers or in different batches by the same manufacturer must be uniformly pure and potent. The United States Pharmacopeial Convention is a nongovernment organization that promotes public health by establishing state-of-the-art standards to ensure the quality of medicines and other health care technologies. These standards are developed by a unique process of public involvement, and they are accepted worldwide. The convention publishes a single-volume text, the *United States Pharmacopeia (USP)/National Formulary (NF),* which is revised annually. The primary purpose of this volume is to provide standards for the identity, quality, strength, and purity of substances used in the practice of health care. The standards described in the *USP/NF* are enforced by the FDA as the official standards for the manufacture and quality control of medicines and nutritional supplements produced in the United States. The *USP/NF* is also recognized by the Canadian Food and Drugs Act as an authoritative source of drug standards in Canada.

Table 1-1 lists and describes the common sources of drug information available for the professional healthcare provider; additional resources are described in the following sections.

PACKAGE INSERTS

Manufacturers of drugs are required to develop a comprehensive but concise description of the drug, indications and precautions for clinical use, recommendations for dosage, known adverse reactions, contraindications, and other pharmacologic information relating to the drug. Federal law mandates that this material be approved by the FDA before the product is released for marketing and that it be presented on an insert that accompanies each package of the product.

In 2006, the FDA adopted a new format for package inserts to help reduce medication errors and to improve patient education. The new labeling reduces practitioners' time looking for information, decreases the number of preventable medical errors, and improves treatment effectiveness and patient education. Because these labeling revisions represent considerable effort and are most critical for newer and less familiar drugs, the program applies only to relatively new prescription drug products.

FIGURE 1-1 Ampicillin, an antibiotic.

Table 1-1   Sources of Drug Information for Healthcare Providers

SOURCES OF DRUG INFORMATION	DESCRIPTION
USP Dictionary of United States Adopted Names (USAN) and International Drug Names	Published annually Compilation of more than 10,000 drug names Describes the criteria by which drugs are named Online version available
American Drug Index	Index of medicines available in the United States Useful for quickly comparing brand names and generic names and for checking available strengths and dosage forms
American Hospital Formulary Service, Drug Information	Contains monographs about virtually every single-entity drug available in the United States Describes therapeutic uses of drugs, including approved and unapproved uses Online version available
Drug Interaction Facts	Currently considered the most comprehensive book available about drug interactions
Drug Facts and Comparisons	Contains drug monographs that describe all drugs in a therapeutic class Monographs are formatted as tables to allow comparison of similar products, brand names, manufacturers, cost indices, and available dosage forms Online version available
ASHP's Handbook on Injectable Drugs: IV Decision Support	Collection of monographs about 332 injectable drugs with sections on available concentrations, compatibility with other drugs, dosage and rate of administration, stability, pH, and other useful information Interactive version available
Handbook of Nonprescription Drugs: An Interactive Approach to Self-Care	Most comprehensive text available about over-the-counter medications that can be purchased in the United States Online version available
Martindale: The Complete Drug Reference	Considered one of the most comprehensive texts available for information about drugs in current use throughout the world Contains extensive referenced monographs about the international names, pharmacologic activity, and side effects of more than 5500 drugs Online subscription available
Physicians' Desk Reference (PDR)	Discusses more than 3000 therapeutic agents Divided into six sections: (1) manufacturers' index; (2) brand and generic name index; (3) product category index; (4) product identification guide; (5) product information section; and (6) dietary supplements Includes a tear-out form for the MedWatch program for use by health professionals to voluntarily report adverse effects of drugs
Natural Medicines Comprehensive Database	Scientific gold standard for evidence-based information about herbal medicines and combination products involving herbal medicines Only available in an online database available by subscription or at libraries
LactMed a Toxnet Database	Contains information on drugs and other chemicals to which breastfeeding mothers may be exposed Includes information on the levels of such substances in breast milk and infant blood, and the possible adverse effects in the nursing infant Provides suggested therapeutic alternatives to those drugs, where appropriate All data are derived from the scientific literature and are fully referenced A peer-review panel evaluates the data to ensure scientific validity and currency Database is updated monthly *http://toxnet.nlm.nih.gov/newtoxnet/lactmed.htm*
Developmental and Reproductive Toxicology Database (DART)	Provides more than 200,000 journal references covering teratology and other aspects of developmental and reproductive toxicology Funded by several federal agencies Contains references from the early 1900s to the present *http://toxnet.nlm.nih.gov/newtoxnet/dart.htm*

Continued

Table 1-1	Sources of Drug Information for Healthcare Providers—cont'd

SOURCES OF DRUG INFORMATION	DESCRIPTION
Canadian Drug Standards	
European Pharmacopoeia *Pharmacopée Française* *The International Pharmacopoeia (Ph. Int.)* *British Pharmacopoeia* *Canadian Formulary* *The National Formulary* *Pharmaceutical Codex* *United States Pharmacopeia*	All recognized by the Canadian Food and Drugs Act as authoritative sources of drug standards
Canadian Drug Information	
Compendium of Pharmaceuticals and Specialties (CPS)	Published annually by the Canadian Pharmacists Association Comprehensive list of the pharmaceutical products distributed in Canada, as well as other practical information e-CPS available
Patient Self-Care: Helping Patients Make Therapeutic Choices	Published by the Canadian Pharmacists Association Provides comprehensive information for health professionals and consumers about nonprescription drug products available in Canada e-Therapeutics available
Compendium of Self-Care Products (CSCP)	Nonprescription companion to *CPS* and *Patient Self-Care* Offers at-a-glance comparative tables for thousands of products and monographs about hundreds of commonly used nonprescription products

Clinical Goldmine

DailyMed (see Online Resources), which is sponsored by the National Library of Medicine, provides a database for new package inserts that is searchable by product name, indications, dosage and administration, warnings, description of drug product, active and inactive ingredients, and how the drug is supplied. See the section Electronic Databases.

NURSING JOURNALS

Many specialty journals have articles about drug therapy as it relates to a specific field of interest (e.g., *Geriatric Nursing, American Journal of Critical Care*). Nursing journals such as *RN* and *American Journal of Nursing* provide drug updates and articles that discuss nursing considerations related to drug therapy and drugs. Nurses must keep in mind that the purpose of using resources like journals is for professional knowledge of current evidence-based practice changes and not as a primary source for drug information; they must be mindful of the accuracy of the information contained and should check the dates on articles to validate the currency of the information.

ELECTRONIC DATABASES

With the exponential growth of information about medicines and health, it is almost impossible to make the information available without the use of electronic databases. The U.S. National Library of Medicine provides Medline and other searchable databases at no cost. Most of the drug information sources listed in Table 1-1 are also available via electronic retrieval from libraries. Many college libraries subscribe to CINAHL (Cumulative Index to Nursing and Allied Health Literature). These sources give nurses access to a wealth of information from sources published in the United States and other countries.

Databases for practitioners are also available by subscription. UpToDate, Lexi-Comp, and ePocrates are three vendors with several different packages of regularly updated information (see Online Resources). Lexi-Comp has a particularly strong database because the American Hospital Formulary Service is available through its portal.

The DailyMed system (see Online Resources) was developed in collaboration with federal agencies—including the FDA, the National Library of Medicine, the Agency for Healthcare Research and Quality, the National Cancer Institute in the Department of Health and Human Services, and the Department of Veterans Affairs—to provide high-quality information about marketed drugs. DailyMed makes available to healthcare providers and the public a standard, comprehensive, up-to-date resource about medicines.

UNITED STATES DRUG LEGISLATION

Drug legislation provides a legal basis for drug treatments and protects the consumer from false claims made by the drug manufacturer. The need for such protection is great, because manufacturers and advertisers may make unfounded claims about the benefits of their products.

FEDERAL FOOD, DRUG, AND COSMETIC ACT

The Federal Food, Drug, and Cosmetic Act of 1938 requires the FDA to determine the safety of drugs before marketing and to ensure that certain labeling specifications and standards in advertising are met in the marketing of products. Manufacturers are required to submit new drug applications to the FDA for the review of safety studies before the products can be released for sale.

There are two key amendments to the 1938 act. The Durham Humphrey Amendment of 1952 divides medicines into prescription and nonprescription (OTC) categories based on safety. Prescription medicine labels are required to contain the statement "Caution: Federal Law prohibits dispensing without a prescription" or "Prescription only." The Kefauver-Harris Drug Amendment was brought about in 1962 as a result of the thalidomide tragedy. Thalidomide was an incompletely tested drug that had been approved for use as a sedative-hypnotic during pregnancy. Fetuses exposed to thalidomide were born with serious birth defects. This amendment provides greater control and

surveillance of the distribution and clinical testing of investigational drugs and requires that a product be proven both safe and effective before release for sale.

CONTROLLED SUBSTANCES ACT

The Comprehensive Drug Abuse Prevention and Control Act, which is commonly referred to as the *Controlled Substances Act,* was passed by Congress in 1970. This statute repealed almost 50 other laws written between 1914 and 1970 that related to the control of drugs. The new composite law was designed to improve the administration and regulation of the manufacturing, distribution, and dispensing of drugs that require control by the government because of their high incidence of abuse. The basic structure of the Controlled Substances Act consists of five classifications, or **schedules,** of controlled substances. The degree of control, the conditions of record keeping, the particular order forms required, and other regulations depend on these classifications (Box 1-1).

Drug Enforcement Administration

The U.S. Drug Enforcement Administration (DEA) was organized to enforce the Controlled Substances Act, to gather intelligence, to train its officers, and to conduct research in the area of dangerous drugs and drug abuse. The DEA is a bureau of the Department of

---

Box 1-1   Controlled Substance Drug Schedules*

SCHEDULE I DRUGS
1. Very high potential for abuse
2. Not currently accepted for medical use in the United States
3. Lack of accepted safety for use under medical supervision

Examples: lysergic acid diethylamide (LSD), peyote, heroin, hashish

SCHEDULE II DRUGS
1. High potential for abuse
2. Currently accepted for medical use in the United States
3. Abuse potential that may lead to severe psychological or physical dependence
4. Requires new prescription; no refills

Examples: amphetamines, morphine, Vicodin, methadone, Percodan, methylphenidate (Ritalin), Adderall

SCHEDULE III DRUGS
1. High potential for abuse but less so than drugs in Schedules I and II
2. Currently accepted for medical use in the United States
3. Abuse potential that may lead to moderate or low physical dependence or high psychological dependence
4. Prescription outdates in 6 months; no more than five refills in that 6 months

Examples: Empirin with codeine, Lortab, Fiorinal, Tylenol with codeine, Norco

SCHEDULE IV DRUGS
1. Low potential for abuse compared with drugs in Schedule III
2. Currently accepted for medical use in the United States
3. Abuse potential that may lead to limited physical or psychological dependence compared with drugs in Schedule III
4. Prescription outdates in 6 months; no more than five refills in that 6 months

Examples: phenobarbital, chlordiazepoxide, diazepam, flurazepam, temazepam

SCHEDULE V DRUGS
1. Low potential for abuse compared with drugs in Schedule IV
2. Currently accepted for medical use in the United States
3. Abuse potential of limited physical or psychological dependence liability compared with drugs in Schedule IV; because abuse potential is low, a prescription may not be required
4. Prescription outdates in 6 months, no more than five refills in that 6 months

Examples: Lomotil, Robitussin AC

*Drugs that are listed in Schedule I are not available for other than highly controlled research purposes. Drugs in Schedule II are available by prescription only in limited quantities, usually no more than a 30-day supply. The prescription cannot be refilled. A new prescription must be issued for continued use. Drugs categorized as Schedule III, IV, or V may be ordered by prescription with a maximum supply of 30 days of medicine. The prescription may be refilled up to five times, but outdates at 6 months, at which time a new prescription is required if the medicine is to be continued. Prescription medicines that are not classified as controlled substances may be refilled for up to 1 year, if approved by the prescriber. Most state laws mandate that a prescription outdates in 1 year.

Justice, and the director of the DEA reports to the Attorney General of the United States. The U.S. Attorney General, after public hearings, has the authority to reschedule a drug, to bring an unscheduled drug under control, or to remove controls on scheduled drugs.

Every manufacturer, physician, nurse practitioner, physician assistant, dentist, pharmacy, and hospital that manufactures, prescribes, or dispenses any of the drugs listed in the five schedules must register biannually with the DEA. A healthcare provider's prescription for substances named in this law must contain the healthcare provider's name, address, DEA registration number, and signature; the patient's name and address; and the date of issue. The pharmacist cannot refill such prescriptions without the approval of the healthcare provider.

Controlled Substances in Hospitals

All controlled substances kept in hospitals for unit stock must be ordered on special forms that are used to help maintain the inventory and dispersion control records of the scheduled drugs. When a nurse administers a Schedule II drug from a healthcare provider's order, the name of the patient, the date and time of administration, the drug administered, and the drug dosage must be entered on the controlled substances record.

Possession of Controlled Substances by Individuals

Federal and state laws make the possession of controlled substances without a valid prescription a crime, except in specifically exempted cases. The law makes no distinction between professional and practical nurses with regard to the possession of controlled drugs. Nurses may give controlled substances only under the direction of a healthcare practitioner who has been licensed to prescribe or dispense these agents. Nurses may not have controlled substances in their possession unless the following conditions are met: (1) they are giving them to a patient under a physician's order; (2) the nurse is a patient for whom a physician has prescribed scheduled drugs; or (3) the nurse is the official custodian of a limited supply of controlled substances on a unit or for a department of the hospital. Controlled substances that are ordered for patients but not used must be returned to the source from which they were obtained (i.e., the physician or pharmacy). Violation or failure to comply with the Controlled Substances Act is punishable by fine, imprisonment, or both and by the possible loss of professional licensing.

EFFECTIVENESS OF DRUG LEGISLATION

Enforcing the laws regarding the proper distribution and use of drugs is dependent on many organizations working together to ensure the understanding of the reasons for the drug legislation. The National Coordi-

nating Council on Patient Information and Education (NCCPIE) is a driving force behind the effort to educate healthcare professionals and the public with regard to the possible consequences of indiscriminant use of drugs. Other organizations involved in this very important effort are the American Medical Association; the American Dental Association; the American Pharmacists Association; the American Society of Health-System Pharmacists; and local, county, and state health departments.

NEW DRUG DEVELOPMENT

It currently takes an average of 8 to 15 years and more than $2 billion in research and development costs to bring a single new drug to market; healthcare professionals and consumers alike often have a lack of understanding about this process. The Pharmaceutical Manufacturers Association estimates that only 1 out of 10,000 chemicals investigated is actually found to be "safe and effective" and ultimately brought to the pharmacist's shelf.

The Food, Drug, and Cosmetic Act of 1938 charged the FDA with the responsibility of regulating new drugs. Rules and regulations evolved by the FDA divide new drug development into four stages: (1) preclinical research and development; (2) clinical research and development; (3) New Drug Application (NDA) review; and (4) postmarketing surveillance (Figure 1-2).

PRECLINICAL RESEARCH AND DEVELOPMENT STAGE

The preclinical research phase of new drug development begins with the discovery, synthesis, and purification of the drug. The goal at this stage is to use laboratory studies to determine whether the experimental drug has therapeutic value and whether the drug appears to be safe in animals. Enough data must be gained to justify testing the experimental drug in humans.

The preclinical phase of data collection may require 1 to 3 years, although the average length of time is 18 months. Near the end of this phase, the investigator (often a pharmaceutical manufacturer) submits an Investigational New Drug (IND) application to the FDA; this application describes all of the studies completed to date, discusses the expected safety of the drug, and explains the testing that is planned for human subjects. Within 30 days, the FDA must make a decision on the basis of safety considerations about whether to allow the human study to proceed. Only about 20% of the chemicals tested in the preclinical phase advance to the clinical testing phase.

CLINICAL RESEARCH AND DEVELOPMENT STAGE

The stage in which humans are first tested (i.e., the clinical research or IND stage) is usually subdivided

| Preclinical Research and Development | FDA | Clinical Research and Development | NDA Review | Postmarketing Surveillance |

FIGURE 1-2 The new drug review process.

into three phases. Phase 1 studies determine an experimental drug's pharmacologic properties, such as its pharmacokinetics, metabolism, safe dosage range, potential for toxicity at a certain dosage, and safe routes of administration. The study population is comprised of normal volunteers or the intended treatment population, such as those patients for whom the standard treatments of certain cancers or dysrhythmias have been ineffective. Phase 1 studies usually require 20 to 100 subjects who are treated for 4 to 6 weeks.

If phase 1 trials are successful, the drug is moved to phase 2, which involves a smaller population of patients who have the condition that the drug is designed to treat. Studies at various dosages are conducted to determine the success rate and safety of a drug for its intended use. If successful, the drug is advanced to phase 3 trials, in which larger patient populations are used to ensure the statistical significance of the results. Phase 3 studies also provide additional information about proper dosing and safety.

The entire clinical research phase may require 2 to 10 years, with the average experimental drug requiring 5 years. Each study completed is reviewed by the FDA to help ensure patient safety and efficacy. Only one out of five drugs that enter clinical trials makes it to the marketplace. The others are eliminated because

of efficacy or safety problems or a lack of commercial interest.

Fast Tracking

To expedite the development and approval of drugs for the treatment of life-threatening illnesses (e.g., acquired immunodeficiency syndrome), the FDA has drafted rules that allow certain INDs to receive the highest priority for review within the agency. This procedure is sometimes known as *fast tracking*. Additional rules allow INDs to be used for the treatment of a life-threatening disease in a particular patient—even if the patient does not fit the study protocol for the drug—when there is no alternative therapy. These cases are known as *treatment INDs*. A potentially lifesaving drug may be allowed for treatment IND status during late phase 2 studies, phase 3 studies, or after all clinical studies have been completed but before marketing approval.

Parallel Tracking

Another mechanism to make INDs available to patients with life-threatening illnesses is known as *parallel tracking*. With this procedure, an IND may be used for patients who cannot participate in controlled clinical trials and when there is no satisfactory standard therapeutic alternative. Parallel track studies are conducted along with the principal controlled clinical trials; however, unlike a controlled study, the parallel track study does not involve a concurrent control group.

Investigators and patients must realize that there may be greater uncertainty regarding the risks and benefits of therapy with agents that are in relatively early stages of testing and development. Parallel tracking is similar to the treatment IND process, but allows for access to investigational agents when there is less accumulated evidence of efficacy than required for a treatment IND. A drug may be released through the parallel track mechanism when phase 2 trials have been given approval to proceed but have not necessarily been started.

NEW DRUG APPLICATION REVIEW

When sufficient data have been collected to demonstrate that the experimental drug is both safe and effective, the investigator submits an NDA to the FDA to formally request approval to market a new drug for human use. Thousands of pages of NDA data are reviewed by a team of pharmacologists, toxicologists, chemists, physicians, and others (as appropriate), who then make a recommendation to the FDA about whether the drug should be approved for use. The average NDA review takes 17 months. After a drug is approved by the FDA, it is the manufacturer's decision as to when to bring a product to the marketplace.

POSTMARKETING SURVEILLANCE STAGE

If the manufacturer decides to market the medicine, the postmarketing surveillance stage begins; this is the fourth stage of drug product development. This process consists of an ongoing review of adverse effects of the new drug and periodic inspections of the manufacturing facilities and the resulting products. Other studies completed during the fourth stage include identifying other patient populations for whom the drug may be useful, refining dosing recommendations, and exploring potential drug interactions.

 Clinical Goldmine

Healthcare practitioners make a significant contribution to the knowledge of drug safety by reporting adverse effects to the FDA using the MedWatch program for the voluntary reporting of adverse events and product problems (see Online Resources).

BLACK BOX WARNING

Although the FDA's drug-approval process is one of the most stringent in the world, a study has demonstrated the value of the ongoing safety review of medicines and the use of the MedWatch program. Of the 548 new chemical entities approved by the FDA from 1975 to 1999, a total of 56 drugs (10.2%) acquired new **black box warnings** (which indicate very serious or potentially life-threatening problems) or were withdrawn from the market because of serious or fatal complications (Lasser et al, 2002).

The probability of a drug acquiring a new black box warning or being withdrawn from the market within 25 years of being released is estimated at 20%. Consequently, it is the responsibility of all healthcare professionals to constantly monitor their patients for adverse effects of drugs and to complete a MedWatch form when adverse effects are suspected. More than 200,000 MedWatch forms are filed with the FDA annually.

From a safety standpoint, prescribers, other healthcare practitioners, and patients should be aware that recently marketed medicines carry a risk of causing unsuspected serious adverse effects. One could make the point that there is a 90% probability that there will be no serious complications, but the devastating—and sometimes fatal—consequences cannot be ignored. When choosing medicines for treatment, it becomes important to consider whether an equally effective alternative drug is already available. At a minimum, this reduces the risk of an undiscovered adverse drug reaction, and it is often less expensive. At a maximum, the patient, his or her family, and the prescriber are saved the anguish of an avoidable adverse drug reaction.

RARE DISEASES AND THE DEVELOPMENT OF ORPHAN DRUGS

The National Organization for Rare Disorders, which is a coalition of 140 rare-disease groups, estimates that more than 6000 rare health conditions exist in about 20 million Americans. Examples of these rare diseases are cystic fibrosis, Hansen's disease (leprosy), sickle cell anemia, blepharospasm, infant botulism, and *Pneumocystis jiroveci* pneumonia (see Online Resources). Historically, pharmaceutical manufacturers have been reluctant to develop products that could be used to treat these illnesses. The medicines that are developed for these conditions are known as *orphan drugs,* because the manufacturers have been unable to recover the costs of the research due to the very limited use of the final product. Because no companies were willing to "adopt" the diseases to complete extensive research to develop products for treatment, the diseases became known as *health orphans.*

In 1983, Congress passed the Orphan Drug Act to stimulate the development and market availability of products that are used for the treatment of rare diseases. The act defines the term *rare disease* as a condition that affects fewer than 200,000 people in the United States. The FDA's Office of Orphan Products Development (OOPD) promotes the development of products that demonstrate promise for the diagnosis or treatment of rare diseases or conditions.

The OOPD interacts with medical and research communities, professional organizations, academia, and the pharmaceutical industry, as well as with rare-disease groups. The OOPD administers the major provisions of the Orphan Drug Act, which provide incentives for sponsors to develop products for rare diseases.

The law provides research grants, protocol development assistance by the FDA, special tax credits for the cost of clinical trials, and 7 years of exclusive marketing rights after the product has been approved. On average, an orphan drug receives FDA approval 10 to 11 months sooner than a non-orphan drug. The act has been quite successful: more than 200 new drugs have been approved by the FDA for the treatment of rare diseases, benefiting several million people. Examples include pentamidine and atovaquone for *Pneumocystis jiroveci* pneumonia, thalidomide for Hansen's disease, zidovudine for the human immunodeficiency virus, DNase (Pulmozyme) for cystic fibrosis, and Leustatin for hairy cell leukemia.

DRUG NAMES, STANDARDS, AND LEGISLATION IN CANADA

CANADIAN DRUG NAMES

OFFICIAL DRUG

The term *official drug* pertains to any drug for which a standard is described specifically in the Food and Drug Regulations or in any publication named in the Food and Drugs Act as being satisfactory for officially meeting the standards for drugs in Canada.

CHEMICAL NAME

The *chemical name* is most meaningful to the chemist. By means of the chemical name, the chemist understands the exact chemical constitution of the drug and exact placing of its atoms or molecular groupings. The chemical name is the same in both Canada and the United States.

PROPER NAME OR GENERIC NAME

The *proper name* is the nonproprietary (generic) name, which is used to identify an official drug in Canada. The *generic name* is the same in both Canada and the United States.

BRAND NAME

The *brand name* (or proprietary name) is the name assigned to the drug by its manufacturer to distinguish the drug for advertisement and sale. Brand names for the same generic drug product are frequently different between Canada and the United States. Figure 1-3 depicts the application of terminology to drug nomenclature.

FIGURE 1-3 Tetracycline, an antibiotic.

EXAMPLE: See Figure 1-3.

Chemical name: 4-dimethylamino-1,4,4a,5,5a,6,11,12a-octahydro-3,6,10,12,12a-pentahydroxy-6-methyl-1,11,dioxo-2-napthacenecarboxamide
Proper name: tetracycline
Official name: Tetracycline, USP
Brand names: Apo-Tetra; Nu-Tetra

SOURCES OF CANADIAN DRUG STANDARDS

The Food and Drugs Act recognizes the standards described by international authoritative books as being acceptable for official drugs in Canada (see Table 1-1).

CANADIAN DRUG LEGISLATION

FOOD AND DRUGS ACT AND REGULATIONS

The **Food and Drugs Act** (1927) **and Regulations** (1953, 1954, 1979) empower Health Canada to protect the public from foreseeable risks related to the manufacture and sale of drugs, cosmetics, food, and therapeutic devices. The legislation provides for a review of the safety and efficacy of drugs before their clearance for marketing in Canada and determines whether the medicine is *prescription* or *nonprescription*. Also included in this legislation are requirements for good manufacturing practices, adequate labeling, and fair advertising.

In Canada (as in the United States), an effort has been made to align the provincial drug schedules so that the conditions for the sale of medicines are consistent across Canada. The National Association of Pharmacy Regulatory Authorities (NAPRA) proposed a new national drug scheduling model. This model is in various stages of implementation across the provinces and territories of Canada. With the use of this model, all medicines in Canada are assigned to one of four categories:

Schedule I: All prescription drugs, including narcotics
Schedule II: Restricted-access nonprescription drugs
Schedule III: Pharmacy-only nonprescription drugs
Unscheduled: Drugs that are not assigned to the previous categories

Schedule II drugs are available for sale directly from the pharmacist and are kept "behind the counter." Examples include insulin, pseudoephedrine, glucagon, loperamide (for children under age 12), and nitroglycerin sublingual spray and tablets (other dosage forms are Schedule I). These medications are in two categories: (1) those that patients may require urgently and cannot delay taking until after an appointment with a prescriber (insulin, nitroglycerin, glucagon); and (2) those that require appropriate counseling to avoid improper use (loperamide, pseudoephedrine). Placement with a pharmacist does not allow for patient self-selection and allows for pharmacist intervention for these medications. This restriction is meant to ensure the following: (1) that patients are not self-diagnosing medically serious diseases (e.g., diabetes mellitus, angina); and (2) that patients are educated about the proper use of these drugs through appropriate counseling from the pharmacist.

Schedule III drugs are pharmacy-only nonprescription drugs. These medicines can be sold only through pharmacies and include levonorgestrel emergency contraception, diphenhydramine, child preparations of antihistamines, and the low-dose histamine-2 antagonists. It is expected that if clients have questions, they could easily consult with a pharmacist.

Medicines that are not categorized in Schedule I, II, or III are considered to be "unscheduled" (e.g., nicotine gum and patches, acetylsalicylic acid, lower-dose ibuprofen, some lower-dosage "cough and cold" preparations) and can be sold at any retail outlet. Adequate information is available for the patient to make a safe and effective choice, and labeling is sufficient to ensure the appropriate use of the drug without professional supervision.

Drugs requiring a prescription—except for controlled drugs—are listed on Schedule F of the Food and Drug Regulations. Schedule F drugs may be prescribed only by qualified practitioners because they would normally be used most safely under supervision. Most antibiotics, antineoplastics, corticosteroids, cardiovascular drugs, and antipsychotics are Schedule F drugs.

CONTROLLED DRUGS AND SUBSTANCES ACT

The **Controlled Drugs and Substances Act** (1997) establishes the requirements for the import, production, export, distribution, and possession of substances classified as narcotics and substances of abuse in Canada. The Controlled Drugs and Substances Act describes eight schedules of controlled substances. Assignment to a schedule is based on the potential for abuse and the ease with which illicit substances can be manufactured in illegal laboratories. The degree of control; the conditions of record keeping; assignment of penalties for possession, trafficking, and manufacturing; and

other regulations depend on these classifications. (Note that the Schedules I, II and III under the Food and Drugs Act are different from the Schedules I-VIII of the Controlled Drugs and Substances Act). Examples of schedule assignment are as follows:

Schedule I: Opium poppy and its derivatives (e.g., heroin, morphine); coca and its derivatives (e.g., cocaine), pethidine (meperidine), methadone, fentanyl

Schedule II: Cannabis

Schedule III: Amphetamines, methylphenidate, lysergic acid diethylamide (LSD), methaqualone, psilocybin, mescaline

Schedule IV: Sedative-hypnotic agents (e.g., barbiturates, benzodiazepines); butorphanol, anabolic steroids

Schedule V: Propylhexedrine, phenylpropanolamine, pyrovalerone

Schedule VI: Part I class A precursors (e.g., ephedrine, pseudoephedrine, norephedrine [phenylpropanolamine], ergotamine) and part II precursors (e.g., acetone, ethyl ether, hydrochloric acid, sulfuric acid, toluene)

Schedule VII: Cannabis resin (3 kg); cannabis (marijuana) (3 kg) (must be read in conjunction with Schedule II)

Schedule VIII: Cannabis resin (1 g); cannabis (marijuana) (30 g) (must be read in conjunction with Schedule II)

The Controlled Drugs and Substances Act and accompanying regulations provide for the nonprescription sale of certain codeine preparations (e.g., Tylenol No. 1 with codeine, Benylin with codeine). The content must not exceed the equivalent of 8 mg of codeine phosphate per solid dosage unit or 20 mg per 30 mL of a liquid preparation, and the preparation must also contain two additional nonnarcotic medicinal ingredients. These preparations may not be advertised or displayed, and they may be sold only by pharmacists (see previous discussion of Schedule II drugs). In hospitals, the pharmacy usually requires strict inventory control of these products and other narcotics.

Requirements for the legitimate administration of drugs to patients by nurses are generally similar in Canada and the United States. Individual hospital policy determines specific record-keeping requirements on the basis of federal and provincial laws. Violations of these laws will result in fines or imprisonment in addition to the loss of professional licensing.

NONPRESCRIPTION DRUGS

The NAPRA drug schedules list three categories of nonprescription drugs, including Schedule II, III, and unscheduled drugs. See discussion under Food and Drugs Act and Regulations.

Get Ready for the NCLEX® Examination!

Key Points

- In the classification system used in the United States, each drug has three names: a *chemical* name, a *generic* name, and a *brand* name. The chemical name is most meaningful to the chemist. The generic name is simpler than the chemical name. The first letter of the generic name is not capitalized. The brand names are selected by the manufacturer and deliberately made easier to pronounce, spell, and remember. A brand name is followed by the symbol ®. The first letter of the brand name is capitalized.
- Drugs may be classified by a variety of methods according to the *body system* that they affect (e.g., the central nervous system, the cardiovascular system, the gastrointestinal system); their *therapeutic use* or *clinical indications* (e.g., antacids, antibiotics, antihypertensives, diuretics, laxatives); and their *physiologic* or *chemical action* (e.g., anticholinergic agents, beta-adrenergic blockers, calcium channel blockers, cholinergic agents).
- Table 1-1 lists and describes the common sources of drug information available for the healthcare provider; additional resources are described in the following sections.
- Prescription drugs require an order by a health professional who is licensed to prescribe drugs, such as a physician, a nurse practitioner, a physician assistant, a pharmacist, or a dentist. Nonprescription or OTC drugs are sold without a prescription in a pharmacy or in the health section of department or grocery stores.
- Rules and regulations evolved by the FDA divide new drug development into four stages: (1) preclinical research and development; (2) clinical research and development; (3) NDA review; and (4) postmarketing surveillance (see Figure 1-2).
- In Canada, the *proper name* is the nonproprietary (generic) name, which is used to identify an official drug. The *generic name* is the same in both Canada and the United States.

Additional Learning Resources

SG Go to your Study Guide for additional Review Questions for the NCLEX® Examination, Critical Thinking Clinical Situations, and other learning activities to help you master this chapter content.

evolve Go to your Evolve website (http://evolve .elsevier.com/Clayton) for additional online resources.

🌐 Online Resources
- DailyMed: http://dailymed.nlm.nih.gov/dailymed/about.cfm
- ePocrates: www.epocrates.com
- iPharmacy: http://itunes.apple.com/us/app/id348702163?mt=8&ign-mpt=uo%3D6; https://market.android.com/details?id=com.sigmaphone.topmedfree

- Lexi-Comp: http://online.lexi.com
- MedicinesComplete: http://www.medicinescomplete.com
- MedWatch: www.fda.gov/Safety/MedWatch/default.htm
- National Organization for Rare Disorders: www.rarediseases.org
- UpToDate: www.uptodate.com
- U.S. National Library of Medicine: www.nlm.nih.gov

Online Resources for Canadian Practitioners
- Canadian drug names: http://www.hc-sc.gc.ca/dhp-mps/prodpharma/databasdon/index-eng.php
- National Association of Pharmacy Regulatory Authorities (NAPRA) proposal for drug schedule outlines: http://napra.ca/Content_Files/Files/Schedules-Outline.pdf
- Controlled Substances and Drugs Act: http://laws-lois.justice.gc.ca/eng/acts/c-38.8/

Review Questions for the NCLEX® Examination

1. A patient has received a prescription from his primary care provider for the drug metoprolol (Lopressor). He asks the nurse why there are three names for the same drug. The nurse responds with which statements(s)? *(Select all that apply.)*
   1. "One of the names is the brand name of the drug, and the other is the generic name and the last is the chemical name."
   2. "When drugs are discovered, all drugs are given a detailed chemical name and a simple generic name. If the company that discovered the drug brings it to the marketplace for sale, the manufacturer will give it a distinctive brand name."
   3. "Lopressor is the generic name, and metoprolol is the brand name."
   4. "The two names are used to determine whether the drug is a Schedule III or a Schedule IV drug."
   5. "Generally, the generic form of the drug is less expensive."

2. Antacids, antibiotics, antihypertensives, diuretics, and laxatives are examples of drugs that are categorized by which factor?
   1. Nonprescription status
   2. Body system
   3. Chemical action
   4. Clinical indication

3. Which electronic database(s) provide(s) drug information for healthcare providers? *(Select all that apply.)*
   1. Lexi-Comp
   2. CINAHL
   3. Medline
   4. DailyMed
   5. Health on the Net

4. A patient asked the nurse what would be an example of an appropriate source for drug information on the Internet. The nurse responds:
   1. "The Internet is not an appropriate place to look up any drug information; you need to ask your physician or pharmacist."
   2. "There are several reliable sites for drug information that are from official sources, for example, DailyMed."
   3. "The Internet is reliable for any drug information that you search for."
   4. "The only acceptable drug information sources are the package inserts."

5. The nurse knows that the difference between prescription and nonprescription drugs involves: *(Select all that apply.)*
   1. Nonprescription drugs are available over-the-counter.
   2. Prescription drugs are those drugs that may be prescribed by dentists, pharmacists, nurse practitioners, and physicians.
   3. Recreational drugs are available by prescription only.
   4. Over-the-counter drugs are available at a pharmacy or health section of grocery stores.
   5. Prescription drugs have been approved for use by the FDA.

6. During which stage of the process of new drug development does testing on humans start?
   1. The preclinical research and development stage
   2. The postmarketing surveillance stage
   3. The postclinical research and development stage
   4. The clinical research and development stage

7. A nurse was teaching a patient from Canada the names of her medications and reviewed the differences between Canadian names. Which statement indicates the patient understands the instructions?
   1. "The proper name of the medication is the same as the brand name in Canada."
   2. "The proper name of the medication is the same as the generic name in Canada."
   3. "The chemical name is the one used the most when buying medications in Canada."
   4. "The chemical names and the brand names are the only names used in Canada."

Basic Principles of Drug Action and Drug Interactions

Objectives

1. Identify common drug administration routes.
2. Identify the meaning and significance of the term *half-life* when used in relation to drug therapy.
3. Describe the process of how a drug is metabolized in the body.
4. Compare and contrast the following terms that are used in relationship to medications: *desired action, common adverse effects, serious adverse effects, allergic reactions,* and *idiosyncratic reactions.*
5. Identify what is meant by a drug interaction.
6. Differentiate among the terms *additive effect, synergistic effect, antagonistic effect, displacement, interference,* and *incompatibility.*
7. Identify one way in which alternatives in metabolism create drug interactions.

Key Terms

receptors (rē-SĔP-tĕrz) (p. 13)
pharmacodynamics (făr-mă-kō-dī-NĂM-ĭks) (p. 13)
agonists (ĂG-ŏ-nĭsts) (p. 13)
antagonists (ăn-TĂG-ŏ-nĭsts) (p. 13)
partial agonists (PĂR-shŭl ĂG-ŏ-nĭsts) (p. 13)
enteral (ĔN-tĕr-ăl) (p. 14)
parenteral (pă-RĔN-tĕr-ăl) (p. 14)
percutaneous (pĕr-kū-TĀ-nē-ŭs) (p. 14)
pharmacokinetics (făr-mă-kō-kĭ-NĔT-ĭks) (p. 14)
absorption (ăb-sŏrp-shŭn) (p. 14)
distribution (dis-trib-byü-shan) (p. 15)
drug blood level (p. 15)
metabolism (mĕ-TĂ-bō-lĭ-sm) (p. 15)
excretion (ĕks-KRĒ-shŭn) (p. 15)
half-life (p. 15)
onset of action (p. 16)
peak action (p. 16)

duration of action (p. 17)
desired action (p. 17)
side effects (p. 17)
common adverse effects (ĂD-vŭrs ĕf-FĔCTS) (p. 17)
serious adverse effects (p. 17)
idiosyncratic reaction (ĭd-ē-ō-sĭn-KRĂT-ĭk rē-ĂK-shŭn) (p. 18)
allergic reactions (ă-LŬR-jĭk) (p. 18)
drug interaction (p. 18)
unbound drug (ŭn-BŎWND) (p. 18)
additive effect (ĂD-ĭ-tĭv) (p. 19)
synergistic effect (sĭn-ĕr-JĬS-tĭk) (p. 19)
antagonistic effect (ăn-tăg-ŏ-NĬST-ĭk) (p. 19)
displacement (dĭs-PLĀS-mĕnt) (p. 19)
interference (ĭn-tŭr-FĔR-ĕns) (p. 19)
incompatibility (ĭn-kŏm-păt-ĭ-BĬL-ĭ-tē) (p. 19)

BASIC PRINCIPLES RELATED TO DRUG THERAPY

DRUG RESPONSES IN THE BODY

When administered to the body, drugs do not create new responses, but rather alter existing physiologic activity in several different ways. Usually the drug forms chemical bonds with specific sites, called *receptors*, within the body. This bond forms only if the drug and its receptor have similar shapes and if the drug has a chemical affinity for the receptor. The relationship between a drug and a receptor is similar to that seen between a key and lock (Figure 2-1, *A*). The study of the interactions between drugs and their receptors and the series of events that result in a pharmacologic response is called *pharmacodynamics*. Most drugs have several different atoms within each molecule that interlock into various locations on a receptor. The better the fit between the receptor and the drug molecule, the better the response from the drug. The intensity of a drug response is related to how well the drug molecule fits into the receptor and to the number of receptor sites that are occupied. Drugs that interact with a receptor to stimulate a response are known as *agonists* (Figure 2-1, *B*). Drugs that attach to a receptor but do not stimulate a response are called *antagonists* (Figure 2-1, *C*). Drugs that interact with a receptor to stimulate a response but inhibit other responses are called *partial agonists* (Figure 2-1, *D*).

FIGURE 2-1 **A,** Drugs act by forming chemical bonds with specific receptor sites, similar to a key and lock. **B,** The better the fit, the better the response. Drugs with complete attachment and response are called *agonists.* **C,** Drugs that attach but do not elicit a response are called *antagonists.* **D,** Drugs that attach and elicit a small response but also block other responses are called *partial agonists.*

Drug response must be stated in relation to the physiologic activity expected in response to the drug therapy (e.g., an antihypertensive agent is successful if the patient's blood pressure is lower after receiving the drug than it was before the drug was started). Therefore it is important to perform a thorough nursing assessment to identify the baseline data. After that is done, results from regular assessments can be compared with the baseline data by the physician, the nurse, and the pharmacist to evaluate the effectiveness of the drug therapy.

ROUTES OF DRUG ADMINISTRATION

The most common routes of drug administration are the enteral, parenteral, and percutaneous routes. When using the **enteral** route, the drug is administered directly into the gastrointestinal (GI) tract by the oral, rectal, or nasogastric route. The **parenteral** route bypasses the GI tract with the use of subcutaneous, intramuscular, or intravenous injection. The **percutaneous** route involves drugs being absorbed through the skin and mucous membranes. Methods of the percutaneous route include inhalation, sublingual (under the tongue), and topical (on the skin) administration.

LIBERATION, ABSORPTION, DISTRIBUTION, METABOLISM, AND EXCRETION

After they have been administered, all drugs go through five stages: *l*iberation, *a*bsorption, *d*istribution, *m*etabolism, and *e*xcretion (LADME). After liberation from the dosage form, each drug has its own unique ADME characteristics. The study of the mathematic relationships among the ADME features of individual medicines over time is called *pharmacokinetics.*

Liberation

Regardless of the route of administration, a drug must be released from the dosage form (i.e., liberated) and dissolved in body fluids before it can be absorbed into body tissues. For example, before a solid drug that is taken orally can be absorbed into the bloodstream for transport to the site of action, the dosage form (usually a capsule or tablet) must disintegrate, and the active drug must dissolve in the GI fluids so that it can be transported across the stomach or intestinal lining into the blood. The process of converting the drug into a form that will activate a response can be partially controlled by the pharmaceutical dosage form used (e.g., solution, suspension, capsule, tablet [with various coatings]). This conversion process can also be influenced by administering the drug with or without water or food in the patient's stomach.

Absorption

Absorption is the process whereby a drug is transferred from its site of entry into the body to the circulating fluids of the body (i.e., blood and lymph) for distribution around the body. The rate at which this occurs depends on the route of administration, the blood flow through the tissue where the drug is administered, and the solubility of the drug. It is therefore important to do the following: (1) administer oral drugs with an adequate amount of fluid (usually a large [8-oz] glass of water); (2) give parenteral forms properly so that they are deposited in the correct tissue for enhanced absorption; and (3) reconstitute and dilute drugs only with the diluent recommended by the manufacturer in the package literature so that drug solubility is not impaired. Equally important are nursing assessments that reveal poor absorption (e.g., if insulin is administered subcutaneously and a lump remains at the site of injection 2 to 3 hours later, absorption from that site may be impaired).

The rate of absorption when a drug is administered by a parenteral route depends on the rate of blood flow through the tissues. Circulation or blood flow must be determined before the administration of drugs by the parenteral route to identify any circulatory insufficiency. If any such insufficiency is noted, injections will not be absorbed properly, and the drug will not be effective. Subcutaneous (subcut) injections have the slowest absorption rate, especially if peripheral circulation is impaired. Intramuscular (IM) injections are more rapidly absorbed because of greater blood flow per unit weight of muscle compared with subcutaneous tissue. Cooling the area of injection slows the rate of absorption, whereas heat or massage hastens the rate of absorption. Drugs are dispersed throughout the body most rapidly when they are administered by intravenous (IV) injection. The nurse must be thoroughly educated regarding the responsibilities and techniques associated with administering IV medications. It is important to remember that after a drug enters the patient's bloodstream, it cannot be retrieved.

The absorption of topical drugs that have been applied to the skin can be influenced by the drug concentration, the length of contact time, the size of the affected area, the thickness of the skin surface, the hydration of the tissue, and the degree of skin disruption. Percutaneous (i.e., across-the-skin) absorption is greatly increased in newborns and young infants, who have thin, well-hydrated skin. When drugs are inhaled, their absorption can be influenced by the depth of the patient's respirations, the fineness of the droplet particles, the available surface area of the patient's mucous membranes, the contact time, the hydration state, the blood supply to the area, and the concentration of the drug itself.

Distribution

The term *distribution* refers to the ways in which drugs are transported throughout the body by the circulating body fluids to the sites of action or to the receptors that the drug affects. *Drug distribution* refers to the transport of the drug throughout the entire body by the blood and lymphatic systems and the transport from the circulating fluids into and out of the fluids that bathe the receptor sites. Organs with the most extensive blood supplies (e.g., heart, liver, kidneys, brain) receive the distributed drug most rapidly. Areas with less extensive blood supplies (e.g., muscle, skin, fat) receive the drug more slowly.

After a drug has been dissolved and absorbed into the circulating blood, its distribution is determined by the chemical properties of the drug and how it is affected by the blood and tissues that it contacts. Two factors that influence drug distribution are protein binding and lipid (fat) solubility. Most drugs are transported in combination with plasma proteins (especially albumin), which act as carriers for relatively insoluble drugs. Drugs that are bound to plasma proteins are pharmacologically inactive because the large size of the complex keeps them in the bloodstream and prevents them from reaching the sites of action, metabolism, and excretion. Only the free, or *unbound*, portion of a drug is able to diffuse into tissues, interact with receptors, and produce physiologic effects; it is also only this portion that can be metabolized and excreted. The same proportions of bound and free drug are maintained in the blood at all times. Thus, as the free drug acts on receptor sites or is metabolized, the decrease in the serum drug level causes some of the bound drug to be released from protein to maintain the ratio between bound and free drug.

When a drug leaves the bloodstream, it may become bound to tissues other than those with active receptor sites. The more lipid-soluble drugs have a high affinity for adipose tissue, which serves as a repository site for these agents. Because there is a relatively low level of blood circulation to fat tissues, the more lipid-soluble drugs tend to stay in the body much longer. Equilibrium is established between the repository site (i.e., lipid tissue) and the circulation so that as the **drug blood level** drops as a result of binding at the sites of physiologic activity, metabolism, or excretion, more drug is released from the lipid tissue. By contrast, if more drug is given, a new equilibrium is established among the blood, the receptor sites, the lipid tissue repository sites, and the metabolic and excretory sites.

Distribution may be general or selective. Some drugs cannot pass through certain types of cell membranes, such as the blood-brain barrier (i.e., the central nervous system) or the placental barrier (i.e., the placenta), whereas other types of drugs readily pass into these tissues. The distribution process is very important because the amount of drug that actually gets to the receptor sites determines the extent of pharmacologic activity. If little of the drug actually reaches and binds to the receptor sites, the response will be minimal.

Metabolism

Metabolism is the process whereby the body inactivates drugs. The enzyme systems of the liver are the primary sites for the metabolism of drugs, but other tissues and organs (e.g., white blood cells, GI tract, lungs) metabolize certain drugs to a minor extent. Genetic, environmental, and physiologic factors are involved in the regulation of drug metabolism reactions. The most important factors for the conversion of drugs to their metabolites are genetic variations of enzyme systems, the concurrent use of other drugs, exposure to environmental pollutants, concurrent illnesses, and age. (For more information, see Chapter 3.)

Excretion

The elimination of drug metabolites and, in some cases, of the active drug itself from the body is called *excretion*. The two primary routes of excretion are through the GI tract into the feces and through the renal tubules into the urine. Other routes of excretion include evaporation through the skin, exhalation from the lungs, and secretion into saliva and breast milk.

Because the kidneys are major organs of drug excretion, the nurse should review the patient's chart for the results of urinalysis and renal function tests. A patient with renal failure often has an increase in the action and duration of a drug if the dosage and frequency of administration are not adjusted to allow for the patient's reduced renal function.

Figure 2-2 shows a schematic review of the ADME process of an oral medication. It is important to note how little of the active ingredient actually reaches the receptor sites for action.

HALF-LIFE

Drugs are eliminated from the body by means of metabolism and excretion. A measure of the time required for elimination is the half-life. The **half-life** is defined as the amount of time required for 50% of the drug to be eliminated from the body. For example, if a patient is given 100 mg of a drug that has a half-life of 12 hours, the following would be observed:

TIME (HOURS)	HALF-LIFE	DRUG REMAINING IN BODY (%)
0	—	100 mg (100)
12	1	50 mg (50)
24	2	25 mg (25)
36	3	12.5 mg (12.5)
48	4	6.25 mg (6.25)
60	5	3.12 mg (3.12)

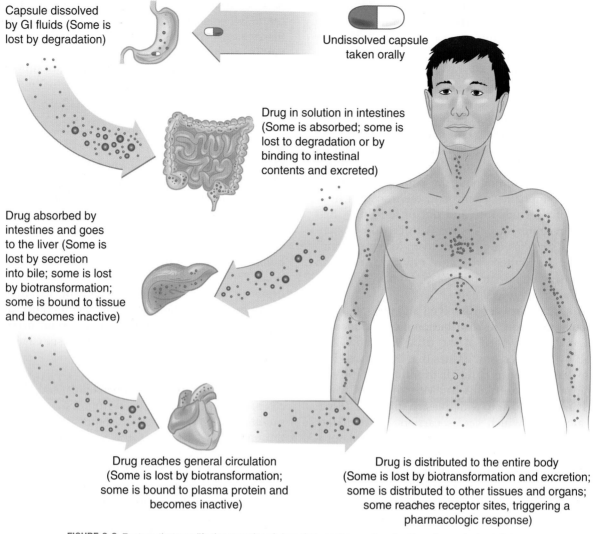

Capsule dissolved by GI fluids (Some is lost by degradation)

Undissolved capsule taken orally

Drug in solution in intestines (Some is absorbed; some is lost to degradation or by binding to intestinal contents and excreted)

Drug absorbed by intestines and goes to the liver (Some is lost by secretion into bile; some is lost by biotransformation; some is bound to tissue and becomes inactive)

Drug reaches general circulation (Some is lost by biotransformation; some is bound to plasma protein and becomes inactive)

Drug is distributed to the entire body (Some is lost by biotransformation and excretion; some is distributed to other tissues and organs; some reaches receptor sites, triggering a pharmacologic response)

FIGURE 2-2 Factors that modify the quantity of drug that reaches a site of action after a single oral dose.

Note that as each 12-hour period (i.e., one half-life) passes, the amount remaining is 50% of what was there 12 hours earlier. After six half-lives, more than 98% of the drug has been eliminated from the body.

The half-life is determined by an individual's ability to metabolize and excrete a particular drug. Because most patients metabolize and excrete a particular drug at approximately the same rate, the approximate half-lives of most drugs are now known. When the half-life of a drug is known, dosages and frequency of administration can be calculated. Drugs with long half-lives (e.g., digoxin, with a half-life of 36 hours) need to be administered only once daily, whereas drugs with short half-lives (e.g., aspirin, with a half-life of 5 hours) need to be administered every 4 to 6 hours to maintain therapeutic activity. For patients who have impaired hepatic or renal function, the half-life may become considerably longer because of their reduced ability to metabolize or excrete the drug. For example, digoxin has a half-life of about 36 hours in a patient with normal renal function; however, it has a half-life of

about 105 hours in a patient with complete renal failure. Monitoring diagnostic tests that measure renal or hepatic function is important. Whenever laboratory data reflect impairment of either function, the nurse should notify the healthcare provider.

DRUG ACTIONS

All drug actions have an onset, peak, and duration of action. The **onset of action** is when the concentration of a drug at the site of action is sufficient to start a physiologic (pharmacologic) response. Many factors—such as the route of administration, the rate of absorption, distribution, and binding to receptor sites—affect the onset of action. In general, increasing the dose of the drug hastens the onset of action by shortening the time required to achieve the necessary concentration of drug at the target site. **Peak action** is the time at which the drug reaches the highest concentrations on the target receptor sites, thereby inducing the maximal pharmacologic response for the dose given.

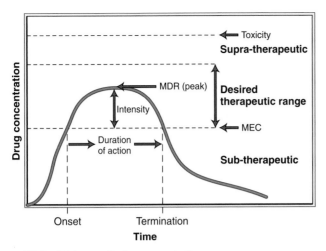

MEC = Minimum effective concentration
MDR = Maximum drug response (peak effect)

FIGURE 2-3 A time-response curve, which is also known as a *drug concentration–time profile*, demonstrates the relationship between the administration of a drug and the patient's response. If the drug level does not reach the minimum effective concentration, there will be no pharmacologic effect. If the peak level exceeds the toxicity threshold, toxic effects will result. The optimal drug concentration is in the middle of the therapeutic range.

The **duration of action** is how long the drug has a pharmacologic effect. The onset, peak, and duration of action of a drug are often illustrated by a time-response curve, which is also known as a drug concentration–time profile (Figure 2-3). A time-response curve demonstrates the relationship between the administration of a drug and the associated response. If the drug level does not reach the minimum effective concentration, there will be no pharmacologic effect. If the peak level exceeds the toxicity threshold, toxic effects will result. Generally, the drug concentration is targeted to be in the middle of this range, between the minimum effective response and the toxic response; this is referred to as the *therapeutic range.*

DRUG BLOOD LEVEL

When a drug is circulating in the blood, a blood sample may be drawn and assayed to determine the amount of drug present. This is known as a *drug blood level.* It is important for certain drugs (e.g., anticonvulsants, aminoglycoside antibiotics) to be measured to ensure that the drug blood level is within the therapeutic range. If the drug blood level is low, the dosage must be increased, or the medicine must be administered more frequently. If the drug blood level is too high, the patient may develop signs of toxicity; in this case, the dosage must be reduced or the medicine administered less frequently.

ADVERSE EFFECTS OF DRUGS

No drug has a single action. When a drug enters a patient and is then absorbed and distributed, the **desired action** (i.e., the expected response) usually occurs. However, all drugs have the potential to affect more than one body system simultaneously, thereby producing responses that are known as *side effects* or *common adverse effects*, which are mild, or *serious adverse effects*, which can lead to toxicity. The World Health Organization's definition of an adverse drug reaction (ADR) is "any noxious, unintended, and undesired effect of a drug, which occurs at dosages used in humans for prophylaxis, diagnosis, or therapy." A more common definition is as follows: "Right drug, right dose, right patient, bad effect." Adverse drug reactions should not be confused with medication errors or adverse drug events (ADEs), which are defined as "an injury resulting from medical intervention related to a drug." (For more information, see Chapter 6.)

Recent studies have indicated the following:
- Adverse drug reactions may be responsible for more than 100,000 deaths among hospitalized patients per year, which makes them one of the top six leading causes of death in the United States.
- An average of 6% of hospitalized patients experience a significant ADR at some point during their hospitalizations.
- Between 5% and 9% of hospitalization costs are attributable to ADRs.
- The most commonly seen ADRs are rash, nausea, itching, thrombocytopenia, vomiting, hyperglycemia, and diarrhea.
- The classes of medicines that account for the largest number of ADRs are antibiotics, cardiovascular medicines, cancer chemotherapy agents, analgesics, and antiinflammatory agents.

Most ADEs are predictable because of the pharmacologic effects of a drug, and patients should be monitored so that dosages can be adjusted to allow for the maximum therapeutic benefits with a minimum of adverse effects. As described in Units III through X of this text, each drug has a series of parameters (e.g., therapeutic actions to expect, adverse effects, probable drug interactions) that should be monitored by the nurse, physician, pharmacist, and patient to optimize therapy while reducing the possibility of serious adverse effects.

Accurate and appropriate drug-drug interaction information must be available to prescribers, and continual attention is currently focused on this issue. Further population-based studies still need to be conducted to meet federal initiatives to promote the meaningful use of information technologies and to integrate knowledge databases with clinical decision systems. Ideally, clinical decision systems and the databases of drug interactions that interface with them help the prescriber to identify and avoid potential medication interactions (Hines et al, 2011).

All hospitals have internal mechanisms for reporting suspected ADRs, and health professionals should not hesitate to report possible reactions. By monitoring and tracking the occurrences of ADRs, clinical protocols and improved patient screening will reduce the frequency of recurrence. The U.S. Food and Drug Administration's MedWatch program is also available for the voluntary reporting of adverse events. (For more information, see MedWatch on Evolve.)

Idiosyncratic Reaction

Two other types of drug actions are much more unpredictable: idiosyncratic reactions and allergic reactions. An **idiosyncratic reaction** occurs when something unusual or abnormal happens when a drug is first administered. The patient usually demonstrates an unexpectedly strong response to the action of the drug. This type of reaction is generally the result of a patient's inability to metabolize a drug because of a genetic deficiency of certain enzymes. Fortunately, this type of reaction is rare.

Allergic Reaction

Allergic reactions, which are also known as *hypersensitivity reactions,* occur in about 6% to 10% of patients who are taking medications. Allergic reactions occur among patients who have previously been exposed to a drug and whose immune systems have developed antibodies to the drug. Upon re-exposure to the drug, the antibodies cause a reaction; this reaction is most commonly seen as raised, irregularly shaped patches on the skin known as *hives,* which cause severe itching, known as *urticaria.*

Occasionally, a patient has a severe, life-threatening reaction that causes respiratory distress and cardiovascular collapse; this is known as an *anaphylactic reaction.* This condition is a medical emergency, and it must be treated immediately. Fortunately, anaphylactic reactions occur much less often than the more mild urticarial reactions.

If a patient has a mild reaction, it should be understood as a warning to not take the medication again. The patient is much more likely to have an anaphylactic reaction during his or her next exposure to the drug. Patients should receive information about the drug name and be instructed to tell healthcare practitioners that they have had such reactions and that they must not receive the drug again. In addition, patients should wear a medical alert bracelet or necklace that explains the allergy.

DRUG INTERACTIONS

A **drug interaction** is said to occur when the action of one drug is altered or changed by the action of another drug. Drug interactions are elicited in two ways: (1) by agents that, when combined, *increase* the actions of one or both drugs; and (2) by agents that, when combined, *decrease* the effectiveness of one or both drugs. Some drug interactions are beneficial, such as the use of caffeine, a central nervous system stimulant, with an antihistamine, a central nervous system depressant. The stimulatory effects of the caffeine counteract the drowsiness caused by the antihistamine without eliminating the antihistaminic effects. The mechanisms of drug interactions can be categorized as those that change the absorption, distribution, metabolism, or excretion of a drug and those that enhance the pharmacologic effect of a drug.

CHANGES IN ABSORPTION

Most drug interactions that change absorption take place in the GI tract, usually the stomach. Examples of this type of interaction include the following:

- Antacids inhibit the dissolution of ketoconazole tablets by increasing the gastric pH. The interaction is managed by giving the antacid at least 2 hours after ketoconazole administration.
- Aluminum-containing antacids inhibit the absorption of tetracycline. Aluminum salts form an insoluble chemical complex with tetracycline. The interaction is managed by separating the administration of tetracycline and antacids by 3 to 4 hours.

CHANGES IN DISTRIBUTION

Drug interactions that cause a change in distribution usually affect the binding of a drug to an inactive site (e.g., circulating plasma albumin, muscle protein). When a drug is absorbed into the blood, it is usually transported throughout the body bound to plasma proteins. It often binds to other proteins, such as those in muscle. A drug that is highly bound (e.g., >90% bound) to a protein-binding site may be displaced by another drug that has a higher affinity for the binding site. Significant interactions can take place this way because little displacement is required to have a major impact. Remember, only the **unbound drug** is pharmacologically active. If a drug is 90% bound to a protein, then 10% of the drug is providing the physiologic effect. If another drug is administered with a stronger affinity for the protein-binding site and displaces just 5% of the bound drug, there is now 15% unbound for physiologic activity; this is the equivalent of a 50% increase in dosage (i.e., from 10% to 15% active drug). For example, the anticoagulant action of warfarin is increased by administration with furosemide, which is a loop diuretic. Furosemide displaces warfarin from albumin-binding sites, thereby increasing the amount of unbound anticoagulant. This interaction is managed by decreasing the warfarin dosage.

CHANGES IN METABOLISM

Drug interactions usually result from a change in metabolism that involves inhibiting or inducing (stimulating) the enzymes that metabolize a drug. Medicines known to bind to enzymes and to slow the metabolism of other drugs include verapamil, chloramphenicol, ketoconazole, amiodarone, cimetidine, and erythromycin. Serum drug levels usually increase as a result of inhibited metabolism when these drugs are given concurrently, and the dosages usually must be reduced to prevent toxicity. For example, erythromycin inhibits the metabolism of theophylline; therefore the dose of theophylline must be reduced on the basis of theophylline serum levels and signs of toxicity. Because erythromycin (an antibiotic) is usually administered only in short courses, the theophylline dosage usually needs to be increased when the erythromycin is discontinued.

Common drugs that bind to an enzyme that increases its metabolism of the drug (enzyme inducers) are phenobarbital, carbamazepine, rifampin, and phenytoin. Rapidly metabolized drugs include disopyramide, doxycycline, griseofulvin, warfarin, metronidazole, mexiletine, quinidine, theophylline, and verapamil. When administered with enzyme inducers, the dosage of the more rapidly metabolized drug should generally be increased to provide therapeutic activity. The patient must be monitored closely for adverse effects, especially if the enzyme inducer is discontinued. The metabolism of the induced drug decelerates, thus leading to accumulation and toxicity if the dosage is not reduced. For example, if a woman who is taking oral contraceptives (e.g., Ortho-Novum [norethindrone and ethinyl estradiol], Lo/Ovral [ethinyl estradiol and norgestrel]) requires a course of rifampin antimicrobial therapy, the rifampin will induce the enzymes that metabolize both the progesterone and estrogen components of the contraceptive, thereby causing an increased incidence of menstrual abnormalities and reduced effectiveness of conception control. This interaction is managed by advising the patient to use an additional form of contraception while she is receiving rifampin therapy.

CHANGES IN EXCRETION

Drug interactions that cause a change in excretion usually act in the kidney tubules by changing the pH to enhance or inhibit excretion. The classic example of altered urine pH is with acetazolamide (which elevates urine pH) and quinidine. The alkaline urine produced by acetazolamide causes quinidine to be reabsorbed in the renal tubules, which potentially increases the physiologic and toxic effects of quinidine. The frequent monitoring of quinidine serum levels and assessments for signs of quinidine toxicity are used as guides for reducing quinidine dosage.

DRUGS THAT ENHANCE THE PHARMACOLOGIC EFFECTS OF OTHER DRUGS

Major drug interactions also occur between drugs. This may occur when one drug enhances the physiologic effects of another drug. Alcohol and sedative-hypnotic agents both cause sedation, but when used together can cause significant central nervous system depression. Another drug interaction that can have serious consequences is the interaction between aminoglycoside antibiotics (gentamicin, tobramycin) and a neuromuscular blocking agent such as pancuronium. When used together, the antibiotic increases the neuromuscular blockade prolonging return to normal respirations and recovery time. Table 2-1 defines drug-drug interactions.

Because it is impossible to memorize all possible drug interactions, the nurse must check for drug interactions when they are suspected. The nurse must take the time to consult drug resource books and pharmacists to ensure that a patient who is receiving multiple medications does not experience unanticipated drug interactions.

Table 2-1   Terminology Related to Drug-Drug Interactions

TERM	DEFINITION	EXAMPLE
Additive effect	Two drugs with similar actions are taken for an increased effect	hydrocodone + acetaminophen = added analgesic effect
Synergistic effect	The combined effect of two drugs is greater than the sum of the effect of each drug given together	aspirin + codeine = much greater analgesic effect
Antagonistic effect	One drug interferes with the action of another	tetracycline + antacid = decreased absorption of the tetracycline
Displacement	The displacement of the first drug from protein-binding sites (i.e., bound drugs are inactive) by a second drug increases the activity of the first drug because more unbound drug is available	warfarin + valproic acid = increased anticoagulant effect
Interference	The first drug inhibits the metabolism or excretion of the second drug, thereby causing increased activity of the second drug	probenecid + ampicillin = prolonged antibacterial activity of ampicillin because probenecid blocks the renal excretion of ampicillin
Incompatibility	The first drug is chemically incompatible with the second drug, thereby causing deterioration when the drugs are mixed in the same syringe or solution or are administered together at the same site; signs include haziness, formation of a precipitate, or a change in the color of the solution when the drugs are mixed	ampicillin + gentamicin = ampicillin inactivates gentamicin

Get Ready for the NCLEX® Examination!

Key Points

- The most common routes of drug administration are the enteral, parenteral, and percutaneous routes.
- The half-life of a drug is defined as the amount of time required for 50% of the drug to be eliminated from the body.
- After administration, all drugs go through five stages: *l*iberation, *a*bsorption, *d*istribution, *m*etabolism, and *e*xcretion (LADME). The enzyme systems of the liver are the primary sites for the metabolism of drugs, but other tissues and organs (e.g., white blood cells, GI tract, lungs) metabolize certain drugs to a minor extent.
- When a drug enters a patient and is absorbed and distributed, the desired action usually occurs. However, all drugs have the potential to affect more than one body system simultaneously, causing common adverse effects, which are mild or severe and can lead to toxicity.
- Drug interactions are elicited in two ways: (1) by agents that, when combined, *increase* the actions of one or both drugs; and (2) by agents that, when combined, *decrease* the effectiveness of one or both of the drugs.

Additional Learning Resources

SG to your Study Guide for additional Review Questions for the NCLEX® Examination, Critical Thinking Clinical Situations, and other learning activities to help you master this chapter content.

evolve Go to your Evolve website (http://evolve .elsevier.com/Clayton) for additional online resources.

Review Questions for the NCLEX® Examination

1. A nurse was reviewing the drug route for an order written to be given via nasogastric tube and understood that this meant the drug would be administered by this route:
   1. enteral.
   2. parenteral.
   3. percutaneous.
   4. intramuscular.

2. A patient takes 50 mg of a drug that has a half-life of 12 hours. What percentage of the dose remains in the body 36 hours after the drug is administered?
   1. 50 mg (100%)
   2. 25 mg (50%)
   3. 12.5 mg (25%)
   4. 6.25 mg (12.5%)

3. What is the portion of a drug that is pharmacologically active called?
   1. Protein-bound drug
   2. Unbound drug
   3. Drug tolerance level
   4. Incompatibility factor

4. When a drug that is considered an antihypertensive causes a drop in blood pressure to the normal range, this effect is called:
   1. antagonistic effect.
   2. desired effect.
   3. side effect.
   4. additive effect.

5. After the nurse injects the patient with the morning insulin dose, when will the action of the drug reach its highest physiologic effect?
   1. During peak action
   2. During displacement
   3. During the half-life
   4. During onset of action

6. When a patient has taken a drug and a rash appears along with severe itching, this reaction is called:
   1. idiosyncratic reaction.
   2. antagonistic effect.
   3. allergic reaction.
   4. displacement effect.

7. When a patient who was prescribed warfarin and valproic acid begins experiencing an increased effect of warfarin, this is known as:
   1. synergistic effect.
   2. antagonistic effect.
   3. idiosyncratic effect.
   4. displacement effect.

8. A person who has an increased metabolic rate (e.g., hyperthyroidism) generally requires what type of dosage?
   1. Normal dosage
   2. Lower-than-normal dosage
   3. Higher-than-normal dosage
   4. A dosage that is based on his or her thyroid function levels

objectives should state the purpose of the activities and the expected outcomes. Objectives may be developed in conjunction with a nursing diagnosis statement (e.g., Imbalanced nutrition: Less than body requirements), or they can be developed for common conditions that require care delivery (e.g., care of the patient who is receiving chemotherapy). Regardless of the format used, these instructional materials have established content that is given in outline form, and they are arranged so that one nurse can initiate the teaching and document the degree of understanding, and then another nurse can continue the teaching during a different shift or on a different day. The first nurse should check off what has been accomplished so that the next nurse knows where to resume the lesson.

At the start of each subsequent teaching session, it is important to review what has been covered previously and to affirm the retention of information from the previous lessons. The method known as *teach back* refers to asking the patient to explain in his or her own words what instruction was just received. This is an important part of patient education that will identify gaps in learning and help focus the nurse on what needs to be instructed. When psychomotor skills are being taught, return demonstrations by the patient are key to helping the patient practice and gain confidence in performing the task. Giving the patient immediate feedback about the skills and then giving him or her time to practice the skills that are more difficult allows the patient time to improve on mastering the procedure. If appropriate, equipment may be left with the patient for practice before the next session.

Sometimes it is particularly useful to set up a video of skill demonstrations for the patient to view alone at a convenient time. At the next meeting, the video can be reviewed together with the nurse, and important points can be discussed and clarified if the patient expresses confusion or uncertainty. This technique reinforces what has been said, reviews what has been learned, and provides the learner with repetition, which is necessary for learning.

MOTIVATE THE INDIVIDUAL TO LEARN

Before initiating a teaching plan, the nurse should be certain that the patient can focus and concentrate on the tasks and materials to be learned. The patient's basic needs (e.g., food, oxygen, pain relief) must be met before he or she can focus on learning. The nurse must recognize the individual's health beliefs when trying to motivate the patient. Because health teaching requires the integration of the patient's beliefs, attitudes, values, opinions, and needs, an individualized teaching plan must be developed based on the patient's beliefs and needs (Box 5-2).

Teaching does not require a formal setting. Some of the most effective teaching can be done while care is being delivered. The patient can be exposed to a skill, a treatment, or facts that must be comprehended in small increments. The nurse who explains a procedure and informs the patient why a certain procedure is being performed reinforces the need for it and motivates the patient to learn. When the patient understands the personal benefits of performing a task, his or her willingness to do it is strengthened.

DETERMINE READINESS TO LEARN

A patient's perception of his or her health and health status may differ from the nurse's judgment; therefore the values of health to each patient may differ greatly. The patient may not realize that a healthy lifestyle will provide significant benefits. A person who commonly indulges in alcohol, smoking, or a high-fat diet and leads a sedentary lifestyle may not consider the consequences of these practices in relation to health. Not everyone is interested in the concept of healthy living. The nurse must respect the individuality of the patient, family, or group being treated; he or she should accept that not everyone is motivated by the possibility of a higher level of wellness.

The nurse can positively influence the learning process by being enthusiastic about the content to be taught. A patient's response to the new information will vary and depends on several factors, including the following: the need to know, the patient's life experiences and self-concept, the effect of the illness on the patient's lifestyle, the patient's experience with learning new materials, and the patient's readiness to learn. Consideration must be given to the patient's psychosocial adaptation to illness and his or her ability to focus on learning. For example, during the denial, anger, or bargaining stages of grieving, the patient usually is neither prepared nor willing to accept the limitations imposed by the disease process. During the resolution and acceptance stages of the grieving process, the patient moves toward accepting responsibility and develops a willingness to learn what is necessary to attain an optimal level of health. The nurse can use encouragement and support the patient's attempts to learn new, challenging, or difficult procedures (Figure 5-2).

For teaching activities that are conducted with children, psychosocial, cognitive, and language abilities must be considered. Cognitive and motor development, as well as the patient's language usage and understanding, must be assessed. Age definitely influences the types and amounts of self-care activities that the child is capable of learning. The nurse should consult a text that addresses developmental theory for further information.

Adult education is usually oriented toward learning what is necessary to maintain a particular lifestyle. In general, adults need to understand why they must learn something before they undertake the effort to learn it. When planning the educational needs of the patient, the nurse must assess what the patient already knows and what additional information is desired.

Box 5-2	Sample Teaching Plan for a Patient With Diabetes Mellitus Taking One Type of Insulin*

UNDERSTANDING OF HEALTH CONDITION
- Assess the patient's and the family's understanding of diabetes mellitus.
- Clarify the meaning of the disease in terms that the patient is able to understand.
- Establish learning goals through mutual discussion. Teach the most important information first. Set dates for the teaching of content after discussion with the patient.

FOOD AND FLUIDS
- Arrange for the patient and his or her family members and significant others to attend nutrition lectures and demonstrations about food preparation.
- Reinforce knowledge of exchange lists (or other dietary methods) with the use of tactful questioning and by giving the patient a chance to practice food selections for daily meals from the menus provided.
- Explain how to manage the diabetic diet during illness (e.g., with nausea and vomiting, patient should increase fluid intake) and when to contact the healthcare provider.
- Stress the interrelationship of food with the onset, peak, and duration of the prescribed insulin.

MONITORING TESTS
- Demonstrate how to collect and test blood glucose samples and, as appropriate, urine.
- Validate understanding by having the patient collect, test, and record the results of the testing for the remainder of the hospitalization.
- Stress serum glucose testing before meals and at bedtime.
- Explain the importance of regular follow-up laboratory studies (e.g., fasting plasma glucose testing, postprandial Hb A_{1c}) to monitor the patient's degree of control.

MEDICATIONS AND TREATMENTS
- Teach the name, dosage, route of administration, desired action, and storage and refilling procedures for the type of insulin prescribed.
- Explain the principles of insulin action, onset, peak, and duration (see Chapter 35).
- Demonstrate how to prepare and administer the prescribed dose of insulin.
- Teach site location and self-administration of insulin.
- Give specific instructions that address the reading of the syringe to be used at home.
- Teach the patient how to obtain supplies (e.g., disposable syringes, needles, glucometer, glucose monitoring strips, insulin pen).
- Discuss the usual timing of reactions, the signs and symptoms of hypoglycemia or hyperglycemia, and the management of each complication.
- Validate the patient's understanding of common adverse effects and serious adverse effects.
- Teach and validate family members' and significant others' understanding of the signs and symptoms of hypoglycemia and hyperglycemia and the management of each complication.

- Teach a general approach to the management of illnesses (e.g., the actions required if nausea and vomiting or fever occur; stress glucose monitoring before meals and at bedtime; discuss the situations when there is a need to call a healthcare provider).

PERSONAL HYGIENE
- Discuss the great importance of managing personal hygiene, and emphasize the need to consult a healthcare provider for guidance and discussion:
  - Regular foot care
  - Meticulous oral hygiene and dental care
  - Care of cuts, scratches, and minor and major injuries
  - Stress management and needed alterations in insulin dosage during an illness

ACTIVITIES
- Help the patient develop a detailed time schedule for usual activities of daily living. Incorporate diabetic care needs into this schedule.
- Encourage maintaining all usual activities of daily living. Discuss anticipated problems and possible interventions.
- Discuss personal care needs not only at home, but also in the work setting, as appropriate. (Consider involving the industrial nurse, if available, in the work setting.)
- Discuss the effects of an increase or decrease in activity level on the management of diabetes mellitus.

HOME OR FOLLOW-UP CARE
- Arrange for outpatient or healthcare provider follow-up appointments and schedule ordered laboratory tests.
- Advise the patient to seek assistance from the healthcare provider or from the nearest emergency department service for problems that may develop.
- Arrange appropriate referrals to community health agencies, if needed.
- Complete a diabetic alert card or another means (e.g., an identification necklace or bracelet) of alerting people to the individual's needs in case of an emergency.
- Discuss an exercise program with the healthcare provider.

SPECIAL EQUIPMENT AND INSTRUCTIONAL MATERIAL
- Develop a list of equipment and supplies to be purchased; have a family member purchase and bring these to the hospital for use during teaching sessions (e.g., blood glucose monitoring supplies, syringes, insulin pen, needles, alcohol wipes).
- Show audiovisual materials that address insulin preparation, storage, and administration, as well as serum glucose testing.
- Develop a written record (see Chapter 35), and assist the patient with maintaining data during hospitalization.

OTHER
- Teach measures to make travel easier.
- Tell the patient about the American Diabetes Association and about the materials available from this resource.

*Each item listed must be assessed for the individual's current knowledge base and level of understanding throughout the course of teaching. The process is reassessed and the teaching continued until the patient masters all facets of self-care needs. With the advent of shorter hospitalizations, inpatient and outpatient teaching may be necessary, and it may include referral to community-based healthcare agencies, as needed. Discharge charting and referral should carefully document those facets of the teaching plan that have been mastered and those that need to be taught. The healthcare provider should be notified of deficits in the patient's learning ability or in his or her mastery of needed elements in the teaching plan.

FIGURE 5-2 A patient does a return demonstration of an insulin injection after being taught by the nurse. (Courtesy Jim Varney, North Yorkshire, UK.)

Life Span Considerations
Older Adults

Teaching Older Adults

The older adult needs to be further assessed before the implementation of health teaching; these assessments should include vision, hearing, and short- and long-term memory. If a task is to be taught, fine and gross motor abilities need to be evaluated as well. An older patient may also have major concerns regarding the cost of the proposed treatments in relation to available resources. A patient will often evaluate the benefits of planned medical interventions and their overall effect on the quality of life. Any of these situations can affect the ability of the patient to focus on the new information to be taught, thus influencing his or her response to and the overall outcome of the teaching. Older adults have often experienced losses and may be facing social isolation, physical (functional) losses, and financial constraints. Because older adults often have more chronic health problems, a new diagnosis, an exacerbation of a disease, or a new crisis may be physically and emotionally overwhelming. Therefore the timing of patient instruction is of great significance.

When teaching an older patient, it is prudent to slow the pace of the presentation and to limit the length of each session to prevent overtiring. Older adults can learn the material, but they often process things more slowly than younger people do because their short-term memory may be more limited. The nurse must work with the patient to develop ways to remember what is being taught. The more that the older person is involved in forming the associations that will be used to remember new ideas and to connect these ideas with past experiences, the better the outcome.

Many patients are embarrassed by their inability to master a task. Asking them if they understand is not going to be effective because they will not admit their embarrassment or that they do not understand. The nurse should provide information in small increments and allow for practice, review, practice, review, and practice until success is achieved. The nurse can stop at appropriate intervals and reschedule sessions to meet the patient's learning needs. *Teach back* can be used as an important tool to help the nurse verify the information understood.

When the patient becomes anxious, the presentation of new information can be slowed, repeated, or stopped and the session rescheduled. Fear and anxiety often impair a person's ability to focus on the task or content being presented, so creating an environment that is conducive to learning is important.

When anxiety is high, the ability to focus on details is reduced. The nurse should anticipate periods during hospitalization when teaching can be more effective. Some teaching is most successful when it is done spontaneously, such as when the patient asks direct questions about his or her progress toward discharge. The nurse also must learn to anticipate inopportune times to initiate teaching, such as when a patient becomes withdrawn after learning about a diagnosis with a poor prognosis. With reduced hospital stays, the ability to time patient education ideally and to perform actual teaching is a challenge. It is imperative that the nurse document those aspects of health teaching that have been mastered and—of equal importance—those that have not been; he or she must then request referral to an appropriate agency for follow-up teaching and assistance.

Clinical Goldmine

Consider the lighting so that there is no glare on reading materials; face the learner for better eye contact; and speak directly and in a clear tone, without shouting. Be calm, use tact and diplomacy if frustrations develop, and try to instill confidence in the learner's ability to surmount any problems.

SPACE THE CONTENT

Spacing or staggering the amount of material given during one session should be considered, regardless of the age of the person being taught. People tend to remember what is learned first. With this principle in mind, the nurse can provide multiple short sessions rather than a few longer sessions that may overwhelm the patient.

USE REPETITION TO ENHANCE LEARNING

It is important for the nurse to recognize that patients need repetition to learn new content. The nurse needs to repeat what was previously taught to help the patient understand what is important to remember and build on it to the next level.

CONSIDER EDUCATION LEVEL

An important consideration to keep in mind when teaching adult patients is their literacy level. Just giving the patient a pamphlet to read may not be appropriate if the patient cannot read. Instead, the nurse could review the pamphlet with the patient and then determine the level of the patient's understanding of the information.

Medical terms may not be understood, and written instructions left at the bedside may be misinterpreted or not read at all. Some patients may be illiterate, whereas others may read at a first-grade, seventh-grade, or collegiate level. Therefore if written materials are used, it is important to consider these wide variations in literacy.

INCORPORATE CULTURE AND ETHNIC DIVERSITY

Many healthcare providers have a limited understanding of what other cultures believe and the importance of these benefits to the learning process. **Ethnocentrism** is the assumption that one's culture provides the right way, the best way, and the only way to live. Briefly, people who believe in the theory of ethnocentrism assume that their way of viewing the world is superior to that of others (Leininger, 2002). As an understanding of cultural diversity increases, healthcare providers must expand their knowledge of the basic tenets of the belief systems that they may encounter among their patients.

Because there are differing beliefs, it is important that the nurse explore the meaning of an illness with the patient. Members of other cultures do not always express themselves when their views are in conflict with those of another culture. Unless a careful assessment of psychosocial needs is performed, the true meaning of an illness or the proposed intervention may never be uncovered. Even the assessment process has obstacles attached. Patients in some cultures do not believe that family information should be shared outside of the family. For example, some Eastern European cultures prefer not to reveal any history of psychiatric illness or treatment and are usually reluctant to share any sexual history. Others, such as the Native American culture, believe that only the affected individual may reveal information.

Communication is vitally important within any cultural group. However, verbal and nonverbal types of communication mean different things to different cultures. For example, whites tend to value eye contact, whereas in other cultures (e.g., Native Americans, Asians) direct eye contact is a sign of disrespect or rudeness. As a part of communication, knowing how to address the patient is also important. African American patients often prefer to have their formal names used rather than their first names, especially older family members. Chinese people tend to be more formal than Americans, and husbands and wives do not necessarily have the same last name. The simple gesture of asking the patient how he or she prefers to be addressed is both helpful and respectful.

Working with an interpreter when a language barrier exists presents several additional challenges to understanding. The nurse should first explain the educational session to the interpreter and then discuss the types of questions that will be asked of the patient. Whenever a third person enters into the communication cycle, a lack of clarity and misinterpretation can occur. The nurse should keep questions brief and ask them one at a time to give the interpreter an opportunity to rephrase the question and obtain a response. Sometimes supplementing questions with pictures and pantomime gestures may be helpful. When using an interpreter, the nurse should look directly at the patient (not at the interpreter) while conversing.

The members of the health team should always try to ascertain the patient's beliefs about illness. The following should be taken into consideration:

- Is "good health" defined as the ability to work or to fulfill family roles, or is it a reward from God or a balance with nature?
- Does the patient believe that healthcare can improve health outcomes, or does fate determine the outcome?
- Are any cultural or religious disease prevention approaches used in the household?
- Do family members wear talismans or charms for protection against illness?
- Are cultural healers important (e.g., Chinese herbalists, Native American medicine men)?

As part of the *cultural assessment,* the nurse should determine factors that relate to the cultural beliefs of the family. Inquire as to whether other family members should be included in the discussion of the patient's medical care. Be sure to include the decision makers in the teaching session so that the teaching will not be wasted. Always remain sensitive to the patient's and family's cultural beliefs and practices. Nurses can demonstrate understanding, empathy, respect, and patience for the patient's cultural values through their communication and actual delivery of healthcare. Consult assessment textbooks for more extensive coverage of ethnic and cultural issues.

As cultural mixes become more common, educational materials are being adapted to meet a variety of cultural considerations. Unfortunately, this does not solve all of the problems. Interpreting written materials still leaves room for misunderstanding, because many people cannot read or do not read at the level of the provided materials.

STRATEGIES FOR HEALTH TEACHING

TEACH APPROPRIATE USE OF THE INTERNET

It has become common for consumers to access the Internet for healthcare inquiries, including medical consultation from an online physician or another healthcare professional about a particular healthcare concern. Consumers can purchase medications online and research healthcare treatments. The convenience of accessing electronic healthcare information is a powerful resource for consumers, and it is one that provides anonymity and that may serve to empower the patient. Valid healthcare information can assist patients with the making of informed healthcare decisions (Table 5-1).

Today, many patients present to the healthcare provider's office with some knowledge of their disease, treatment, and medications. This has altered the nurse's role as a provider of healthcare education to resemble that of a consultant. It is the nurse's role to teach patients to use the Internet effectively, to evaluate websites for validity, and to assist patients with understanding the information that they have accessed. The nurse should also provide patients with the tools to evaluate websites for validity and to tell them about reputable sites that are specific to their healthcare needs. With the abundance of health- and disease-related information on the Internet, the quality of information varies. Therefore it is essential that the nurse maintain an educational partnership with the patient and his or her caregivers.

ENCOURAGE ADHERENCE

Healthcare providers and educators tend to think that a patient should change behaviors and adhere to a new therapeutic regimen simply because the nurse said so. However, patients do have the right to make their own life choices, and they often do. Unfortunately, there is no way to ensure adherence unless the patient recognizes its value.

Success with a health regimen is enhanced when the nurse conveys an enthusiastic attitude, appears positive about the subject matter, and shows confidence in the abilities of the patient to understand the lesson. Reinforcing positive accomplishments fosters successful achievement.

The patient's response to the therapeutic regimen (including medications) and his or her degree of compliance are influenced by several variables, including the following:
- Beliefs about the seriousness of the illness
- Perceptions of the benefits of the proposed treatment plans

Table 5-1 Sources of Patient Information

SOURCE	DESCRIPTION
Health on the Net Foundation (http://www.hon.ch)	Leading organization that promotes and guides the deployment of useful and reliable online medical and health information and its appropriate and efficient use
Healthcare institution intranet	Data available through an institution-specific intranet Provides an online resource for drug information (e.g., Micromedex) Often includes information about diseases and diagnostic testing Information may be printed by the nurse and used for patient education
Krames Online (http://nih.kramesonline.com)	Patients access this site on their own Includes information about diseases, conditions, treatments, procedures, surgeries, and medications, including prescription medications and over-the-counter products
Therapeutic Choices	Published by the Canadian Pharmacists Association 1200-page handbook that describes major diseases and their treatment Discussions of medical conditions are brief Focuses on goals of therapy, management algorithms, and the discussion of nonpharmacologic and pharmacologic therapies

- Personal beliefs, values, and attitudes toward health, the provider of the medication, and the healthcare system, including prior experience with the system
- Effects of the proposed changes on personal lifestyle
- Acceptance (or denial) of the illness and its associated problems; other psychological issues, such as anger about the illness, apathy, depression, forgetfulness, and confusion
- High stress or daily stresses, such as dysfunctional families, difficult living situations, poverty, long working hours in a tense environment, and problematic parenting issues
- Comprehension and understanding of the health regimen or frequent changes in the regimen; the inability to read written instructions

- Multiple physicians or healthcare providers prescribing medications
- Costs of treatment in relation to resources and possible difficulty with getting prescriptions filled
- Support of significant others or problems with assistance needed in the home
- Amount of control that the patient experiences with regard to the disease or condition
- Side effects of the treatment and the degree of inconvenience, annoyance, or impairment in functioning that they produce
- Degree of positive response achieved
- Physical difficulties that limit access to or use of medication, such as swallowing tablets, difficulty with opening containers or handling small tablets, or the inability to distinguish colors or identifying markings on different medications
- Concerns about taking drugs and the fear of addiction

Evaluating the ability of a patient to comply with a proposed health regimen is a complex process that involves using established criteria to reach a conclusion. The ultimate goal is to assist patients with achieving the greatest degree of control possible within the context of their beliefs, values, and needs. Healthcare professionals can offer support and encouragement, be complimentary about positive achievements, and encourage an examination of the available options and the benefits of a healthy lifestyle. It is vital to assist patients with exploring options when a problem or complication arises rather than giving up on the treatment because information about alternatives is lacking. Financial considerations may also affect the patient's decisions.

Strategies for Increasing Adherence

The challenge for nursing is to increase the adherence of patients to their healthcare regimen and to minimize hospital readmission and suffering from complications. It is estimated that poor adherence to medical therapy accounts for about $300 billion in unnecessary healthcare expenses each year. One model that has been used to induce behavioral change in patients is called the *Case Management Adherence Guidelines, version 1*. This project, developed by Pfizer and the Case Management Society of America, is a series of tools that are used by case managers (many of whom are nurses) to assess the patient's motivation level and his or her knowledge of prescribed medications and other therapies. It also assesses a patient's social support system. The tools help to identify those who are more at risk for nonadherence so that interventions can be initiated early during the care process. A key principle of this model is that the nurse must recognize that the patient will make the final decisions. The nurse must negotiate with (not dictate to) the patient to implement actions that may result in positive change. This approach gives the nurse and patient ownership of the goals to be achieved.

Another type of research technique used to study adherence is **ethnography**. When a patient is not meeting expected outcomes, an ethnographer may visit the patient at home to observe how the patient administers his or her healthcare regimen. Observations are made with regard to how and which procedures are accomplished and what errors are being made. Industry has used these methods for many years to help design work flow for production, and it has been discovered that this is also a valuable tool in health care for improving patient outcomes. It is important to remember that the patient may not be purposefully nonadherent; rather, the home environment may not be set up to allow the patient to follow care instructions.

USE RELEVANT CONTENT

Nurses tend to think that patients will do what is suggested simply because they have been told that it will be beneficial. In the hospital, the nurse and other healthcare members reinforce the basic therapeutic regimen; at discharge, however, the patient leaves the controlled environment and is free to choose to follow the prescribed treatment or to alter it as deemed appropriate on the basis of personal values and beliefs. For learning to take place, the patient must perceive the information as being relevant. Whenever possible, start with simple and attainable goals to build the patient's confidence. It is important to correlate the teaching with the patient's perspective of the illness and his or her ability to control the signs and symptoms or the course of the disease process.

COMMUNICATE GOALS AND EXPECTATIONS OF THERAPY

Before discharge, reasonable responses to the planned therapy should be discussed. The patient should know what signs and symptoms may be altered by the prescribed medications. The precautions necessary when taking a medication must be explained by the nurse and understood by the patient (e.g., to use caution when operating power equipment or a motor vehicle, to avoid direct sunlight, to ensure that follow-up laboratory studies are carried out).

Changes in Expectations

Changes in the patient's expectations should be assessed as therapy progresses and as the patient gains understanding and skill with regard to managing the diagnosis. The expectations of therapy for patients with acute illnesses may vary widely from those of patients with chronic illnesses.

Cooperative Goal Setting

An attitude of shared input into goals and outcomes can encourage the patient to enter into a therapeutic alliance. Therefore the patient should be taught to help monitor the parameters that are used to evaluate therapy. It is imperative that the nurse nurture a cooperative environment that encourages the patient to do the following: (1) keep records of the essential data that are needed to evaluate the prescribed therapy; and (2) contact the healthcare provider for advice rather than alter the medication regimen or discontinue the medication entirely. For each major class of drugs in this book, written records (located on Evolve) are provided to help the nurse identify essential data that the patient needs to understand and record. In the event that the patient and his or her family or significant others do not understand all aspects of the continuing therapy prescribed, they may be referred to a community-based agency for help with achieving long-term healthcare requirements.

Discharge Planning and Teaching

A summary statement of the patient's unmet needs must be written and placed in the medical chart. The healthcare provider should be consulted about the possibility of a referral to a community-based agency for continued monitoring or treatment. The nurse's discharge notes must identify the nursing diagnoses that have not been met and the potential collaborative problems that require continued monitoring and intervention. All counseling information should be carefully drafted in a manner that the patient can read and understand.

Get Ready for the NCLEX® Examination!

Key Points

- The three domains of learning are the cognitive, affective, and psychomotor domains.
- The main principles of learning include the patient's attitudes toward learning, readiness to learn, and individual learning style.
- Patient education in relation to medications includes understanding the benefits of the medications, the common adverse effects, and potential drug interactions.
- Nurses play an important role in teaching patients about how they can maintain and improve their own well-being by understanding the intent of the therapies prescribed.
- The types of information discussed with the patient and his or her family include the medications and treatments to be continued after discharge and activities, special equipment, and follow-up care.
- Specific techniques used to facilitate patient education include determining the patient's readiness to learn, repetition of information, motivating the patient, and understanding the patient's culture.

Additional Learning Resources

SG Go to your Study Guide for additional Review Questions for the NCLEX® Examination, Critical Thinking Clinical Situations, and other learning activities to help you master this chapter content.

evolve Go to your Evolve website (http://evolve .elsevier.com/Clayton) for additional online resources.

Review Questions for the NCLEX® Examination

1. Which statement is an example of an objective or outcome of health teaching that involves the cognitive domain of learning?
   1. The patient will demonstrate the correct way to use a peak flow meter.
   2. The patient will verbalize an understanding of the potential side effects of digoxin.
   3. The patient will correctly place medications in the proper box when filling the drug box.
   4. The patient will discuss with his or her spouse how the treatment proposal will affect their lives.

2. The nurse is developing a teaching plan for a patient who will have limited activity at home after a recent fall. What principle of learning is involved when teaching this patient?
   1. The timing of the teaching is important for learning to take place.
   2. Teaching is effective when all family members are present.
   3. The affective domain is particularly useful when dealing with the grieving process.
   4. Financial considerations are not part of the issues involved in patient teaching.

3. The nurse was reviewing the discharge medication list with the patient who recently had been hospitalized for heart failure. The patient stated that the medications were not new and that everything was fine. The nurse made the following correct reply:
   1. "Your medications are important to understand so that you will not have to come back to the hospital frequently."
   2. "The doctor wants you to remember all your medications so when you go back to the clinic you will know the list."
   3. "Your medication list is not as important as remembering to take your doses every day."
   4. "I have to tell you all these medications before you can go home."

4. Which patient is most ready to begin a patient teaching session?
   1. A patient who has had nausea and vomiting for the past 24 hours
   2. A patient who has just been told that he needs to have major surgery
   3. A patient who has voiced a concern about how insulin injections will affect her lifestyle
   4. A patient who is complaining bitterly about a low-fat, low-cholesterol diet after his heart attack

5. The following information about medications is important to teach patients: (Select all that apply.)
   1. The name, dosage, and route of administration of the medication
   2. The laboratory studies that need to be monitored while on the medication
   3. The common adverse effects and possible serious adverse effects to watch for
   4. The correct pharmacy to obtain the medication from
   5. The correct schedule or timing of the medication to follow

6. The patient presents with educational information about medication that has been obtained from the Internet. What does the role of the nurse as consultant include? (Select all that apply.)
   1. Evaluating websites for validity
   2. Assisting the patient with purchasing medications online
   3. Assisting the patient with understanding the information accessed
   4. Providing the patient with tools to evaluate websites for validity
   5. Encouraging the use of one search engine

chapter

Principles of Medication Administration and Medication Safety

6

http://evolve.elsevier.com/Clayton

Objectives

1. Identify the legal and ethical considerations for medication administration.
2. Compare and contrast the various systems used to dispense medications.
3. Identify what a narcotic control system entails.
4. Define the four categories of medication orders.
5. Identify common types of medication errors and actions that can be taken to prevent them.
6. Identify precautions used to ensure the right drug is prepared and given to the right patient.
7. List the seven rights of medication administration.
8. Identify the appropriate nursing documentation of medications, including the effectiveness of each medication.

Key Terms

nurse practice act (p. 60)
standards of care (p. 60)
summary sheet (SŬM-ă-rē SHĒT) (p. 61)
consent form (kŏn-SĔNT) (p. 61)
order form (ŌR-dŭr) (p. 61)
history and physical examination form (HĬS-tō-rē and FĬZ-ĭ-kŭl ĕgz-ăm-ĭ-NĀ-shŭn) (p. 61)
progress notes (PRŎ-grĕs) (p. 61)
nurses' notes (p. 61)
nursing care plan (p. 61)
laboratory tests record (LĂB-ōr-ă-tōr-ē) (p. 63)
graphic record (GRĂ-fĭk) (p. 63)
medication administration record (MAR) (p. 63)
flow sheets (FLŌ SHĒTS) (p. 63)
consultation reports (kŏn-sŭl-TĀ-shŭn) (p. 63)
medication profile (PRŌ-fīl) (p. 64)
PRN (p. 65)
patient education record (PĀ-shĕnt ĕd-jū-KĀ-shŭn) (p. 65)
Kardex (KĂR-dĕks) (p. 65)
floor or ward stock system (FLŌR or WŌRD STŎK SĬS-tĕm) (p. 67)
individual prescription order system (ĭn-dĭ-VĬD-jū-ăl prē-SKRĬP-shŭn) (p. 68)

unit-dose drug-distribution systems (YŪ-nĭt DŌS DRŬG dĭs-trĭ-BYŪ-shŭn) (p. 68)
computer-controlled dispensing system (kŏm-PYŪ-tŭr kŏn-TRŌLD dĭ-SPĔN-sĭng) (p. 68)
bar codes (BĂR KŌDZ) (p. 69)
long-term care unit-dose system (p. 69)
narcotic control systems (năr-KŎ-tĭk kŏn-TRŌL) (p. 70)
disposal of unused medicines (dĭs-PŌ-zŭl of ŭn-YŪZD MĔD-ĭ-sĕnz) (p. 72)
stat order (STĂT ŌR-dŭr) (p. 72)
single order (SĬN-gŭl) (p. 73)
standing order (STĂN-dĭng) (p. 73)
PRN order (p. 73)
computerized provider order entry (CPOE) systems (p. 73)
medication safety (p. 73)
medication errors (ĀR-ŭrz) (p. 73)
adverse drug events (p. 73)
high-alert medications (HĪ-ă-LŬRT) (p. 74)
medication reconciliation (rĕ-kŏn-sĭl-ē-Ă-shĕn) (p. 74)
handoffs (HĂND-ŏfs) (p. 74)
verification (văr-ĭ-fĭ-KĀ-shĕn) (p. 75)
transcription (trăn-SKRĬP-shĕn) (p. 75)
variance (VĀR-ē-ăns) (p. 75)

Before medications are administered, the nurse must understand the professional responsibilities associated with medication administration, drug orders, medication delivery systems, and the nursing process as it relates to drug therapy. Ignorance of the nurse's overall responsibilities as part of the system may result in delays in the receiving and administering of medications and serious administration errors. In either case, care is compromised, and the patient may suffer unnecessarily.

LEGAL AND ETHICAL CONSIDERATIONS

The practice of nursing under a professional license is a privilege, not a right. When accepting this privilege, the nurse must understand that this responsibility includes accountability for one's actions and judgments during the execution of professional duties. An understanding of the **nurse practice act** and the rules and regulations established by the state boards of nursing for the various levels of entry (i.e., practical nurse, registered nurse, and nurse practitioner) is a solid foundation for beginning practice. Many state boards have developed specific guidelines for nurses to use when practicing nursing.

STANDARDS OF CARE

Standards of care are guidelines that have been developed for the practice of nursing. These guidelines are defined by the nurse practice act of each state, by state and federal laws that regulate health care facilities, by The Joint Commission, and by professional organizations such as the American Nurses Association and other specialty nursing organizations (e.g., the Intravenous Nurses Society). Nurses must also be familiar with the established policies of the employing health care agency. Policies developed by the health care agency must adhere to the minimum standards of state regulatory authorities; however, agency policies may be more stringent than those that are recognized by the state. Employment by the agency implies the willingness of the nurse to adhere to established standards and to work within established guidelines. Examples of policy statements that are related to medication administration include the following:

1. *Educational requirements for professionals who are authorized to administer medications.* Many health care facilities require the passing of a written test to confirm the knowledge and skills needed for medication calculation, preparation, and administration before granting approval to an individual to administer any medications.
2. *Approved lists of intravenous solutions and medications that the nurse can start or add to an existing infusion.*
3. *Lists of restricted medications (e.g., antineoplastic agents, magnesium sulfate, allergy extracts, lidocaine, RhoGAM [Rh$_o$ (D) immune globulin], heparin) that may be administered only by certain staff members with specific credentials or training.*
4. *Lists of abbreviations that are not to be used in documentation to avoid medication errors* (see the page facing the inside back cover of this book).

Before administering any medication, the nurse must have a current license to practice, a clear policy statement that authorizes the act, and a medication order signed by a practitioner who is licensed with prescriptive privileges at that institution. The nurse must understand the individual patient's diagnosis and symptoms that correlate with the rationale for drug use. The nurse should also know why a medication is ordered and its expected actions, usual dosing, proper dilution, route and rate of administration, adverse effects, and the contraindications for the use of a particular drug. If drugs are to be administered with the use of the same syringe or at the same intravenous (IV) site, drug compatibility should be confirmed before administration. If the nurse is unsure about any of these key medication points, then he or she must consult an authoritative resource or the hospital pharmacist before administering a medication. The nurse must be accurate when calculating, preparing, and administering medications. The nurse must assess the patient to be certain that therapeutic and adverse effects associated with the medication regimen are reported. Nurses must be able to collect patient data at regularly scheduled intervals and to record observations in the patient's chart when evaluating a treatment's effectiveness. Claiming unfamiliarity with any of these nursing responsibilities when an avoidable complication arises is unacceptable; in fact, it is considered negligence of nursing responsibility.

Nurses must take an active role in educating the patient, the family, and significant others in preparation for the patient's discharge from the health care environment. A person's health will improve only to the extent that the patient understands how to care for himself or herself. Specific teaching goals should be developed and implemented. Nursing observations and the patient's progress toward the mastery of skills should be charted to document the patient's degree of understanding.

PATIENT CHARTS

The patient's chart or the electronic medical record is a primary source of information that is necessary for the patient assessment so that the nurse can create and implement plans for patient care. It is also where the nurse provides the documentation of the nursing assessments performed, the observations reported to the physician for further verification, the basic nursing measures implemented (e.g., daily treatments), the patient teaching performed, and the observed responses to therapy.

This record serves as the communication link among all members of the health care team regarding the patient's status, the care provided, and the patient's progress. The chart is a legal document that describes the patient's health, that lists diagnostic and therapeutic procedures initiated, and that describes the patient's response to these measures. The chart must be kept current as long as the patient is in the hospital. After the patient's discharge, this record is maintained according to policies within the institution. The patient record may be used for research to compare responses to selected therapies in a sampling of patients with similar diagnoses.

CONTENTS OF PATIENT CHARTS

Although each health care facility uses a slightly different format, the basic patient chart consists of the following elements. The different forms are often printed on different colored paper, or dividers with tabs separate the different sections.

Summary Sheet

The **summary sheet** gives the patient's name, address, date of birth, attending physician, gender, marital status, allergies, nearest relative, occupation and employer, insurance carrier and other payment information, religious preference, date and time of admission to the hospital, previous hospital admissions, and admitting problem or diagnosis. The date and time of discharge are added when appropriate.

Consent Forms

The admission **consent form** grants permission to the health care facility and the health care provider to provide treatment. Other types of consent forms are used during the course of a hospitalization, such as an operative procedure permit or consent, an invasive procedure consent, a blood-product consent, and a consent to bill the patient's insurance carrier.

Physician's Order Form

All procedures and treatments are ordered by the health care provider on the **order form**. These orders include general care (e.g., activity, diet, frequency of vital signs), laboratory tests to be completed, other diagnostic procedures (e.g., radiography, electrocardiography, computed tomography), and all medications and treatments (e.g., physical or occupational therapy).

History and Physical Examination Form

During admission to the hospital, the patient is interviewed by a healthcare provider and given a physical examination. The healthcare provider records the findings on the **history and physical examination form** and lists the problems to be corrected (e.g., the diagnoses). The history and physical examination form is often referred to as "the H&P."

Progress Notes

The attending healthcare provider records frequent observations of the patient's health status in the **progress notes**. In most hospitals, other health professionals (e.g., pharmacists, dietitians, physical and respiratory therapists) may record observations and suggestions.

Nurses' Notes

Although the format varies among institutions, the **nurses' notes** generally start with the nursing history. On admission, the nurse performs a complete health assessment of the patient. This process includes a head-to-toe physical assessment, and it also incorporates a patient and family history that provides insights into individual and family needs, life patterns, psychosocial and cultural data, and spiritual needs. This assessment will serve as the basis for the development of the individualized care plan and as a baseline for comparison when ongoing assessment data are gathered.

Nurses record the following in their notes: ongoing assessments of the patient's condition; responses to nursing interventions ordered by the physician (e.g., treatments or medications) or to those initiated by the nurse (e.g., skin care, patient education); evaluations of the effectiveness of nursing interventions; procedures completed by other healthcare professionals (e.g., wound cleaning by a physician, fitting for a prosthesis by a prosthetician); and other pertinent information (e.g., physician or family visits, patient's responses after these visits). Entries may be made on the nurses' notes or flow sheets throughout a shift, but general guidelines include the following: (1) completing records, including vital signs, immediately after assessing the patient, whether when he or she is first admitted or after he or she returns from a diagnostic procedure or therapy; (2) recording all "as needed" (PRN) medications immediately after administration and addressing the effectiveness of the medication; (3) recording change in the patient's status and who was notified (e.g., healthcare provider, manager, patient's family); (4) discussing the treatment of a sudden change in the patient's status; and (5) recording information about the transfer, discharge, or death of a patient. In addition to the accurate charting of the observations in a clear and concise form, the nurse should report significant changes in a patient's status to the charge nurse. The charge nurse then makes a nursing judgment regarding the notification of the attending healthcare provider. Nurses' notes are quickly being replaced by computerized charting methods that allow the nurse to document findings and basic care delivered using multiple screens of data and checklist-type formats.

Nursing Care Plans

After the initial data collection, the nurse develops an individualized **nursing care plan**. Care plans incorporate nursing diagnoses, critical pathway information, and physician-ordered and nursing-ordered care (see Nursing Care Plan). Most acute care facilities require the nurse to chart against each identified nursing diagnosis stated in the care plan every 8 hours. Care plans are evaluated and modified on a continuum throughout the course of treatment. The plan should be shared with the health care team to ensure an interdisciplinary approach to care. Many institutions have developed standardized care plans for the various nursing diagnoses. It is the nurse's responsibility to identify those

⭐ Nursing Care Plan | Risk for Infection

ASSESSMENT

Mrs. Spicer was admitted to the medical nursing unit 3 days ago with a diagnosis of lymphoma. She received her first dose of multiagent chemotherapy yesterday. Jess Ralston is the student nurse who is caring for Mrs. Spicer. He begins his shift by conducting a focused assessment.

Assessment Activities	Findings/Defining Characteristics
Review the patient's chart for laboratory data that reflect immune function.	The data show a reduction in the number of white blood cells (i.e., leukopenia).
Ask the patient to describe her appetite and to review her food intake for the last 24 hr. Weigh the patient and measure her height.	The patient reports that she has not had an interest in eating for a couple of weeks. She has lost approximately 6 lb. Her current weight is 125 lb, and her height is 5'7". Her food intake yesterday consisted of a small cup of applesauce, half of a bowl of soup, some crackers, and two glasses of juice. The patient states, "I get full easily and lose interest in food."
Palpate the patient's cervical and clavicular lymph nodes.	Her lymph nodes are enlarged and painless.
Review the effects of chemotherapy in a drug reference.	Multiagent chemotherapy causes drug-induced pancytopenia.

NURSING DIAGNOSIS

Risk for infection related to chemotherapy and reduced food intake

PLANNING

Goal	Expected Outcomes*
RISK CONTROL: INFECTIOUS PROCESS, IMMUNE STATUS	
Patient will remain free from symptoms of infection.	Patient will observe and report signs of infection (i.e., fever, shaking, chills).
KNOWLEDGE: INFECTION CONTROL	
Patient will become knowledgeable about infection risks.	Patient will identify routines to follow in the home to reduce the transmission of microorganisms.
	Patient will identify signs and symptoms that indicate infection needing to be reported to the healthcare provider.
	Patient will demonstrate appropriate hand hygiene, and verbalize oral care and perineal care.

INTERVENTIONS

Nursing Actions	Rationale
INFECTION PROTECTION AND CONTROL	
Monitor the patient's body temperature routinely, inspect her oral cavity for lesions, inspect her IV access site for drainage, and observe her for evidence of cough, ask her about any unusual discharge or burning on urination.	Interventions are designed to prevent infection and ensure the early detection of infection in a patient who is at risk.
Teach the patient how to perform hand hygiene by handwashing or the use of alcohol-based hand rubs.	Rigorous hand hygiene reduces bacterial counts on the hands.
	The patient can easily come in contact with infectious agents that can cause infection.
Consult with a dietitian about providing a high-calorie, high-protein, low-bacteria diet. Minimize the patient's intake of salads, raw fruits and vegetables, undercooked meat, pepper, and paprika. Offer the patient small, frequent meals.	Maintaining calorie and protein intake will prevent weight loss. Foods high in bacteria should be avoided because they increase risk for gastrointestinal infection.
Instruct the patient to report any of the following to the healthcare provider:	Signs of infection are indicative of local or systemic infection.
• A temperature of >100° F (38° C)	
• A persistent cough with or without sputum, pus or foul-smelling drainage from a body site	
• The presence of an abscess	
• Urine that is cloudy or foul smelling	
• Burning during urination	

*Outcome classification labels and interventions from Moorhead S, Johnson M, Maas M, Swanson E: *Nursing outcomes classification (NOC)*, ed. 4, St. Louis, 2008, Elsevier.

⭐ Nursing Care Plan   Risk for Infection—cont'd

Nursing Actions	Rationale
Teach the patient to do the following activities at home: • Avoid crowds and large gatherings of people. • Bathe daily. • Do not share personal toiletry items (e.g., toothbrush, washcloth, deodorant stick) with family members. • Practice hand hygiene. • Do not drink water that has been standing for >15 min. • Do not reuse cups or glasses without washing them first.	These measures are designed to prevent infection in those patients with impaired immune function.

EVALUATION

Nursing Actions	Patient Response/Finding	Achievement of Outcome
Compare the patient's body temperature and other physical findings with baseline data.	The patient remains afebrile and denies having a cough or burning during urination. There are no signs of drainage or discharge from body sites.	The patient has no active infection at this time.
Ask the patient to describe the signs and symptoms that should be reported to a health care provider.	The patient is able to identify the temperature range to report. She was able to describe a cough but unable to identify signs of urinary infection or local discharge.	The patient has a partial understanding of the signs and symptoms to report. She will require additional instruction and should be offered an information sheet.
Ask patient to explain the measures to take at home to reduce exposure to infectious agents.	The patient is able to discuss the need to avoid sharing personal hygiene articles. She asked for a listing of other precautions and requested that her husband be included in the discussion.	The patient has a partial understanding of restrictions. The nurse will obtain printed guidelines to give to the patient and include the patient's husband in a discussion this evening.

Adapted from Ackley BJ, Ladwig GB: *Nursing diagnosis handbook: An evidence-based guide to planning care,* ed. 10, St. Louis, 2014, Mosby.

diagnoses, interventions, and outcomes that are appropriate for the patient.

Laboratory Tests Record

The **laboratory tests record** has all the laboratory test results in one section of the chart. Hospitals that use computerized reports may list consecutive values of the same test if that test has been repeated several times (e.g., electrolytes). Computerized laboratory data access provides online laboratory results as soon as the tests are completed. Other hospitals may attach small report forms to a full-sized backing sheet as each report returns from the laboratory. Because some medication doses are based on daily blood studies, it is important to be able to locate these data within the patient's chart.

Graphic Record

The **graphic record** (Figure 6-1, *A*) is an example of the manual recording of temperature, pulse, respiration, and blood pressure. Figure 6-1, *B*, is a computer-database–generated example of the vital signs, fluid intake and output, glucose, dietary intake, and other information to be used for the ongoing assessment of the patient's status.

Pain assessment, which is now considered the fifth vital sign, can also be recorded in a graphic form. In addition to the graphic recording of pain, assessments of pain can be found under other flow sheets in the chart that will record the details of the pain events. The **medication administration record (MAR)** details the pain medications that the patient received.

Flow Sheets

Flow sheets are a condensed form for recording information for the quick comparison of data. Examples of flow sheets in common use are diabetic, pain and neurologic flow sheets. The graphic record that is used for recording vital signs is another type of flow sheet (see Figure 6-1, *A*).

Consultation Reports

When other physicians or health professionals are asked to consult about a patient, the specialist's summary of findings, diagnoses, and recommendations for treatment are recorded in the **consultation reports** section.

Other Diagnostic Reports

Reports of surgery, electroencephalography, electrocardiography, pulmonary function tests, radioactive scans, and radiography are usually recorded in the other diagnostic reports section of the patient's chart.

Medication Profile and Medication Administration Record

The **medication profile**, also called the medication worklist when in an electronic format, lists all medications to be administered and is printed from the computerized patient database, thereby ensuring that the pharmacist and the nurse have identical medication profiles for the patient. The medications are usually grouped according to the following categories: those scheduled to be given on a regular basis (e.g., every 6 hours, twice daily), parenteral, stat (from the Latin *statim*, meaning "immediately"), and preoperative orders. PRN medications are those medications that are given on an "as needed" basis and are usually listed at the bottom of the profile, or they may be found on a separate page as unscheduled medication orders.

The *medication administration record (MAR)* is a record of the time that the medication was administered and identifies who gave it (Figure 6-2, *A*). Generally, the nurse records and initials the time that the medication was given. Medication profiles are kept in a notebook or clipboard file on the medication cart for the 24-hour period that they are in use; they then become a permanent part of the patient's chart. In the

FIGURE 6-1 A, Manual vital signs record. (**A,** Courtesy St. Mary's Health Center, St. Louis, Mo.)

B

FIGURE 6-1, cont'd   B, Electronic charting of vital signs and intake and output. (**B,** Courtesy Creighton University Medical Center, Omaha, Neb.)

acute care setting, a new profile is generated every 24 hours at the same time that the unit-dose cart is refilled. Figure 6-2, *B*, is an example of an electronic-database–generated MAR that lists all scheduled medications for an 8-hour shift. By clicking the cursor on the highlighted area (i.e., regular insulin in this illustration), a window opens to reveal details of the order.

In the long-term care setting, the MAR uses the same principles; however, it generally provides a space for medications to be recorded for up to 1 month. The MAR also includes the name of the pharmacy that dispensed the prescribed medications and the assigned prescription number. Medications that are prescribed for residents in the long-term care setting must be reviewed on a scheduled basis; therefore the MAR identifies the reviewer and the date of review.

PRN or Unscheduled Medication Record

Some clinical settings use a separate **PRN** (from the Latin *pro re nata*, meaning "as circumstances require") medication record rather than the MAR to record the date, the time, the PRN medication administered, the dose, the reason for administering the PRN medication, and the patient's response to the drug given. In most clinical settings that involve the use of electronic forms of charting, the PRN medications are recorded on the same MAR.

Patient Education Record

The **patient education record** provides a means of documenting the health teaching provided to the patient, the family, or significant others, and it includes statements about the patient's mastery of the content presented.

Additional forms included in a patient's chart depend on the therapy prescribed. These may include the following: separate medication administration records; health teaching records; operative and anesthesiology records; recovery room records; physical, occupational, or speech therapy records; inhalation therapy reports; and a diabetic's daily record of insulin dosage and blood glucose (sugar) test results. Each page that is placed in the patient's chart is imprinted with the patient's name, registration number, and unit or room number. Nurses often use data from all of these sections to formulate a plan of nursing care.

KARDEX RECORDS

The **Kardex** is a large index-type card that is usually kept in a flip file or a separate holder that contains pertinent information such as the patient's name, diagnosis, allergies, treatments, and the nursing care plan. When the unit-dose system is used, medications are not listed on the Kardex; rather, they are listed separately on the medication profile. Although the Kardex is used primarily by nurses, patient data can be quickly accessed by all members of the health care team. The Kardex is often completed in pencil and updated regularly. Because it is not a legal document, it is destroyed when the patient is discharged from the institution. Traditional Kardex information is evolving into an electronic database format that is continually updated throughout each shift.

EVOLVING CHARTING METHODOLOGIES

Regardless of the method of charting used, the documentation process needs to adhere to The Joint Commission standards that incorporate established standards of care. The Joint Commission requires that all charting methodologies incorporate nursing process criteria and evidence of teaching and discharge planning. When more than one health discipline is providing patient care, a multidisciplinary care plan must be completed. This facilitates communication among interdisciplinary team members and healthcare providers. Improving patient safety at the point of care has become standard in every health care institution.

The format and extent of use of electronic database charting vary widely among institutions, but each method incorporates the standards of care and The Joint Commission requirements. Some clinical sites

MARTINDALE HOMETOWN HOSPITAL

MEDICATION ADMINISTRATION RECORD

NAME: Joseph Lorenzo RM-BD: 621-2
ID NO: 016-28-3978 AGE: 62
DIAGNOSIS: Myocardial Infarction SEX: M
PHYSICIAN: M. Martin, M.D. Ht: 6' Wt: 200 lb

		Init	Signature	Title

	SCHEDULED MEDICATIONS			
DATES:	MEDICATION—STRENGTH—FORM—ROUTE	0030-0729	0730-1529	1530-0029
1/25/yr	RANITIDINE ZANTAC 150 MG TABLET ORAL TWICE A DAY		0900	1800
1/25/yr	DILTIAZEM HYDROCHLORIDE CARDIZEM 90 MG TABLET ORAL 4 TIMES DAILY		0900 1300	1800 2100
1/25/yr	WARFARIN SODIUM COUMADIN 1 MG TABLET ORAL EVERY OTHER DAY	NOT GIVEN	TODAY	
	IV AND PIGGYBACK ORDERS			
1/25/yr	CEFTAZIDIME (FORTAZ) 1 G IV SODIUM CHLORIDE 0.9% 50 ML EVERY 8 HOURS INFUSE: 20 MIN	0200	1000	1800
1/25/yr	GENTAMICIN PREMIX 80 MG IV ISO-OSMOTIC SOLN 100 ML BY IV PUMP EVERY 12 HOURS INFUSE: 30 MIN	0200	1400	
1/25/yr	BY IV PUMP 1 IV DSW-5/0.2 NACl 1000 ML RATE: 100 ML/HR			
	PRN MEDICATIONS			
1/25/yr	ACETAMINOPHEN TYLENOL 650 MG (23325) TABLET ORAL EVERY 4 HOURS AS NEEDED PRN			
1/25/yr	MAGNESIUM HYDROXIDE MILK OF MAGNESIA 60 ML (CONC) ORAL CONC AS NEEDED PRN			
1/25/yr	ALBUTEROL PROVENTIL INHALER 90 MCG/INH AEROSOL INH AS NEEDED PRN SEE RESPIRATORY THERAPY NOTES AT BEDSIDE			

Age/Sex HT WT Date 62/ M 6'0" 200 lb 1/25/yr Room-Bd Name 621 2 Joseph Lorenzo	ALLERGIES: CODEINE

A

FIGURE 6-2 A, Medication profile. Note the separation of scheduled orders, IV, and PRN medications.

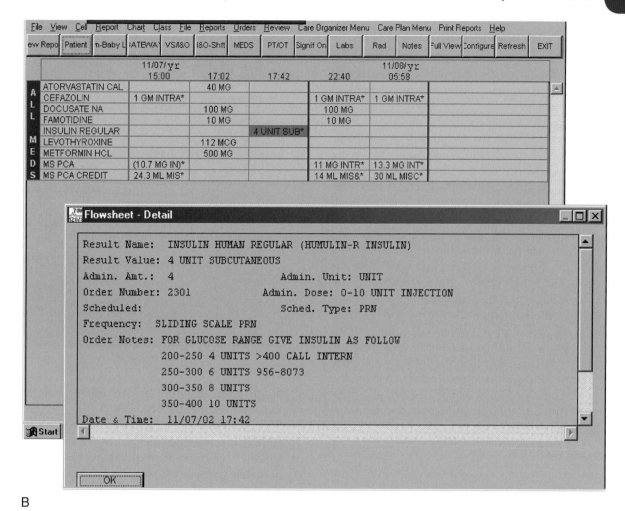

FIGURE 6-2, cont'd B, Electronically generated medication sheet listing all scheduled medications for an 8-hour shift. By clicking the cursor on the highlighted area ("4 UNIT SUB" in this illustration), a window opens to reveal details of the order. (Courtesy Creighton University Medical Center, Omaha, Neb.)

have extensive online electronic charting developed, whereas others have little or none. For example, one hospital may elect to combine all of the elements formerly found in the Kardex, the care plan, the MAR, and the critical pathways into one document known as a *patient profile* that the nurse can access for each 8-hour shift. Regardless of the methodology used, the adage "If you didn't chart it, it didn't happen" still holds true.

DRUG DISTRIBUTION SYSTEMS

Before administering medications, it is important that the nurse understand the overall medication delivery system that is used at the employing health care agency. Although no two drug distribution systems function in exactly the same way, the following general types are used.

FLOOR OR WARD STOCK SYSTEM

In the **floor or ward stock system,** all but the most dangerous or rarely used medications are stocked at the nursing station in stock containers. This system has generally been used in very small hospitals and hospitals in which there are no direct charges to the patient for medications (e.g., in some government hospitals). Some advantages of this system are the ready availability of most drugs, fewer inpatient prescription orders, and the minimal return of medications. The disadvantages are as follows:
- Increased potential for medication errors because of the large array of stock medications from which to choose and the lack of review by the pharmacist of a patient's medication order
- Increased danger of the unnoticed passing of expiration dates and drug deterioration, as well as increased quantities of expired drugs to be discarded
- Economic loss caused by misplaced or forgotten charges and the misappropriation of medication by hospital personnel
- Need for larger stocks and frequent total drug inventories
- Storage problems on the nursing units of many hospitals

INDIVIDUAL PRESCRIPTION ORDER SYSTEM

With the **individual prescription order system**, medications are dispensed from the pharmacy with the receipt of a prescription or drug order for an individual patient.

The pharmacist usually sends a 3- to 5-day supply of medication in a bottle that is labeled for a specific patient. After the prescriptions are received at the nurses' station, medications are placed in the medication cabinet in accordance with institutional practices. Generally, the medication containers are arranged alphabetically by the patient's name, but they may be arranged numerically by the patient's room or bed number. This system provides greater patient safety because of the review of prescription orders by the pharmacist and nurse before administration; it also involves less danger of drug deterioration, easier inventory control, smaller total inventories, and reduced revenue loss because of improved charging systems and less pilferage. Although dispensing medication to individual patients is better than the floor or ward stock system, the major disadvantages of this system are the time-consuming procedures that are used to schedule, prepare, administer, control, and record the drug distribution and administration process.

UNIT-DOSE SYSTEM

Unit-dose drug-distribution systems use single-unit packages of drugs that are dispensed to fill each dose requirement as it is ordered. Each package is labeled with the drug's generic and brand names, the manufacturer, the lot number, and the expiration date. When they are dispensed by the pharmacy, the individual packages are placed in labeled drawers that are assigned to individual patients. The drawers are kept in a large unit-dose cabinet (Figure 6-3) that is kept at the nurses' station; in some institutions, individualized containers or envelopes may be locked in a cabinet in the patient's room. With most unit-dose systems, a pharmacist refills the drawers every 24 hours. In long-term care facilities, these drawers are usually exchanged on a 3- or 7-day schedule.

Advantages of the system include the following:
- The time that is normally spent by nursing personnel preparing drugs for administration is drastically reduced.
- The pharmacist has a profile of all medications for each patient and is therefore able to analyze the prescribed medications for drug interactions or contraindications. This method increases the pharmacist's involvement and makes better use of his or her extensive drug knowledge.
- Counting drugs from multidose packets is no longer necessary as a result of unit-dose packaging, thereby reducing errors.
- It is the nurse's responsibility to check drugs and calculate dosages (see the information under the

FIGURE 6-3 Unit-dose cabinet.

"Right Dose" heading later in this chapter), thereby reducing errors.
- There is less waste and misappropriation because single units are dispensed.
- Credit is given to the patient for unused medications because each dose is individually packaged. (Under the individual prescription order system, returned bottles of unused medications are destroyed out of fear of contamination.)

The unit-dose medication is prepared under rigid controls, and it is dispensed only after pharmacists have completed quality control procedures. Nurses should always check medications before administration. If there is a discrepancy between the Kardex (i.e., the medication profile) and the medication in the cart, then the pharmacist and the original prescriber's order should be consulted.

At the time of administration, the nurse should check all aspects of the medication order as stated on the medication profile against the medication container removed from the patient's drawer for administration. The number of doses remaining in the drawer for the shift should also be checked. If the number of remaining doses is incorrect, the medication order should be checked before continuing with the drug administration. It is always possible that the drug has been discontinued or that someone else has given the dose, omitted a dose, or given the wrong patient the wrong medication. If an error has been made, it should be reported in accordance with hospital policies.

COMPUTER-CONTROLLED DISPENSING SYSTEM

A common system for medication ordering and administration is a **computer-controlled dispensing system**

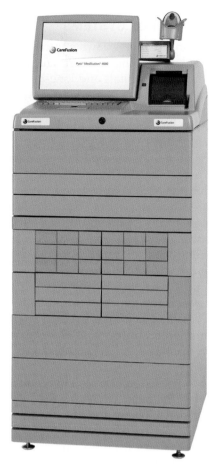

FIGURE 6-4 Electronic dispensing system: the Pyxis system. (Courtesy and © Becton, Dickinson and Company.)

FIGURE 6-5 **A,** The nurse removes a single dose of medicine from the electronic dispensing system. **B,** A single-dose, bar-coded medication package is scanned by the nurse before it is administered. (Courtesy and © Becton, Dickinson and Company.)

that uses the unit-dose system described earlier. It is resupplied by the pharmacy daily and is stocked with single-unit packages of medicines (i.e., the Pyxis system, Figure 6-4). When a drug order is received in the pharmacy for a patient, it is entered into the computerized system. The nurse—who is using a security code and password and, with newer systems, a fingerprint—accesses the system and selects the patient's name, the medication profile, and the drugs that are due for administration. The drug order appears on the screen, and a specific section of the cart opens so that the nurse can take a single dose of medicine out of the cart (Figure 6-5, *A*). This process continues until all drugs ordered for a specific time of administration are retrieved. During the actual administration process at the bedside, the nurse uses a handheld scanner that reads the **bar codes** on the nurse's identification badge, the patient's wristband, and the unit-dose medication packet, thereby linking this information with the patient database (Figure 6-5, *B*). If there is an error (e.g., wrong dose, wrong time of administration, wrong patient), an alert pops up on the computer and the user is unable to continue until the error is corrected. If the process is correct and the medicine is administered, there is automatic documentation in the patient's MAR of the administration.

Controlled drugs are also kept in this automated dispensing cart. The system provides a detailed record of the controlled substance dispensed, including the date, the time, and by whom it was accessed. A second qualified nurse must witness the disposal of a portion of a dose of a controlled substance or the return to the automated dispensing cart of any controlled substance that is not used. The automated dispensing system is currently the safest and most economical method of drug distribution in hospitals and long-term care facilities.

Long-Term Care Unit-Dose System

The **long-term care unit-dose system** is an adaptation of the system that is used in the acute care setting. The unit-dose cart is designed with individual drawers to hold one resident's medication containers for 1 week. The drawer is labeled with the resident's name and room number, the pharmacy's name and telephone number, and the name of the health care facility. The pharmacist fills the medication container with the prescribed drug. Each container has enough compartments to contain the prescribed number of doses of the drug for each day of the week. The individual compartments may be labeled with the days of the week. The medication cart has other compartments for storing bottles of medication that cannot be placed in patients' drawers. The cart has a storage area for medication cups, a medicine crusher, drinking cups, straws, alcohol wipes, syringes, and other necessities for the preparation and administration of the medications prescribed. The entire cart has a locking system that should be secured when the medication cart is not in use or when it is unattended while medications are being dispensed.

The unit-dose system may involve the use of a color-coding system to simplify finding the medication holder for a specific time of day; for example, purple = 6 AM (0600); pink = 8 AM (0800); yellow = noon (1200); green = 2 PM (1400) or 4 PM (1600); orange = early evening; and red = PRN. Using this method to organize the medications allows the nurse or medication aide to remove all of the pink holders for administering the prescribed 8 AM (0800) tablets or capsules. Each medication holder is also labeled with the resident's name, the physician's name, the prescription number, the generic or brand name of the drug (or both), the dose, the frequency of the drug order (e.g., four times daily), and the actual time that the drug in this holder is to be administered (e.g., 8 AM, or 0800). This system is easy to use unless the user is color blind. By using military time to mark the individual containers, the individual who is color blind can use the military time as a guideline.

At the time of administration, the nurse or medication aide checks all aspects of the medication order (as stated on the medication profile) against the medication container that has been removed from one of the drawers. The number of doses remaining in the holder is checked against the days of the week that remain for the medication to be administered. If the resident refuses the medication, it must be charted on the record with the reason that the medication was refused. In a long-term care setting, a resident seldom wears an identification band; therefore third-party identification of the resident must be relied on until the nurse or medication aide is able to identify the resident. If pictures of the residents are used as identifiers, the institution should have a policy in place to update the photos on a regular basis. Medications should be charted as soon as they are administered. The medication aide has specific limitations on the types of medications that he or she can administer; therefore nurses should be thoroughly familiar with the laws and guidelines of their state. The nurse is ultimately responsible for verifying the qualifications of the individual who is being supervised in the medication-aide capacity and for the medications that the medication aide is administering.

NARCOTIC CONTROL SYSTEMS

As described in Chapter 1, laws regulating the use of controlled substances have been enacted and are rigidly enforced in hospitals and long-term care facilities with the use of **narcotic control systems**. It is a standard policy that controlled substances are issued in single-unit packages and kept in a locked cabinet. If the automated dispensing system is not available, a designated individual is responsible for the key to the cabinet. When controlled substances are issued to a nursing unit, they are accompanied by an inventory sheet (Figure 6-6) that lists each type of controlled substance being supplied. This record is used to account for the disposition of each type of medication issued. When the controlled substance supply is dispensed to the nursing unit by the pharmacist, the nurse receiving the drug supply is responsible for counting and verifying the number and types of controlled substances received. The nurse then signs a record attesting to the accuracy and receipt of the controlled substances and locks them in the controlled substances (narcotic) cabinet.

When a controlled substance is ordered for a particular patient, the nurse caring for the patient uses a key to the cabinet to obtain and prepare the medication for administration. At the time of removal from the cabinet, the inventory control record (see Figure 6-6) must be completed; it must indicate the time, the patient's name, the drug, and the dose, and it must include the signature of the nurse who is responsible for checking out the controlled substance. If a portion of the medication is to be discarded because of a smaller prescribed dose, two nurses must check the dose, the preparation, and the portion discarded. Both nurses must then cosign the inventory control record to verify the transaction. The cabinet is relocked, the medicine is administered, and the documentation is completed.

Before the administration of any controlled substance, the patient's chart should be checked to verify that the time interval since the last use of the drug has elapsed as specified in the physician's orders (see Chapter 19 for details about the monitoring of pain and the use of analgesics). Immediately after the administration of a controlled substance, the nurse who is administering the medication should complete the charting. At appropriate intervals after the administration of a controlled substance, the degree and duration of effectiveness should be recorded in the nurse's notes or the pain flow sheet.

At the end of each shift, the contents of the controlled substances cabinet or the controlled substances cart are counted (inventoried) by two nurses: one from the shift that is about to end and the other from the oncoming shift. Each container is counted, and the remaining numbers of tablets, ampules, and prefilled syringes are added to the amount used in accordance with the inventory control record. The amount of each

FIGURE 6-6 Controlled substances inventory form. (Courtesy University Hospital, The University of Nebraska Medical Center; ©Board of Regents of the University of Nebraska, Lincoln, Neb.)

drug remaining plus the amount recorded as being administered to individual patients should equal the total number issued. During the counting procedure, packages of unopened prefilled syringes are visually inspected to verify that the seal and cellophane coverings are intact. If the package seal is broken, closer scrutiny of the package is required. These observations should include tilting a package of prefilled syringes to observe the rate of air bubble movement inside the barrel, the uniformity of color of the solutions in each of the barrels, and the similarity in fluid levels in each of the barrels. The same medication in the same type of syringe should be the same color and travel through the barrel at the same rate, and all fluid levels should be similar.

Discrepancies in the number of remaining doses are checked with nursing personnel on the unit to see if all controlled substances used have been charted. If this does not reveal the source of the inaccuracy, each

patient's chart is checked to be certain that all controlled substances recorded on the individual patient's chart for the shift coincide with the controlled substances inventory record. If the error is still not found, the pharmacy and the nursing service office should be contacted in accordance with institution policy. If the count appears to be accurate but tampering with the contents of the containers is suspected, a report should be made to the pharmacy and the nursing service office. When the controlled substances inventory is complete, the two nurses who are counting sign the inventory control shift record to verify that the records and inventory are accurate at that time. With the controlled substance cart, the computer generates an end-of-shift report that also identifies discrepancies so that the staff involved can account for the use of controlled substances.

When an automated dispensing cart such as Pyxis (see Figure 6-4) is used, the shift change narcotic check is not done. At the time of administration, the nurse will verify the correct count of the drug desired before removing the drug from the cart. At that time, the system will be activated if a discrepancy occurs. Discrepancies are tracked by nursing and pharmacy, and they are resolved as soon as they are discovered. The pharmacy also checks for discrepancies when controlled substances are restocked in the automated dispensing system. Reconciliation sheets must be completed if there are inaccuracies in the count.

DISPOSAL OF UNUSED MEDICINES

In recent years, environmental concerns have arisen about the proper **disposal of unused medicines**, because trace levels of medicines have been found in rivers, lakes, and community water supplies. Concerns have been expressed about the appropriateness of the common practice of flushing unused medicines down the toilet, because many people assume that this is the primary source of water contamination. However, the U.S. Food and Drug Administration's Center for Drug Evaluation and Research has stated that drugs found in ground water are primarily drugs that have been incompletely absorbed and metabolized by the body after human consumption and that have entered the environment after passing through waste-water treatment plants. Scientists from the Environmental Protection Agency have found no evidence of adverse human health effects from unmetabolized drugs in the environment.

The U.S. Food and Drug Administration, working in conjunction with the White House Office of National Drug Control Policy, issued the guidelines addressing prescription and nonprescription medication disposal:

- Follow specific disposal instructions on the drug label or in the patient information leaflet that accompanies the medication. Do not flush prescription drugs down the toilet unless specifically instructed to do so by the manufacturer.
- If no instructions are given, throw the drugs in the household trash, but first:
  - Empty the drugs from the container, and then mix them with an undesirable substance, such as used coffee grounds or kitty litter. This makes the product considerably less appealing to children and pets and less recognizable to people who may intentionally go through trash (e.g., dumpster divers).
  - Put this mixture in a sealable bag, an empty can, or another container to prevent the medication from leaking out of the garbage bag.
- Use community drug take-back programs that allow the public to bring unused drugs to a central location for proper disposal. The drugs are often destroyed using a biohazard-controlled incinerator.

- Before throwing out an empty prescription bottle, scratch out all identifying information on the label to make it unreadable. This will help to protect patient identity and health information.
- Controlled substances (e.g., opiate analgesics) should be flushed down the toilet to reduce the danger of unintentional use or overdose and illegal abuse. An example is the fentanyl patch, which, even after it has been used by the patient for 3 days, can still contain enough medicine to cause severe respiratory depression in babies, children, and pets.
- Additional guidelines for the disposal of drugs that are classified as hazardous medications (e.g., chemotherapeutic agents) have also been defined.

MEDICATION ORDERS

Medications for patient use must be ordered by licensed physicians or dentists (or, in some states, by nurse practitioners and physician assistants) acting within their areas of professional training. Placing an order for a medication or treatment is known as *issuing a prescription*. Initially, a prescription may be issued verbally or in written form. Prescriptions that are issued for nonhospitalized patients use a form that is similar to that shown in Figure 6-7, whereas prescriptions for hospitalized patients are written on the order form. All prescriptions must contain the following elements: the patient's full name, the date, the drug name, the route of administration, the dose, the duration of the order, and the signature of the prescriber. Additional information may be required for certain types of medications (e.g., for IV administration, the concentration, dilution, and rate of flow should be specified in addition to the method [i.e., "IV push" or "continuous infusion"]).

TYPES OF MEDICATION ORDERS

Medication orders fall into four categories: stat, single, standing, and PRN orders. The **stat order** is generally

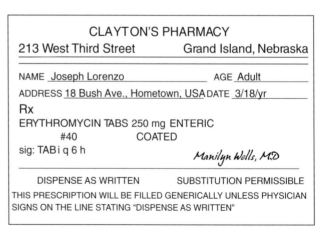

FIGURE 6-7 Prescription showing patient name, patient address, date, drug and strength, number of tablets, directions for use, and the healthcare provider's signature.

used on an emergency basis. It means that the drug is to be administered as soon as possible, but only once. For example, if a patient is having a seizure, the physician may order "diazepam 10 mg IV stat," which means that the drug is to be given immediately and one time only.

The **single order** means administration at a certain time but only one time. For example, a one-time order may be written for "furosemide 20 mg IV to be given one time at 7 AM." Furosemide would then be administered at that time, but once only.

The **standing order** indicates that a medication is to be given for a specified number of doses: for example, "cefazolin 1 g q6h × 4 doses." A standing order may also indicate that a drug is to be administered until it is discontinued at a later date: for example, "ampicillin 500 mg PO q6h." In the interest of patient safety, however, all accredited health care agencies have policies that automatically cancel an order after a certain number of doses is administered or after a certain number of days of therapy have passed (e.g., surgery, after 72 hours for narcotics, after one dose only for anticoagulants, after 7 days for antibiotics).

A **PRN order** means "administer if needed." This order allows a nurse to judge when a medication should be administered on the basis of the patient's need and when it can be safely administered.

Verbal Orders

Health care agencies have policies regarding who may accept verbal orders and under what circumstances they should be accepted. The practice is strongly discouraged and should be avoided whenever possible to prevent medication errors. However, when a verbal order is accepted, the person who took the order is responsible for accurately entering it on the order sheet and signing it. The prescriber must cosign and date the order, usually within 24 hours.

Electronic Transmission of Patient Orders

Many physicians' offices fax new orders to the area where the patient is admitted or transferred. These fax transmissions must have an original signature within a specified time, often 24 hours. Hospital units also find it useful to fax orders to the nursing home where the individual is being transferred. This allows the receiving agency to prepare for the patient or resident, and the original orders, which have been signed by the physician, then accompany the individual at the time of transfer.

Computerized provider order entry (CPOE) systems are used to transmit orders electronically. Software has been developed that allows for the use of CPOE and clinical decision-making support systems (CDSSs). The computerized system integrates the ordering system with the pharmacy, the laboratory, and the nurses' station, thereby providing access instantly to online information that may affect a patient's care needs.

MEDICATION SAFETY

Medication safety is freedom from accidental injury from medications. The nurse should be aware of how to properly handle certain medications (e.g., chemotherapy drugs, topical hormones), which can cause a reaction when they come in contact with the skin. The nurse also needs to be aware of how to correctly prepare and administer medications to prevent injury (e.g., a needlestick).

Medication errors can be defined as the failure of a planned action to be completed as intended or the use of a wrong plan to achieve a goal. Medication errors include prescribing errors, transcription or order communication errors, dispensing errors, administration errors, and errors of monitoring or education for proper use (Box 6-1). Medication errors can result in serious complications known as *adverse drug events*. In 2000 the National Academy of Science's Institute of Medicine estimated the number of lives lost as a result of preventable medication errors to be more than 7000 deaths in hospitals annually (Lasser et al, 2000). The Institute of Medicine has further estimated that the additional costs of adverse drug events annually are $2 billion in hospitals and more than $3 billion in extended-care facilities (National Research Council, 2000).

Box 6-1 Examples of Medication Errors

PRESCRIBING ERRORS
- Suboptimal drug therapy decisions
- Drug for patient with known allergy or intolerance
- Incorrect dose for diagnosis
- Unauthorized drug prescribed

TRANSCRIPTION ERRORS
- Misinterpretation or misunderstanding of drug ordered or any directions listed
- Illegible handwriting
- Unapproved abbreviations
- Omission of orders

DISPENSING
- Wrong drug or dose sent to nursing unit
- Wrong formulation or dosage form

ADMINISTRATION
- Incorrect strength (dose) given
- Extra dose given or missed dose
- Wrong administration time
- Incorrect administration technique

MONITORING
- Suboptimal monitoring
- Suboptimal assessment of drug response or revision of regimen
- Suboptimal patient education

TECHNOLOGY AND PREVENTION OF ADVERSE DRUG EVENTS

Adverse drug events occur most commonly during ordering and at the administration stage. Therefore, preventive measures are being implemented that include substantial changes in the ordering system used for medications and laboratory studies. The use of the CPOE technology checks for potential drug interactions and the appropriateness of drug dosages ordered, as well as for laboratory findings (e.g., therapeutic drug levels at the time of order entry).

Automated ordering and dispensing systems have been developed to minimize medication errors. Automated systems use robotics and bar-coding technology to fill the orders entered by the physician. Robotics in the pharmacy can free some of the pharmacists for deployment to clinical units, where they can make patient rounds; check for medication response; review current laboratory data; and work with the prescriber to select, dose, and monitor drug therapy.

HIGH-ALERT MEDICATIONS

The Institute for Safe Medication Practices (ISMP) has conducted a survey of several acute-care hospitals to determine which medications cause serious patient harm or death. As a result of this study, medications and classifications that pose significant risk in the acute clinical setting were identified. These are now known as *high-alert medications*, and they include insulin, heparin, opioids, injectable potassium or potassium phosphate concentrate, neuromuscular blocking agents, and chemotherapeutic agents. Although mistakes may or may not be more common with these medicines, the consequences of an error are much more devastating to patients. The ISMP continues to monitor the frequency of drug errors in the clinical literature to update the list of high-alert medications.

Cohen (2008) has discussed high-alert medications and the role that they play in medication errors, and practices to aid in prevention have been recommended, including the following: (1) standardizing processes within the institution; (2) developing processes to make errors stand out (i.e., making staff more alert and aware to catch errors before they reach the patient); and (3) developing methods to minimize the consequences of errors that reach the patient. Cohen also discusses several practices to promote medication safety, including the following: (1) the use of technology, including CPOE, bar-coded drug administration, and smart pumps for controlled administration; (2) the restriction of high-alert medications during the dispensing process (e.g., removing neuromuscular blocking agents from readily available floor stock); (3) the avoidance of verbal orders for high-alert medicines; (4) the use of checklists for high-alert drugs; (5) the use of generic and brand names on the MAR to avoid errors with sound-alike drugs; (6) the standardizing of drug concentrations and dosing infusion charts; and (7) the performance of double-checking before administration and patient education.

MEDICATION RECONCILIATION

Another process that involves the goal of eliminating medication errors is **medication reconciliation**, which involves comparing a patient's current medication orders with all of the medications that the patient is actually taking. This process makes use of a single, shared, and updated medication and allergy list for patients across the continuum of inpatient and outpatient care that is to be used during **hand-offs** or the transition of patients during care. Reconciliation aims to prevent omissions, duplications, differences in dosing, and drug interactions. It should be completed as part of every transition of care during which new medications are ordered or existing orders are rewritten. Transitions in care include changes in setting, service, practitioner, or level of care (e.g., critical care to general care to rehabilitation services).

Medication reconciliation is a five-step process: (1) develop a list of current medications being administered; (2) develop a list of medications that were prescribed; (3) compare the medications on the two lists; (4) make clinical decisions on the basis of this comparison; and (5) communicate the new list to appropriate caregivers and to the patient. Accurate and complete medication reconciliation can prevent many prescribing and administration errors. Failure to reconcile medications may be compounded by the practice of writing blanket orders (e.g., "resume preop medications"), which are known to result in adverse drug events. Such orders are explicitly prohibited by The Joint Commission's medication management standards.

SOUND-ALIKE MEDICATIONS

The ISMP regularly reports medication errors that are the result of the similarity of sound-alike names (e.g., Mucomyst and Mucinex; Evista and Avinza). Manufacturers have a responsibility to avoid using brand names that are similar to other medicines to help avoid errors. As recommended by the ISMP, include both the generic name and the brand name on the computer order entry screen.

Most products with sound-alike names are used for different purposes. It is important for the nurse to be familiar with patients' diagnoses and to know what medicines are used for these conditions so that they are able to question why a particular medicine may have been prescribed when a patient does not have a diagnosis that requires that medicine. For example, the generic name for Evista is raloxifene, which is used to prevent osteoporosis in postmenopausal women; alternatively, Avinza is an extended-release form of creams with a gloved hand using firm but gentle strokes. Creams are to be gently rubbed into the area.

5. *Dressings:* Check specific orders regarding the type of dressing to be used. If a dressing is to be applied, spread the prescribed amount of ointment directly onto the dressing material with a tongue blade; the impregnated dressing material can then be applied to the affected skin surface. Secure the dressing in place.

6. *Wet dressings:* Always completely remove the previous dressing. Wring out wet dressings to prevent dripping, and apply the gauze in a single layer directly to the wound surface. For deeper wounds, pack the wound loosely with moist gauze sponges so that all surfaces are in contact with the moisture. Apply a layer of dry gauze sponges and an absorbent pad to the area. To secure a dressing that requires repeated changes, apply a binder, or use Montgomery tapes.

7. Clean the area and the equipment used, and make sure that the patient is comfortable after the application procedure. (NOTE: Sterile supplies, gloves, and equipment are used for some wounds; however, clean rather than sterile items [e.g., gauze, gloves] may be used when applying most types of dressings [e.g., to a pressure ulcer]. Always check institutional policies and use clinical judgment.)

8. Perform hand hygiene.

PATIENT TEACHING

1. If appropriate, teach the patient to apply the medication and dressings.
2. Teach personal hygiene measures that are appropriate to the underlying cause of the skin condition (e.g., acne, contact dermatitis, infection).
3. When dressings are ordered, suggest the purchase of gauze and other necessary supplies.
4. Stress gentleness and moderation with regard to the amount of medication to be applied.
5. Emphasize that the patient must avoid touching or scratching the affected area.
6. Tell the patient to wash his or her hands before and after touching the affected area or applying the medication. Stress the prevention of the spread of infection.

DOCUMENTATION

Provide the right documentation of the medication administered and the patient's response to drug therapy.

1. Chart the date, time, drug name, dosage, and route of administration.
2. Perform and record regular patient assessments for the evaluation of the treatment's therapeutic effectiveness (e.g., change in size of affected area, reduced drainage, decreased itching, lowered temperature with an infection).

3. On the patient's record, document any signs and symptoms of adverse drug effects, and provide a narrative description of the area being treated.

4. Develop a written record for the patient to use when charting progress for the evaluation of the effectiveness of the treatments being used. List the patient's symptoms (e.g., rash on the lower leg with redness and vesicles present, decubitus ulcer on the sacrum). List the data to be collected regarding the medication prescribed and its effectiveness (e.g., vesicles now crusted, weeping, or appear to be drying; redness in lower leg is lessening; measure the area of decubitus in cm and indicate if the wound is extending, remaining the same, or shrinking).

5. Educate the patient on what to expect and what to do if adverse symptoms develop.

PATCH TESTING FOR ALLERGENS

Patch testing is a method that is used to identify a patient's sensitivity to contact materials (e.g., soaps, pollens, dyes). The suspected **allergens** (antigens) are placed in direct contact with the skin surface and covered with nonsensitizing, nonabsorbent tape. Unless pronounced irritation appears, the patch is usually left in place for 48 hours and then removed. The site is left open to air for 15 minutes and then "read." A positive reaction is noted by the presence of redness and swelling, called a *wheal,* which indicates an allergy to the specific allergen. It may be necessary to read the areas after 3 days and again after 7 days to detect delayed reactions.

Intradermal tests may also be used to determine the patient's allergy to specific antigens. See Chapter 10 for more information about the intradermal administration of allergens.

Perform premedication assessments. See individual drug monographs.

EQUIPMENT

- Alcohol for cleansing the area
- Solutions of suspected antigens
- 1 × 1-inch gauze pads
- Droppers
- Mineral or olive oil
- Water
- Clippers
- Hypoallergenic tape
- Record for charting data about the substances applied and the patient's responses
- MAR, computer profile, or order sheet

SITES

The back, arms, or thighs are commonly used. (*Do not* apply to the face or areas that are susceptible to friction from clothing.) Selected areas are spaced 2 to 3 inches apart. The type of allergen applied and the site of application are documented on the patient's chart

FIGURE 7-1 Patch test for contact dermatitis. **A,** Reading chart, patch testing. **B,** Patch testing sites.

(Figure 7-1). Hair is clipped from sites to ensure that the allergen is kept in close contact with the skin surface, thereby preventing a false-negative reaction.

TECHNIQUE

CAUTION: Emergency equipment must be available before starting allergy testing in case of an anaphylactic response. Personnel should be familiar with the procedure to follow if an emergency does arise.

1. Follow the Procedure Protocol described previously. Check with the patient before starting the testing to ensure that no antihistamines or anti-inflammatory agents (e.g., aspirin, ibuprofen, diphenhydramine, corticosteroids) have been taken for 24 to 48 hours before the test. If the patient has taken an antihistamine or an anti-inflammatory agent, consult the healthcare provider before proceeding with the testing. Review the chart to ensure that the patient is not in an immunocompromised state as a result of disease or treatments such as chemotherapy or radiation therapy.
2. Follow the procedure protocol described earlier.
3. Position the patient so that the surface on which the test materials are to be applied is horizontal. Provide for patient's comfort before beginning the testing.
4. Cleanse the selected area thoroughly with the use of an alcohol wipe. Use circular motions, starting at the planned site of application and continuing outward to the periphery. Allow the area to air-dry.
5. Prepare the designated solutions using aseptic technique.
6. Follow the specific directions of the employing healthcare agency regarding the application of liquid and solid forms of suspected allergens. A dropper is usually used to apply suspected liquid contact-type materials; solid materials are applied directly to the skin surface and then moistened with mineral or olive oil.
7. The following methods may be used:
   - After application, follow institutional policy for covering the test site.
   - Designated amounts of standardized-strength chemical solutions are arranged in metal receptacles that are backed with hypoallergenic adhesive. These solutions are then applied to the selected site. It is important to identify the contents of each receptacle correctly.
   - Patches that are impregnated with designated allergens are available for direct application to the prepared sites.
   - A patch test series kit is available that contains nonirritating concentrations of allergens that are packaged in syringes for dispersal. Although the kit contains 20 allergens, any number of them may be applied to individual patches or holding devices, which are then applied to the patient's skin.
8. Chart the times, agents, concentrations, and amounts applied. Make a diagram in the patient's chart, and number each location. Record which agent and concentration were placed at each site. Subsequent readings of each area are then performed and charted on this record.
9. Follow directions regarding the time of the reading of the skin testing being performed. The testing sites should be inspected in good light. Generally, a positive reaction (i.e., the development of a wheal) to a dilute strength of a suspected allergen is considered clinically significant. Measure the diameter of erythema in millimeters, and palpate and measure the size of any induration (i.e., the hardening of an area of the body that has reacted to

FIGURE 8-20 Administering a disposable enema (Fleet enema). **A,** Place the patient in a left lateral position, unless a knee–chest position has been specified. **B,** Remove the protective covering from the rectal tube and lubricate the tube. **C,** Insert the lubricated rectal tube into the patient's rectum and dispense the solution by compressing the plastic container. **D,** Replace the used container in its original wrapping for disposal.

Get Ready for the NCLEX® Examination!

Key Points

- Solid dose forms of medications include capsules, timed-release capsules, lozenges, tablets, caplets, and orally disintegrating tablets and films.
- Liquid dose forms for medications include elixirs, emulsions, suspensions, and syrups.
- The unit-dose system uses individual packaged medications that are distributed to each patient using a medication cart. The electronic controlled system uses unit-dose medications distributed in a locked password-protected medication system using a computer and bar code scanner system.
- Liquid forms of medications are administered by oral syringe or by gastric tube.

- Nasogastric tube medication administration requires checking placement of the tube before administration and correct technique to ensure all medication is given accurately.
- Rectal suppositories and enemas are administered with the patient positioned on his or her left side and inserted with a water-based lubricant.

Additional Learning Resources

SG Go to your Study Guide for additional Review Questions for the NCLEX® Examination, Critical Thinking Clinical Situations, and other learning activities to help you master this chapter content.

evolve Go to your Evolve website (http://evolve.elsevier.com/Clayton) for additional online resources.

Review Questions for the NCLEX® Examination

1. The prescriber has changed the route of the patient's medication from an intravenous route to an oral route. What effect (in general) does the change in route have on the drug dosage and the absorption time?
   1. Decreased dosage and increased absorption time
   2. Increased dosage and increased absorption time
   3. Increased dosage and decreased absorption time
   4. Decreased dosage and decreased absorption time

2. With regard to the administration of oral medications, put the following actions that the nurse takes in chronologic order.
   1. Give the patient water to drink.
   2. Identify the patient.
   3. Check all aspects of the medication order.
   4. Sit the patient upright.
   5. Document the administration.

3. The nurse knows that when administering guaifenesin syrup to a 5-year-old child that the following principles apply. (Select all that apply.)
   1. The correct amount of liquid should be measured in a medicine cup by reading the meniscus at eye level.
   2. Hold the bottle containing the liquid so the label is covered with the palm of the hand.
   3. Use a syringe that compares closely to the volume to be measured.
   4. The expiration date does not need to be checked on liquids.
   5. A syringe can be used when giving an infant medications.

4. The nurse is to administer several medications to the patient via an NG tube. What is the nurse's first action?
   1. Add the medication to the tube feeding being given.
   2. Crush all tablets and capsules before administration.
   3. Administer all of the medications mixed together.
   4. Check for the placement of the tube.

5. When administering an intermittent enteral feeding to an adult patient, the nurse finds that the residual aspirate obtained is 150 mL. What does the nurse do?
   1. Administers the next scheduled feeding
   2. Stops feeding the patient for 30 minutes
   3. Reinstills the aspirate and starts a new feeding
   4. Notifies the healthcare provider

6. When administering a rectal suppository, the patient needs to be in this position:
   1. Semi-Fowler's
   2. Lithotomy
   3. Sims'
   4. Right side-lying

Objectives

1. Identify the parts of a syringe and needle, as well as examples of the safety-type syringes and needles.
2. Describe how to select the correct needle gauge and length and how the needle gauge is determined.
3. List the advantages and disadvantages of using a glass syringe versus a plastic syringe.
4. Compare and contrast the volumes of medications that can be measured in a tuberculin syringe and those of larger-volume syringes.
5. Compare and contrast the advantages and disadvantages of using prefilled syringes.
6. Differentiate among ampules, vials, and Mix-O-Vials.
7. Describe the technique used to prepare two different drugs in one syringe (e.g., insulin).

Key Terms

barrel (BĂ-rŭl) (p. 116)
plunger (PLŬN-jŭr) (p. 116)
tip (p. 116)
milliliter scale (MĬL-ĭ-lē-tŭr) (p. 116)
tuberculin syringe (tū-BĔR-kū-lĭn sĭ-RĬNJ) (p. 117)
insulin syringe (ĬN-sŭ-lĭn) (p. 117)
prefilled cartridges and syringes (prē-FĬLD) (p. 118)

insulin pen (p. 118)
needle gauge (NĒ-dŭl GĀJ) (p. 120)
safety devices (SĂF-tē dě-VĪ-sĕz) (p. 122)
ampules (ĀM-pyūlz) (p. 124)
vials (VĪ-ălz) (p. 124)
Mix-O-Vials (MĬKS Ō VĪ-ălz) (p. 124)

The routes of drug administration can be classified into three categories: enteral, parenteral, and percutaneous. The term *parenteral* means administration by any route other than the enteral—or gastrointestinal—tract. As ordinarily used, the term *parenteral route* refers to intradermal, subcutaneous (subcut), intramuscular (IM), or intravenous (IV) injections.

When drugs are given parenterally rather than orally, the following factors are involved: (1) the onset of drug action is generally more rapid but of shorter duration; (2) the dosage is often smaller because drug potency tends not to be altered immediately by the stomach or liver; and (3) the cost of drug therapy is often higher. Drugs are administered by injection when all of the drug must be absorbed as rapidly and completely as possible, when the drug must be absorbed at a steady and controlled rate, or when a patient is unable to take a medication orally because of nausea and vomiting.

SAFE PREPARATION, ADMINISTRATION, AND DISPOSAL OF PARENTERAL MEDICATIONS AND SUPPLIES

Drug preparation and administration errors have been identified as contributing factors to the high incidence of adverse drug events as discussed in Chapter 6. The actual rate of errors that occur during the preparation and administration of medications is not known, but the potential is high. Thus the nurse must be diligent to prevent errors from occurring.

The role of the nurse in providing accurate drug administration requires attention to detail in all facets of pharmacotherapy. It is essential that nurses who are preparing and administering medications focus on the following: (1) the basic knowledge needed regarding the individual drugs being ordered, prepared, and administered; (2) the symptoms for which the medication is prescribed and the collection of baseline data to be used for the evaluation of the therapeutic outcomes desired for the prescribed medicine; and (3) the nursing assessments necessary to detect, prevent, or ameliorate adverse events. Finally, the nurse must exercise clinical judgment regarding the scheduling of new drug orders, missed doses, modified drug orders, the substitution of therapeutically equivalent medicines by the pharmacy, or changes in the patient's condition that require consultation with a physician, healthcare provider, or pharmacist.

Injection of drugs requires skill and special care because of the trauma at the site of needle puncture, the possibility of infection, the chance of allergic reaction, and the fact that, after it is injected, the drug is irretrievable. Therefore medications must be prepared and administered carefully and accurately. Aseptic technique is used to avoid infection, and accurate drug dosing—along with the correct rate and site of injection—is followed to avoid injuries such as abscess formation, necrosis, skin sloughing, nerve injuries, and prolonged pain. Thus the parenteral administration of medications requires specialized knowledge and manual skills to ensure safety and therapeutic effectiveness for patients.

Healthcare professionals place the safety of their patients first, but the Occupational Safety and Health Administration (OSHA) has reported that more than 5 million workers in the healthcare industry and related occupations are at risk for occupational exposure to blood-borne pathogens, including such devastating diseases as human immunodeficiency virus, hepatitis B virus, and hepatitis C virus. It is estimated that there are 600,000 to 800,000 needlesticks and percutaneous injuries involving healthcare workers annually. Studies have indicated that nurses sustain the majority of these injuries and that as many as one third of all sharps injuries (i.e., from needles, lancets, and scalpels) are related to the disposal process. Consequently, nurses have three primary safety concerns: for the patient, for themselves, and for other healthcare workers. Paramount to the safe administration of medicines is the need for nurses to follow established policies and procedures while checking and transcribing orders; preparing, administering, recording, and monitoring therapeutic responses to drug therapy; and disposing of parenteral supplies and equipment.

EQUIPMENT USED FOR PARENTERAL ADMINISTRATION

SYRINGES

Syringes are made of glass or hard plastic; glass syringes are rarely used in clinical practice. A syringe has three parts (Figure 9-1). The **barrel** is the outer portion on which the calibrations for the measurement of the drug volume are located (Figure 9-2). The **plunger** is the inner cylindrical portion that fits snugly into the barrel. This portion is used to draw up and eject the solution from the syringe. The **tip** is the portion that holds the needle. Syringes are considered to be sterile when the package is still intact from the manufacturer. The nurse will remove the outer sheath that covers the syringe and then hold the barrel; the barrel is then

considered unsterile or contaminated, whereas the inside of the barrel remains sterile. Nurses must keep the tip of the syringe sterile when connecting needles.

All syringes, regardless of their manufacturer, are available with a Luer-Slip or Luer-Lok tip. The Luer system consists of two parts: the male tapered end (Figure 9-3, *A*) and the reverse tapered female connector with an outer flange (see Figure 9-3, *B*).

The two types of syringe tips are the Luer-Slip, which has a male tapered end (Figure 9-4, *A*), and the Luer-Lok (see Figure 9-4, *B*), which has a threaded locking collar outside of the male Luer-Slip that will lock the flange of the female connector securely. When the female connector is placed on a male Luer-Slip with a locking collar and given a half twist, it is securely locked in place (see Figure 9-3, *C* or Figure 9-4, *B*). However, if a female adapter is placed on a male Luer-Slip without a collar (see Figure 9-4, *A*), the connection is only relatively secure.

Syringe Calibration

A syringe is calibrated in milliliters (mL) (see Figure 9-2). The most commonly used syringes are 1, 3, and 5 mL, but syringes of 10, 20, and 50 mL are also available. (NOTE: Technically, the milliliter is a measure of volume.)

Reading the Calibration of the Syringe

Milliliter (mL) scale. The **milliliter scale** represents the units whereby medications are routinely ordered. For volumes of 1 mL or less, use a 1-mL or tuberculin

FIGURE 9-2 Reading the calibrations of a 3-mL syringe.

FIGURE 9-1 Parts of a syringe.

FIGURE 9-3 The Luer system consists of two parts: **A,** the male tapered end, and **B,** the reverse-tapered female connector with an outer flange. **C,** The two components are joined together. The hub of the female connector slips over the male tapered end and is twisted so that the flange on the hub locks into the threads of the locking collar.

FIGURE 9-4 **A,** Male slip adapter tip (Luer-Slip). **B,** Male slip adapter with outer locking collar (Luer-Lok). (Courtesy and © Becton, Dickinson and Company.)

syringe for the more precise measurement of the drug. Milliliters are read on the scale marked "mL" (see Figures 9-2 and 9-6). The shorter lines represent 0.1 mL, and the longer lines each represent 0.5 mL.

Tuberculin syringe. The **tuberculin syringe,** or 1-mL syringe, was originally designed to administer tuberculin inoculations (see Figure 9-4, *A* and *B;* Figure 9-5). Today, it is used to measure small volumes of medication accurately. This type of syringe holds a total of 1 mL; each of the longest lines represents 0.1 ($\frac{1}{10}$) mL, the intermediate lines represent 0.05 ($\frac{5}{100}$) mL, and the shortest lines represent 0.01 ($\frac{1}{100}$) mL.

The volumes within glass syringes are read at the point where the plunger is directly parallel with the calibration on the syringe (Figure 9-6). Volumes in disposable plastic syringes are read at the point where the rubber flange of the syringe plunger is parallel to the calibration scale of the barrel (Figure 9-7). In addition, note the area of the needle to keep sterile and the area on the syringe plunger to avoid touching.

Insulin syringe. The **insulin syringe** has a scale that has been specifically calibrated for the measurement of insulin. Insulin is now manufactured with a U-100 concentration in the United States. The U-100 syringe

FIGURE 9-5 Tuberculin syringe calibration.

(Figure 9-8, *A*) holds 100 units of insulin per milliliter. Variations may be noticed in the way that units are marked on the scale, but, in general, the shorter lines represent 2 units of insulin, whereas the longer lines measure 10 units of insulin. Low-dose insulin syringes (see Figure 9-8, *B*) may be used for patients who are receiving 50 units or less of U-100 insulin. The shorter lines on the scale of the low-dose insulin syringe measure 1 unit, whereas the longer lines each represent 5 units. When traveling abroad, be aware that U-40 concentration insulin (i.e., 40 units of

FIGURE 9-6 Reading the measured amount of medication in a glass syringe.

FIGURE 9-7 Reading the measured amount of medication in a plastic syringe.

FIGURE 9-8 Calibration of insulin syringes. **A,** U-100 insulin syringe. **B,** Low-dose insulin syringe. Low-dose syringes are available in 25-, 30-, and 50-unit sizes to measure U-100 insulin more accurately.

insulin/mL) is commonly available. A specific insulin syringe that has been calibrated for U-40 insulin should be used with the U-40 insulin.

Insulin delivery aids (e.g., nonvisual insulin measurement devices, syringe magnifiers, needle guides, vial stabilizers) are available for people with visual impairments. Information about these products is available in the American Diabetes Association's annual diabetes resource guide, which is published each January.

Life Span Considerations

Tuberculin Syringe

The tuberculin syringe (see Figure 9-5), which makes use of the metric system of measurement, will provide the most accurate measurement for doses of parenteral medications of 1 mL or less. The practice of adding 0.2 mL of air bubbles to empty all of the medication contained in the needle of a syringe thoroughly can significantly increase a drug dose, especially when small volumes of medicine are being administered to neonates or infants. Check institutional policy regarding medication administration for the procedure to be used.

Prefilled Cartridges and Syringes

Several manufacturers supply a premeasured amount of medication in either presealed cartridge-needle units or in prefilled complete syringes. Both are used once and then discarded. Advantages of the **prefilled cartridges and syringes** include the time saved in preparing a standard amount of medication for one injection and the diminished chance of contamination between patients and hospital personnel. Disadvantages include additional expense and the limitation of the volume if a second medication is be added to the cartridge or syringe.

The prefilled cartridge units are marketed under the brand name Carpuject. The cartridge contains the amount of drug for one standard dose of medication. The drug name, concentration, and volume are clearly printed on the cartridge. The Carpuject prefilled cartridges require a holder that corresponds with the type of cartridge used (Figure 9-9). Examples of drugs dispensed in prefilled cartridges are morphine, ketorolac, hydromorphone, ondansetron and heparin. Other medicines (e.g., specific vaccines, enoxaparin, dalteparin, diclofenac, amiodarone) are shipped from the manufacturer in a syringe for ease of use. Many hospital pharmacies prefill syringes for specific doses of medication for patients with specific conditions. The syringe is labeled with the drug name and dosage, the patient's name and room number, and the dates of preparation and expiration.

Insulin is also available in a prefilled syringe known as an **insulin pen** (Figure 9-10). When capped, these pens look very much like ink pens, which allows the patient to carry insulin in a discreet manner. When needed, the cap is removed, a needle is attached, air bubbles are removed, the dose is dialed in, the needle is inserted into the subcut tissue, and a trigger is pushed to inject the measured dose. When finished, the needle is removed and the cap replaced, and the device again takes on the appearance of a pen. These pens are available in a variety of colors and styles, including a prefilled, disposable model; a smaller, low-dose model; and a refillable model into which a new cartridge can be inserted when needed. The patient should be instructed regarding the correct method of holding the pen and reading the dosing dial as

FIGURE 9-9 A, Carpuject cartridge holder and prefilled sterile cartridge with needle. **B,** Assemble the Carpuject by inserting the pre-filled cartridge inside the Carpuject holder; lay the white flange of the syringe over one end and lock the blue end down to keep the syringe in place. **C,** Twist the white end to screw into the pre-filled cartridge. **D** and **E,** Remove the green cover from the tip of the cartridge; keeping this end sterile, attach the needle to the cartridge. **F,** Needle is now attached to the pre-filled cartridge in a Carpuject cartridge holder.

FIGURE 9-10 Elements of the insulin pen. *A,* Pen cap. *B,* Measuring device. *C,* Prefilled syringe to be covered by the protective cap. (Copyright Eli Lilly and Co. All rights reserved. Used with permission.)

indicated by the manufacturer; this will help to prevent dosing errors.

Another type of prefilled syringe is the EpiPen (Figure 9-11). This syringe is a disposable automatic injection device that has been prefilled with epinephrine for use in an emergency, such as that caused by an allergic reaction to insect stings or bites, foods, or drugs. When held perpendicularly against the thigh and activated, a needle penetrates the skin into the muscle, and a single dose of epinephrine is injected into the muscle. This product is available in adult and pediatric dosages for use at home or when traveling for those who have strong reactions when they are

FIGURE 9-11 Prefilled syringe and needle containing epinephrine for use during emergencies. (From Mylan Inc., Canonsburg, PA.)

Beveled tip

Shaft

Hub

FIGURE 9-12 Parts of a needle.

FIGURE 9-13 Needle length and gauge.

exposed to allergens. It is important to educate those who are carrying these prefilled syringes to monitor the expiration date of this medication on a regular basis. After the epinephrine has been administered, the person should go to a hospital emergency department because additional treatment may be necessary. Another recently released product of injectable epinephrine for allergies is Auvi-Q.

THE NEEDLE

Parts of the Needle

The needle parts are the hub, the shaft, and the beveled tip (Figure 9-12). The angle of the bevel can vary; the longer the bevel, the easier the needle penetration.

Needles are sterile when they arrive from the manufacturer. Nurses must pay careful attention to keep the parts of the needle sterile and to avoid contamination. If contamination is suspected during the process of withdrawing medications, discard the needle in a sharps container and start again with a new one.

Needle Gauge

The **needle gauge** is the diameter of the hole through the needle. The larger the gauge number, the smaller the hole. The gauge number is marked on the hub of the needle and on the outside of the disposable package. The proper needle gauge is usually selected on the basis of the viscosity (thickness) of the solution to be injected. A thicker solution requires a larger diameter, so a smaller gauge number is chosen (Figure 9-13). Finer needles (e.g., 27, 29, 31, and 32 gauge) are available for specialty use.

SELECTION OF THE SYRINGE AND NEEDLE

The size of the syringe used is determined by the volume of medication to be administered, the degree of accuracy needed for the measurement of the dose, and the type of medication to be administered.

Needle selection should be based on the correct gauge for the viscosity of the solution and the correct needle length for the delivery of the medication to the correct site (e.g., intradermal, subcut, IM, or IV). Table 9-1 may be used as a guide to select the proper volume of syringe and the length and gauge of needle for adult patients.

In small children and older infants, the usual maximum volume for an IM injection at one site is 1 mL. In small infants, the muscle mass may only be able to tolerate a volume of 0.5 mL using a ½-inch–long needle. For older children, the volume should be individualized; generally, the larger the muscle mass, the greater the similarity to the adult volume for one injection site. Pediatric IM injections routinely use a 25- to 27-gauge needle that is 1 to 1½ inches long, depending on the assessment of the depth of the muscle mass of the child. Also available for pediatric use are 31-gauge, ½-inch needles.

Selection of Needle Length

Assess the depth of the patient's tissue for administration (e.g., muscle tissue for IM administration, subcutaneous tissue for subcut injection), and choose a needle length that corresponds to the findings.

Table 9-1 Selection of Syringe and Needle

ROUTE	VOLUME (ML)	GAUGE	LENGTH*
Intradermal	0.01-0.1	26-29	⅜ to ½ inch
Subcutaneous	0.5-2	25-27	Individualized on the basis of the depth of the appropriate tissue at the site
Intramuscular	0.5-2†	20-23	Individualized on the basis of the depth of the appropriate tissue at the site

*When judging the needle length, allow an extra ¼ to ½ inch to remain above the skin surface when the injection is administered. In the rare event of a needle breaking, this allows a length of needle to protrude above the skin to grasp for removal.
†Divided doses are generally recommended for volumes that exceed 2 to 3 mL, particularly for medications that are irritating to the tissues.

FIGURE 9-14 Use body size **(A)** to estimate needle length for an intramuscular injection **(B)**.

EXAMPLE:

Compare the muscle depth of a 250-pound, obese, sedentary woman with the muscle depth of a 105-pound, debilitated adult patient. The obese individual may require a 1½- to 2-inch needle, and the frail person may need a 1- to 1½-inch needle. A child may require a 1-inch needle (Figure 9-14).

PACKAGING OF SYRINGES AND NEEDLES

The sterility of the syringe and needle to be used should always be inspected and verified when preparing and administering a parenteral medication. Wrappers should be checked for holes, signs of moisture penetrating the wrapper, and the expiration date.

With prepackaged disposable items, the continuity of the wrapper, loose lids or needle guards, and any penetration of the paper or plastic container by the needle should also be checked. Should contamination be suspected, do not use the syringe; return it to the pharmacy for replacement.

SAFETY SYSTEMS FOR PARENTERAL PREPARATION, ADMINISTRATION, AND DISPOSAL

The Centers for Disease Control and Prevention estimates that 62% to 88% of sharps injuries can potentially be prevented with the use of medical devices. In response to this important public health concern, the U.S. Congress passed the Needlestick Safety and Prevention Act in 2000. This act required OSHA to revise its standards on blood-borne pathogens for the closer monitoring and reporting of needlestick injuries and to mandate the development of new safety equipment for the healthcare industry. One of the major developments has been the broader use of needleless systems. In accordance with OSHA regulations, needleless systems are required for the following: (1) for the collection of body fluids or the withdrawal of body fluids after initial venous or arterial access is established; (2) for the administration of medication or fluids; or (3) for any other procedure involving the potential for occupational exposure to blood-borne pathogens as a result of percutaneous injuries from contaminated sharps. Needleless systems provide an alternative to needles for routine procedures, thereby reducing the risk of percutaneous injury involving contaminated sharps. Another delivery system under development is a jet injection system that delivers subcut injections of liquid medication (e.g., insulin, vaccine) through the skin without requiring the use of a needle.

BLUNT ACCESS DEVICES

The blunt access device (e.g., the spike) is a safety innovation that was created to reduce the frequency of needle injuries. Note in Figure 9-15, *A* that needleless access devices do not have a stainless steel needle that is suitable for injection. The spike is used when drawing liquid from a rubber-diaphragm–covered vial. Another type of blunt access device that is more commonly known as a *filter needle* looks similar to other spikes, but it contains an internal filter. This device is used to withdraw liquid from a glass ampule. The filter screens out glass particles that may have fallen into the ampule when the top was broken off (see Figure 9-24). In addition to preventing needlestick injuries, these blunt access devices have the advantage of drawing larger fluid volumes from the container more rapidly. After the spike is used to draw up a medication, it is removed, and the appropriately sized needle is attached to the syringe if the medication is intended for injection directly into the patient.

FIGURE 9-15 Needle-free access devices. **A,** INTERLINK Vial Access Cannula entering a universal vial adapter. **B,** CLAVE Access System: *a,* a needle-free multidose vial adapter; *b,* the device snaps onto the top of a standard 20-mm medication vial; *c,* a single-dose vial adapter. (*A,* Courtesy Baxter Healthcare Corp. All rights reserved. *B,* Courtesy ICU Medical Inc.)

SAFETY DEVICES

Safety devices have been developed for syringes and needles. Some products have a sleeve that is stored around the syringe barrel while the syringe is being filled through the needle (Figure 9-16). After administration, the sleeve is pulled forward fully to lock the shield permanently in place to cover the needle. Another type of safety shielding device attaches to the needle hub (Figure 9-17). After the medicine is injected, the healthcare provider pushes the hinged shield forward, thereby covering the needle. Other safety shield devices are also available for short needles (Figure 9-18). The BD Integra Syringe System is a spring-loaded syringe that retracts the needle into the syringe after injection. This system also uses a technology called Tru-Lok Technology, which involves an apparatus that is similar to Luer-Lok technology. It allows for the changing of the needle between aspiration and administration, it locks the syringe and needle together securely, and it has a very low waste space in the hub and the safety device can be closed "hands-free" (Figure 9-19). Like all safety-designed syringes and needles, it is necessary to read the accompanying literature for adjustments that need to be made when operating these devices.

Flanges   Safe lock indicator   Sleeve

A

B   C   D   E

FIGURE 9-16 An example of a safety syringe that includes a full protective sheath. **A,** Syringe showing a sheath that covers the needle with a safe lock indicator. **B,** Assemble the device by holding the needle and the syringe by the flanges (wings) and twisting the needle until it is firmly seated. **C,** During aspiration, press the index finger against the flanges to prevent sleeve movement. (NOTE: If it is necessary to transport a filled syringe to the point of administration, use a safe, passive, one-handed recapping technique, per Occupational Safety and Health Administration standards, to cover the needle before transporting it to the point of use.) **D,** After injection, grasp the sleeve firmly, and twist the flanges to loosen the sleeve. **E,** Fully retract the needle into the sleeve until it locks in the protected position. When the green band fully covers the red band and an audible click is heard, the sleeve is locked into position. Place in sharps container.

Bevel up = Lever arm up

A   B

C   D

FIGURE 9-17 An example of a safety syringe that includes a shielding mechanism. **A,** Attach the needle and shield assembly to any standard Luer-Lok or Luer-Slip syringe. Twist it until it is firmly seated, and then pull the shield straight off of the needle to avoid damaging the needle's point. **B,** Aspirate the medication into the syringe per the usual technique. (NOTE: If it is necessary to transport a filled syringe to the point of administration, use a safe, passive, one-handed recapping technique, per Occupational Safety and Health Administration standards, to cover the needle before transporting it to the point of use.) **C,** Administer the injection in accordance with established technique. **D,** After injection, immediately apply a single finger stroke to the activation-assist lever arm to activate the shielding mechanism. Place in sharps container. (NOTE: Activate the device away from yourself and others, listen for the click, and visually confirm that the needle tip is fully covered.)

A   B

C   D

FIGURE 9-18 Another example of a safety syringe that includes a shielding mechanism. **A,** Aspirate the medication into the syringe per the usual technique. The safety arm can be rotated for scale readability. **B,** Administer the injection. To facilitate a low angle of injection, the safety arm can be rotated so that it is oriented to the needle bevel. **C,** After injection, apply a single finger stroke to activate the safety arm by moving it completely forward. **D,** The safety arm is locked and fully extended when you hear the click and the needle tip is covered.

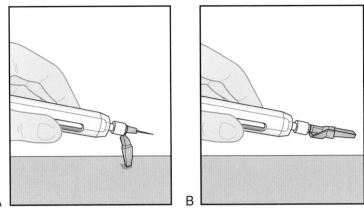

FIGURE 9-19 Hands-free safety device.

FIGURE 9-20 Needle disposal container also known as a sharps container.

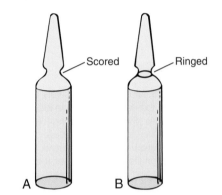

FIGURE 9-21 A, Scored ampule. **B,** Ringed ampule.

APPROPRIATE DISPOSAL

The appropriate disposal of used syringes and needles—including those with needle protection devices—is crucial to the prevention of needle injury and the transfer of blood-borne pathogens. To help minimize accidental needlesticks, a needle disposal container is commonly used for all sharps (Figure 9-20). When the container is full, the lid stays in place, and the entire container is disposed of in a specific manner to comply with OSHA standards. It is important to teach self-injecting patients how to protect themselves and others from accidental stick injury. Patients are encouraged to purchase a Sharps Disposal by Mail System at their pharmacy for the disposal of syringes, needles, and lancets. It is critical that patients use these systems to prevent the accidental exposure of sanitation workers to needles. The mail system includes a sharps container, an outer shipping box, and a prepaid postage label so that, when the container is filled, it can be mailed to an appropriate disposal center. If a patient is uncertain about the safest procedure for the disposal of used syringes and needles, he or she should contact the local sanitation service or department.

PARENTERAL DOSE FORMS

All parenteral drug dose forms are packaged so that the drug is sterile and ready for reconstitution (if needed) and administration.

AMPULES

Ampules are glass containers that usually contain a single dose of a medication. The container may be scored (Figure 9-21, *A*) or have a darkened ring around the neck (see Figure 9-21, *B*) to indicate where the ampule should be broken open for withdrawing the medication.

VIALS

Vials are glass or plastic containers that contain one or more doses of a sterile medication. Before use, the rubber diaphragm is sealed with a metal lid to ensure sterility (Figure 9-22, *A*). The mouth of the vial is covered with a thick rubber diaphragm through which a needle is passed to remove the medication (see Figure 9-22, *B*). The medication in the vial may be in solution, or it may be a sterile powder to be reconstituted just before administration. The drug also can be withdrawn from the vial using a spike attached to the syringe (see Figure 9-15).

MIX-O-VIALS

Mix-O-Vials are glass containers with two compartments (Figure 9-23). The lower chamber contains the drug (solute), and the upper chamber contains a sterile diluent (solvent); between the two areas is a rubber stopper. A single dose of medication is normally contained in the Mix-O-Vial. At the time of use, pressure is applied to the top rubber diaphragm

FIGURE 9-22 **A,** Vial protected by metal lid. **B,** Rubber diaphragm exposed when lid removed.

FIGURE 9-23 Mix-O-Vial.

plunger. This forces the solvent and the rubber stopper to fall into the bottom chamber where the diluent mixes with the powder, thereby dissolving the drug.

PREPARATION OF PARENTERAL MEDICATION

EQUIPMENT

- Drug in a sterile, sealed container
- Syringe of the correct volume
- Needles of the correct gauge and length
- Needleless access device
- Antiseptic alcohol wipe
- Medication profile

TECHNIQUE

Procedure Protocol

The standard procedures for preparing all parenteral medications are as follows:

1. Perform hand hygiene *before* preparing any medication or handling sterile supplies. During the actual preparation of a parenteral medication, the primary rule to remember is "sterile to sterile" and "unsterile to unsterile" when handling the syringe and the needle.

2. Use the *seven rights* of medication preparation and administration throughout the procedure.
3. Check the drug dose form ordered against the source available.
4. Check compatibility charts or contact the pharmacist before mixing two medications or before adding medication to an IV solution.
5. Check medication calculations. When in doubt about a dose, check it with another qualified nurse. (Most hospital policies require fractional doses of medications and doses of heparin and insulin to be checked by two qualified personnel before administration.)
6. Know the institutional policy regarding limitations on the types of medications to be administered by nursing personnel.
7. Prepare the drug in a clean, well-lit area, and use aseptic technique throughout the entire procedure.
8. After completing the standard procedures for preparing all parenteral medications, concentrate on the procedure at hand to ensure accuracy during preparation.
9. Check the expiration date on the medication container.

GUIDELINES FOR PREPARING MEDICATIONS

Preparing a Medication From an Ampule

1. Move all the solution to the bottom of the ampule, and flick the side of the glass container with the fingers to displace the medication from the top portion of the ampule (Figure 9-24, *A*).
2. Cover the ampule neck area with an antiseptic alcohol wipe in its sleeve while breaking the top off (see Figure 9-24, *B*, *C*, and *D*). Discard the wipe and the top in a sharps container.
3. With the use of a filter needle, withdraw all the medication from the ampule (see Figure 9-24, *E* and *F*).
4. Remove the filter needle from the ampule, and point vertically. Pull back on the plunger (this allows air to enter the syringe), and then replace the filter needle with a new sterile needle of the appropriate gauge and length for administration.
5. Push the plunger slowly until the medication appears at the tip of the needle or measure the amount of air to be included to allow for the total clearance of the medication from the needle when injected. (Never add air to a syringe that is to be used to administer an IV medication.)

Drugs in a vial may be in solution ready for administration, or they may be in powdered form for reconstitution before administration.

Preparing a Medication From a Vial
Reconstitution of a Sterile Powder

1. Read the accompanying literature from the medication's manufacturer, and follow specific instructions for reconstituting the drug that has been

FIGURE 9-24 Withdrawing from an ampule with a filter needle. **A,** Obtain a filter needle and displace the medication from the top portion of the ampule. **B,** Cover the ampule neck area with an antiseptic alcohol wipe remaining in its cover. **C** and **D,** Snap off the top of the ampule sharply in one swift motion. **E,** Using a filter needle withdraw the medication from the ampule. **F,** Note that the needle must be lowered to withdraw all of the solution from the ampule.

ordered. Add only the diluent specified by the manufacturer.

2. Cleanse the rubber diaphragm of the vial of diluent with an antiseptic alcohol wipe (Figure 9-25, *A*).

3. Pull back on the plunger of the syringe to fill it with an amount of air equal to the volume of solution to be withdrawn (see Figure 9-25, *B*).

4. Insert the needle or needleless access device through the rubber diaphragm, and inject the air (see Figure 9-25, *C*).

5. Withdraw the measured volume of diluent required to reconstitute the powdered drug (see Figure 9-25, *D* and *E*). Remove the needle from the diaphragm of the diluent container.

6. Recheck the type and volume of diluent to be injected against the type and amount required.

7. Tap the vial containing the powdered drug to break up the caked powder (see Figure 9-25, *F*). Wipe the rubber diaphragm of the vial of powdered drug with a new alcohol wipe (see Figure 9-25, *G*).

8. Insert the needle or needleless access device in the diaphragm, and inject the diluent into the powder (see Figure 9-25, *H*).

9. Remove the syringe and needle from the rubber diaphragm.

10. *Mix thoroughly* to ensure that the powder is entirely dissolved *before* withdrawing the dose (see Figure 9-25, *I*).

11. Label the reconstituted medication, and include the date and time of reconstitution, the volume and type of diluent added, the name of the reconstituted drug, the concentration of the reconstituted drug, the expiration date and time, and the name of the person who reconstituted the drug. Store the medication in accordance with the manufacturer's instructions.

12. Change the needle (as described previously), or remove the needleless access device. Attach a needle of the correct gauge and length to administer the medication to the patient.

Removal of a Volume of Liquid From a Vial
(see Figure 9-25)

1. Calculate the volume of medication required for the prescribed dose of medication to be administered.

2. Cleanse the rubber diaphragm of the vial of diluent with an antiseptic alcohol wipe.

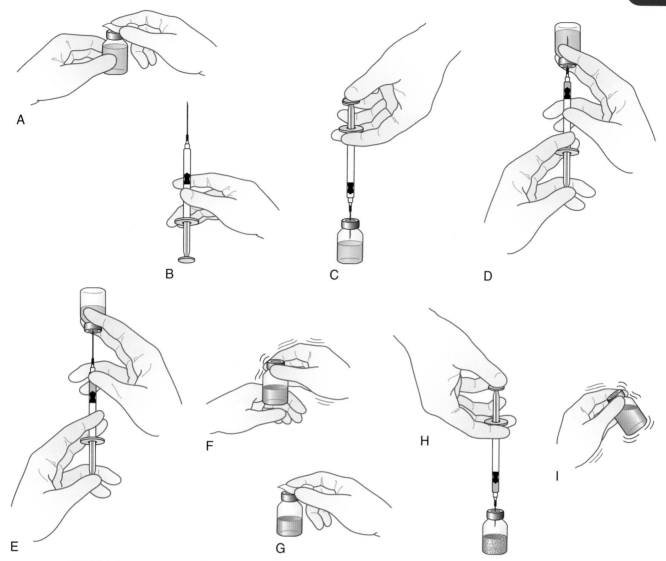

FIGURE 9-25 Removal of a volume of liquid from a vial: reconstitution of a powder. **A,** Cleanse the rubber diaphragm of the vial. **B,** Pull back on the plunger of the syringe to fill with an amount of air that is equal to the volume of the solution to be withdrawn. **C,** Insert the needle through the rubber diaphragm; inject the air with the vial sitting in a downward position. **D,** Withdraw the volume of diluent required to reconstitute the drug. **E,** Move the needle downward to facilitate the removal of all of the diluent. **F,** Tap the container with the powdered drug to break up the caked powder. **G,** Wipe the rubber diaphragm of the vial of the powdered drug with a new antiseptic alcohol wipe. **H,** Insert the needle with the diluent in the syringe into the rubber diaphragm, and inject the diluent into the powdered drug. **I,** Mix thoroughly to ensure that the powdered drug is dissolved before withdrawing the prescribed dose.

3. Pull back on the plunger of the syringe to fill it with an amount of air equal to the volume of solution to be withdrawn.
4. Insert the needle or needleless access device through the rubber diaphragm, and inject the air.
5. Withdraw the volume of drug required to administer the prescribed dose.
6. Recheck all aspects of the drug order.
7. Change the needle or remove the needleless access device. Attach a needle of the correct gauge and length to administer the medication to the patient.

Preparing a Drug From a Mix-O-Vial
1. Check the drug order against the medication available for administration.

2. To mix the drug, do the following:
   - Tap the container in the hand a few times to break up the caked powder.
   - Remove the plastic lid protector (Figure 9-26, *A*).
   - Push firmly on the diaphragm/plunger. The downward pressure will dislodge the divider between the two chambers (see Figure 9-26, *B* and *C*).
   - Mix thoroughly to ensure that the powder is *completely dissolved* before drawing up the medication for administration.
   - Cleanse the rubber diaphragm, and remove the drug in the same manner as described for the removal of a volume of liquid from a vial (see Figure 9-25, *A* through *E*).

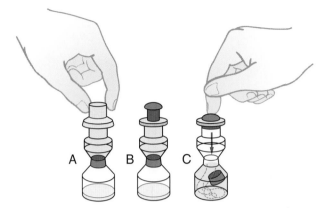

FIGURE 9-26 Using a Mix-O-Vial. **A,** Remove the plastic lid protector. **B,** The powdered drug is in the lower half; the diluent is in the upper half. **C,** Push firmly on the diaphragm plunger; downward pressure dislodges the divider between the two chambers.

Preparing Two Medications in One Syringe

Occasionally, two medications may be drawn into the same syringe for a single injection. This is usually done when preparing a preoperative medication or when two types of insulin are ordered to be administered at the same time. Mixing insulin is a routine procedure, so it will be used to illustrate this technique (Figure 9-27). Before administering insulin, the nurse always evaluates the patient's blood glucose level.

1. Check the compatibility of the two drugs to be mixed before starting to prepare the medications.
2. Check the labels of the medications against the medication order.
3. Check the following:
   - *Type:* NPH, regular, Humulin, other
   - *Concentration:* U-100 (U-100 = 100 units per mL)
   - *Expiration date:* Do NOT use the insulin if the expiration date has passed.
   - *Appearance:* Clear? Cloudy? Precipitate present?
   - *Temperature:* The insulin should be at room temperature.
4. The American Diabetes Association's 2003 guidelines state that "when mixing rapid- or short-acting insulin with intermediate or long-acting insulin, the clear rapid- or short-acting insulin should be drawn into the syringe first." When teaching a patient to mix insulin for self-administration, using a consistent method of preparing the mixture should be stressed so that this becomes a habit for the patient. This can help to prevent the patient from inadvertently reversing the dose of short- and long-acting insulin in the mixture.
5. Procedure:
   - Check the expiration date on the vial of insulin.
   - To resuspend the insulin, roll the vial or pen between the palms of the hands or invert the vial several times to mix the contents thoroughly.
   - Check the insulin order and the calculations of the preparation with another qualified nurse in accordance with institutional policy.
   - Cleanse the top of *both* vials with separate antiseptic alcohol wipes (see Figure 9-27, *A*).
   - Pull back the plunger on the syringe to an amount that is equal to the volume of the longer-acting insulin that has been ordered (see Figure 9-27, *B*).
   - Insert the needle through the rubber seal of the longer-acting insulin bottle, and inject the air (see Figure 9-27, *C*). Do not bubble air through the insulin solution, because it might break up insulin particles.
   - Remove the needle and the syringe. Do not withdraw insulin at this time.
   - Pull back the plunger on the syringe to an amount that is equal to the volume of the shorter-acting insulin that has been ordered (see Figure 9-27, *D*).
   - Insert the needle through the rubber seal of the second bottle, and inject the air (see Figure 9-27, *E*). Invert the bottle, and withdraw the volume of shorter-acting insulin (see Figure 9-27, *F*).
   - NOTE: Check for bubbles in the insulin in the syringe. Flick the side of the syringe with the fingers to displace the bubbles, and then recheck the amount of insulin in the syringe.
   - Check the medication order against the label of the container and the amount in the syringe.
   - Wipe the lid of the longer-acting insulin container again (see Figure 9-27, *G*). Recheck the drug order against this container, insert the needle of the syringe containing the shorter-acting insulin, and withdraw the specified amount of longer-acting insulin (see Figure 9-27, *H*). Be careful *not* to inject any of the first type of insulin already in the syringe into the vial.
   - Remove the needle and syringe. Recheck the drug order against the label on the insulin container and the amount in the syringe (see Figure 9-27, *I*).
   - Withdraw a small amount of air into the syringe, and then mix the two medications. Remove air

FIGURE 9-27 Preparing two drugs in one syringe. **A,** Check the insulin order, and then cleanse the tops of both vials with an antiseptic alcohol wipe. **B,** Pull back on the plunger to an amount that is equal to the volume of the longer-acting insulin. **C,** Insert the needle through the rubber diaphragm of the longer-acting insulin, and inject the air. Remove the needle and the syringe; do not remove the insulin. **D,** Pull back the plunger on the syringe to a point that is equal to the volume of the shorter-acting insulin ordered. **E,** Insert the needle through the rubber diaphragm, and inject the air. **F,** Invert the bottle, and withdraw the volume of the shorter-acting insulin ordered. Check the amount withdrawn against the amount ordered. **G,** Rewipe the lid of the longer-acting insulin. **H,** Insert the needle; withdraw the specified amount of longer-acting insulin. **I,** Remove the needle and the syringe; recheck the drug order against the labels on the insulin containers and the amount in the syringe.

carefully so that part of the medication is not displaced.
- Administer the insulin to the patient by the subcut route.

Preparing Medications for Use in the Sterile Field During a Surgical Procedure
Drugs Used in the Operating Room
- All medications used during an operative procedure must remain sterile.

- All medication containers (e.g., ampules, vials, piggyback containers, blood bags) used during the surgical procedure should remain in the operating room until the entire procedure is completed. If a question arises, the container is then available.
- *Do not save* any unused portion of medication for use during another surgical procedure. Discard this medication at the end of the surgical procedure, or send the patient's medication to the patient care unit with the patient, if appropriate (e.g., antibiotic

ointment for a patient who is having ophthalmic surgery).

- Adhere to hospital policies that address the handling and storage of medications in the operating room.
- *Always* tell the surgeon the name and dosage or concentration of the medication or solution that is being handed to him or her.
- *Always* repeat the entire medication order back to the surgeon when the request is made to verify all aspects of the order. If in doubt, repeat this information again until accuracy is certain.

Drugs Used in the Sterile Surgical Field

- Prepare the drug prescribed in accordance with the directions.
- Always check the accuracy of the drug order against the medication being prepared at least three times during the preparation phase: (1) when it is first removed from the drug storage area; (2) immediately before removing the solution for use in the sterile field; and (3) immediately after completing the transfer of the medication or solution to the sterile field. *Always* tell the surgeon the name and dose or concentration of the medication or solution when passing it to him or her for use.
- The circulating (nonsterile) nurse retrieves the medication from storage, reconstitutes it as needed, and turns the medication container so that the scrubbed (sterile) person can read the label. It is best to read the label aloud to ensure that both individuals are verifying the contents against the verbal order from the surgeon.

Method 1

1. The circulating (nonsterile) nurse cleanses the top of the vial or breaks off the top of the ampule, as described previously.
2. The scrubbed (sterile) person chooses a syringe of the correct volume for the medication to be withdrawn and attaches a large-bore needle to facilitate the removal of the solution from the container.
3. The circulating (nonsterile) nurse holds the ampule or vial in such a way that the scrubbed (sterile) person can easily insert the sterile needle tip into the medication container (Figure 9-28, *A*).

FIGURE 9-28 Preparing a medication in the operating room. **A,** The circulating (nonsterile) nurse holds the vial to facilitate the scrubbed (sterile) person inserting the sterile needle tip into the medication container. **B,** The needle is disconnected from the syringe and left in the vial.

4. The scrubbed person pulls back the plunger on the syringe until all of the medication prescribed has been withdrawn from the container and from the needle used to withdraw the medication.
5. The needle is disconnected from the syringe and left in the vial or ampule (see Figure 9-28, *B*).
6. The medication container is again shown to the scrubbed person and read aloud to verify all components of the drug prepared against the medication or solution requested.

Method 2

1. The circulating (nonsterile) nurse removes the entire lid of the vial with a bottle opener, cleanses the rim of the vial, and pours the medication directly into a sterile medicine cup held by the scrubbed nurse.
2. The scrubbed person continues drug preparation on the sterile field in accordance with the intended use (e.g., irrigation, injection).

Regardless of the method used to transfer the medication to the sterile field, both the sterile scrubbed person and the nonsterile circulating nurse should know the location and the exact disposition of each medication on the sterile field.

Get Ready for the NCLEX® Examination!

Key Points

- A syringe has three parts: the barrel, the plunger, and the tip that holds the needle. Types of safety syringes and needles include the Luer-Lok and needleless systems of blunt needles and shields over the needles.

- To correctly determine the gauge and length of the needle to use, the site of injection and the size of the patient are factored in, as well as the volume of medication to be administered.
- The tuberculin syringe is used to measure volumes of less than 1 mL; the standard syringe sizes are 1, 3, and 5 mL.

- Prefilled cartridge-needle units and syringes contain a standard dose of a medication and are a time saver for the nurse, but more expensive than a multidose vial of medication. Cartridges require a special cartridge holder to administer the medication. *Ampules* are glass containers of medications that need to be opened by snapping (breaking) the neck of the ampule before use. *Vials* have a rubber diaphragm that a needle passes through to access the medication. *Mix-O-Vials* are glass containers with two compartments. The lower compartment contains the medicine in powder form, and the upper compartment contains the diluent needed to dissolve the medicine. The two chambers are separated by a rubber plug. To mix the medicine, a rubber stopper on the top chamber is pushed, forcing the rubber stopper between the chambers to drop into the lower chamber, along with the diluent. Shaking the container dissolves the medicine, allowing it to be drawn up into a syringe for administration.
- Insulin can be mixed in one syringe by drawing up the short-acting insulin first, then adding the longer-acting insulin to the same syringe using a specific method.

Additional Learning Resources

SG Go to your Study Guide for additional Review Questions for the NCLEX® Examination, Critical Thinking Clinical Situations, and other learning activities to help you master this chapter content.

evolve Go to your Evolve website (http://evolve .elsevier.com/Clayton) for additional online resources.

Review Questions for the NCLEX® Examination

1. Which parts of the syringe and needle are considered sterile? *(Select all that apply.)*
   1. The tip of the needle
   2. The outer barrel of the syringe
   3. The plunger tip of the syringe
   4. The Luer-Lok end
   5. The inner barrel of the syringe

2. The nurse was preparing to give an injection into her patient's abdomen for his early morning insulin dose. Which needle length and gauge are appropriate to use?
   1. 18 gauge, 1½ inch
   2. 20 gauge, 1 inch
   3. 22 gauge, ⅝ inch
   4. 25 gauge, ⅝ inch

3. The nurse is preparing an IM injection of 1 mL of flu vaccine for an average adult patient and will be using this needle length and syringe size when administering the dose:
   1. ⅝ inch, 3 mL
   2. 1 inch, 3 mL
   3. 1½ inch, 5 mL
   4. ⅝ inch, 5 mL

4. The tuberculin syringe can be used for medications that are: *(Select all that apply.)*
   1. volumes less than 1 mL.
   2. for pediatric patients.
   3. for diabetic patients with insulin if a syringe marked in units is not available.
   4. highly viscous solutions.
   5. volumes greater than 1 mL.

5. Prefilled cartridge-needle units and syringes have many advantages that include: *(Select all that apply.)*
   1. they require special cartridge holders.
   2. they diminish the chance of contamination of the medication.
   3. they are cheaper than the multidose vials.
   4. they save the nurse the time it takes to prepare the injection.
   5. they contain a standard amount of medication.

6. When removing a parenteral medication from an ampule, what must the nurse do?
   1. Inject air equal to the amount of medication to be removed.
   2. Use a needleless spike for removing the medication.
   3. Use a filter needle or filter straw to ensure that no glass is drawn into the syringe.
   4. Depress the top rubber diaphragm to displace the stopper.

7. The nurse is teaching the patient how to prepare 10 units of regular insulin and 5 units of NPH insulin for injection. List in the correct order the proper sequence for preparation that the nurse will describe to the patient.
   1. Inject appropriate volumes of air into the NPH vial and the regular insulin vial.
   2. Withdraw 10 units of regular insulin into the syringe.
   3. Wipe the tops of the insulin vials with alcohol.
   4. Withdraw 5 units of NPH insulin into the syringe to mix with the regular insulin.
   5. Inject the insulin in the proper subcut site.

Objectives

1. Describe the technique that is used to administer a medication via the intradermal route.
2. List the equipment needed, and describe the technique that is used to administer a medication via the subcutaneous route.
3. Describe the technique used to administer medications intramuscularly.
4. Describe the landmarks that are used to identify the vastus lateralis muscle, the rectus femoris muscle, the ventrogluteal area, and the deltoid muscle site before medication is administered.
5. Identify suitable sites for the intramuscular administration of medication in an infant, a child, an adult, and an older adult.

Key Terms

intradermal (ĭn-tră-DŬR-măl) (p. 132)
erythema (ĕr-ĭ-THĒ-mă) (p. 134)
induration (in-dĕ-RĀ-shĕn) (p. 134)
anergic (ăn-ĔR-jĭk) (p. 134)
subcutaneous (sŭb-kū-TĀ-nē-ŭs) (p. 134)
intramuscular (ĭn-tră-MŬS-kyū-lăr) (p. 136)

vastus lateralis (VĂS-tŭs lăt-ĕr-Ă-lĭs) (p. 136)
rectus femoris (RĔK-tŭs FĔ-mŭr-ĭs) (p. 137)
ventrogluteal area (vĕn-trō-GLOO-tē-ăl) (p. 137)
deltoid muscle (DĔL-tŏyd MŬS-ŭl) (p. 138)
Z-track method (ZĒ TRĂK MĔTH-ĭd) (p. 140)

ADMINISTRATION OF MEDICATION BY THE INTRADERMAL ROUTE

Intradermal injections are made into the dermal layer of skin just below the epidermis (Figure 10-1). Small volumes, usually 0.1 mL, are injected. The absorption from intradermal sites is slow, thereby making it the route of choice for allergy sensitivity tests, desensitization injections, local anesthetics, and vaccinations.

Perform premedication assessments. See individual drug monographs.

EQUIPMENT

- Medication to be injected (see the medication profile)
- Tuberculin syringe with 26-gauge, ¼-inch, or 28-gauge, ½-inch needle, or a special needle and syringe for allergens
- Metric ruler, if performing skin testing procedure
- Gloves
- Antiseptic alcohol wipe
- Prescriber's order

SITES

Intradermal injections may be made on any skin surface, but the site should be hairless and receive little friction from clothing. The upper chest, the scapular areas of the back, and the inner aspect of the forearms are the most commonly used areas (Figure 10-2, A and B).

TECHNIQUE

This example of an intradermal injection technique involves allergy sensitivity testing. (CAUTION: Do not start any type of allergy testing unless emergency equipment [including epinephrine] is available in the immediate area in case of an anaphylactic response. Nurses should be familiar with the procedure to follow if an emergency does arise.)

1. Follow the procedure protocol.
2. Verify the identity of the patient using two identifiers. Check with the patient before starting the testing to ensure that he or she has not taken any antihistamines or antiinflammatory agents (e.g., aspirin, ibuprofen, corticosteroids) and that he or she has not received immunosuppressant therapy for 24 to 48 hours before the tests. If the patient has taken antihistamines, certain sleep medications (e.g., doxylamine, diphenhydramine), or antiinflammatory agents, check with the healthcare provider before proceeding with the testing.
3. Provide for patient privacy. Cleanse the area selected for testing thoroughly with an antiseptic alcohol wipe. Use circular motions, starting at the planned site of injection and continuing outward in circular motions to the periphery. Allow the area to air-dry.
4. Two methods can be used to administer allergy testing. One method requires the intradermal

132

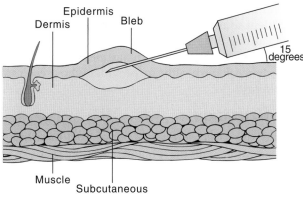

FIGURE 10-1 Intradermal injection technique.

injection of the allergens; the other is completed by using the skin prick method.

Intradermal Injection Method

1. Perform hand hygiene, and apply clean gloves.
2. Prepare the designated solutions for injection using aseptic technique. Usual volumes to be injected range between 0.01 and 0.05 mL. A positive-control solution that contains histamine and a negative-control solution that contains saline or the diluent of the allergen are also administered.
3. Insert the needle at a 15-degree angle with the needle bevel upward. (NOTE: There is a controversy regarding whether the needle bevel should be upward or downward. Check the procedure manual for facility policy.) The solution being injected is

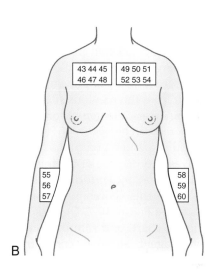

Reading Chart for Intradermal Testing

Patient Name:_____

Identification Number:_____

Physician Name:_____

DATE:	TIME:	AGENT	CONCENTRATION	DOSAGE	SITE NUMBER*	Reading Time in Hours or Minutes, 30 min or 24, 48, or 72 hr		

*Refer to diagram of sites, Figure 11-2, A and B
- Follow directions for the "reading" of the skin testing performed.
- Inspect sites in a good light.
- Record reaction in upper half of box using the following guidelines, e.g.,
  + (1+)   No wheal, 3 mm flare
  ++ (2+)   2 to 3 mm wheal with flare
  +++ (3+)   3 to 5 mm wheal with flare
  ++++ (4+) >5 mm wheal
- Record measurement of induration (process of hardening) in mm in lower half of box, e.g.,

FIGURE 10-2 Intradermal sites. **A,** Posterior view. **B,** Anterior view. **C,** Reading a chart for intradermal testing.

deposited in the space immediately below the skin; remove the needle quickly. A small bleb will appear on the surface of the skin as the solution enters the intradermal area (see Figure 10-1). Be careful not to inject into the subcutaneous space, and do not wipe the site with alcohol after injection.

4. *Do not* recap any needles that have been used. Activate the safety device if on the syringe. Dispose of used needles and syringes into a puncture-resistant needle disposal container in accordance with institutional policy.

Skin Prick Test Method

1. Perform hand hygiene, and apply clean gloves.
2. Make a grid of at least four squares, more if needed, on the test site at 2-cm intervals with a pen.
3. Place a drop of each allergen in one of the grid squares of the testing site. A positive-control solution that includes histamine and a negative-control solution that includes saline or the diluent of the allergen are also administered.
4. Using a lancet with a 1-mm point, prick the skin through the allergen drop. Wipe the lancet with dry gauze between each prick to prevent the carryover of the allergen from the previous site.
5. Gently blot the excess allergen off of the site.
6. The skin prick test can be read 10 to 20 minutes after administration, depending on protocol.
7. Remove gloves and dispose of them in accordance with institutional policy. Perform hand hygiene.
8. Chart the times, agents, concentrations, and amounts administered (see Figure 10-2, C). Make a diagram in the patient's chart, and number each location. Record what agent at what concentration was injected at each site. (Subsequent readings of each area are then performed and charted on this record.)
9. Follow the directions regarding the time of the reading of the skin testing being performed. The inspection of the injection sites should be performed in good light. Generally, a positive reaction (i.e., the development of a wheal) to a diluted strength of suspected allergen is considered clinically significant. Measure the diameter of the wheal in millimeters and **erythema** (i.e., redness at the site of injection), and palpate and measure the size of any **induration.** No reaction to the allergens, especially to the positive control, is known as an *anergic reaction.* Anergy is associated with immunodeficiency disorders. Record this information in the patient's chart.

The injection technique can easily be modified for desensitization injections and vaccinations.

PATIENT TEACHING

Tell the patient the time, date, and place to return to have the test sites read, if necessary. Tell the patient not to wash or scrub the area until the injections have been read. If the patient develops an area of severe burning or itching, he or she should try not to scratch it. Tell the patient to report immediately the development of any breathing difficulty, severe hives, or rashes and to go to the nearest emergency department if he or she is unable to reach the healthcare provider who prescribed the skin tests.

DOCUMENTATION

Provide the *right documentation* of the medication administration and the patient's responses to drug therapy.

1. Chart the date, time, drug name (including agent, concentration, and amount), dosage, and site of administration (see Figure 10-2).
2. Perform a reading of each site after the application of the test as directed by the healthcare provider or the policy of the healthcare agency.
3. Chart and report any signs and symptoms of adverse drug effects.
4. Perform and validate essential patient education about the drug therapy and other essential aspects of intervention for the disease process that is affecting the individual.

The following is a list of commonly used readings of reactions and their appropriate symbols:

+ (1+)	No wheal, 3-mm flare
++ (2+)	2- to 3-mm wheal with flare
+++ (3+)	3- to 5-mm wheal with flare
++++ (4+)	>5-mm wheal

Generally, a positive reaction to delayed hypersensitivity skin testing (to evaluate in vivo cell-mediated immunity) requires an induration of at least 5 mm in diameter.

ADMINISTRATION OF MEDICATION BY THE SUBCUTANEOUS ROUTE

Subcutaneous (subcut) injections are made into the loose connective tissue between the dermis and the muscular layer (Figure 10-3). Absorption is slower and drug action is generally longer with subcut injections as compared with intramuscular (IM) or intravenous injections. If the patient's circulation is adequate, then the drug is completely absorbed from the tissue.

Many drugs cannot be administered by this route because no more than 2 mL can ordinarily be deposited at a subcut site. The drugs must be quite soluble and potent enough to be effective in a small volume without causing significant tissue irritation. Drugs commonly injected into the subcut tissue are heparin, enoxaparin, and insulin.

Perform premedication assessments. See the individual drug monographs.

EQUIPMENT

- Medication to be injected (see the medication profile)

FIGURE 10-3 Subcutaneous injection. Inject at a 45- to 90-degree angle depending on the depth of subcutaneous tissue, the length of the needle, and the volume to be injected.

FIGURE 10-4 Subcutaneous injection sites and rotation plan. **A,** Posterior view. **B,** Anterior view. This illustrates commonly used subcutaneous sites for self-administration, and it provides an example of a rotation schedule for insulin injection using one site systematically before proceeding to the next site of administration.

Syringe Size

Choose a syringe that corresponds with the volume of drug to be injected at one site. The usual amount injected subcutaneously at one site is 0.5 to 2 mL. Correlate the syringe size with the size of the patient and the tissue mass.

Needle Length

Assess each patient so that the needle length selected will deposit the medication into the subcut tissue rather than the muscle tissue. Needle lengths of $\frac{3}{8}$-, $\frac{1}{2}$-, and $\frac{5}{8}$-inch are routinely used. It is prudent to leave an extra $\frac{1}{4}$-inch of needle extending above the skin surface in case the needle breaks.

Needle Gauge

Commonly used gauges for subcut injections are 25 to 29 gauge.

SITES

Common sites used for the subcut administration of medications include the upper arms, the anterior thighs, and the abdomen (Figure 10-4). Less common areas are the buttocks and the upper back or scapular region.

A plan for rotating injection sites should be developed for all patients who require repeated injections (see Figure 10-4). The anterior view (see Figure 10-4, *B*) illustrates areas that are easily accessible for self-administration. The posterior view (see Figure 10-4, *A*) illustrates less commonly used areas that may be used by a caregiver who is injecting the medication into the patient.

When administering insulin subcutaneously, it is important to rotate the injection sites to prevent lipohypertrophy or lipoatrophy, which slows the absorption rate of the insulin. The American Diabetes Association Clinical Practice Recommendations state that insulin injection sites should be rotated systematically within one area before progressing to a new site for injection (see Figure 10-4); it is thought that this will decrease variations in insulin absorption. Absorption is known to be fastest when the insulin is administered in the abdomen; this is followed by the arms, thighs, and buttocks. Because exercise is also known to affect the rate of insulin absorption, site selection should take this factor into consideration.

TECHNIQUE

1. Follow the procedure protocol.
2. Verify the identity of the patient using two identifiers. Ensure that the patient does not have an allergy to the medication.
3. Check the accuracy of the drug order against the medication being prepared at least three times during the preparation phase: (1) when first removing the drug from the storage area; (2) immediately after preparation; and (3) immediately before administration.
4. Consult the master rotation schedule for the patient so that the drug is administered at the correct site.
5. Explain carefully to the patient what to expect.
6. Provide for the patient's privacy, and position the patient appropriately.
7. Apply clean gloves.
8. Expose the selected site, and locate the landmarks.
9. Cleanse the skin surface with an antiseptic alcohol wipe starting at the injection site and working outward in a circular motion toward the periphery.
10. Allow the area to air-dry.
11. View the site of injection and the length of the needle. Assess whether the injection is most appropriately administered at a 45- to 90-degree angle for subcutaneous delivery.

Method

1. Insert the needle quickly at a 45- to 90-degree angle; slowly inject the medication. The American Diabetes Association Clinical Practice Recommendations state that "thin individuals or children may need to pinch the skin and inject at a 45-degree angle to avoid IM injection, especially in the thigh area."
2. Withdraw the needle; gentle pressure may be applied to the site with an antiseptic alcohol wipe, but *do not* rub.
3. *Do not* recap any needles that have been used. Activate the safety device. Dispose of used needles and syringes into a puncture-resistant needle disposal container in accordance with institutional policy.
4. Remove gloves and dispose of them according to facility policy. Perform hand hygiene.

PATIENT TEACHING

Perform appropriate patient teaching as described in the related drug monographs.

DOCUMENTATION

Provide the *right documentation* of the medication administration and the patient's response to drug therapy.

1. Chart the date, time, drug name, dose, site, and route of administration.
2. Perform and record regular patient assessments for the evaluation of the therapeutic effectiveness (e.g., blood pressure, pulse, output, improvement or quality of cough and productivity, degree and duration of pain relief).
3. Chart and report any signs and symptoms of adverse drug effects.
4. Perform and validate essential patient education about the drug therapy and other essential aspects of intervention for the disease process that is affecting the individual.

ADMINISTRATION OF MEDICATION BY THE INTRAMUSCULAR ROUTE

Intramuscular injections are made by penetrating a needle through the epidermis, dermis and the subcut tissue into the muscle layer. The injection deposits the medication deep within the muscle mass (Figure 10-5). Absorption is more rapid than that associated with subcut injections because muscle tissue has a greater blood supply. Site selection is especially important with IM injections because the incorrect placement of the needle may cause damage to nerves or blood vessels. Complications from improper technique of IM injections include hematoma, (when a vein is punctured) and pain (when a nerve is touched). A large, healthy muscle that is free from infections and wounds should be used.

Perform premedication assessments. See the individual drug monographs.

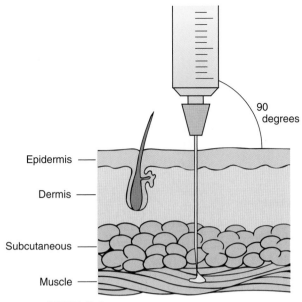

FIGURE 10-5 Intramuscular injection technique.

EQUIPMENT

- Medication to be injected (see the medication profile)

Syringe Size

Choose a syringe that corresponds with the volume of drug to be injected at one site. The usual amount injected intramuscularly at one site is 0.5 to 2 mL. In infants and children, the amount should range between 0.5 and 1 mL, and it should not exceed 1 mL. Correlate the syringe size with the size of the patient and the tissue mass. In adults, divided doses are generally recommended for amounts in excess of 3 mL; 1 mL is the maximum amount to be injected in the deltoid area. Other factors that influence syringe size and needle gauge include the type of medication, the site of administration, the thickness of the subcut fatty tissue, and the age of the individual.

Needle Length

Assess each patient so that the needle length selected will deposit the medication into the muscular tissue (Figure 10-6). There is a significant difference among the needle lengths that are appropriate for an obese patient, an infant, or an emaciated or debilitated patient. Needles that are commonly used are 1 to 1½ inches long, although longer lengths may be required for obese patients.

Needle Gauge

Commonly used gauges for IM injections are 20 to 23 gauge.

SITES

Vastus Lateralis Muscle

The **vastus lateralis** muscle is located on the anterior lateral thigh, away from nerves and blood vessels. The

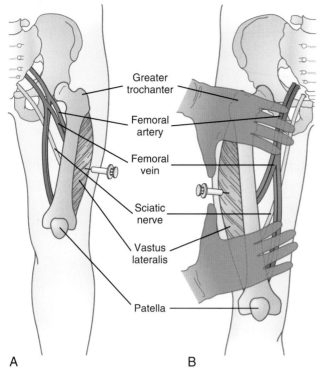

A **B**

FIGURE 10-6 Vastus lateralis muscle. **A,** Child or infant. **B,** Adult.

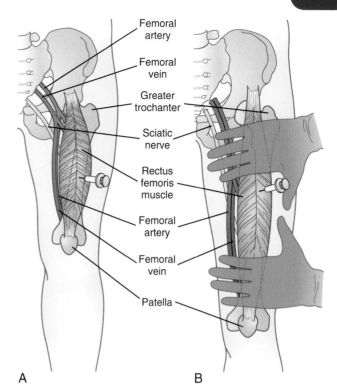

A **B**

FIGURE 10-7 Rectus femoris muscle. **A,** Child or infant. **B,** Adult.

midportion is one handbreadth below the greater trochanter and one handbreadth above the knee (see Figure 10-6). This is generally the preferred site for IM injections in infants because it has the largest muscle mass for that age group. This muscle is also a good choice for an injection site in healthy, ambulatory adults (see Figure 10-6, *B*). It accommodates a large volume of medication, and it allows for good drug absorption. In the older, debilitated, or nonambulatory adult, the muscle should be carefully assessed before injection because significantly less muscle mass may be present. If muscle mass is insufficient, an alternative site should be selected.

Rectus Femoris Muscle

The **rectus femoris** muscle (Figure 10-7) lies just medial to the vastus lateralis muscle, but it does not cross the midline of the anterior thigh. The injection site is located in the same manner as is used for the vastus lateralis muscle. This muscle may be used in both children and adults when other sites are unavailable. A primary advantage to its use is that it may be used more easily by patients for self-administration. A disadvantage is that the medial border is close to the sciatic nerve and major blood vessels (see Figure 10-7). If the muscle is not well developed, injections into this site may also cause considerable discomfort and potential injury.

Gluteal Area

The gluteal area is a commonly used site of injection because it is free of major nerves and blood vessels.

Life Span Considerations

Injection Sites

- The *vastus lateralis* site is preferred in infants. In the older, debilitated, or nonambulatory adult, carefully assess the sufficiency of the muscle mass before using this site for injection.
- The *ventrogluteal* site is also appropriate for infants and adults, and it may be used as often as needed because of the convenience of the thigh muscle.
- The *deltoid* site is preferred when administering 1 mL or less because of the convenience of the arm muscle.

The dorsogluteal area must not be used in children who are less than 3 years old because the muscle has not yet been well developed from walking. The ventrogluteal area is an appropriate site for injections in children who are less than 3 years old; however, this site is not used as often as the thigh muscle because of the convenience of the thigh muscle. The area may be divided into two distinct injection sites: (1) the ventrogluteal area; and (2) the dorsogluteal area.

Ventrogluteal Area. The **ventrogluteal area** is easily accessible when the patient is in a prone, supine, or side-lying position. It is located by placing the palm of the hand on the lateral portion of the greater trochanter with the thumb pointing toward the groin, the index finger on the anterior superior iliac spine, and the middle finger extended to the iliac crest. The injection

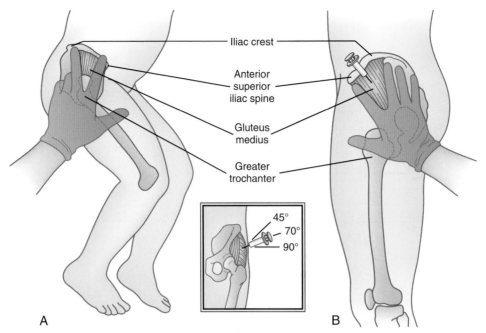

FIGURE 10-8 Ventrogluteal site. **A,** Child or infant. **B,** Adult.

FIGURE 10-9 Prone position. The toes are pointed to promote muscle relaxation.

FIGURE 10-10 Patient lying on the side. Flexing the upper leg promotes muscle relaxation.

is made into the center of the "V" that is formed between the index and middle fingers, with the needle directed slightly upward toward the crest of the ilium (Figure 10-8). Pain on injection can be minimized if the muscle is relaxed. The patient can help with this relaxation by pointing the toes inward while lying in a prone position (Figure 10-9) or by flexing the upper leg if lying on his or her side (Figure 10-10).

Dorsogluteal Area. The use of this site is discouraged and not practiced to any great extent because of the possible damage to the sciatic nerve.

Deltoid Muscle

The **deltoid muscle** is often used because of the ease of access to this area when the patient is in the standing, sitting, or prone position. However, it should be used in infants only when the volume to be injected is small, the drug is nonirritating, and the dose will be quickly absorbed. In adults, the volume should be limited to 1 mL or less, and the substance must not cause irritation. Caution must also be exercised to avoid the clavicle, the humerus, the acromion, the brachial vein and artery, and the radial nerve. The injection site (Figure 10-11) of the deltoid muscle is located by palpating the acromion process or top of the shoulder and measuring down two to three fingerbreadths. It is advisable to palpate the muscle of the deltoid, which is roughly triangular shaped, to determine the thickest part of the muscle, which will then be the area for the injection.

SITE ROTATION

A master plan for site rotation should be developed and used for all patients who require repeated injections (Figure 10-12).

TECHNIQUE

1. Follow the procedure protocol.
2. Verify the identity of the patient using two identifiers. Ensure that the patient does not have an allergy to the medication.
3. Check the accuracy of the drug order against the medication being prepared at least three times during the preparation phase: (1) when first removing the drug from the storage area; (2) immediately after preparation; and (3) immediately before administration.

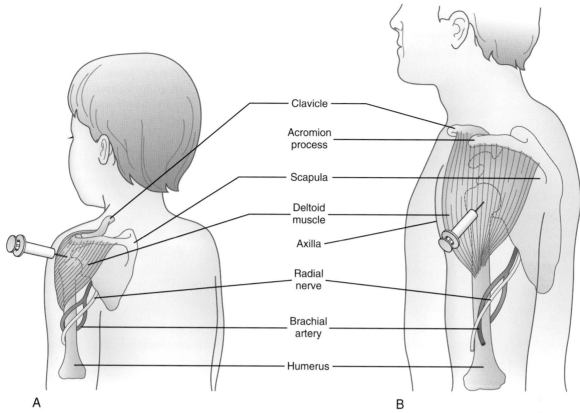

FIGURE 10-11 Deltoid muscle site. **A,** Child or infant. **B,** Adult.

4. Check the institutional policy regarding whether 0.1 or 0.2 mL of air should be added to the syringe *after* accurately measuring the prescribed volume of drug for administration. NOTE: The rationale for adding the air is that it will result in the needle being completely cleared of all medication at the time of injection. Conversely, if the volume is completely drawn into the syringe before changing the needle, then the drug volume ordered will still be administered as long as the same size needle is used for drawing up and injection. Thus the needle should not need to be completely cleared of medication by air during administration. This issue can be critical when small volumes of potent drugs are repeatedly administered to infants.

5. Consult the master rotation schedule for the patient so that the drug is administered at the correct site (see Figure 10-12).

6. Explain carefully to the patient what will be done.

7. Provide for the patient's privacy; position the patient appropriately (see Figures 10-9 and 10-10 for relaxation techniques).

8. Apply clean gloves. Expose the selected site, and locate the landmarks.

9. Cleanse the skin surface with an antiseptic alcohol wipe starting at the injection site and working outward in a circular motion toward the periphery.

10. Allow the area to air-dry.

11. Using the nondominant hand, spread the skin and hold down to push subcut tissue away and allow greater needle penetration.

12. Insert the needle at a 90-degree angle using a quick, dart-throwing action.

13. Inject the medication using gentle, steady pressure on the plunger and wait for a count of 3 before removing needle. This will ensure all the medication has been delivered. (NOTE: The need to aspirate before injection is no longer practiced; it has been found to cause more damage and is considered unnecessary.)

14. After removing the needle, apply gentle pressure to the site. Massage can increase the pain if the muscle mass is stressed by the amount of medication given.

15. *Do not* recap any needles that have been used. Activate the safety device. Dispose of used needles and syringes into a puncture-resistant needle disposal container in accordance with institutional policy.

16. Apply a small bandage to the site.

17. Provide emotional support to the patient. Children should be comforted during and after the injection. Sometimes letting a child hold your hand or say "ouch" helps. Praise the patient for his or her assistance and cooperation.

18. Remove gloves and perform hand hygiene.

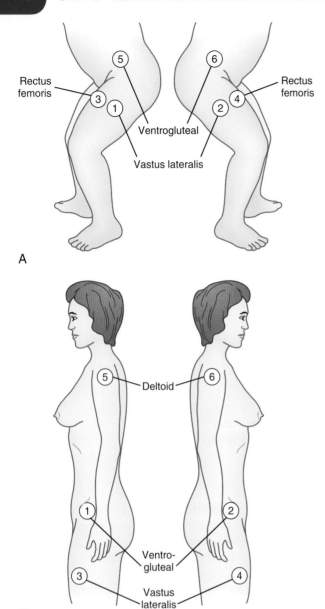

FIGURE 10-12 Intramuscular master rotation plan. **A,** Infant or child. Note that the deltoid site may also be used in an infant or child; however, the volume of medication must be small and the drug nonirritating. **B,** Adult. In an adult, avoid using the rectus femoris site because of the pain produced.

PATIENT TEACHING

Perform appropriate patient teaching as described in related drug monographs.

DOCUMENTATION

Provide the *right documentation* of the medication administration and the patient's response to drug therapy.

1. Chart the date, time, drug name, dose, site, and route of administration.
2. Perform and record regular patient assessments for the evaluation of the therapeutic effectiveness (e.g., blood pressure, pulse, output, improvement or quality of cough and productivity).
3. Chart and report any signs and symptoms of adverse drug effects.
4. Perform and validate essential patient education about the drug therapy and other essential aspects of intervention for the disease process that is affecting the individual.

Z-TRACK METHOD

The use of a **Z-track method** (Figure 10-13) may be appropriate for medications that are particularly irritating or that stain the tissue. Check facility policy regarding which personnel may administer medications using this method.

1. Provide for patient privacy.
2. Apply clean gloves.
3. Expose the ventrogluteal site or vastus lateralis site (Figure 10-13, *A*).
4. Calculate and draw up the medication; add 0.5 mL of air to ensure that the drug will clear the needle.
5. Position the patient, and cleanse the area for injection as previously described. Never inject into the patient's arm.
6. Stretch the patient's skin approximately 1 inch to one side (see Figure 10-13, *B*).
7. Insert the needle. Choose a needle of sufficient length to ensure deep muscle penetration.
8. Gently inject the medication, and then wait approximately 10 seconds (see Figure 10-13, *C*).
9. Remove the needle, and allow the skin to return to its normal position (see Figure 10-13, *D*).
10. *Do not* massage the injection site.
11. If further injections are to be made, alternate among sites.
12. *Do not* recap any needles that have been used. Dispose of used needles and syringes into a puncture-resistant needle disposal container in accordance with institutional policy.
13. Remove gloves, and dispose of them according to facility policy. Perform hand hygiene.
14. Walking will help with the medication's absorption. Vigorous exercise or pressure on the injection site (e.g., tight-fitting clothing) should be temporarily avoided.

Documentation and patient teaching are the same as for other IM injections.

volume of medicine over a set time. Syringe pumps are more commonly used when small volumes need to be administered. Examples of small syringe pumps are those that continually infuse insulin into the subcutaneous tissue of patients with diabetes mellitus and patient-controlled analgesia pumps, which allow patients who are receiving pain medications to administer continual infusions and intermittent boluses of the medicine for comfort.

Syringe pumps are easy to use, and their use is taught to patients needing home infusion therapy, when patients self-administer medications through an implanted infusion port. It is important that the nurse become familiar with the specific devices that are used in the clinical setting for safe and efficient patient care.

INTRAVENOUS ACCESS DEVICES

Intravenous access devices are often subdivided into four groups on the basis of the location of the terminal tip of the access device: (1) **peripheral devices** are for short-term use in peripheral veins in the hand or forearm; (2) **midline catheters** are for use over 2 to 4 weeks, and are inserted into intermediate-sized veins and advanced into larger vessels; (3) **central devices** are inserted into intermediate-sized vessels and advanced into central veins where the tip of the catheter typically will be in the superior vena cava to allow for maximal mixing with large volumes of blood; and (4) **implantable venous infusion ports**, which are placed into central veins for long-term therapy.

Peripheral Access Devices

All needles—if they are long enough—may be used to administer medications or fluids intravenously. However, special equipment has been designed for this purpose. **Winged needles**, which are also known as *butterfly* or *scalp needles*, are short, sharp-tipped needles (Figure 11-5) that were originally designed for venipuncture of small veins in infants and for geriatric use. These needles are available in sizes that range

from 17 to 29 gauge, and have been designed to minimize tissue injury during insertion. The winged area is pinched together to form a handle while the needle is being inserted. The wings are then laid flat against the skin to form a base that can be anchored with tape. Two types of these needles are now available: one with a short length of plastic tubing and a permanently attached resealable injection port and one with a variable length of plastic tubing with a female Luer adapter for the attachment of a syringe or an administration set (see Figure 11-5). The patency of the needle is maintained with the use of a heparin or saline flush routine in accordance with facility policy.

Over-the-needle catheters, which are also known as *short peripheral venous catheters,* are recommended for routine peripheral infusion therapy. The needles are stainless steel and coated with a Teflon-like plastic catheter (Figure 11-6, *A*). After the needle penetrates the vein in the hand or forearm, the catheter is advanced into the vein, and the metal needle is removed, thereby leaving the plastic catheter in place. An IV administration set is then attached to the catheter for continuous infusion. This unit is used when IV therapy is expected to continue for a few days. The rationale for the use of the plastic catheter is that it does not have a sharp tip that could cause venous irritation and extravasation.

When a patient no longer requires IV fluid therapy but venous access is still needed for medication administration, an extension tube with an injection port is

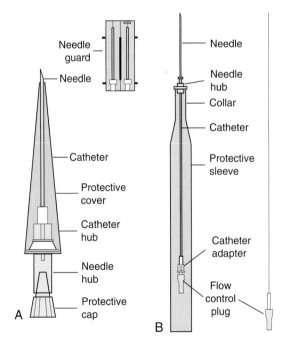

FIGURE 11-6 A, Over-the-needle catheter. This unit is the most commonly used type of catheter when intravenous therapy is expected to continue for several days. **B,** In-the-needle catheters make use of a large-bore needle for venipuncture. A 4- to 6-inch sterile, small-gauge, plastic catheter is then advanced through the needle and into the vein. The needle is withdrawn, and the skin forms a seal around the plastic catheter. The intracatheter is infrequently used today.

FIGURE 11-5 Winged needle with a female Luer adapter. (Courtesy Narang Medical Limited.)

attached to the catheter and the IV fluid is discontinued. This type of IV access device is called a *saline lock* or a *medlock* (i.e., *medication lock*). Normal saline flushing rather than heparin is sufficient to prevent clotting and maintain the peripheral catheter integrity. Generally, peripheral catheters should be changed every 72 to 96 hours to prevent infection and phlebitis. Blood samples should not be drawn from peripheral catheters. If sites for venous access are limited and no evidence of infection is present, peripheral venous catheters can remain in place, although the patient and the insertion site should be monitored closely for signs and symptoms of phlebitis, infiltration, and infection. The Centers for Disease Control (CDC) recommends that peripheral catheters not be changed for pediatric patients unless this is clinically indicated.

In-the-needle catheters make use of large-bore needles for venipuncture (see Figure 11-6, *B*). A 4- to 6-inch sterile, smaller-gauge, plastic catheter is then advanced through the needle into the vein. The needle is withdrawn, and the skin forms a seal around the plastic catheter. The IV administration set is attached directly to the plastic catheter. In-the-needle catheters are seldom used today for peripheral IVs because of the risk of shearing the through-the-needle catheter.

Midline access catheters are selected for use if it is anticipated that IV access will be needed for 7 days or more. These catheters are often left in place for 2 to 4 weeks. Midline catheters are flexible and 3 to 8 inches long, and are inserted at the antecubital fossa into the cephalic or basilic vein and advanced to the distal subclavian vein. They do not enter the superior vena cava. Midline catheters appear to be associated with lower rates of phlebitis than short peripheral catheters; they have a lower rate of infection, and they cost less than central venous catheters. The CDC recommends the replacement of the catheter and the rotation of the injection site no more frequently than every 72 to 96 hours, but the CDC does not provide recommendations regarding the maximum length of time that the catheter may remain in place. Many institutions require that the healthcare provider write an order that indicates that the IV may be left in place for more than 72 hours. Midline catheters are used for continuous access, repeated access, or IV solutions with high flow rates. This type of catheter needs to be flushed with saline and heparin solution after each use, or at least once daily if it is not in use. Blood should not be drawn through this catheter.

Central Access Devices

Central IV access devices, which are also known as *indwelling catheters,* are used in the following situations: when the purpose of therapy dictates their use (e.g., large volumes of medication, for irritating medicine such as chemotherapy, or when hypertonic solutions such as total parenteral nutrition [TPN] are to be infused); when peripheral sites have been exhausted as a result of repeated use or the condition of the veins for access is poor; when long-term or home therapy is required; or when emergency conditions mandate adequate vascular access.

The central venous sites that are most commonly used for central venous catheters are the subclavian and jugular veins. When the upper body veins are not acceptable, the femoral veins may be accessed for short-term or emergency use. A physician can also elect to perform a venisection or a cutdown to insert this type of catheter into the basilic or cephalic veins in the antecubital fossa. Three types of devices, based on the placement of the catheter's proximal tip, are routinely used for central catheters: peripheral devices, tunneled devices, and implantable devices.

Peripherally inserted central venous catheters (PICCs) are inserted into the superior vena cava or just outside the right atrium by way of the cephalic or basilar veins of the antecubital space, thereby providing an alternative to subclavian or jugular venous catheterization. Peripherally inserted central venous catheters are available in sizes that range from 14 to 28 gauge, with various lengths, thereby making them available for pediatric use. The catheter itself can have an open tip or a valved (Groshong) tip, and it comes with a single or double lumen. The PICC line has the advantage of ease of insertion because the procedure can be performed at the bedside by a qualified nurse. Peripherally inserted central venous catheters are associated with fewer mechanical complications (e.g., thrombosis, hemothorax); they cost less than other central venous catheters, they are easier to maintain than short peripheral catheters (because there is less frequent infiltration and phlebitis), and they require less frequent site rotation. Peripherally inserted central venous catheter lines routinely remain in place for 1 to 3 months, but they can last for 1 year or more if they are cared for properly. When the device is not in use, the IV is disconnected and the catheter is flushed and capped. The line should be flushed with a saline-heparin solution after every use or daily, if not used, in accordance with institutional policy.

Tunneled central venous catheters are surgically placed during an outpatient procedure with the patient under local anesthesia. The terminal tip of the catheter is inserted through an incision and into the subclavian vein, where it is then advanced to the superior vena cava. The proximal end of the catheter is tunneled about 6 inches away under the skin on the chest to exit near a nipple. A Dacron cuff is often placed around the catheter under the skin, which anchors the catheter and forms a seal around the catheter as the skin heals, thereby helping to keep the tunnel sterile.

Three types of catheters that are frequently used are the Hickman, Broviac, and Groshong catheters (Figure 11-7). The Broviac catheter is a single-lumen catheter with a larger external diameter and a standard end hole. The Hickman catheter is larger in diameter than

Table 12-2   Adrenergic Agents

GENERIC NAME	BRAND NAME	AVAILABILITY	ADRENERGIC RECEPTOR	ACTION	CLINICAL USES
albuterol*	Proventil HFA; Ventolin HFA; ProAir HFA	Aerosol: 108 mcg/puff Tablets: 2, 4 mg Syrup: 2 mg/5 mL Tablets, extended release: 4, 8 mg Nebulizer solution: 0.083%/3-mL ampule, 0.5%/0.5-mL ampule and 20-mL bottle; 0.63-mg/3-mL ampule, 1.25-mg/3-mL ampule	β_2	Bronchodilator	Asthma, emphysema
arformoterol*	Brovana	Nebulizer: 15 mcg/2 mL in 2-mL vials	β_2	Bronchodilator	Emphysema, chronic bronchitis
dopamine ●	—	IV: 40, 80, 160 mg/mL in 5-, 10-, 20-mL ampules; 200, 400, and 800 mg in D5W (various volumes available)	α, β_1, dopaminergic	Vasopressor	Shock, hypotension; inotropic agent
dobutamine ●	—	IV: 12.5 mg/mL in 250-mg/20-mL vial; 500-mg/40-mL vial	β_1	Cardiac stimulant	Inotropic agent
ephedrine* ●	—	Subcut, IM, IV: 50 mg/mL in 1-mL ampules	α, β	Bronchodilator, vasoconstrictor	Nasal decongestant, hypotension
epinephrine* ●	Adrenalin	IV:1:1000 in 1-mL ampules; 1:10,000 in 10-mL prefilled syringes	α, β	Allergic reactions, vasoconstrictor, bronchodilator, cardiac stimulant	Anaphylaxis, cardiac arrest; topical vasoconstrictor
formoterol*	Foradil, Perforomist, Oxeze ♣	Capsule for inhalation: 12 mcg Nebulizer: 20 mcg/2 mL in 2-mL container	β_2	Bronchodilator	Asthma, emphysema, chronic bronchitis
indacaterol*	Arcapta Neohaler; Onbrez Breezhaler ♣	Capsule for inhalation: 75 mcg	β_2	Bronchodilator	Emphysema, chronic bronchitis
isoproterenol ●	Isuprel	Subcut, IM, IV: 0.2 mg/mL solution; 1-, 5-mL vials	β	Bronchodilator, cardiac stimulant	Shock, digitalis toxicity, bronchospasm
metaproterenol	—	Tablets: 10, 20 mg Syrup: 10 mg/5 mL Nebulizer solution: 0.4%/2.5-mL ampule, 0.6%/2.5-mL ampule	β_2	Bronchodilator	Bronchospasm
norepinephrine (levarterenol) ●	Levophed	IV: 1 mg/mL in 4-mL ampules	α_1	Vasoconstrictor	Shock, hypotension
phenylephrine†	Neo-Synephrine	Subcut, IM, IV: 10 mg/mL in 1-mL ampules ● Ophthalmic drops: 0.12%, 2.5%, 10% Nasal solutions: 0.125%, 0.25%, 0.5%, 1% Tablets: 5, 10 mg Syrup: 2.5 mg/5 mL, 7.5 mg/5 mL	α_1	Vasoconstrictor	Shock, hypotension, nasal decongestant; ophthalmic vasoconstrictor, mydriatic
salmeterol	Serevent Diskus	Aerosol powder: 50 mcg/dose	β_2	Bronchodilator	Asthma, emphysema, chronic bronchitis
terbutaline*	Bricanyl ♣	Tablets: 2.5, 5 mg Subcut: 1 mg/mL in 1-mL ampules	β_2	Bronchodilator, uterine relaxant	Emphysema, asthma

α, alpha; β, beta; *IM*, intramuscular; *IV*, intravenous; *Subcut*, subcutaneous.
♣ Available in Canada.   ● High-alert medication.
*See also Bronchodilators (Chapter 30).
†See also Decongestants (Chapter 29).

amitriptyline, imipramine), atropine, and halothane anesthesia may increase both therapeutic and toxic effects. Many over-the-counter medications (e.g., cold remedies, appetite suppressants/diet pills [e.g., pseudoephedrine, ephedrine, ma huang]) contain adrenergic medicines that can have an additive effect when they are taken with a prescribed adrenergic agent. Monitor patients for tachycardia, serious dysrhythmias, hypotension, hypertension, and chest pain.

Agents That Inhibit Therapeutic Activity. The concurrent use of beta-adrenergic blocking agents (e.g., propranolol, nadolol, timolol, pindolol, atenolol, metoprolol), alpha-adrenergic blocking agents (e.g., phenoxybenzamine, phentolamine), and reserpine with adrenergic agents is not recommended.

DRUG CLASS: ALPHA- AND BETA-ADRENERGIC BLOCKING AGENTS

ACTIONS

The alpha- and beta-adrenergic blocking agents act by plugging the alpha or beta receptors, which prevents other agents—usually the naturally occurring catecholamines—from stimulating the specific receptors.

The beta blockers can be subdivided into nonselective and selective beta antagonists. The nonselective blocking agents have an equal affinity for beta-1 and beta-2 receptors, and they inhibit both. These agents are propranolol, nadolol, pindolol, penbutolol, carteolol, sotalol, and timolol. The selective beta-1 blocking agents exhibit action against the heart's beta-1 receptors (cardioselective) and do not readily affect the beta-2 receptors of the bronchi. The selective beta-1 antagonists are esmolol, metoprolol, acebutolol, betaxolol, bisoprolol, and atenolol. This selective action is beneficial for patients in whom nonselective beta blockers may induce bronchospasm (e.g., those with asthma). However, it is important to note that the selectivity of these agents is only relative. In larger doses, these agents will also inhibit the beta-2 receptors. There are no selective beta-2 blockers available. Labetalol and carvedilol exhibit selective alpha-1 and nonselective beta-adrenergic blocking activity. The alpha and beta blockers are listed in Figure 12-1.

USES

Because one of the primary actions of the alpha-receptor stimulants is vasoconstriction, it would be expected that alpha-blocking agents are indicated for patients with diseases that are associated with vasoconstriction. Alpha blockers (e.g., prazosin, terazosin, doxazosin) are sometimes used to treat hypertension (see Chapter 22). Alfuzosin, doxazosin, and tamsulosin are used to relax the smooth muscle of the bladder and prostate; they are used to treat urinary obstruction caused by benign prostatic hyperplasia (see Chapter 40).

Beta-adrenergic blocking agents (e.g., beta blockers) are used extensively to treat hypertension, post–myocardial infarction, angina pectoris, cardiac dysrhythmias, symptoms of hyperthyroidism, and stage fright. Nonselective beta blockers must be used with extreme caution in patients with respiratory conditions such as bronchitis, emphysema, asthma, or allergic rhinitis. A beta blockade produces severe bronchoconstriction and may aggravate wheezing, especially during pollen season.

Beta blockers should be used with caution in patients with diabetes and in those who are susceptible to hypoglycemia. Beta blockers further induce the hypoglycemic effects of insulin and reduce the release of insulin in response to hyperglycemia. All beta blockers mask most of the signs and symptoms of acute hypoglycemia.

Beta-adrenergic blocking agents should be used only in patients with controlled heart failure. Further hypotension, bradycardia, or heart failure may develop.

❖ NURSING IMPLICATIONS FOR BETA-ADRENERGIC BLOCKING AGENTS

See also the nursing implications for patients with antidysrhythmic therapy (Chapter 23, pp. 365-367) and for those with hypertension (Chapter 22, pp. 342-344).

■ Premedication Assessment

1. Obtain baseline vital signs: heart rate and blood pressure.
2. See also the premedication assessments for patients with antidysrhythmic therapy (Chapter 23) and for those with hypertension (Chapter 22).

■ Availability, Dosage, and Administration

See Table 12-3.

Individualization of Dosage. Although the onset of activity is fairly rapid, it may take several days to weeks for a patient to show optimal improvement and to become stabilized on an adequate maintenance dosage. Patients must be periodically reevaluated to determine the lowest effective dosage that is necessary to control the disorder.

Sudden Discontinuation. Patients must be counseled against poor adherence or the sudden discontinuation of therapy without a healthcare provider's advice. Sudden discontinuation has resulted in an exacerbation of anginal symptoms, and this has been followed in some cases by myocardial infarction. When discontinuing chronically administered beta blockers, the dosage should be gradually reduced over 1 to 2 weeks, with careful patient monitoring. If anginal symptoms develop or become more frequent, beta blocker therapy should be restarted temporarily.

■ Common Adverse Effects

Most of the adverse effects associated with beta-adrenergic blocking agents are dose related. Response

Table 12-3 Beta-Adrenergic Blocking Agents

GENERIC NAME	BRAND NAME	AVAILABILITY	CLINICAL USES	DOSAGE RANGE
acebutolol	Sectral, Apo-acebutolol ✦	Capsules: 200, 400 mg	Hypertension, ventricular dysrhythmias	PO: initial, 400 mg daily; maintenance, 600-1200 mg daily
atenolol	Tenormin, Apo-Atenol ✦	Tablets: 25, 50, 100 mg	Hypertension, angina pectoris, after myocardial infarction	PO: initial, 50 mg daily; maintenance, ≤200 mg daily
betaxolol	Kerlone	Tablets: 10, 20 mg	Hypertension	PO: initial, 10 mg daily; maintenance, 20 mg daily
bisoprolol	Zebeta, PMS-Bisoprolol ✦	Tablets: 5, 10 mg	Hypertension	PO: initial, 5 mg daily; maintenance, 10-20 mg daily
carvedilol	Coreg, Coreg CR, Apo-Carvedilol ✦	Tablets: 3.125, 6.25, 12.5, 25 mg Capsules, extended release: 10, 20, 40, 80 mg	Hypertension, heart failure, myocardial infarction	PO: initial, 6.25 mg twice daily; maintenance, ≤50 mg daily
esmolol ❶	Brevibloc	Injection: 10 mg/mL in 10-mL ampules; 20 mg/mL in 100-mL bag	Supraventricular tachycardia, hypertension	IV: initial, 500 mcg/kg/min for 1 min followed by 50 mcg/kg/min for 4 min and then adjusted to patient's needs
labetalol ❶	Trandate	Tablets: 100, 200, 300 mg Injection: 5 mg/mL in 4-, 20-, 40-mL vials	Hypertension	PO: initial, 100 mg twice daily; maintenance, ≤2400 mg daily
metoprolol ❶	Lopressor, Toprol XL, Betaloc ✦	Tablets: 25, 50, 100 mg Tablets, extended release: 25, 50, 100, 200 mg Injection: 1 mg/mL in 5-mL ampules	Hypertension, myocardial infarction, angina pectoris, heart failure	PO, extended release: initial, 50 mg daily; maintenance, 100-450 mg daily PO, not extended release: 50 mg twice daily
nadolol	Corgard, Apo-Nadol ✦	Tablets: 20, 40, 80 mg	Angina pectoris, hypertension	PO: initial, 40 mg daily; maintenance, 40-80 mg daily; maximum, 320 mg daily for hypertension; maximum, 240 mg for angina.
nebivolol	Bystolic	Tablets: 2.5, 5, 10, 20 mg	Hypertension	PO: initial, 5 mg daily; maintenance, ≤40 mg daily
penbutolol	Levatol	Tablets: 20 mg	Hypertension	PO: initial, 20 mg daily; maintenance, 20-40 mg daily Maximum: 80 mg daily
pindolol	Apo-Pindol ✦	Tablets: 5, 10 mg	Hypertension	PO: initial, 5 mg twice daily; maintenance, 10-30 mg daily; maximum, 60 mg daily
propranolol ❶	Inderal, Inderal LA, Teva-propranolol ✦	Tablets: 10, 20, 40, 60, 80 mg Solution: 20, 40 mg/5 mL Capsules, sustained release: 60, 80, 120, 160 mg IV: 1 mg/mL in 1-mL ampules	Dysrhythmias, hypertension, angina pectoris, myocardial infarction, migraine, tremor, hypertrophic subaortic stenosis	PO, immediate release: initial, 40 mg twice daily; maintenance, 120-640 mg daily in two to four divided doses PO, sustained release: 80-160 mg daily; maximum 640 mg daily IV: 1-3 mg with close electrocardiographic monitoring
sotalol	Betapace, Sorine, Riva-Sotalol ✦	Tablets: 80, 120, 160, 240 mg	Dysrhythmias	PO: initial, 80 mg twice daily; maintenance, ≤320 mg daily
timolol	Mylan-Timolol ✦	Tablets: 5, 10, 20 mg	Hypertension, myocardial infarction, migraine	PO: initial, 10 mg twice daily; maintenance, ≤30 mg twice daily

IV, intravenous; PO, by mouth.
✦ Available in Canada. ❶ High-alert medication.

by individual patients is highly variable. Many of these adverse effects may occur, but they may be transient. Strongly encourage patients to see their healthcare providers before discontinuing therapy. Minor dosage adjustment may be all that is required to eliminate most adverse effects.

Endocrine

Patients with diabetes. Monitor for symptoms of hypoglycemia, including headache, weakness, decreased coordination, general apprehension, diaphoresis, hunger, or blurred or double vision. Many of these symptoms may be masked by beta-adrenergic blocking agents. Notify the healthcare provider if any of the symptoms described appear intermittently.

■ **Serious Adverse Effects**

Cardiovascular

Bradycardia, peripheral vasoconstriction (e.g., purple, mottled skin). Discontinue further doses until the patient is evaluated by a healthcare provider.

Heart failure. Monitor patients for an increase in edema, dyspnea, crackles, bradycardia, and orthopnea. Notify the healthcare provider if these symptoms develop.

Respiratory

Bronchospasm, wheezing. Withhold additional doses until the patient has been evaluated by a healthcare provider.

■ **Drug Interactions**

Antihypertensive Agents. All beta-blocking agents have hypotensive properties that are additive with antihypertensive agents (e.g., angiotensin-converting enzyme inhibitors, calcium channel blockers, diuretics, angiotensin-receptor blockers, methyldopa, hydralazine, clonidine, reserpine). If it is decided to discontinue therapy in patients who are receiving beta blockers and clonidine concurrently, the beta blocker should be withdrawn gradually and discontinued several days before gradually withdrawing the clonidine.

Beta-Adrenergic Agents. Depending on the dosage, the beta stimulants (e.g., isoproterenol, metaproterenol, terbutaline, albuterol) may inhibit the action of beta-blocking agents and vice versa.

Lidocaine, Phenytoin, Disopyramide, Digoxin. When these drugs are occasionally used concurrently, the patient must be monitored carefully for additional arrhythmias, bradycardia, and signs of heart failure.

Enzyme-Inducing Agents. Enzyme-inducing agents (e.g., cimetidine, phenobarbital, pentobarbital, rifampin, phenytoin) enhance the metabolism of propranolol, metoprolol, pindolol, and timolol. This reaction probably does not occur with nadolol or atenolol because they are not metabolized, but rather are excreted unchanged. The dosage of the beta blocker may have to be increased to provide therapeutic activity. If the enzyme-inducing agent is discontinued,

the dosage of the beta blocker will also require reduction.

Nonsteroidal Anti-Inflammatory Agents. Indomethacin, salicylates, and possibly other prostaglandin inhibitors reduce the antihypertensive activity of propranolol and pindolol. This results in a loss of hypertensive control. The dose of the beta blocker may have to be increased to compensate for the antihypertensive inhibitory effect of indomethacin and perhaps other prostaglandin inhibitors.

DRUG CLASS: CHOLINERGIC AGENTS

ACTIONS

Cholinergic agents, which are also known as *parasympathomimetic agents,* produce effects that are similar to those of acetylcholine. Some cholinergic agents act by directly stimulating the parasympathetic nervous system, whereas others inhibit acetylcholinesterase, which is the enzyme that metabolizes acetylcholine after it has been released by the nerve ending. These latter agents are known as *indirect-acting cholinergic agents.* Some of the cholinergic actions are slow heartbeat; increased GI motility and secretions; increased contractions of the urinary bladder, with relaxation of the muscle sphincter; increased secretions and contractility of the bronchial smooth muscle; sweating; miosis (constriction) of the pupil, which reduces intraocular pressure; increased force of the contraction of skeletal muscle; and, sometimes, decreased blood pressure.

USES

See Table 12-4.

❖ **NURSING IMPLICATIONS FOR CHOLINERGIC AGENTS**

See also the nursing implications for patients with disorders of the eyes (Chapter 42), glaucoma (Chapter 42), urinary system disease (Chapter 41), and respiratory tract disease (Chapters 29 and 30).

■ **Premedication Assessment**

1. Obtain baseline vital signs: heart rate and blood pressure.
2. See also the premedication assessments for patients with disorders of the eyes (Chapter 42), glaucoma (Chapter 42), urinary system disease (Chapter 41), and respiratory tract disease (Chapters 29 and 30).

■ **Dosage and Administration**

See Table 12-4.

■ **Common Adverse Effects**

Because cholinergic fibers innervate the entire body, effects in most body systems can be expected. Fortunately, because all receptors do not respond to the same dosage, adverse effects are not always seen. The

Table 12-4   Cholinergic Agents

GENERIC NAME	BRAND NAME	AVAILABILITY	CLINICAL USES
bethanechol	Urecholine; Duvoid ❖	Tablets: 5, 10, 25, 50 mg	Urinary retention
edrophonium	Enlon	Injection: 10 mg/mL in 15-mL vial	Diagnosis of myasthenia gravis; reverse nondepolarizing muscle relaxants (e.g., tubocurarine)
guanidine	Guanidine	Tablets: 125 mg	Treatment of myasthenia gravis
neostigmine	Prostigmin	Tablets: 15 mg Injection: 0.5, 1 mg/mL	Treatment of myasthenia gravis; reverse nondepolarizing muscle relaxants (e.g., tubocurarine)
physostigmine	—	Injection: 1 mg/mL in 2-mL ampules	Reverse toxicity of overdoses of anticholinergic agents (e.g., pesticides, insecticides)
pilocarpine	Isopto Carpine, Pilopine HS ❖	Tablets: 5, 7.5 mg Ophthalmic solution: 1, 2, 4%	Treat symptoms of dry mouth due to salivary gland hypofunction due to radiation therapy Glaucoma
pyridostigmine	Mestinon; Mestinon-SR ❖	Tablets: 60 mg Syrup: 60 mg/5 mL Tablets, sustained release: 180 mg	Treatment of myasthenia gravis

❖ Available in Canada.

higher the dosage, however, the greater the likelihood of adverse effects.

Gastrointestinal

Nausea, vomiting, diarrhea, abdominal cramping. These symptoms are extensions of the pharmacologic effects of the medication, and they are dose related. Reducing the dosage may be effective for controlling adverse effects without eliminating the desired pharmacologic effect.

Cardiovascular

Dizziness, hypotension. Monitor the patient's blood pressure and pulse. To minimize hypotensive episodes, instruct the patient to rise slowly from a supine or sitting position, and have him or her perform exercises to prevent blood from pooling while he or she is standing or sitting in one position for a prolonged period. Teach the patient to sit or lie down if he or she feels faint.

- **Serious Adverse Effects**

Respiratory

Bronchospasm, wheezing. Withhold the next dose until the patient is evaluated by a healthcare provider.

Cardiovascular

Bradycardia. Withhold the next dose until the patient is evaluated by a healthcare provider.

- **Drug Interactions**

Atropine, Antihistamines. Atropine, other anticholinergic agents, and most antihistamines antagonize the effects of cholinergic agents.

DRUG CLASS: ANTICHOLINERGIC AGENTS

ACTIONS

Anticholinergic agents, which are also known as *cholinergic blocking agents* or *parasympatholytic agents*, block the action of acetylcholine in the parasympathetic nervous system. These drugs act by occupying receptor sites at parasympathetic nerve endings, which prevent the action of acetylcholine. The parasympathetic response is reduced, depending on the amount of anticholinergic drug that is blocking the receptors. The inhibition of cholinergic activity (e.g., anticholinergic effects) includes the following: mydriasis (dilation) of the pupil with increased intraocular pressure in patients with glaucoma; dry, tenacious secretions of the mouth, nose, throat, and bronchi; decreased secretions and motility of the GI tract; increased heart rate; and decreased sweating.

USES

See Table 12-5.

❖ NURSING IMPLICATIONS FOR ANTICHOLINERGIC AGENTS

See also the nursing implications for patients with Parkinson's disease (Chapter 14), disorders of the eyes (Chapter 42), and for antihistamines (Chapter 29).

- **Premedication Assessment**

1. All patients should be screened for closed-angle glaucoma because anticholinergic agents may precipitate an acute attack. Patients with open-angle

Table 12-5   Anticholinergic Agents

GENERIC NAME	BRAND NAME	AVAILABILITY	CLINICAL USES
atropine	Atropine Sulfate	Injection: 0.05, 0.1, 0.4, 0.8, 1 mg/mL	Presurgery: to reduce salivation and bronchial secretions; to minimize bradycardia during intubation; for the treatment of pylorospasm and spastic conditions of the gastrointestinal tract; for the treatment of urethral and biliary colic
dicyclomine	Bentyl, Bentylol ♣	Tablets: 20 mg Capsules: 10 mg Syrup: 10 mg/5 mL Injection: 10 mg/mL Solution: 1 mg/5 mL	Irritable bowel syndrome; infant colic
glycopyrrolate	Robinul	Tablets: 1, 2 mg Injection: 0.2 mg/mL	Peptic ulcer disease; presurgery: to reduce salivation and bronchial secretions and to minimize bradycardia during intubation
mepenzolate	Cantil	Tablets: 25 mg	An aid in treatment of peptic ulcer disease
propantheline	—	Tablets: 15 mg	An aid in treatment of peptic ulcer disease

♣ Available in Canada.

glaucoma can safely use anticholinergic agents in conjunction with miotic therapy.

2. Check for the patient's history for an enlarged prostate. If this condition is present, anticholinergic agents may cause the patient to have the temporary inability to void.

3. Obtain baseline vital signs: heart rate and blood pressure. See also the premedication assessments for patients with Parkinson's disease (Chapter 14), disorders of the eyes (Chapter 42), and antihistamines (Chapter 29).

▪ Availability
See Table 12-5.

▪ Common Adverse Effects
Because cholinergic fibers enervate the entire body, effects from blocking this system occur throughout most systems. Fortunately, because all receptors do not respond to the same dose, all adverse effects are not seen to the same degree with all cholinergic blocking agents. The higher the dosage, however, the greater the likelihood of more adverse effects. The following symptoms are the anticholinergic effects that are produced by these agents. Patients who are taking these medications should be monitored for the development of these adverse effects.

Sensory

Blurred vision. Warn the patient that blurred vision may occur, and make appropriate suggestions for the patient's personal safety.

Gastrointestinal

Constipation; dryness of the mucosa of the mouth, nose, and throat. Mucosa dryness may be alleviated by sucking hard candy or ice chips or by chewing gum.

Give the patient stool softeners as prescribed. Encourage adequate fluid intake and the eating of foods that provide sufficient bulk.

Genitourinary

Urinary retention. If the patient develops urinary hesitancy, assess him or her for bladder distention. Contact the healthcare provider for further evaluation.

▪ Serious Adverse Effects
Sensory

Glaucoma. All patients should be screened for closed-angle glaucoma before the initiation of therapy. Patients with open-angle glaucoma can safely use anticholinergic agents. Monitor the patient's intraocular pressures regularly.

Psychological

Confusion, depression, nightmares, hallucinations. Perform a baseline assessment of the patient's degree of alertness and orientation to name, place, and time before initiating therapy. Make regularly scheduled subsequent evaluations of the patient's mental status, and compare findings. Report the development of alterations, and provide for patient safety during these episodes. A reduction in the daily medication dosage may control these adverse effects.

Cardiovascular

Orthostatic hypotension. Although orthostatic hypotension occurs infrequently and is generally mild, all anticholinergic agents may cause some degree of this condition, which is manifested by dizziness and weakness, particularly when therapy is initiated. Monitor the patient's blood pressure daily in both the supine and standing positions. Anticipate the development of postural hypotension, and take measures to prevent it.

Teach the patient to rise slowly from a supine or sitting position, and encourage the patient to sit or lie down if he or she feels faint.

Palpitations, dysrhythmias. Contact the healthcare provider for further evaluation.

■ Drug Interactions

Amantadine, Tricyclic Antidepressants, Phenothiazines. These agents may potentiate anticholinergic adverse effects. Confusion and hallucinations are characteristic of excessive anticholinergic activity.

Get Ready for the NCLEX® Examination!

Key Points

- The nervous system is one of two primary regulators of body homeostasis and defense. The CNS is composed of the brain and the spinal cord.
- The peripheral nervous system is subdivided into the afferent and efferent nerve pathways. The afferent (peripheral) nerves conduct signals from sensory receptors (e.g., vision, pressure, pain, cold, warmth, touch, smell) throughout the body to the CNS. The CNS processes these signals and controls the body's response by sending signals back through the efferent nerves of the peripheral nervous system. The efferent nervous system is subdivided into the motor nervous system, which controls skeletal muscle, and the autonomic nervous system, which regulates smooth muscle and heart muscle and which controls secretions from certain glands.
- Nerve impulses are passed between neurons and from neurons to end organs by neurotransmitters. The main neurotransmitters of the autonomic nervous system are acetylcholine and norepinephrine. Nerve endings that liberate acetylcholine are called *cholinergic fibers;* those that secrete norepinephrine are called *adrenergic fibers.*
- The CNS is composed of systems of different types of neurons that secrete separate neurotransmitters, such as acetylcholine, norepinephrine, epinephrine, dopamine, serotonin, and GABA.
- The control of neurotransmitters is a primary way to alleviate the symptoms that are associated with many diseases. As shown in Table 12-1, the administration of one type of autonomic nervous system drug can affect several organ systems, and adverse effects can be numerous. Therefore the use of these drugs requires the monitoring of more than just the symptoms for which the medicine was prescribed.

Additional Learning Resources

SG Go to your Study Guide for additional Review Questions for the NCLEX® Examination, Critical Thinking Clinical Situations, and other learning activities to help you master this chapter content.

evolve Go to your Evolve website (http://evolve .elsevier.com/Clayton) for additional online resources.

Review Questions for the NCLEX® Examination

1. The peripheral nervous system includes the following components: (*Select all that apply.*)
   1. afferent nerves.
   2. brain.
   3. efferent nerves.
   4. spinal cord.
   5. skeletal muscles.

2. The two major neurotransmitters of the autonomic nervous system are:
   1. norepinephrine and epinephrine.
   2. dopamine and serotonin.
   3. acetylcholine and norepinephrine.
   4. endorphins and enkephalins.

3. Cholinergic agents are drugs that have this effect: (*Select all that apply.*)
   1. slowing the heart rate.
   2. increasing the heart rate.
   3. dilating the pupils.
   4. constricting the pupils.
   5. increased gastric motility.

4. The two broad classes of drugs used to stimulate the adrenergic nervous system are:
   1. dopamine and norepinephrine.
   2. epinephrine and serotonin.
   3. catecholamines and noncatecholamines.
   4. dopaminergic receptors and beta blockers.

5. Adrenergic agents that stimulate the beta receptors of the autonomic nervous system have the following effects: (*Select all that apply.*)
   1. constriction of the coronary arterioles.
   2. relaxation of the urinary bladder.
   3. increased renal perfusion.
   4. increased heart rate.
   5. increased blood glucose.

6. A patient who has recently been prescribed a beta-adrenergic blocking agent presents to the emergency department with a serious adverse effect. Which adverse effect is the patient likely exhibiting?
   1. Hypertension
   2. Angina pectoris
   3. Bronchoconstriction
   4. Cardiac dysrhythmias

7. Which data in the patient's history and physical examination cause the nurse to question a preoperative medication order for atropine sulfate and morphine?
   1. Excessive oral secretions
   2. Bradycardia
   3. Increased gastric motility
   4. Prostatic enlargement

8. The anticholinergic agent atropine is used for the following conditions: (*Select all that apply.*)
   1. dilation of the pupils.
   2. constriction of the pupils.
   3. decreased oral secretions (saliva).
   4. increased GI motility.
   5. decreased sweating.

Drugs Used for Sleep

Objectives

1. Differentiate among the terms sedative and hypnotic; initial, intermittent, and terminal insomnia; transient, short-term and chronic insomnia and rebound sleep and paradoxical excitement.
2. Identify alterations found in the sleep pattern when hypnotics are discontinued.
3. Cite nursing interventions that can be implemented as an alternative to administering a sedative-hypnotic medication.
4. Compare the effects of barbiturates and benzodiazepines on the central nervous system.
5. Identify the antidote drug used for the management of benzodiazepine overdose.
6. Identify laboratory tests that should be monitored when benzodiazepines or barbiturates are administered for an extended period.

Key Terms

rapid eye movement (REM) sleep (p. 187)
insomnia (ĭn-SŎM-nē-ă) (p. 188)
hypnotic (hĭp-NŎT-ĭk) (p. 188)

sedative (SĔD-ă-tĭv) (p. 188)
rebound sleep (RĒ-bŏwnd SLĒP) (p. 188)

SLEEP AND SLEEP PATTERN DISTURBANCE

Sleep is a state of unconsciousness from which a patient can be aroused by an appropriate stimulus. It is a naturally occurring phenomenon that occupies about one third of an adult's life.

Adequate sleep that progresses through the normal stages is important to maintain body function, including psychiatric equilibrium and the strengthening of the immune system to ward off disease. A normal sleep duration of 7 to 8 hours per night is thought to be optimal for good health. Studies also show that a reduced amount of sleep is associated with overweight and obesity, as well as the development of metabolic syndrome (see Chapter 20). Obesity itself is also detrimental to healthy sleep patterns, and it can contribute to the development of sleep apnea. Other studies show a strong connection between a shortened duration of sleep and cardiovascular disease. Individuals who sleep less than 5 hours per night have a threefold increased risk of heart attacks. The National Health Interview Survey also demonstrates a close relationship between symptoms of insomnia and common adverse physical and mental health conditions, including obesity, diabetes mellitus, hypertension, heart failure, anxiety, and depression. *Healthy People 2020* has as one of its objectives the promotion of sleep health, which includes promoting optimal sleep durations and reducing the prevalence and effect of sleep disorders.

Natural sleep rhythmically progresses through phases that provide both physical and mental rest. On the basis of brain-wave activity, muscle activity, and eye movement, normal sleep can be divided into two phases: non–rapid eye movement (NREM) sleep and rapid eye movement (REM) sleep. The NREM phase can be further divided into four stages, each of which is characterized by a specific set of brain-wave activities. Stage 1 is a transition phase between wakefulness and sleep that lasts only a few minutes. Some people experience it as wakefulness, whereas others feel it as drowsiness. Approximately 2% to 5% of sleep is stage 1 sleep. Stage 2 sleep comprises about 50% of normal sleep time. People often experience a drifting or floating sensation, and if they are awakened during this stage, they will often deny being asleep, responding, "I was just resting my eyes." Stages 1 and 2 are light sleep periods from which a person is easily aroused. Stage 3 is a transition from the lighter to deeper sleep state of stage 4. Stage 4 sleep is dreamless, very restful, and associated with a 10% to 30% decrease in blood pressure, respiratory rate, and basal metabolic rate. Stage 4 sleep is also referred to as *delta sleep* on the basis of the pattern of brain waves that are observed during this stage. Stage 4 sleep comprises 10% to 15% of sleep time in young, healthy adults. Stage 4 sleep diminishes in length as people age, and many people who are more than 75 years old do not demonstrate any stage 4 sleep patterns. Older adults also take longer to cycle through the relaxation stages of NREM sleep, with an increased frequency and duration of awakenings.

During a normal night of sleep, a person will rhythmically cycle from wakefulness through stages 1, 2, 3, and 4; he or she will then go back to stage 3, then to stage 2, and then to REM sleep over the course of about 90 minutes. The early episodes of REM sleep last only a few minutes. However, as sleep progresses, the amount of REM sleep increases, with REM periods becoming longer and more intense around 5 AM. This type of sleep represents 20% to 25% of sleep time, and it is characterized by REM, dreaming, increased heart rate, irregular breathing, the secretion of stomach acids, and some muscular activity. REM sleep appears to be an important time for the subconscious mind to release anxiety and tension and reestablish a psychiatric equilibrium.

Insomnia is the most common sleep disorder known; 95% of all adults experience insomnia at least once during their lives, and up to 35% of adults will have insomnia during a given year. The term insomnia is defined as the inability to sleep. In general, insomnia is not a disease but rather a symptom of physical or mental stress. It is usually mild and lasts only a few nights. Common causes are changes in lifestyle or environment (e.g., hospitalization), pain, illness, the excess consumption of products that contain caffeine (e.g., coffee, energy drinks) or alcohol, eating large or rich meals shortly before bedtime, and stress. *Initial insomnia* is the inability to fall asleep when desired, *intermittent insomnia* is the inability to stay asleep, and *terminal insomnia* is characterized by early awakening with the inability to fall asleep again. Insomnia is also classified in accordance with its duration. A sleep disturbance that lasts only a few nights is considered to be *transient insomnia*. A sleep disturbance that lasts less than 3 weeks is referred to as *short-term insomnia*, and it is usually associated with travel across time zones, illness, or anxiety (e.g., job-related changes, financial stress, examinations, emotional relationships). *Chronic insomnia* requires at least 1 month of sleep disturbance before the individual is diagnosed with a sleep disorder. About 10% of adults and up to 20% of older people report having chronic insomnia. Women report experiencing insomnia twice as frequently as men. A higher incidence of insomnia is reported by older adults, the unemployed, those of lower socioeconomic status, and the recently separated or widowed. As many as 40% of patients with chronic insomnia also have psychiatric disorders (e.g., anxiety, depression, substance abuse). People with chronic insomnia often develop fatigue or drowsiness that interferes with daytime functioning and employment responsibilities.

SEDATIVE-HYPNOTIC THERAPY

Drugs that are used in conjunction with altered patterns of sleep are known as *sedative-hypnotic agents*. A hypnotic is a drug that produces sleep; a sedative quiets the patient and gives him or her a feeling of relaxation and rest, but this is not necessarily accompanied by sleep. A good hypnotic should provide the following actions within a short period of time: the onset of restful, natural sleep; a duration of action that allows a patient to awaken at the usual time; a natural awakening with no "hangover" effects; and no danger of habit formation. Unfortunately, the ideal hypnotic is not available; however, for short-term use, benzodiazepines and three benzodiazepine receptor agonists—zolpidem, zaleplon, and eszopiclone—are available. The most commonly used sedative-hypnotic agents increase total sleeping time, especially the time spent in stage 2 sleep (i.e., light sleep); however, they also decrease the number of REM periods and the total time spent in REM sleep. Rapid eye movement sleep is needed to help maintain a mental balance during daytime activities. When REM sleep is decreased, there is a strong physiologic tendency to make it up. Compensatory REM sleep, or rebound sleep, seems to occur even when hypnotic agents are used for only 3 or 4 days. After the chronic administration of sedative-hypnotic agents, REM rebound may be severe and accompanied by restlessness and vivid nightmares. Depending on the frequency of hypnotic administration, normal sleep patterns may not be restored for weeks. The effects of REM rebound may enhance an individual's chronic use of and dependence on these agents to avoid the unpleasant consequences of rebound sleep. Because of this, a vicious cycle occurs as the normal physiologic need for sleep is not met and the body attempts to compensate.

Because sedative-hypnotic agents have many adverse effects, especially with long-term use, medications that are recognized for other primary uses are being used by healthcare providers for the treatment of insomnia. Antidepressants such as amitriptyline, trazodone, and mirtazapine are prescribed in lower dosages for their sedative effects to assist patients with getting to sleep (see Chapter 16). Anticonvulsants that are used in this way include gabapentin and topiramate (see Chapter 18). Antipsychotic agents such as quetiapine and olanzapine are prescribed for patients with psychoses who also have insomnia (see Chapter 17). However, it is important to note that no extensive studies have been completed regarding the use of these antidepressants, antipsychotics, and anticonvulsants for insomnia, so their long-term effects are unknown, and their use for treating chronic insomnia cannot be recommended.

ACTIONS

Sedatives, which are used to produce relaxation and rest, and hypnotics, which are used to produce sleep, are not always different drugs. Their effects may depend on the dosage and the condition of the patient. A small dose of a drug may act as a sedative, whereas a larger dose of the same drug may act as a hypnotic and produce sleep.

Sedative-hypnotic medications may be classified into three groups: barbiturates; benzodiazepines; and nonbarbiturate, nonbenzodiazepine sedative-hypnotic medications.

USES

The primary uses of sedative-hypnotic medications are as follows: (1) to improve sleep patterns for the temporary treatment of insomnia; and (2) to decrease the level of anxiety and increase relaxation or sleep before diagnostic or operative procedures.

❖ NURSING IMPLICATIONS FOR SEDATIVE-HYPNOTIC THERAPY

■ Assessment

Central Nervous System Function. Because sedative-hypnotic drugs depress overall central nervous system (CNS) function, identify the patient's level of alertness and orientation, as well as his or her ability to perform various motor functions.

Vital Signs. Obtain the patient's current blood pressure, pulse, and respiration rates before initiating drug therapy.

Sleep Pattern. Assess the patient's usual pattern of sleep, and obtain information about the pattern of sleep disruption (e.g., difficulty falling asleep, inability to remain asleep the entire night, awakening during the early morning hours and unable to return to a restful sleep).

Ask about the amount of sleep (i.e., number of hours) that the patient considers normal and how his or her insomnia is managed at home. Does the patient have a regular time to go to bed and wake up? If the patient is taking medications, determine the drug, dosage, and frequency of administration and whether this may be contributing to sleeplessness. (Medicines that may induce or aggravate insomnia include theophylline, caffeine, pseudoephedrine, ephedrine, nicotine, levodopa, corticosteroids, and selective serotonin reuptake inhibitor antidepressants.)

Patients with persistent insomnia should be carefully monitored for the number of naps taken during the day. Investigate the type of activities that the patient performs immediately before going to bed.

Anxiety Level. Assess the patient's exhibited degree of anxiety. Is it really a sedative-hypnotic medication that the patient needs, or does the patient just need someone to listen to him or her? Ask about the stressors that the patient has been experiencing in his or her personal and work environments.

Environmental Control. Obtain data related to possible disturbances present in the individual's sleeping environment that may interfere with sleep (e.g., room temperature, lights, noise, traffic, restlessness, a snoring partner).

Nutritional Needs. Obtain a dietary history to identify sources of caffeinated products that may act as stimulants.

Alcohol Intake. Although alcohol causes sedation, it disrupts sleep patterns and may cause early-morning awakening.

Exercise. Obtain data related to the patient's usual degree of physical activity and at what times during the day he or she is most active.

Respiratory Status. People with respiratory disorders and those who snore heavily may have low respiratory reserves and should not receive hypnotic agents because of their potential to cause respiratory depression.

■ Implementation

Vital Signs. Obtain the patient's vital signs periodically as the situation indicates.

Preoperative Medication. Give the patient preoperative medications at the specified time.

Monitoring Effects. When a medication is administered, carefully assess the patient at regular intervals for the drug's therapeutic and adverse effects.

As-Needed Medications. If giving the patient as-needed (PRN) medications, ask the patient about the effectiveness of previously administered therapy. It is sometimes necessary to repeat a medication if an order permits doing so. This is done at the nurse's discretion on the basis of the evaluation of a particular patient's needs.

■ Patient Education: Promote Good Sleep Hygiene

Bedtime. Encourage the patient to choose a standard time to go to bed to help the body establish a rhythm and routine.

Nutrition. Teach the patient appropriate nutrition information concerning the Food and Drug Administration's (FDA's) recommendations of MyPlate, adequate fluid intake, and vitamin use. Communicate the information at the educational level of the patient.

Avoid Heavy Meals During the Evening. Alcohol and caffeine consumption should be reduced or discontinued, especially within several hours of bedtime. Educate the patient about decaffeinated or herbal products that can be substituted for caffeinated foods. Help the patient to avoid products that contain caffeine, such as coffee, tea, energy drinks, soft drinks, and chocolate. Limit the total daily intake of these items, and provide the patient with warm milk and crackers as a bedtime snack. Protein foods and dairy products contain an amino acid that synthesizes serotonin, which is a neurotransmitter that has been found to increase sleep time and decrease the time required to fall asleep.

For insomnia, suggest that the patient drink warm milk about 30 minutes before going to bed.

Personal Comfort. Position the patient for maximum comfort, provide a back rub, encourage the patient to empty the bladder, and be certain that the bedding is clean and dry. Take time to meet the patient's individual needs and to calm his or her fears. Foster a trusting relationship.

Environmental Control. Tell the patient to sleep in an environment that promotes sleep, such as a quiet, darkened room free from distractions and to avoid using the bedroom for watching television, responding to e-mails, preparing work for the following day, eating, and paying bills. Provide adequate ventilation, subdued lighting, and a comfortable room temperature and control traffic in and out of the patient's room.

For safety, instruct the patient to leave a nightlight on and not smoke in bed after taking medication.

Activity and Exercise. Suggest the inclusion of exercise in the patient's daily activities so that the patient obtains sufficient exercise and is tired enough to sleep. For some individuals, plan a quiet "unwinding" time before retiring for the night. For children, assist with sleep by providing a warm bath and structure before bedtime. Try a bedtime story that is pleasant and soothing (rather than one that may cause anxiety or fear).

Stress Management

- Explore personal and work stressors that could have a bearing on the patient's insomnia. Some stressors may exist in the work environment; therefore the involvement of the occupational health nurse, along with a thorough exploration of work factors, may be appropriate. Stress produced within the dynamics of the family may require professional counseling.
- Teach the patient relaxation techniques and personal comfort measures (e.g., a warm bath) to relieve stress. Playing soft music may also promote relaxation.
- Make referrals for the mastery of biofeedback, meditation, or other techniques to reduce stress levels.
- Encourage the patient to openly express feelings about his or her stress and insomnia. The adjustment to this situation involves working through great personal fears, frustrations, hostilities, and resentments.
- Explore the coping mechanisms that the person uses in response to stress, and identify methods of channeling these toward positive realistic goals and alternatives to the use of medication.

Fostering Health Maintenance. Throughout the course of treatment, discuss medication information and how it will benefit the patient. Stress the importance of nonpharmacologic interventions and the long-term effects that compliance with the treatment regimen can provide.

Provide the patient or the patient's significant others with important information that is contained in the specific drug monographs for the medicines prescribed. Additional health teaching and nursing interventions for the common adverse effects and serious adverse effects that require contact with the healthcare provider are described in the following drug monographs (e.g., barbiturates, benzodiazepines, miscellaneous sedative-hypnotic medications).

Patient Self-Assessment. Enlist the patient's help with developing and maintaining a written record of monitoring parameters (e.g., extent and frequency of insomnia); see the Patient Self-Assessment Form for Sleeping Medication on the Evolve website. Complete the Premedication Data column for use as a baseline to track the patient's response to drug therapy. Ensure that the patient understands how to use the form, and instruct the patient to bring the completed form to follow-up visits. During these follow-up visits, focus on issues that will foster the patient's adherence with the therapeutic interventions that have been prescribed.

DRUG THERAPY FOR SLEEP DISTURBANCE

DRUG CLASS: BARBITURATES

The first barbiturate went on the market as a sedative-hypnotic product in 1903. It became so successful that chemists identified some 2500 compounds, of which more than 50 went on to be distributed commercially. Barbiturates became such a mainstay of therapy that fewer than a dozen other sedative-hypnotic agents were successfully marketed through 1960. The release of the first benzodiazepine—chlordiazepoxide—in 1961 started the decline in the use of barbiturates. However, several barbiturate compounds are still prescribed (Table 13-1).

ACTIONS

Barbiturates can reversibly depress the activity of all excitable tissues. The CNS is particularly sensitive, but the degree of CNS depression—ranging from mild sedation to deep coma and death—depends on the dose, the route of administration, the degree of tolerance from any previous use, the degree of excitability of the CNS at the time of administration, and the condition of the patient. When used for hypnosis, barbiturates suppress REM and the sleep patterns of stages 3 and 4. Because barbiturates have long half-lives, residual daytime sedation is a common adverse effect.

USES

Barbiturates are now rarely used for sedation and hypnosis, but when they are used, therapy should be limited to 2 weeks because tolerance to sedation and hypnosis develops during this time. The ultra–short-acting agent, methohexital, may be administered intravenously as a general anesthetic. Short-acting barbiturates (e.g., pentobarbital, secobarbital) are used for sedation before diagnostic procedures; intermediate-acting barbiturates (e.g., amobarbital, butalbital) are used as sedative-hypnotic agents; and the long-acting

Table 13-1 Barbiturates

GENERIC NAME	BRAND NAME	AVAILABILITY	ADULT ORAL DOSAGE RANGE	COMMENTS
amobarbital ❶	Amytal	Injection: 500-mg vials	Sedation: 30-50 mg IM two or three times daily Insomnia: 65-200 mg IM 30 min before bedtime; maximum 500 mg	Intermediate acting; schedule II; used primarily as a sedative before anesthesia or during labor
butabarbital	Butisol	Tablets: 30, 50 mg Elixir: 30 mg/5 mL	Sedation: 15-30 mg three or four times daily Hypnosis: 50-100 mg at bedtime	Intermediate acting; schedule III; elixir contains 7.5% alcohol; used primarily as a daytime sedative and a bedtime hypnotic
pentobarbital ❶	Nembutal	Injection: 50 mg/mL	Insomnia: 150-200 mg IM at bedtime Sedation: 2-6 mg/kg IV (maximum 100 mg)	Short acting; schedule II; used primarily as a preanesthetic sedative for pediatric patients
phenobarbital ❶	Luminal, Solfoton	Tablets: 15, 16, 16.2, 30, 32.4, 60, 97.2, 100 mg Elixir: 20 mg/5 mL Injection: 65, 130 mg/mL	Sedation: 30-120 mg daily in 2-3 divided doses Hypnosis: 100-200 mg Anticonvulsant: 1-3 mg/kg/day in 1-2 divided doses	Long acting; schedule IV; currently used most commonly as an anticonvulsant; may also be used as a daytime sedative, preanesthetic, or hypnotic agent; also available for use IM and IV; elixir contains 13.5% alcohol
secobarbital	Seconal	Capsules: 100 mg	Hypnosis: 100 mg at bedtime	Short acting; schedule II; used primarily as a daytime sedative or a bedtime hypnotic; therapy not recommended for more than 14 days

❶ High-alert medication.

barbiturate phenobarbital is used primarily as an anticonvulsant drug.

❖ NURSING IMPLICATIONS OF BARBITURATE THERAPY

▪ Premedication Assessment
1. Seek information from the patient regarding any prior use of sedative-hypnotic medications.
2. Obtain information related to the patient's baseline neurologic function (e.g., degree of alertness).
3. Obtain the vital signs (e.g., blood pressure, pulse, respirations, pain rating using a scale of 0 to 10).

▪ Availability, Dosage, and Administration
See Table 13-1. Rapidly discontinuing barbiturates after the long-term use of high dosages may result in symptoms that are similar to those of alcohol withdrawal. These may vary from weakness and anxiety to delirium and grand mal seizures. Discontinuation of barbiturates consists of cautious and gradual withdrawal over 2 to 4 weeks.

▪ Common Adverse Effects
General adverse effects of barbiturates include drowsiness, lethargy, headache, muscle or joint pain, and mental depression.

Neurologic

Hangover, sedation, lethargy, diminished alertness. Patients may complain of "morning hangover," blurred vision, and transient hypotension on arising. The hangover feeling commonly occurs after the administration of hypnotic doses of long-acting barbiturates. Patients may display a dulled affect, a subtle distortion of mood, and impaired coordination. Explain to the patient the need to first rise to a sitting position, stay sitting for several moments until any dizziness or lightheadedness passes, and then standing slowly. Assistance with ambulation may be required. If the hangover effect becomes troublesome, there should be a reduction in the dosage, a change in the medication, or both. People who work around machinery, drive a car, pour and give medicines, or perform other duties for which they must remain mentally alert should not take these medications while working.

■ Serious Adverse Effects

Psychological

Excessive use or abuse. The habitual use of barbiturates may result in physical dependence. Discuss the issue with the healthcare provider, and make plans to cooperatively approach the gradual withdrawal of the medications being abused. Help the patient to recognize the abuse problem. Identify the patient's underlying needs, and plan for the more appropriate management of those needs. Provide for the emotional support of the individual; display an accepting attitude and be kind but firm.

Paradoxical response. Older patients and those who are in severe pain may respond paradoxically to barbiturates by demonstrating excitement, euphoria, restlessness, and confusion. Provide supportive physical care and safety during these responses. Assess the level of the patient's excitement, and deal calmly with the individual. During periods of excitement, protect the patient from harm and provide for the physical channeling of energy (e.g., walking). Seek a change in the patient's medication order.

Hypersensitivity. Reactions to barbiturates are infrequent, but they may be serious. Report symptoms of hives, pruritus, rash, high fever, or the inflammation of the mucous membranes for evaluation by a healthcare provider. Withhold further barbiturate administration until the healthcare provider's approval has been granted.

Blood dyscrasias. Blood dyscrasias are rare; however, laboratory studies (e.g., red and white blood cell counts, differential counts, platelets) should be scheduled when symptoms warrant. Stress the importance of the patient returning for this laboratory work. Monitor the patient for the development of sore throat, fever, purpura, jaundice, or excessive and progressive weakness.

■ Drug Interactions

Antihistamines, Alcohol, Analgesics, Anesthetics, Tranquilizers, Valproic Acid, Monoamine Oxidase Inhibitors, and Other Sedative-Hypnotics. These agents increase the toxic effects of barbiturates. Monitor the patient for excessive sedation, and reduce the dosage of the barbiturate, if necessary.

Phenytoin. The effects of barbiturates on phenytoin are variable. Serum levels may be ordered, and a change in phenytoin dosage may be required. Observe patients for increased seizure activity and for signs of phenytoin toxicity (e.g., nystagmus, sedation, lethargy).

Reduced Effects. Barbiturates reduce the effects of the following medicines:

- *Warfarin:* Monitor the patient's prothrombin time, and increase the dosage of warfarin, if necessary.

- *Estrogens:* This drug interaction may be critical in patients who are receiving oral contraceptives that contain estrogen. If patients develop spotting and breakthrough bleeding, a change in oral contraceptives and the use of alternative forms of contraception should be considered.

- *Corticosteroids, beta-adrenergic blockers, metronidazole, doxycycline, antidepressants, quinidine, and chlorpromazine:* The patient should be monitored for signs of increased activity of the illness for which the medication was prescribed. Dosage increases may be necessary, or the barbiturate may have to be discontinued.

DRUG CLASS: BENZODIAZEPINES

Benzodiazepines have been extremely successful products from both the therapeutic and safety standpoints. A major advantage of these drugs compared with the barbiturate and other nonbarbiturate sedative-hypnotic agents is the wide safety margin between therapeutic and lethal doses. Intentional and unintentional overdoses well above the normal therapeutic doses are well tolerated and not fatal.

More than 2000 benzodiazepine derivatives have been identified, and more than 100 have been tested for sedative-hypnotic or other therapeutic activity. Although there are many similarities among the benzodiazepines, they are difficult to characterize as a class. Some benzodiazepines are effective anticonvulsants, others serve as antianxiety and muscle-relaxant agents, and others are used as sedative-hypnotic drugs.

ACTIONS

Benzodiazepines exert their effects through stimulation of the gamma-aminobutyric acid (GABA)-benzodiazepine receptor complex. GABA is an inhibitory neurotransmitter that exerts its effects at specific receptor subtypes designated GABA-A and GABA-B. GABA-A is the primary receptor subtype in the CNS. Specific benzodiazepine (BZD) receptor subtypes are thought to be coupled to GABA-A receptors. The BZD_1 receptors are located in the cerebellum and cerebral cortex, the BZD_2 receptors are located in the cerebral cortex and spinal cord, and the BZD_3 receptors in the peripheral tissues. Activation of the BZD_1 receptors is thought to mediate sleep, and the BZD_2 receptor affects muscle relaxation, anticonvulsant activity (see Chapter 18), motor coordination, and memory.

USES

Estazolam, flurazepam, quazepam, temazepam, and triazolam are the benzodiazepines that have been marketed for hypnosis. Triazolam, which is a shorter-acting hypnotic, as well as estazolam and temazepam, which are intermediate-acting hypnotic agents, do not contain active metabolites and therefore do not accumulate as readily after several nights of dosing.

Flurazepam and quazepam have long half-lives and active metabolites, thus making patients much more susceptible to hangovers the day after use. Benzodiazepines that are used as sedative-hypnotic agents increase stage 2 sleep and decrease stages 3 and 4 sleep and, to a lesser extent, REM sleep.

When benzodiazepine therapy is started, patients experience deep and refreshing sleep. However, benzodiazepine-induced sleep varies from normal sleep in that there is less REM sleep. With the chronic administration of benzodiazepines, the amount of REM sleep gradually increases as tolerance develops to the REM-suppressant effects of the drugs. When benzodiazepines are discontinued, a rebound increase in REM sleep may occur despite the patient's tolerance. During the rebound period, the number of dreams stays about the same, but many of the dreams are reported to be bizarre. After long-term use of most benzodiazepines, there is also a rebound in insomnia. Consequently, it is important to use these agents only for short courses (i.e., usually no more than 4 weeks) of therapy.

The short-acting benzodiazepines (e.g., midazolam, lorazepam) are used parenterally as preoperative sedatives and intravenously for conscious sedation before short diagnostic procedures or for the induction of general anesthesia. Midazolam has a more rapid onset of action, produces a greater degree of amnesia, and has a much shorter duration compared with diazepam. Lorazepam is used as an antianxiety agent in general, but it is particularly useful before diagnostic procedures when a longer duration of action is required; a parenteral dosage form is available. It also has no active metabolites that may prolong sedation.

Flumazenil (Romazicon) is an antidote that is administered intravenously for the complete or partial reversal of the effects of benzodiazepines that are used as general anesthetics or during diagnostic or therapeutic procedures. Flumazenil is also used for the management of an intentional or accidental overdose of benzodiazepines.

THERAPEUTIC OUTCOMES

The primary therapeutic outcomes sought from benzodiazepine therapy are as follows:
1. To produce mild sedation
2. For short-term use, to produce sleep
3. Preoperative sedation with amnesia

❖ NURSING IMPLICATIONS FOR BENZODIAZEPINES

▪ Premedication Assessment
1. Record the patient's baseline vital signs (e.g., blood pressure, pulse, respirations); measure the patient's blood pressure in both sitting and lying positions.
2. Check for a history of blood dyscrasias or hepatic disease, and determine whether the patient is in the first trimester of pregnancy.
3. Assess the patient's level of pain.

▪ Availability, Dosage, and Administration
See Table 13-2. The habitual use of benzodiazepines may result in physical and psychological dependence. The rapid discontinuance of benzodiazepines after long-term use may result in symptoms that are similar to those of alcohol withdrawal, such as weakness, anxiety, delirium, and grand mal seizures. These symptoms may not appear for several days after discontinuation. Discontinuation of benzodiazepines consists of the gradual withdrawal over 2 to 4 weeks.

Table 13-2   Benzodiazepines Used for Sedation and Hypnosis

GENERIC NAME	BRAND NAME	AVAILABILITY	ADULT ORAL DOSAGE RANGE	COMMENTS
estazolam	—	Tablets: 1, 2 mg	Hypnosis: 1-2 mg at bedtime	Intermediate acting; schedule IV; used to treat insomnia; tapering therapy recommended to reduce rebound insomnia; minimal morning hangover
flurazepam	Flurazepam, Apo-Flurazepam ✤	Capsules: 15, 30 mg	Hypnosis: 15-30 mg at bedtime	Long acting; schedule IV; used for short-term treatment of insomnia for up to 4 wk; morning hangover may be significant; rebound insomnia and rapid eye movement sleep occur less frequently

Continued

Table 13-2 Benzodiazepines Used for Sedation and Hypnosis—cont'd

GENERIC NAME	BRAND NAME	AVAILABILITY	ADULT ORAL DOSAGE RANGE	COMMENTS
lorazepam ❶ ⇄ Do not confuse lorazepam with loperamide.	Ativan, Apo-Lorazepam ♣ ⇄ Do not confuse Ativan with Ambien or Atarax.	Tablets: 0.5, 1, 2 mg Oral solution: 2 mg/mL Injection: 2, 4 mg/mL in 1-, 10-mL vials; 2, 4 mg/mL in prefilled syringes	Hypnosis: 2-4 mg at bedtime	Used primarily to treat insomnia but may also be used for preoperative anxiety, status epilepticus; administration IM and IV also available
midazolam	—	Syrup: 2 mg/mL Injection: 1, 5 mg/mL in 1-, 2-, 5-, 10-mL vials; 2 mg/2 mL in prefilled syringes	Preoperatively: 0.07-0.08 mg/kg IM 1 hr before surgery Induction of anesthesia: 0.2-0.3 mg/kg IV Conscious sedation: 0.5-2 mg IV slowly over 2 min; repeat every 2-3 min as needed	Short acting; schedule IV; causes amnesia in most patients; lower dosages for patients more than 55 yr old Onset: IM, 15 min; IV, 3-5 min Duration: IM, 30-60 min; IV, 2-6 hr
quazepam	Doral	Tablets: 15 mg	Hypnosis: 7.5-15 mg at bedtime	Long acting; schedule IV; used to treat insomnia; tapering therapy recommended to reduce rebound insomnia; morning hangover may be significant
temazepam	Restoril ⇄ Do not confuse Restoril with Remeron, Risperdal, or Vistaril. Novo-Temazepam ♣	Capsules: 7.5, 15, 22.5, 30 mg	Hypnosis: 15-30 mg at bedtime	Intermediate acting; schedule IV; used to treat insomnia; minimal if any morning hangover; rebound insomnia may occur
triazolam	Halcion ⇄ Do not confuse Halcion with Haldol. Apo-Triazo ♣	Tablets: 0.125, 0.25 mg	Hypnosis: 0.125-0.5 mg at bedtime	Short acting; schedule IV; used to treat insomnia but tends to lose effectiveness within 2 wk; tapering therapy recommended to reduce rebound insomnia; rapid onset of action; no morning hangover

♣ Available in Canada; ⇄ do not confuse; ❶ high-alert medication.

5. The nurse was discussing the difference between temazepam (Restoril) and zolpidem (Ambien) with a patient requesting drug therapy for sleep disturbance. Which of the following statements are appropriate? (*Select all that apply.*)
   1. "When you take Restoril, it can cause rebound insomnia if you abruptly stop taking it without tapering the drug."
   2. "There is no difference between these drugs; you can take them without any worries."
   3. "Ambien is also available in a sublingual tablet form, which disintegrates in seconds."
   4. "The side effect of morning drowsiness is only caused by Restoril, not Ambien."
   5. "Ambien is used for short-term treatment of insomnia."

6. The nurse taking care of a patient who was admitted for an overdose of lorazepam (Ativan) knows this antidote will be used:
   1. diphenhydramine (Benadryl).
   2. temazepam (Restoril).
   3. flumazenil (Romazicon).
   4. selegiline (Eldepryl).

7. The nurse is monitoring laboratory results for a patient who has been taking quazepam (Doral) for several years. The following tests need to be followed to monitor for hepatotoxicity: (*Select all that apply.*)
   1. AST.
   2. platelet count.
   3. alkaline phosphatase.
   4. WBC.
   5. ALT.

Drugs Used for Parkinson's Disease

Objectives

1. Identify the signs and symptoms of Parkinson's disease.
2. Identify the neurotransmitter that is found in excess and the neurotransmitter that is deficient in people with parkinsonism.
3. Describe the reasonable expectations of the medications that are prescribed for the treatment of Parkinson's disease.
4. Cite the action of carbidopa, levodopa, and apomorphine on the neurotransmitters involved in Parkinson's disease.
5. Explain the action of entacapone and of the monoamine oxidase inhibitors (selegiline and rasagiline) as it relates to the treatment of Parkinson's disease.
6. Describe the symptoms that can be attributed to the cholinergic activity of pharmacologic agents.
7. Cite the specific symptoms that should show improvement when anticholinergic agents are administered to the patient with Parkinson's disease.

Key Terms

Parkinson's disease (PĂR-kĭn-sĕnz dĭ-ZĒZ) (p. 200)
dopamine (DŌ-pă-mēn) (p. 200)
neurotransmitter (nyū-rō-TRĂNZ-mĭ-tĕr) (p. 200)
acetylcholine (ăs-ē-tĭl-KŌ-lēn) (p. 200)
anticholinergic agents (ĂN-tē-kō-lĭn-ŬR-jĭk) (p. 202)
tremors (TRĔ-mŭrz) (p. 203)

dyskinesia (dĭs-kĭ-NĒ-zhă) (p. 203)
propulsive, uncontrolled movement (prō-PŬL-sĭv ŭn-kŏn-TRŌLD MŬV-mĕnt) (p. 204)
akinesia (ă-kĭ-NĒ-zhă) (p. 204)
livedo reticularis (lĭ-VĒ-dō rĭ-tĭk-yĕ-LĀR-ĭs) (p. 209)

PARKINSON'S DISEASE

Parkinson's disease is a chronic, progressive disorder of the central nervous system. It is the second most common neurodegenerative disease after Alzheimer's disease. An estimated 1% of the U.S. population that is more than 50 years old, 2% of the population that is more than 60 years old, and 4% to 5% of the population 85 years old or older have this disorder. Thirty percent of patients report an onset of symptoms before the age of 50 years; 40% report that the onset occurred between the ages of 50 and 60 years; and the remainder reports that their symptoms began after the age of 60 years. The incidence is slightly higher in men than women, and all races and ethnic groups are affected. Characteristic motor symptoms include muscle tremors, slowness of movement when performing daily activities (i.e., bradykinesia), muscle weakness with rigidity, and alterations in posture and equilibrium. The symptoms associated with parkinsonism are caused by a deterioration of the dopaminergic neurons in the substantia nigra pars compacta, which results in a depletion of dopamine along the nigrostriatal pathway that extends into neurons in the autonomic ganglia, the basal ganglia, and the spinal cord and causes progressive neurologic deficits. These areas of the brain are responsible for maintaining posture and muscle tone, as well as for regulating voluntary smooth muscle activity and other nonmotor activities. Normally, a balance exists between dopamine, which is an inhibitory neurotransmitter, and acetylcholine, which is an excitatory neurotransmitter. With a deficiency of dopamine, a relative increase in acetylcholine activity occurs and causes the symptoms of parkinsonism. About 80% of the dopamine in the neurons of the substantia nigra pars compacta of the brain must be depleted for symptoms to develop.

Whereas the motor symptoms associated with parkinsonism have been considered to be the hallmarks of the disease, subtle nonmotor symptoms are now being recognized as occurring as much as 10 years before the onset of motor symptoms. Nonmotor symptoms usually start with constipation, progressing over the next few years with orthostatic hypotension, nocturnal sleep disturbances with daytime somnolence, depression, and progressing dementia. It is not known yet whether early treatment with medicines that control the symptoms of Parkinson's disease will slow the progression of the disease.

There are two types of parkinsonism. Primary or idiopathic parkinsonism is caused by a reduction in dopamine-producing cells in the substantia nigra pars compacta. The causes are not yet known, but there appear to be both genetic and environmental factors associated with its development. Approximately 10% to 15% of cases appear to be inherited. Secondary parkinsonism is caused by head trauma, intracranial infections, tumors, and recurrent exposure to drugs and pesticides. Medicines that deplete dopamine and thus cause secondary parkinsonism include dopamine antagonists such as haloperidol, phenothiazines, reserpine, methyldopa, and metoclopramide. In most cases of drug-induced parkinsonism, recovery is complete if the drug is discontinued.

 Life Span Considerations

Parkinson's Disease

Parkinson's disease, which is most often seen in geriatric patients, causes a relative excess of acetylcholine as a result of a deficiency of dopamine. Drug therapy with dopaminergic agents increases dopamine availability, whereas anticholinergic medicines may be taken to counterbalance the excess availability of acetylcholine. Approximately 40% of patients with parkinsonism have some degree of clinical depression as a result of the reduced availability of the active metabolites of dopamine in the brain.

All drugs that are prescribed for the treatment of Parkinson's disease produce a pharmacologic effect on the central nervous system. An assessment of the patient's mental status and physical functioning before the initiation of therapy is essential to serve as a baseline so that comparisons can be made with subsequent evaluations.

Parkinson's disease is, at present, both progressive and incurable. The goals of treatment are to moderate the symptoms and to slow the progression of the disease. It is important to encourage the patient to take the medications as scheduled and to stay as active and involved in daily activities as possible.

Orthostatic hypotension is common with most of the medicines that are used to treat Parkinson's disease. To provide for patient safety, teach the patient to rise slowly from a supine or sitting position, and encourage the patient to sit or lie down if he or she is feeling faint.

Constipation is a frequent problem among patients with Parkinson's disease. Instruct the patient to drink six to eight 8-ounce glasses of liquid daily and to increase bulk in the diet to prevent constipation. Bulk-forming laxatives may also need to be added to the daily regimen.

The motor symptoms of parkinsonism start insidiously and are almost imperceptible at first, with weakness and tremors gradually progressing to involve movement disorders throughout the body (Figure 14-1). The symptoms usually begin on one side of the body (i.e., asymmetric onset and progression) as a tremor of a finger or hand, and they then progress to

FIGURE 14-1 Stages of parkinsonism. **A,** Flexion of the affected arm. The patient leans toward the unaffected side. **B,** Slow, shuffling gait. **C,** The patient has increased difficulty walking and looks for sources of support to prevent falls. **D,** Further progression of weakness. The patient requires assistance from another person for ambulation. **E,** Profound disability. The patient may be confined to a wheelchair as a result of increasing weakness.

become bilateral. The upper part of the body is usually affected first. Eventually, the individual has postural and gait alterations that result in the need for assistance with total care needs. Varying degrees of depression are the most common (i.e., 40% to 50%) nonmotor symptom associated with Parkinson's disease. Most patients with depression also develop feelings of anxiety, and this sometimes includes panic attacks. Those who develop anxiety before depression are very susceptible to depressive episodes after the anxiety. Apathy or depressed emotions with a lack of willpower or the inability to make decisions often accompany depression. Chronic fatigue, which is another common symptom, may also contribute to depression. Dementia, which resembles Alzheimer's disease, occurs in a significant number of patients, but there is continuing debate as to whether it is part of the Parkinson's disease process or if it is caused by concurrent drug therapy, Alzheimer's disease, or other factors. Dementia is characterized by the slowing of the thought processes, lapses in memory, and a loss of impulse control. The diagnosis of Parkinson's disease is based on a careful history taking, a physical examination, and a positive response to dopaminergic treatment. There are no laboratory tests or imaging studies that can confirm the diagnosis.

The patient and the family should understand that Parkinson's disease often has a course that takes place over decades, that the rate of progression varies greatly from one person to another, and that many approaches are available to reduce symptoms. Patients should be counseled about exercise, including stretching, strengthening, cardiovascular fitness, and balance training. Patients and their families often need assistance to learn about the medical regimen that is used to control the disease's symptoms and about how to maintain the patient at an optimal level of participation in activities of daily living (ADLs). Drug therapy presents the potential for many adverse effects that all involved parties must understand.

Nurses can have a major influence in the positive use of coping mechanisms as the patient and family express varying degrees of anxiety, frustration, hostility, conflict, and fear. The primary goal of nursing intervention should be to keep the patient socially interactive and participating in daily activities. This can be accomplished through physical therapy, adherence to the drug regimen, and management of the course of treatment.

DRUG THERAPY FOR PARKINSON'S DISEASE

ACTIONS

The goal of the treatment of parkinsonism is minimizing the symptoms because there is no cure for the disease. Nonpharmacologic therapy focuses on education, support services, exercise, and nutrition. Pharmacologic goals are to relieve symptoms and to restore dopaminergic activity and neurotransmitter function to as close to normal as possible. Treatment is usually started when symptoms progress to the point that they interfere with the patient's ability to perform at work or to function in social situations or impair quality of life. The goal is to improve motor and nonmotor symptoms to optimize quality of life. Drug therapy includes the use of the following: monoamine oxidase inhibitor-type B agents (rasagiline, selegiline), possibly to slow the deterioration of dopaminergic nerve cells; dopamine agonists (carbidopa-levodopa, ropinirole, pramipexole, amantadine [dopamine reuptake inhibitor that increases dopamine release and may have anticholinergic properties]); apomorphine, or entacapone (reduces metabolism of dopamine) in various combinations to enhance dopaminergic activity; and anticholinergic agents to inhibit the relative excess of

cholinergic activity (e.g., tremor). Therapy must be individualized, and realistic goals must be set for each patient. It is not possible to eliminate all symptoms of the disease because the medications' adverse effects would not be tolerated. The trend is to use the lowest possible dose of medication so that, as the disease progresses, dosages can be increased and other medicines added to obtain a combined effect. Unfortunately, as the disease progresses, drug therapy becomes more complex in terms of the number of medicines, dosage adjustments, the frequency of dosage administration, and the frequency of adverse effects. Therapies often have to be discontinued because of the impact of adverse effects on the quality of life. Other drug therapy may also be necessary for the treatment of the nonmotor symptoms of Parkinson's disease.

USES

Rasagiline or selegiline may be used to slow the course of Parkinson's disease by possibly slowing the progression of the deterioration of dopaminergic nerve cells. A dopamine receptor agonist—often carbidopa-levodopa—is initiated when the patient develops functional impairment. Carbidopa-levodopa continues to be the most effective drug for the relief of symptoms; however, after 3 to 5 years, the drug's effect gradually wears off and the patient suffers from "on-off" fluctuations in levodopa activity. A catechol-*O*-methyltransferase (COMT) inhibitor (entacapone) may be added to carbidopa-levodopa therapy to prolong the activity of the dopamine by slowing its rate of metabolism. Apomorphine may also be administered to treat off periods. **Anticholinergic agents** provide symptomatic relief from excessive acetylcholine. These agents are often used in combination to promote optimal levels of motor function (e.g., to improve gait, posture, or speech) and to decrease disease symptoms (e.g., tremors, rigidity, drooling). See Figure 14-2 for an algorithm for the treatment for Parkinson's disease.

❖ NURSING IMPLICATIONS FOR PARKINSON'S DISEASE THERAPY

▪ Assessment

Unified Parkinson's Disease Rating Scale. The Unified Parkinson's Disease Rating Scale (UPDRS) is often used to identify the baseline of Parkinson's disease symptoms at the time of diagnosis and to monitor changes in symptoms that may require medicine dosage adjustment. The UPDRS evaluates the following: (1) mentation, behavior, and mood; (2) self-evaluation of ADLs; (3) motor examination; (4) complications of therapy; (5) modified Hoehn and Yahr staging; and (6) the Schwab and England ADL scale.

History of Parkinsonism. Obtain a history of the patient's exposure to known conditions associated with the development of parkinsonian symptoms, such as head trauma, encephalitis, tumors, and drug exposure (e.g., phenothiazines, reserpine, methyldopa,

If a patient discontinues therapy for longer than 1 week and then wishes to go back to the use of apomorphine, therapy should be reinitiated at the starting dose of 0.2 mL, with gradual increases in dosage to optimal therapy.

Use of an Antiemetic. One of the pharmacologic actions of apomorphine is emesis. The antiemetic trimethobenzamide (Tigan) should be administered orally at a dosage of 300 mg three times daily for at least 3 days before the initial dose of apomorphine. It should be continued for at least the first 2 months of therapy. About 50% of patients are able to discontinue the antiemetic while continuing therapy with apomorphine. Do not use prochlorperazine (Compazine) or ondansetron (Zofran) as antiemetics (see "Drug Interactions" for apomorphine below).

■ **Common Adverse Effects**
Most adverse effects observed with apomorphine agents are direct extensions of their pharmacologic properties.
Gastrointestinal
Nausea, vomiting. These effects can be reduced by premedicating the patient with trimethobenzamide and then slowly increasing the dosage.
Cardiovascular
Orthostatic hypotension. Apomorphine commonly causes orthostatic hypotension, which is manifested by dizziness and weakness, particularly when therapy is initiated. Patients with Parkinson's disease are at risk for falling because of the underlying postural instability associated with the disease; apomorphine may increase the risk of falling by lowering blood pressure and altering mobility. Anticipate the development of postural hypotension, and provide assistance when necessary. Monitor the patient's blood pressure before and during apomorphine therapy in both the supine and standing positions. Teach patients to rise slowly from a supine or sitting position; encourage them to sit or lie down if feeling faint.

■ **Serious Adverse Effects**
Neurologic
Chewing motions, bobbing, facial grimacing, rocking movements. These involuntary movements (dyskinesias) occur in some patients, especially if they are also taking levodopa. A reduction in the dosage of the levodopa or apomorphine may be beneficial.
Sudden sleep events. Sleep episodes have been reported with the dopamine agonists (e.g., apomorphine, pergolide, pramipexole, ropinirole). These episodes are described as sleep attacks or sleep episodes that include daytime sleep. Some sleep events have been reported as sudden and irresistible; other sleep events have been preceded by sufficient warning to prevent accidents. Patients who are taking dopamine agonists should be informed about the possibility of daytime sleepiness and outright sleep attacks with

these medicines and allowed to make their own decisions about driving on the basis of their past experiences with the medicines. The assessment of patients who are at risk for sleep attacks is possible with the Epworth Sleepiness Scale.
Psychological
Nightmares, depression, confusion, hallucinations. Perform a baseline assessment of the patient's degree of alertness and orientation to name, place, and time before initiating therapy. Make regularly scheduled subsequent evaluations of mental status, and compare findings. Report alterations in mood. Provide for patient safety during these episodes. Reducing the daily medication dosage may control these adverse effects.
Cardiovascular
Tachycardia, palpitations. Take the patient's pulse at regularly scheduled intervals. Report any changes for further evaluation.
Genitourinary
Penile erection, priapism. Apomorphine may cause penile erection and, rarely, priapism (i.e., prolonged, painful erection). Apomorphine has been overused because of its ability to induce erection and increase libido. Indications of abuse include frequent erections, atypical sexual behavior, heightened libido, dyskinesias, agitation, confusion, and depression.

■ **Drug Interactions**
Serotonin Antagonists (Ondansetron, Dolasetron, Granisetron, Palonosetron, Alosetron). The use of serotonin antagonists with apomorphine is contraindicated. Profound hypotension and loss of consciousness have been reported.
Phenothiazines, Including Prochlorperazine, Butyrophenones (e.g., Haloperidol), Thioxanthenes, Metoclopramide. These medicines are dopamine antagonists. They will block the dopaminergic effect of apomorphine, thereby aggravating parkinsonian symptoms.
Ethanol, Antihypertensive Agents, Vasodilators (e.g., Nitrates). The use of these agents concurrently with apomorphine significantly increases the frequency of orthostatic hypotension. Alcohol should be avoided when taking apomorphine. Dosage adjustment of the antihypertensive agent is often necessary because of excessive orthostatic hypotension.

pramipexole (pră-mĭ-PĚKS-ŏl)
Mirapex (MĬR-ă-pĕks)
Mirapex ER
⇄ *Do not confuse Mirapex with MiraLAX.*

ACTIONS
Pramipexole is a nonergot dopamine agonist that stimulates D_2 and D_3 dopamine receptors.

USES

Pramipexole may be used alone to manage the early signs and symptoms of parkinsonism by improving ADLs and motor manifestations such as tremor, rigidity, bradykinesia, and postural stability. It may also be used in combination with levodopa for advanced parkinsonism to manage similar signs and symptoms of the disease.

THERAPEUTIC OUTCOMES

The primary therapeutic outcomes sought from pramipexole for the treatment of parkinsonism are as follows:
1. Improved motor and ADL scores
2. Decreased off time
3. Reduced dosage of levodopa

❖ NURSING IMPLICATIONS FOR PRAMIPEXOLE THERAPY

■ Premedication Assessment
1. Perform a baseline assessment of parkinsonism with the use of the UPDRS.
2. Obtain a history of GI and cardiovascular symptoms, including baseline vital signs (e.g., blood pressure, pulse).
3. Ask specifically about any symptoms of hallucinations, nightmares, dementia, or anxiety.

■ Availability
PO: tablets: 0.125, 0.25, 0.5, 0.75, 1, and 1.5 mg; tablets, extended-release, 24 hour: 0.375, 0.75, 1.5, 2.25, 3, 3.75, and 4.5 mg.

■ Dosage and Administration
Adult: PO: Initially, give 0.125 mg three times daily for 1 week. If tolerated, increase the dosage to 0.25 mg three times daily the second week. If tolerated, increase by increments of 0.25 mg three times daily through the seventh week. The usual maintenance dosage is 0.5 to 1.5 mg three times daily, with or without levodopa therapy. When pramipexole is used with levodopa, consider reducing the levodopa dose.

Administer medication with food or milk to reduce gastric irritation.

If pramipexole is to be discontinued, the dosage should be gradually reduced over 1 week.

■ Common Adverse Effects
Pramipexole causes many adverse effects, but most are dose related and are reversible. Adverse effects vary greatly, depending on the stage of the disease and the concurrent use of other medicines.

Gastrointestinal

Nausea, vomiting, anorexia. These effects can be reduced by slowly increasing the dosage, dividing the total daily dose into three doses, and administering the medication with food.

Cardiovascular

Orthostatic hypotension. Although it is generally mild, pramipexole may cause some degree of orthostatic hypotension; this is manifested by dizziness and weakness, particularly when therapy is being initiated. Tolerance usually develops after a few weeks of therapy. Monitor the patient's blood pressure daily in both the supine and standing positions. Anticipate the development of postural hypotension, and take measures to prevent such an occurrence. Teach patients to rise slowly from a supine or sitting position, and encourage them to sit or lie down if feeling faint.

■ Serious Adverse Effects
Neurologic

Chewing motions, bobbing, facial grimacing, rocking movements. These involuntary movements occur in some patients, especially if they are also taking levodopa. A reduction in dosage of the levodopa may be beneficial.

Sudden sleep events. Sleep episodes have been reported with the dopamine agonists (e.g., pramipexole, ropinirole). These episodes are described as "sleep attacks" or "sleep episodes," and they may include daytime sleep. Some sleep events have been reported as sudden and irresistible; other sleep events have been preceded by sufficient warning to prevent accidents. Patients who are taking dopamine agonists should be informed about the possibility of daytime sleepiness and outright sleep attacks with these medicines and be allowed to make their own decisions about driving on the basis of their past experiences with the medicines. The assessment of patients who are at risk for sleep attacks is possible with the Epworth Sleepiness Scale.

Psychological

Nightmares, depression, confusion, hallucinations. Perform a baseline assessment of the patient's degree of alertness and orientation to name, place, and time before initiating therapy. Make regularly scheduled subsequent evaluations of mental status, and compare findings. Report alterations in mood. Provide for patient safety during these episodes. Reducing the daily dosage may control these adverse effects.

Cardiovascular

Tachycardia, palpitations. Take the pulse at regularly scheduled intervals. Report any changes for further evaluation.

■ Drug Interactions
Cimetidine, Ranitidine, Diltiazem, Verapamil, Quinidine, Triamterene. These agents inhibit the urinary excretion of pramipexole. A dose reduction of pramipexole is often required to prevent toxic effects.

Dopamine Antagonists. Dopamine antagonists include phenothiazines, butyrophenones, thioxanthenes, and metoclopramide. As dopamine antagonists, these baseline to track the patient's response to drug therapy. Ensure that the patient understands how to use the form, and instruct the patient to bring the completed form to follow-up visits. During follow-up visits, focus on issues that will foster adherence with the therapeutic interventions prescribed.

Clinical Pitfall

Antidepressants may increase the risk of suicidal thinking and behavior (suicidality) in patients of all ages who are experiencing MDD. Patients who are started on antidepressants should be monitored daily by family members and caregivers for the emergence of agitation, irritability, unusual changes in behavior, and suicidality. Such symptoms should be immediately reported to healthcare providers.

DRUG THERAPY FOR DEPRESSIVE DISORDERS

DRUG CLASS: MONOAMINE OXIDASE INHIBITORS

During the early 1950s, isoniazid and iproniazid were developed to treat tuberculosis. It was soon reported that patients treated with iproniazid exhibited mood elevation. After further investigation, it was discovered that iproniazid—in addition to having antitubercular properties, inhibited monoamine oxidase—whereas isoniazid did not. Other MAOIs were synthesized and used extensively to treat depression until the 1960s, when the TCAs became available.

ACTIONS

Monoamine oxidase inhibitors block the metabolic destruction of epinephrine, norepinephrine, dopamine, and serotonin neurotransmitters by the enzyme monoamine oxidase in the presynaptic neurons of the brain. As a result, the concentration of these central nervous system (CNS) neurotransmitters becomes increased. Although MAO inhibition starts within a few days after initiating therapy, the antidepressant effects require 2 to 4 weeks to become evident. Approximately 60% of the clinical improvement of symptoms of depression occurs after 2 weeks, and maximum improvement is usually attained within 4 weeks.

USES

The MAOIs used today are phenelzine, tranylcypromine, isocarboxazid, and selegiline (Table 16-1). They are equally effective, and they have similar adverse effects. They are most effective for atypical depression, panic disorder, obsessive-compulsive disorder, and

Table 16-1   Antidepressants

GENERIC NAME	BRAND NAME	AVAILABILITY	INITIAL ORAL DOSAGE RANGE (UNLESS OTHERWISE NOTED)	DAILY MAINTENANCE DOSAGE RANGE (mg)	MAXIMUM DAILY DOSAGE RANGE (mg)
Monoamine Oxidase Inhibitors					
isocarboxazid	Marplan	Tablets: 10 mg	10 mg twice daily	40	60
phenelzine	Nardil	Tablets: 15 mg	15 mg three times daily	15-60	90
selegiline ⇄ *Do not confuse selegiline with Serentil, sertraline, Serzone, or Salagen.*	Emsam	Patch, transdermal: 6, 9, 12 mg/24 hr	6-mg patch daily	6	12
tranylcypromine	Parnate	Tablets: 10 mg	30 mg daily divided	30	60
Tricyclic Antidepressants					
amitriptyline ⇄ *Do not confuse amitriptyline with aminophylline.*	—	Tablets: 10, 25, 50, 75, 100, 150 mg	25-75 mg daily, divided as needed	75-200	200 (outpatients) 300 (inpatients)
amoxapine	—	Tablets: 25, 50, 100, 150 mg	50 mg two or three times daily	200-300	400 (outpatients) 600 (inpatients)
clomipramine	Anafranil, Apo-Clomipramine ✦	Capsules: 25, 50, 75 mg	25 mg once daily	100-150	250
desipramine	Norpramin	Tablets: 10, 25, 50, 75, 100, 150 mg	50-75 mg daily, divided in one to four doses	75-200	300

Continued

Table 16-1   Antidepressants—cont'd

GENERIC NAME	BRAND NAME	AVAILABILITY	INITIAL ORAL DOSAGE RANGE (UNLESS OTHERWISE NOTED)	DAILY MAINTENANCE DOSAGE RANGE (mg)	MAXIMUM DAILY DOSAGE RANGE (mg)
doxepin ⇄ Do not confuse doxepin with digoxin.	Apo-Doxepin ⇄ Do not confuse Sinequan with Serentil, Serzone, Seroquel, or Singulair.	Capsules: 10, 25, 50, 75, 100, 150 mg Oral concentrate: 10 mg/mL	25 mg three times daily	75-150	300 (inpatients)
imipramine hydrochloride	Tofranil, Apo-Imipramine ♥	Tablets: 10, 25, 50 mg	30-75 mg daily in one to four divided doses	50-150	200 (outpatients) 300 (inpatients)
imipramine pamoate	Tofranil PM	Capsules: 75, 100, 125, 150 mg	75-150 mg daily at bedtime	75-150	200 (outpatients) 300 (inpatients)
nortriptyline	Pamelor, PMS-Nortriptyline ♥	Capsules: 10, 25, 50, 75 mg Solution: 10 mg/5 mL	25-50 mg in one to four divided doses	50-75	150
protriptyline	Vivactil	Tablets: 5, 10 mg	5-10 mg three times daily	20-40	60
trimipramine	Surmontil	Capsules: 25, 50, 100 mg	25 mg three times daily	50-150	200 (outpatients) 300 (inpatients)
Selective Serotonin Reuptake Inhibitors					
citalopram	Celexa ⇄ Do not confuse Celexa with Zyprexa or Celebrex.	Tablets: 10, 20, 40 mg Liquid: 10 mg/5 mL	20 mg daily	20-40	40
escitalopram	Lexapro ⇄ Do not confuse Lexapro with loxapine.	Tablets: 5, 10, 20 mg Liquid: 1 mg/mL	10 mg daily	10-20	20
fluoxetine ⇄ Do not confuse fluoxetine with fluphenazine, fluvoxamine, famotidine, fluvastatin, or paroxetine.	Prozac Riva-Fluoxetine ♥ ⇄ Do not confuse Prozac with Prilosec, Proscar, or ProSom.	Capsules: 10, 20, 40 mg Tablets: 10, 20, 40, 60 mg Solution: 20 mg/5 mL Capsules, delayed release, weekly: 90 mg	20 mg in the morning	20-60	80
fluvoxamine ⇄ Do not confuse fluvoxamine with fluoxetine.	Luvox ⇄ Do not confuse Luvox with Lasix, Levoxyl, or Lovenox.	Tablets: 25, 50, 100 mg Capsules, sustained release: 100, 150 mg	50 mg at bedtime	50-300	300
paroxetine ⇄ Do not confuse paroxetine with fluoxetine, paclitaxel, or pyridoxine.	Paxil ⇄ Do not confuse Paxil with paclitaxel, Plavix, or Taxol. Paxil CR	Tablets: 10, 20, 30, 40 mg Suspension: 10 mg/5 mL Tablets, sustained release: 12.5, 25, 37.5 mg	20 mg daily	20-50	50

■ **Common Adverse Effects**

Neurologic

Dizziness, drowsiness. The patient should be warned to not work with machinery, operate a motor vehicle, administer medication, or perform other duties that require mental alertness until it is known whether this adverse effect impairs judgment.

Restlessness, agitation, anxiety, insomnia. These effects usually occur early in therapy, and the patient may require short-term treatment with sedative-hypnotic agents. Avoiding bedtime doses may help decrease the incidence of insomnia.

Gastrointestinal

Nausea, anorexia. Most of these effects may be minimized by temporarily reducing the dosage and taking with food.

■ **Serious Adverse Effects**

Psychological

Suicidal ideation. Monitor the patient for changes in thoughts, feelings, and behaviors during the initial stages of therapy.

■ **Drug Interactions**

Monoamine Oxidase Inhibitors. Severe reactions—including excitement, diaphoresis, rigidity, convulsions, hyperpyrexia, and death—have been reported with the concurrent use of MAOIs and SNRIs. It is recommended that at least 14 days lapse between discontinuing an MAOI and starting SNRI therapy (and vice versa).

Cimetidine. Cimetidine inhibits the metabolism of venlafaxine and duloxetine. Patients should be closely monitored for excessive effects of these two drugs when cimetidine is added to the therapeutic regimen.

Trazodone. Serotonin syndrome may develop when trazodone is used in conjunction with venlafaxine. Symptoms of serotonin syndrome include irritability, increased muscle tone, shivering, myoclonus, and reduced consciousness. Use trazodone cautiously; initiate therapy at a lower dosage and closely monitor for the adverse effects listed.

Haloperidol. Venlafaxine increases haloperidol levels and increases the frequency of EPSs, such as akathisia, dystonia, pseudoparkinsonism, and dyskinesia (see Chapter 17 for more information). If these drugs are used concurrently, the dosage of haloperidol may need to be decreased.

DRUG CLASS: TRICYCLIC ANTIDEPRESSANTS

ACTIONS

Until recently, TCAs (see Table 16-1) were the most widely used medications for the treatment of depression. Selective serotonin reuptake inhibitors now have that distinction, but their long-term effects are yet to be completely determined. Tricyclic antidepressants prolong the action of norepinephrine, dopamine, and serotonin to varying degrees by blocking the reuptake of these neurotransmitters in the synaptic cleft between neurons. The exact mechanism of action when these drugs are used as antidepressants is unknown.

USES

Tricyclic antidepressants produce antidepressant and mild tranquilizing effects. After 2 to 4 weeks of therapy, these drugs elevate mood, improve appetite, and increase alertness in approximately 80% of patients with endogenous depression. Combination therapy with phenothiazine derivatives may be beneficial for treating depression associated with schizophrenia or moderate to severe anxiety and depression observed with psychosis.

All TCAs are equally effective for treating depression, assuming that appropriate dosages are used for an adequate period. Consequently, the selection of an antidepressant is based primarily on the characteristics of each agent. Sedation is more notable with amitriptyline, doxepin, and trimipramine. Protriptyline has no sedative properties, and it may actually produce mild stimulation in some patients. All tricyclic compounds display anticholinergic activity, with amitriptyline displaying the most and desipramine the least. This factor should be considered in patients with cardiac disease, prostatic hyperplasia, or glaucoma. Other factors to consider are that men tend to respond better to imipramine than women, and older adults tend to respond better to amitriptyline than younger patients.

Doxepin is also approved for treating anxiety, and imipramine is approved for treating enuresis in children who are 6 years old and older. Clomipramine is not used to treat depression, but it is approved for treating obsessive-compulsive disorder.

Selected TCAs are also used to treat phantom limb pain, chronic pain, cancer pain, peripheral neuropathy with pain, postherpetic neuralgia, arthritic pain, eating disorders, premenstrual symptoms, and obstructive sleep apnea.

THERAPEUTIC OUTCOMES

The primary therapeutic outcomes expected from TCAs are elevated mood and reduction of symptoms of depression.

❖ **NURSING IMPLICATIONS FOR TRICYCLIC ANTIDEPRESSANTS**

■ **Premedication Assessment**

1. Note the consistency of the patient's bowel movements; constipation is common when taking TCAs.
2. Obtain the patient's baseline blood pressures in supine and standing positions; record and report significant hypotension to the healthcare provider before administering the drug.

3. Check the patient's history for symptoms of dysrhythmias, tachycardia, or congestive heart failure; if present, consult the healthcare provider before starting therapy (the patient may require electrocardiography before therapy is started).

4. If the patient has a history of seizures, check with the healthcare provider to see if the dosage of anticonvulsant therapy medications needs to be adjusted.

■ **Availability, Dosage, and Administration**

Adult: PO: See Table 16-1. The medication should be initiated at a low dosage level and increased gradually, particularly for older or debilitated patients. Dosage increases should be made in the evening because increased sedation often occurs.

Observation. Symptoms of depression may improve (e.g., increased appetite, sleep, and psychomotor activity) within a few days. However, the depression still exists, and it usually takes several weeks of the patient receiving therapeutic dosing before improvement is noted. Suicide precautions should be maintained during this time.

■ **Common Adverse Effects**

Cardiovascular

Orthostatic hypotension. All TCAs may cause some degree of orthostatic hypotension, manifested by dizziness and weakness, particularly when therapy is first begun. Monitor the patient's blood pressure daily in both the supine and standing positions. Anticipate the development of postural hypotension, and take measures to prevent such an occurrence. Teach the patient to rise slowly from a supine or sitting position, and encourage the patient to sit or lie down if feeling faint.

Neurologic

Sedative effects. Tell the patient about possible sedative effects. These effects usually occur early in therapy. Taking a single dose at bedtime may diminish or relieve the sedative effects.

Sensory

Blurred vision. Caution the patient that blurred vision may occur, and make appropriate suggestions to ensure the patient's personal safety.

Gastrointestinal

Constipation, dryness of mucosa of the mouth, throat, nose. Mucosal dryness may be relieved by sucking hard candy or ice chips or by chewing gum. The use of stool softeners such as docusate or the occasional use of a stimulant laxative such as bisacodyl may be required for constipation.

■ **Serious Adverse Effects**

Neurologic

Tremor. Approximately 10% of patients develop this adverse effect. Tremor can be controlled with small doses of propranolol.

Numbness, tingling. Report these symptoms to the healthcare provider for further evaluation.

Parkinsonian symptoms. If these symptoms develop, the TCA dosage must be reduced or discontinued. Antiparkinsonian medications will not control symptoms induced by TCAs.

Seizure activity. High doses of antidepressants lower the seizure threshold. Adjustment of anticonvulsant therapy may be required, especially for seizure-prone patients.

Cardiovascular

Dysrhythmias, tachycardia, heart failure. Report these symptoms to the healthcare provider for further evaluation.

Psychological

Suicidal ideation. Monitor the patient for changes in thoughts, feelings, and behaviors during the initial stages of therapy.

■ **Drug Interactions**

Enhanced Anticholinergic Activity. Antihistamines, phenothiazines, trihexyphenidyl, and benztropine enhance the anticholinergic activity associated with TCA therapy. The adverse effects are usually not severe enough to warrant discontinuing therapy, but stool softeners may be required.

Enhanced Sedative Activity. Ethanol, barbiturates, narcotics, tranquilizers, antihistamines, anesthetics, and sedative-hypnotics enhance the sedative activity associated with TCA therapy. Concurrent therapy is not recommended.

Barbiturates. Barbiturates may stimulate the metabolism of TCAs. Dosage adjustments of the antidepressant may be necessary.

Bupropion. Bupropion may increase serum levels of TCAs. Dosages may need to be reduced.

Carbamazepine. Tricyclic antidepressants can increase carbamazepine concentrations, resulting in signs of toxicity such as vertigo, tremor, headache, drowsiness, nausea, and vomiting. The dosage of carbamazepine may need to be reduced. Carbamazepine may also reduce serum levels of TCAs. Dosages of the TCA may need to be increased.

Valproic Acid, Methylphenidate. These medications may increase the serum levels of the TCAs. This reaction has been advantageous in attempts to gain a faster onset of antidepressant activity, but an increased incidence of dysrhythmias also has been reported.

Clonidine. Tricyclic antidepressants inhibit the antihypertensive effects of clonidine and may enhance the hypertension seen with the abrupt discontinuation of clonidine. Concurrent therapy should be avoided.

Monoamine Oxidase Inhibitors. Severe reactions—including convulsions, hyperpyrexia, and death—have been reported with concurrent use. It is recommended that 2 weeks lapse between discontinuing an MAOI and starting TCAs.

Selective Serotonin Reuptake Inhibitors. The interaction between SSRIs and TCAs is complex. The net result is that there is an increased toxicity from the TCAs. Observe patients for signs of toxicity, such as dysrhythmias, seizure activity, and CNS stimulation.

Amphetamines, Tryptophan, Dextromethorphan, Ephedrine, Pseudoephedrine, Epinephrine. All of these agents increase serotonin levels, potentially causing serotonin syndrome when taken by a person receiving TCAs. Symptoms of serotonin syndrome include irritability, increased muscle tone, shivering, myoclonus, and reduced consciousness. These medications should be used together only under the supervision of a healthcare provider.

Cimetidine. Cimetidine inhibits the metabolism of TCAs. Patients should be closely monitored for additional anticholinergic symptoms. In general, cimetidine therapy should be avoided in patients taking TCAs. Ranitidine and famotidine may be used without drug interactions.

Smoking. Cigarette smoking enhances the metabolism of TCAs. Dosages of the TCA may need to be increased to achieve a full therapeutic response.

DRUG CLASS: MISCELLANEOUS AGENTS

---

bupropion (byū-PRŌ-pē-ŏn) **hydrochloride**
  ⇄ *Do not confuse bupropion with buspirone.*
Wellbutrin (wĕl-BYŪ-trĭn)
Zyban (ZĪ-băn)
  ⇄ *Do not confuse Zyban with Zagam.*

ACTIONS

Bupropion is a monocyclic antidepressant. Its mechanism of action is not fully known. Compared with TCAs, it is believed to be a weak inhibitor of the reuptake of the neurotransmitters norepinephrine and dopamine. It has no monoamine oxidase inhibition or serotonin reuptake inhibition.

USES

It is approved for use in patients who are unresponsive to TCAs and who cannot tolerate the adverse effects of TCAs. Disadvantages include seizure activity and the requirement of multiple doses daily. It must not be used in patients with psychotic disorders because its dopamine agonist activity causes increased psychotic symptoms.

Bupropion is also approved (as Zyban) as an aid to support someone who is trying to quit smoking. Treatment should be initiated while the patient is still smoking because approximately 1 week of treatment is required to achieve steady-state blood levels of bupropion. Patients should set a target quit date during the first 2 weeks of treatment with bupropion, generally in the second week. Treatment should be continued for 7 to 12 weeks; longer treatment should be guided by the relative benefits and risks for individual patients.

THERAPEUTIC OUTCOMES

The primary therapeutic outcomes expected from bupropion therapy when used for depression are elevated mood and reduction of symptoms of depression. When it is used for smoking cessation, the expected outcome is the termination of smoking.

❖ NURSING IMPLICATIONS FOR BUPROPION THERAPY

■ **Premedication Assessment**
1. Obtain the patient's baseline weight.
2. Use the Dyskinesia Identification System: Condensed User Scale (DISCUS) or the Abnormal Involuntary Movement Scale (AIMS) (see Evolve website) at specified intervals to detect or check up ⓔ on EPSs; record and report in accordance with institutional policy.

■ **Availability**
PO: 75- and 100-mg tablets; 100-, 150-, and 200-mg 12-hour extended-release tablets and 150- and 300-mg 24-hour extended-release tablets.

■ **Dosage and Administration for Depression**
Adult: PO: Initially, 100 mg twice daily. This may be increased to 100 mg three times daily (at least every 6 hours) after several days of therapy. No single dose of bupropion should exceed 150 mg; do not exceed 450 mg daily. Avoid taking a dose shortly before bedtime.

■ **Dosage and Administration for Smoking Cessation**
Adult: PO: Dosing should begin at 150 mg/day given every day for the first 3 days, followed by a dosage increase for most patients to the recommended usual dosage of 300 mg/day. There should be an interval of at least 8 hours between successive doses. Dosages above 300 mg/day should not be used. Bupropion should be swallowed whole, not crushed, divided, or chewed.

Treatment should continue for 7 to 12 weeks; longer treatment should be guided by the relative benefits and risks for individual patients. If a patient has not made significant progress toward abstinence by the seventh week of therapy with bupropion, it is unlikely that he or she will quit during that attempt and treatment should probably be discontinued. Conversely, a patient who successfully quits after 7 to 12 weeks of treatment should be considered for ongoing therapy with bupropion. Dosage tapering of bupropion is not required when discontinuing treatment. The patient should continue to receive counseling and support throughout treatment with bupropion and for a period of time thereafter.

Individualization of Therapy. The patient is more likely to quit smoking and remain abstinent if seen frequently and receiving support from the healthcare provider. Ensure that the patient reads the instructions provided and has any questions answered. The patient's healthcare provider should review the overall smoking cessation program, including treatment with bupropion. The patient should be advised about the importance of participating in the behavioral interventions, counseling, and support services to be used in conjunction with bupropion.

Observation. Symptoms of depression may improve within a few days (e.g., improved appetite, sleep, and psychomotor activity). However, the depression still exists and it usually takes several weeks of the patient receiving therapeutic dosing before improvement is noted. Suicide precautions should be maintained during this time.

▪ Common Adverse Effects
Gastrointestinal
Anorexia, constipation, diarrhea, nausea, vomiting. Most GI effects may be minimized by temporarily reducing the dosage, giving with food, and using stool softeners for constipation.

Neurologic
Restlessness, agitation, anxiety, insomnia. These effects usually occur early in therapy, and the patient may require short-term treatment with sedative-hypnotic agents. Avoiding bedtime doses may help decrease the incidence of insomnia.

▪ Serious Adverse Effects
Neurologic
Seizures. See "Assessment: History of Seizure Activity" (Chapter 18, p. 269).

Psychological
Suicidal ideation. Monitor the patient for changes in thoughts, feelings, and behaviors during the initial stages of therapy.

▪ Drug Interactions
Cimetidine. Cimetidine inhibits the metabolism of bupropion and increases bupropion blood levels. A decrease in the bupropion dosage may be necessary.

Carbamazepine, Phenobarbital, Phenytoin. Carbamazepine, phenobarbital, and phenytoin may decrease bupropion serum levels, leading to decreased pharmacologic effect. It may be necessary to adjust the dosage of bupropion.

Nicotine Replacement. Although bupropion is used in combination with nicotine replacement products to help with smoking cessation, coadministration of nicotine replacement products with bupropion may cause hypertension. Monitor the patient's blood pressure when products such as nicotine patches or nicotine gum are being used.

Ritonavir. Ritonavir may stimulate the metabolism of bupropion, causing a reduction in serum concentrations of bupropion. An increase in the bupropion dosage may be necessary.

Levodopa. Bupropion has some mild dopaminergic activity and may result in an increase in the adverse effects caused by levodopa. If bupropion is to be added to levodopa therapy, it should be initiated at a lower dosage with small increases in the dosage of bupropion.

---

mirtazapine (mĭr-TĂZ-ĕ-pēn)
  Remeron (RĔ-mĕr-ŏn)
  ⇄ *Do not confuse Remeron with Restoril or Zemuron.*

ACTIONS

Mirtazapine is a tetracyclic antidepressant that is a serotonin antagonist. The mechanism of action is unknown, but the pharmacologic response is similar to that of tricyclic antidepressants.

USES

Mirtazapine is used to treat depression.

THERAPEUTIC OUTCOMES

The primary therapeutic outcomes expected from mirtazapine therapy are elevated mood and reduction of symptoms of depression.

❖ NURSING IMPLICATIONS FOR MIRTAZAPINE THERAPY

▪ Premedication Assessment
1. Obtain the patient's baseline blood pressures in the supine, sitting, and standing positions; record and report significant hypotension to the healthcare provider before administering the drug.
2. Obtain the patient's baseline weight, and schedule weekly weights.
3. Check for a history of seizures. If present, notify the healthcare provider before starting therapy.
4. Check the patient's hepatic studies before initiating therapy and periodically throughout the course of administration.
5. Use the DISCUS or the AIMS (see Evolve website) at specified intervals to detect or check up on EPSs; record and report in accordance with institutional policy.
6. Obtain the patient's white blood cell count before and at regular intervals after initiating therapy because agranulocytosis has been reported.

▪ Availability
PO: 7.5-, 15-, 30-, and 45-mg tablets and 15-, 30-, and 45-mg orally disintegrating tablets (SolTab).

▪ Dosage and Administration
Adult: PO: Initially, 15 mg daily. Every 1 to 2 weeks, the dosage may be increased up to a maximum of

45 mg daily. Increases in dosage should be made in the evening because increased sedation is often present.

Observation. See Tricyclic Antidepressants (p. 241). Symptoms of depression may improve (e.g., increased appetite, sleep, and psychomotor activity) within a few days. However, the depression still exists, and it usually takes several weeks of the patient receiving therapeutic dosing before improvement is noted. Suicide precautions should be maintained during this time.

nefazodone (nĕ-FĂZ-ō-dōn)

ACTIONS

Nefazodone is an antidepressant similar in chemical structure to trazodone. It inhibits serotonin and norepinephrine reuptake from the neuronal cleft, thus prolonging its action. It also blocks serotonin-2 receptors and antagonizes alpha-1 adrenergic receptors, which may result in postural hypotension.

USES

Nefazodone is used to treat depression. It appears to have less anticholinergic, hypotensive, and sedative activity than TCAs. A major disadvantage of nefazodone is the potential for life-threatening liver failure.

THERAPEUTIC OUTCOMES

The primary therapeutic outcomes expected from nefazodone therapy are elevated mood and reduction of symptoms of depression.

❖ **NURSING IMPLICATIONS FOR NEFAZODONE THERAPY**

■ **Premedication Assessment**

1. Obtain the patient's blood pressures in the supine, sitting, and standing positions; report any significant lowering to the healthcare provider before administering the medicine.
2. Obtain the patient's heart rate before and at regular intervals after the initiation of therapy. An electrocardiogram may be required for baseline information before starting therapy. Report any significant lowering of blood pressure to the healthcare provider before administering the medicine.
3. Note any GI symptoms present before start of therapy.
4. Monitor any CNS symptoms present (e.g., insomnia, nervousness).
5. Check liver function test results (aspartate aminotransferase [AST], alanine aminotransferase [ALT], gamma-glutamyltransferase [GGT]) before beginning therapy and periodically throughout the course of administration.

■ **Availability**

PO: 50-, 100-, 150-, 200-, and 250-mg tablets.

■ **Dosage and Administration**

Adult: PO: Initially, 100 mg twice daily. At no less than weekly intervals, increase the dosage by 100 to 200 mg, again on a twice-daily schedule as tolerated. Several weeks of adjustment may be required to optimize therapy. The normal dosage range is 300 to 600 mg daily.

Observation. Symptoms of depression may improve (e.g., increased appetite, sleep, and psychomotor activity) within a few days. However, the depression still exists, and it usually takes several weeks of therapeutic dosing before improvement is noted. Suicide precautions should be maintained during this time.

■ **Common Adverse Effects**

Neurologic

Drowsiness, sedation. Nefazodone has mild to moderate sedating effects. These symptoms tend to disappear with continued therapy and possible readjustment of the dosage. Inform the patient of possible sedative effects. The patient should use caution while driving or performing other tasks that require alertness. Consult with the healthcare provider to consider moving the daily dose to bedtime if sedation continues to be a problem.

Sedative effects. Tell the patient about the potential for sedative effects, especially during the onset of therapy. Taking a single dose at bedtime may diminish or relieve these effects.

Cardiovascular

Orthostatic hypotension. Nefazodone may cause some degree of orthostatic hypotension, manifested by dizziness and weakness, particularly when therapy is initiated. Monitor the patient's blood pressure daily in both the supine and standing positions. Anticipate the development of postural hypotension, and take measures to prevent an occurrence. Teach the patient to rise slowly from a supine or sitting position, and encourage the patient to sit or lie down if feeling faint.

These symptoms are the anticholinergic effects produced by these agents. Patients taking these medications should be monitored for the following adverse effects.

Sensory

Blurred vision. Caution the patient that blurred vision may occur, and make appropriate suggestions for the patient's personal safety.

Gastrointestinal

Constipation, dryness of mucosa of the mouth, throat, and nose. Mucosal dryness may be relieved by sucking on hard candy or ice chips or by chewing gum. The use of stool softeners such as docusate or the occasional use of a stimulant laxative such as bisacodyl may be required for constipation.

Genitourinary

Urinary retention. Patients taking this medicine should be monitored for urinary retention.

■ **Serious Adverse Effects**

Gastrointestinal

Hepatotoxicity. Monitor the patient for symptoms of hepatotoxicity, including anorexia, nausea, vomiting, jaundice, hepatomegaly, splenomegaly, and abnormal liver function test results (e.g., elevated bilirubin, AST, ALT, GGT, alkaline phosphatase levels, increased prothrombin time).

Cardiovascular

Bradycardia. Monitor the patient's heart rate as therapy is initiated and when dosing is adjusted. Bradycardias with a drop of 15 beats/min and rates of less than 50 beats/min have been reported. Notify the healthcare provider immediately, and withhold the next dose until it is specifically approved.

Psychological

Suicidal ideation. Monitor the patient for changes in thoughts, feelings, and behaviors during the initial stages of therapy.

■ **Drug Interactions**

Monoamine Oxidase Inhibitors. Severe reactions—including excitement, diaphoresis, rigidity, convulsions, hyperpyrexia, and death—have been reported with concurrent use of MAOIs and nefazodone. It is recommended that at least 14 days lapse between discontinuing an MAOI and starting nefazodone. It is further recommended that there be a 1-week drug-free interval between discontinuing nefazodone and starting MAOI therapy.

Haloperidol. Nefazodone inhibits the metabolism of haloperidol. It apparently does not increase the serum haloperidol level, but it does prolong the action of haloperidol. Doses may have to be given less often to prevent potential toxicity.

Carbamazepine. Nefazodone inhibits the metabolism of carbamazepine. Monitor the patient for signs of toxicity, such as disorientation, ataxia, lethargy, headache, drowsiness, nausea, and vomiting. Concurrent therapy is contraindicated.

Alprazolam, Triazolam. Nefazodone significantly increases the serum levels of these benzodiazepines. Monitor closely for excessive sedation and impaired motor skills.

Digoxin. Nefazodone significantly increases the serum level of digoxin. Monitor the patient's serum level and observe for signs of toxicity (e.g., dysrhythmias, bradycardia).

St. John's Wort. Nefazodone and St. John's wort may stimulate excess serotonin levels, potentially causing serotonin syndrome. Symptoms of serotonin syndrome include irritability, increased muscle tone, shivering, myoclonus, and reduced consciousness. These substances should not be used concurrently.

Sibutramine, Trazodone. Serotonin syndrome may develop when sibutramine or trazodone is used in conjunction with nefazodone. Concurrent therapy is contraindicated.

Cisapride. Nefazodone may significantly increase the serum concentrations of cisapride, causing potentially fatal cardiac toxicities. Concurrent therapy is contraindicated.

 Herbal Interactions

St. John's Wort

St. John's wort may increase the toxic effects of antidepressant medications. The use of St. John's wort with other antidepressants should be done only with close supervision by a healthcare provider.

---

trazodone (TRĂ-zō-dōn) **hydrochloride**
⇌ *Do not confuse trazodone with amiodarone or tramadol.*

ACTIONS

Trazodone was the first of the triazolopyridine antidepressants to be released for clinical use. The triazolopyridines are chemically unrelated to the other classes of antidepressants. The exact mechanisms of action of trazodone are unknown, but it potentiates serotonin activity by inhibiting reuptake and destruction of serotonin. The actions are complex and in some ways resemble those of the TCAs, benzodiazepines, and phenothiazines; however, the overall activity of trazodone is different from that of each of these classes of drugs.

USES

Trazodone has been shown to be as effective as TCAs in treating depression; depression associated with schizophrenia; and depression, tremor, and anxiety associated with alcohol dependence. Compared with other antidepressants, trazodone has a low incidence of anticholinergic adverse effects, which makes it particularly useful in patients whose antidepressant dosages are limited by anticholinergic adverse effects and in patients with severe closed-angle glaucoma, prostatic hyperplasia, organic mental disorders, or cardiac dysrhythmias. Trazodone is commonly used to treat insomnia in patients with substance abuse because it is sedating, improves sleep continuity, and has minimal potential for tolerance and addiction.

THERAPEUTIC OUTCOMES

The primary therapeutic outcomes expected from trazodone therapy are elevated mood and reduction of symptoms of depression.

❖ **NURSING IMPLICATIONS FOR TRAZODONE THERAPY**

■ **Premedication Assessment**

1. Obtain the patient's baseline blood pressures in the supine, sitting, and standing positions.

2. Record and report significant hypotension to the healthcare provider before administering the drug.

■ **Availability**

PO: 50-, 100-, 150-, and 300-mg tablets; 150- and 300-mg 24-hour extended-release tablets.

■ **Dosage and Administration**

Adult: PO: Initially, 150 mg in three divided doses. Increase the dosage in increments of 50 mg daily every 3 to 4 days while monitoring the clinical response. Do not exceed 400 mg daily in outpatients or 600 mg daily in hospitalized patients.

Trazodone therapy should be initiated at a low dosage and increased gradually, particularly in older adults or debilitated patients. Dosage increases should be made in the evening because increased sedation often occurs. Administer the medication shortly after a meal or with a light snack to reduce adverse effects.

Observation. Symptoms of depression may improve (e.g., increased appetite, sleep, and psychomotor activity) within a few days. However, the depression still exists, and it usually takes several weeks of the patient receiving therapeutic dosing before improvement is noted. Suicide precautions should be maintained during this time.

■ **Common Adverse Effects**

Cardiovascular

Orthostatic hypotension. Although episodes are infrequent and generally mild, trazodone may cause some degree of orthostatic hypotension, manifested by dizziness and weakness, particularly when therapy is initiated. Monitor the patient's blood pressure daily in both the supine and standing positions. Anticipate the development of postural hypotension, and take measures to prevent an occurrence. Teach the patient to rise slowly from a supine or sitting position, and encourage the patient to sit or lie down if feeling faint.

Neurologic

Drowsiness. The patient should be warned to not work with machinery, operate a motor vehicle, administer medication, or perform other duties that require mental alertness until it is known whether this adverse effect impairs judgment.

■ **Serious Adverse Effects**

Cardiovascular

Dysrhythmias, tachycardia. Report these symptoms to a healthcare provider for further evaluation.

Neurologic

Confusion. Before initiating therapy, perform a baseline assessment of the patient's degree of alertness and orientation to name, place, and time. Make regularly scheduled subsequent evaluations of the patient's mental status and compare findings. Report any significant alterations to the prescriber.

Dizziness, lightheadedness. Provide for patient safety during episodes of dizziness, and report these symptoms to the prescriber for further evaluation.

■ **Drug Interactions**

Enhanced Sedative Activity. Ethanol, barbiturates, narcotics, tranquilizers, antihistamines, anesthetics, phenothiazines, and sedative-hypnotics enhance the sedative effects associated with trazodone therapy. Concurrent therapy is not recommended.

Nefazodone, MAOIs, SSRIs, SNRIs. Serotonin syndrome may develop when trazodone is used in conjunction with any of these agents. Symptoms of serotonin syndrome include irritability, increased muscle tone, shivering, myoclonus, and reduced consciousness. Use trazodone cautiously; initiate therapy at a lower dosage and closely monitor for the adverse effects listed.

---

vilazodone (vĭl-ĂZ-zō-dōn)

⇄ *Do not confuse vilazodone with trazodone or nefazodone.*

Viibryd (vī-brĭd)

ACTIONS

Vilazodone is newer medication that acts as an SSRI and a partial agonist of serotonin (5-HT$_{1A}$) receptor that enhances serotonin activity.

USES

Vilazodone is approved to treat MDD in adults.

THERAPEUTIC OUTCOMES

The primary therapeutic outcomes expected from vilazodone therapy are elevated mood and reduction of symptoms of depression.

❖ **NURSING IMPLICATIONS FOR VILAZODONE THERAPY**

■ **Premedication Assessment**

1. Note any GI symptoms present before the start of therapy.
2. Monitor any CNS symptoms present (e.g., insomnia, restlessness).

■ **Availability**

PO: 10-, 20-, and 40-mg tablets.

■ **Dosage and Administration**

Adult: PO: Initially, 10 mg once daily with food, followed by 20 mg once daily with food for the next 7 days, and then increased to the recommended dosage of 40 mg once daily. Vilazodone should be taken with food for optimal absorption.

Observation. Symptoms of depression may improve (e.g., increased appetite, sleep, and psychomotor activity) within a few days. However, the depression still exists, and it usually takes several weeks of the patient receiving therapeutic dosing before improvement is noted. Suicide precautions should be maintained during this time.

■ Common Adverse Effects

Gastrointestinal

Diarrhea, nausea, vomiting. These adverse effects should be mild, particularly if the dose is administered with food. They should also resolve with continued therapy. Patients with persistent vomiting should be evaluated for other causes, as well as for the development of electrolyte imbalance.

Neurologic

Dizziness, drowsiness. Provide for patient safety during episodes of dizziness, and report these symptoms to the healthcare provider for further evaluation. The patient should not take these medications while working with machinery, operating a motor vehicle, administering medication, or performing other duties that require mental alertness.

■ Serious Adverse Effects

Neurologic

Confusion. Before initiating therapy, perform a baseline assessment of the patient's degree of alertness and orientation to name, place, and time. Make regularly scheduled subsequent evaluations of the patient's mental status and compare findings. Report any significant alterations to the prescriber.

Dizziness, lightheadedness. Provide for patient safety during episodes of dizziness, and report these symptoms to the healthcare provider for further evaluation.

Psychological

Suicidal ideation. Monitor the patient for changes in thoughts, feelings, and behaviors, especially during the initial stages of therapy.

■ Drug Interactions

Monoamine Oxidase Inhibitors. Severe reactions—including excitement, diaphoresis, rigidity, convulsions, hyperpyrexia, and death—may result from the concurrent use of MAOIs and vilazodone. It is recommended that at least 14 days lapse between discontinuing an MAOI and starting vilazodone. It is further recommended that there be a 14-day drug-free interval between discontinuing vilazodone and starting MAOI therapy.

Enhanced Sedative Activity. Ethanol, barbiturates, narcotics, tranquilizers, antihistamines, anesthetics, phenothiazines, and sedative-hypnotics enhance the sedative effects that are associated with vilazodone therapy. Concurrent therapy is not recommended.

Nefazodone, Trazodone, MAOIs, SSRIs, SNRIs, Tramadol, Triptans. Serotonin syndrome may develop when vilazodone is used in conjunction with any of these agents. Symptoms of serotonin syndrome include irritability, increased muscle tone, shivering,

myoclonus, and reduced consciousness. Use these drugs cautiously; initiate therapy at a lower dosage and closely monitor for the adverse effects listed.

Aspirin, Nonsteroidal Antiinflammatory Drugs, Warfarin. Serotonin release by platelets plays an important role in hemostasis. Selective serotonin reuptake inhibitors may enhance the anticoagulant effects of warfarin and enhance the potential for GI bleeding caused by nonsteroidal antiinflammatory drugs or aspirin. Observe the patient for petechiae, ecchymoses, nosebleeds, bleeding gums, dark tarry stools, and bright red or coffee ground emesis. Monitor prothrombin time and INR, and reduce the dosage of warfarin if necessary.

Phenytoin, Phenobarbital, Carbamazepine. These agents may enhance the metabolism of vilazodone, reducing serum levels and leading to decreased pharmacologic effect.

Erythromycin, Clarithromycin, Fluoxetine, Grapefruit Juice, Ketoconazole, Nefazodone. These drugs inhibit the metabolism of vilazodone, causing an increase in serum levels and the potential for toxicity. Dosages of the antidepressant may need to be reduced by up to 50% to avoid toxicities.

---

vilazodone (võr tē-ŎX-ět-ēn)
  ⇄ *Do not confuse vortioxetine with atomoxetine.*
Brintellix (brĭn-TĚL-ĭx)
  ⇄ *Do not confuse Brintellix with Brilinta.*

ACTIONS

Vortioxetine is a new medication that acts as an SSRI, an agonist of the serotonin (5-HT_{1A}) receptors that enhances serotonin activity and antagonizes the serotonin (5-HT_3) receptors.

USES

Vortioxetine is approved to treat MDD in adults.

THERAPEUTIC OUTCOMES

The primary therapeutic outcomes expected from vortioxetine therapy are elevated mood and reduction of symptoms of depression.

❖ NURSING IMPLICATIONS FOR VORTIOXETINE THERAPY

■ Premedication Assessment

1. Note any GI symptoms present before the start of therapy.
2. Monitor any CNS symptoms present (e.g., insomnia, restlessness).

■ Availability

PO: 5-, 10-, and 20-mg tablets.

■ Dosage and Administration

Adult: PO: Initially, 10 mg once daily, followed by 20 mg once daily as tolerated. For those not tolerating

10 mg daily, therapy may be reduced to 5 mg daily. Maximum daily dose is 20 mg. If well tolerated, patients should remain on therapy for several months.

When discontinuation is planned, the dose should be tapered to monitor closely for development of withdrawal symptoms and to detect the development of depressive symptoms. The manufacturer recommends that doses of 15 mg daily or higher should be reduced to 10 mg daily for 1 week before full discontinuation to prevent withdrawal symptoms.

- ■ **Common Adverse Effects**
  Gastrointestinal

Diarrhea, nausea, vomiting, dry mouth. These adverse effects should be mild and should resolve with continued therapy. Patients with persistent vomiting should be evaluated for other causes, as well as for the development of electrolyte imbalance (syndrome of inappropriate secretion of antidiuretic hormone or serotonin syndrome).

Neurologic

Dizziness, abnormal dreams. Provide for patient safety during episodes of dizziness. Provide comfort and patient safety in those reporting abnormal dreams. Report these symptoms to the healthcare provider for further evaluation. The patient should not take these medications while working with machinery, operating a motor vehicle, administering medication, or performing other duties that require mental alertness.

- ■ **Serious Adverse Effects**
  Psychological

Suicidal actions, hypomania, mania, serotonin syndrome. Monitor the patient for changes in thoughts, feelings, and behaviors, especially during the initial stages of therapy. Symptoms of depression may improve (e.g., increased appetite, sleep, and psychomotor activity) within a few days. However, the depression still exists, and it usually takes several weeks of the patient receiving therapeutic dosing before improvement is noted. Suicide precautions should be maintained during this time.

Review patient history for a personal or family history of bipolar illness, as vortioxetine may induce latent bipolar illness. Vortioxetine is not approved for treatment of bipolar depression.

- ■ **Drug Interactions**
  Monoamine Oxidase Inhibitors. Severe reactions—including excitement, diaphoresis, rigidity, convulsions, hyperpyrexia, and death—may result from the concurrent use of MAOIs and vortioxetine. It is recommended that at least 14 days lapse between discontinuing an MAOI and starting vortioxetine. It is further recommended that there be a 14-day drug-free interval between discontinuing vortioxetine and starting MAOI therapy.

Nefazodone, Trazodone, MAOIs, SSRIs, SNRIs, Tramadol, Triptans, Buspirone, St. John's Wort, Linezolid, Fentanyl. Serotonin syndrome may develop when vortioxetine is used in conjunction with any of these agents. Symptoms of serotonin syndrome include irritability, hallucinations, delirium, reduced consciousness, increased muscle tone, myoclonus, and shivering. Use these drugs cautiously; initiate therapy at a lower dosage and closely monitor for the adverse effects listed.

Aspirin, Nonsteroidal Antiinflammatory Drugs, Warfarin. Serotonin release by platelets plays an important role in hemostasis. Selective serotonin reuptake inhibitors may enhance the anticoagulant effects of warfarin and enhance the potential for GI bleeding caused by nonsteroidal antiinflammatory drugs or aspirin. Observe the patient for petechiae, ecchymoses, nosebleeds, bleeding gums, dark tarry stools, and bright red or coffee ground emesis. Monitor prothrombin time and INR, and reduce the dosage of warfarin if necessary.

Buspirone. Buspirone inhibits the metabolism of vortioxetine, causing an increase in serum levels and the potential for toxicity. Dosages of vortioxetine should be reduced by up to 50% to avoid toxicities.

DRUG CLASS: ANTIMANIC AGENTS

lithium (LĬTH-ē-um) **carbonate**

ACTIONS

Lithium is a monovalent cation that competes with other monovalent and divalent cations (i.e., potassium, sodium, calcium, magnesium) at cellular binding sites that are sensitive to changes in cation concentration. Lithium replaces intracellular and intraneuronal sodium, stabilizing the neuronal membrane. It also reduces the release of norepinephrine and increases the uptake of tryptophan, the precursor to serotonin. It also interacts with second-messenger cellular processes to inhibit intracellular concentrations of cyclic adenosine monophosphate. Because of the complexity of the CNS, the exact mechanisms of action of lithium for treating mood disorders are unknown. It has no sedative, depressant, or euphoric properties, which differentiates it from all other psychotropic agents.

USES

Lithium is used to treat acute mania and for prophylactic treatment of recurrent manic and depressive episodes in patients with bipolar disorder. In patients with bipolar disorder, it is more effective in preventing signs and symptoms of mania than those of depression. It is also effective in some patients for reducing the recurrence of the depressive episodes associated with unipolar disorder.

THERAPEUTIC OUTCOME

The primary therapeutic outcome expected from lithium therapy is maintaining the individual at an optimal level of functioning, with minimal exacerbations of mood swings.

❖ NURSING IMPLICATIONS FOR LITHIUM THERAPY

▪ Premedication Assessment

1. Before initiating lithium therapy, the following laboratory tests should be completed for baseline information: electrolytes, fasting blood glucose, blood urea nitrogen (BUN), serum creatinine, creatinine clearance, urinalysis, and thyroid function.
2. Obtain baseline blood pressures with the patient in the supine, sitting, and standing positions; record and report significant hypotension to the healthcare provider before administering the drug.
3. Weigh the patient daily, check the hydration status (e.g., moistness of mucous membranes, skin turgor, firmness of eyeball), and monitor urine specific gravity.
4. Lithium may enhance sodium depletion, which increases lithium toxicity. Assess for early signs of lithium toxicity before giving the medication, including nausea, vomiting, abdominal pain, diarrhea, lethargy, speech difficulty, mild dizziness, muscle twitching, and tremor.

▪ Availability

PO: Lithium carbonate: 150-, 300-, and 600-mg capsules and tablets; 300- and 450-mg slow-release tablets. Lithium citrate: solution, 8 mEq/5 mL.

▪ Dosage and Administration

Adult: PO: 300 to 600 mg three or four times daily. Administer with food or milk. An adequate diet is important to maintain normal serum sodium levels and to prevent toxicity. The onset of the acute antimanic effect of lithium usually occurs within 5 to 7 days; the full therapeutic effect often requires 10 to 21 days.

Serum Lithium Levels. Lithium levels are monitored once or twice weekly during the initiation of therapy and monthly while the patient is receiving a maintenance dosage. Blood should be drawn approximately 12 hours after the last dose was administered. The normal serum level is 0.4 to 1.2 mEq/L. Promptly report serum levels higher than these values to the healthcare provider.

Good Nutrition. Lithium may enhance sodium depletion, which increases lithium toxicity. The patient should maintain a normal dietary intake of sodium and adequate maintenance fluids (i.e., 10 to 12 eight-ounce glasses of water daily)—especially when initiating therapy—to prevent toxicity.

▪ Common Adverse Effects

Gastrointestinal

Nausea, vomiting, anorexia, abdominal cramps. These adverse effects are usually mild and tend to resolve with continued therapy. Encourage the patient not to discontinue therapy without first consulting the healthcare provider. If gastric irritation occurs, administer the medication with food or milk. If symptoms persist or increase in severity, report them to the healthcare provider for evaluation. These also may be early signs of toxicity.

Excessive thirst. This adverse effect is usually mild and tends to resolve within a week with continued therapy. Encourage the patient not to discontinue therapy without first consulting the healthcare provider. If excessive thirst persists or becomes severe, the patient should consult the healthcare provider.

Neurologic

Fine hand tremor. If fine hand tremor persists or becomes severe, the patient should consult the healthcare provider.

Genitourinary

Excessive urination. This adverse effect is usually mild and tends to resolve within a week with continued therapy. Encourage the patient not to discontinue therapy without first consulting the healthcare provider. If excessive urination persists or becomes severe, the patient should consult the healthcare provider.

▪ Serious Adverse Effects

Gastrointestinal

Persistent vomiting, profuse diarrhea. These are symptoms of impending serious toxicity. Report them immediately, and do not give the next dose of medication until administration has been reconfirmed by the healthcare provider.

Neurologic

Hyperreflexia, lethargy, weakness. These are signs of impending serious toxicity. Report them immediately, and do not give the next dose of medication until administration has been reconfirmed by the healthcare provider.

Endocrine, Metabolic

Progressive fatigue, weight gain. These may be early signs of hypothyroidism. Report these symptoms to the healthcare provider for further evaluation.

Hyperglycemia. Report these symptoms to the healthcare provider for further evaluation.

Genitourinary

Nephrotoxicity. Monitor urinalysis and kidney function tests for abnormal results. Report an increasing BUN level or creatinine level, increasing or decreasing urine output or decreasing specific gravity (despite adequate fluid intake), and casts or protein in the urine.

■ Rare Adverse Effects From Lithium Therapy

Pruritus, Ankle Edema, Metallic Taste. Report these symptoms for further evaluation by the healthcare provider.

■ Drug Interactions

Reduced Serum Sodium Levels. The therapeutic activity and toxicity of lithium are highly dependent on sodium concentrations. Decreased sodium levels significantly enhance the toxicity of lithium, and high sodium levels result in low lithium levels. Patients who are to begin diuretic therapy, a low-sodium diet, or activities that produce excessive and prolonged sweating should be observed particularly closely.

Diuretics. Diuretics may reduce the elimination of lithium, resulting in lithium toxicity. Monitor the patient's lithium serum levels closely. Monitor patients receiving concurrent long-term therapy for signs of the development of lithium toxicity (e.g., nausea, vomiting, abdominal pain, diarrhea, lethargy, speech difficulty, mild dizziness, tremor).

Methyldopa. Monitor patients receiving concurrent long-term therapy for signs of the development of lithium toxicity (e.g., nausea, vomiting, abdominal pain, diarrhea, lethargy, speech difficulty, mild dizziness, tremor).

Indomethacin, Piroxicam. Indomethacin and piroxicam reduce the renal excretion of lithium, allowing the lithium to accumulate to potentially toxic levels.

Get Ready for the NCLEX® Examination!

Key Points

- The new *Diagnostic and Statistical Manual of Mental Disorders,* 5th edition (DSM-5) recognizes major psychiatric disorders on a continuum from depressive disorders and psychotic spectrum at the ends of the continuum, with bipolar disorders serving as a bridge between the two diagnostic classes in terms of symptomatology, family history, and genetics. The common feature among depressive and bipolar disorders is the presence of sad, empty, or irritable mood, accompanied by changes that significantly affect the individual's capacity to function.
- Treatment of mood disorders requires both nonpharmacologic and pharmacologic therapy. Simultaneous psychotherapy and pharmacologic treatment are more successful than either treatment alone.
- Antidepressant medications act on a variety of receptors in the CNS, as well as peripheral tissues, and are associated with many adverse effects and drug interactions. It is the responsibility of the nurse to educate patients about therapy and to monitor for therapeutic benefit and common and serious adverse effects, as well as to intervene whenever possible to optimize therapeutic outcomes.

Additional Learning Resources

SG Go to your Study Guide for additional Review Questions for the NCLEX® Examination, Critical Thinking Clinical Situations, and other learning activities to help you master this chapter content.

evolve Go to your Evolve website (http://evolve.elsevier.com/Clayton) for additional online resources.

Review Questions for the NCLEX® Examination

1. The nurse was assessing the patient who came in with depression. These components are part of the baseline assessment: (*Select all that apply.*)
   1. oral hygiene and number of dental cavities.
   2. history of previous depression episodes and treatments.
   3. sleep pattern.
   4. suicidal ideation.
   5. tattoos present.

2. Patients who are being treated for depression should continually be monitored for thoughts of suicide. Which behavior may indicate suicidal ideation?
   1. Excessive appetite
   2. Poor hygiene
   3. Comments from the patient such as, "Things will get better after I'm gone."
   4. Sleeping throughout the day

3. The nurse knows to assess for a severe reaction such as excitement, diaphoresis, rigidity, and convulsions, which can occur between SSRIs and these drugs:
   1. MAOIs.
   2. birth control pills.
   3. beta blockers.
   4. antihistamines.

4. The nurse is explaining to the patient taking an MAOI of the need to be aware of this condition developing:
   1. blood dyscrasias.
   2. hyperglycemia.
   3. hypertension.
   4. hyperactivity.

5. A patient came into the clinic after being started on duloxetine (Cymbalta) complaining of drowsiness and nausea. The nurse knows this about SNRIs:
   1. these symptoms are serious adverse effects.
   2. these symptoms may represent a drug interaction with haloperidol.
   3. these symptoms indicate the dose needs to be adjusted.
   4. these symptoms are common adverse effects.

6. Patients taking doxepin should be aware of the following adverse effects common to TCAs: (*Select all that apply.*)
   1. orthostatic hypotension.
   2. parkinsonism symptoms.
   3. dry mouth and throat.
   4. seizure activity.
   5. blurred vision.

7. The nurse discussed ways to prevent lithium toxicity with a patient currently on lithium and included the following measures: (*Select all that apply.*)
   1. "Be sure to report symptoms of persistent vomiting and/or profuse diarrhea."
   2. "You need to drink 10 glasses of water (8 ounces each) daily."
   3. "It is important to draw lithium blood levels monthly."
   4. "Because you are taking lithium, we can prevent lithium toxicity with diuretic therapy."
   5. "Be sure to report symptoms of lethargy and weakness."

Drugs Used for Psychoses

Objectives

1. Identify the signs and symptoms of psychotic behavior.
2. Describe the major indications for the use of antipsychotic agents.
3. Discuss the antipsychotic medications that are used for the treatment of psychoses.
4. Identify the common adverse effects that are observed with the use of antipsychotic medications.

Key Terms

psychosis (sī-KŌ-sĭs) (p. 253)
delusion (dĕ-LŪ-zhŭn) (p. 253)
hallucinations (hă-lū-sĭ-NĀ-shŭn) (p. 254)
disorganized thinking (dĭs-ŌR-găn-īzd THĬN-kĭng) (p. 254)
loosening of associations (LŪ-sĕn-ĭng of ăs-sō-sē-Ā-shŭnz) (p. 254)
disorganized behavior (dĭs-ŌR-găn-īzd bē-HĀV-yŭr) (p. 254)
negative symptoms (NĔG-ĕ-tiv SĬMP-tĕmz) (p. 254)
target symptoms (TĂR-gĕt SĬMP-tĕmz) (p. 254)
typical (first-generation) antipsychotic agents (TĬP-ĭ-kŭl ăn-tī-sī-KŌT-ĭk) (p. 255)
atypical (second-generation) antipsychotic agents (ā-TĬP-ĭ-kŭl ăn-tī-sī-KŌT-ĭk) (p. 255)
equipotent doses (ĕk-wē-PŌ-tĕnt DŌS-ĕz) (p. 255)

extrapyramidal symptoms (EPSs) (ĕks-tră-pĭ-RĂM-ĭ-dăl) (p. 255)
dystonias (dĭs-TŌN-ē-ăz) (p. 258)
pseudoparkinsonian symptoms (SŪ-dō-păr-kĭn-SŌ-nē-ĭn) (p. 258)
akathisia (ă-kĕ-THĬ-zhă) (p. 258)
tardive dyskinesia (TĂR-dĭv dĭs-kĭ-NĒ-zē-ă) (p. 258)
Abnormal Involuntary Movement Scale (AIMS) (ăb-NŌR-mŭl ĭn-VŎL-ĕn-tār-ē MŌV-mĕnt SKĀ-ul) (p. 259)
Dyskinesia Identification System: Condensed User Scale (DISCUS) (dĭs-kĭ-NĒ-zē-a ī-dĕn-tĭ-fĭ-KĀ-shŭn SĬS-tĕm: kŏn-DĔNST YŪ-zŭr SKĀ-ŭl) (p. 259)
neuroleptic malignant syndrome (NMS) (nyū-rō-LĔP-tĭk mă-LĬG-nănt SĬN-drōm mă-LĬG-nănt SĬN-drōm) (p. 259)
depot antipsychotic medicine (DĔ-pō ăn-tē-sī-KŌT-ĭk) (p. 259)

PSYCHOSIS

Psychosis does not have a single definition, but is a clinical descriptor applied to someone who is out of touch with reality. Psychotic symptoms can be associated with many illnesses, including dementias and delirium, that may have metabolic, infectious, or endocrinologic causes. Psychotic symptoms are also common in patients with mood disorders such as major depression and bipolar disorder and schizophrenia spectrum. Psychosis can also be caused by many drugs (e.g., phencyclidine, opiates, amphetamines, cocaine, hallucinogens, anticholinergic agents, alcohol). Psychotic disorders are characterized by loss of reality, perceptual deficits such as hallucinations and delusions, and deterioration of social functioning. Schizophrenia is the most common of the several psychotic disorders defined by the American Psychiatric Association in the *Diagnostic and Statistical Manual of Mental Disorders,* 5th edition.

Psychotic disorders are extremely complex illnesses that are influenced by biologic, psychosocial, and environmental circumstances. Some of the disorders require several months of observation and testing before a final diagnosis can be determined. It is beyond the scope of this text to discuss psychotic disorders in detail, but general types of symptoms associated with psychotic disorders will be described.

A delusion is a false or irrational belief that is firmly held despite obvious evidence to the contrary. Delusions may be persecutory, grandiose, religious, sexual, or hypochondriacal. Delusions of reference—in which the patient attributes a special, irrational, and usually negative significance to other people, objects, or events, such as song lyrics or newspaper articles, in relation to self—are common. Delusions may be defined as "bizarre" if they are clearly irrational and do not derive from ordinary life experiences. A common bizarre delusion is the patient's belief that his or her thinking process, body parts, or actions or impulses are controlled or dictated by some external force.

Hallucinations are false sensory perceptions that are experienced without an external stimulus and seem real to the patient. Auditory hallucinations experienced as voices that are characteristically heard commenting negatively about the patient in the third person are prominent among patients with schizophrenia. Hallucinations of touch, sight, taste, smell, and bodily sensation also occur.

Disorganized thinking is commonly associated with psychoses. These thought disorders may consist of a **loosening of associations** or a flight of ideas so that the speaker jumps from one idea or topic to another unrelated one (derailment) in an illogical, inappropriate, or disorganized way. Answers to questions may be obliquely related or completely unrelated (tangentiality). At its most serious, this incoherence of thought extends into pronunciation itself, and the speaker's words become garbled or unrecognizable. Speech may also be overly concrete (loss of ability to think in abstract terms) and inexpressive; it may be repetitive and may convey little or no real information.

Disorganized behavior is another common characteristic of psychosis. Problems may be noted with any form of goal-directed behavior, leading to difficulties with performing activities of daily living (ADLs), such as organizing meals or maintaining hygiene. The patient may appear markedly disheveled, may dress in an unusual manner (e.g., wearing several layers of clothing, scarves, and gloves on a hot day), or may display clearly inappropriate sexual behavior (e.g., public masturbation) or unpredictable, nontriggered agitation (e.g., shouting, swearing). Disorganized behavior must be distinguished from behavior that is merely aimless or generally not purposeful and from organized behavior that is motivated by delusional beliefs.

Negative symptoms, or changes in affect, may also be symptoms of psychosis. Emotional expressiveness is diminished; there is poor eye contact and reduced spontaneous movement. The patient appears to be withdrawn from others, and the face appears to be immobile and unresponsive. Speech is often minimal (alogia), with only brief, slow, monotone replies given in response to questions. There is a withdrawal from areas of functioning that affect interpersonal relationships, work, education, and self-care (asociality), and anhedonia, the decreased ability to experience pleasure from positive stimuli or reduced pleasure from previously positive stimuli.

TREATMENT OF PSYCHOSIS

The importance of the initial assessment for an accurate diagnosis cannot be underestimated for a patient with acute psychosis. A thorough physical and neurologic examination, a mental status examination, a complete family and social history, and a laboratory workup must be performed to exclude other causes of psychoses, including substance abuse. Both drug and nondrug therapies are critical to the treatment of most psychoses. Long-term outcome is improved for patients with an integrated drug and nondrug treatment regimen. Nonpharmacologic interventions beneficial to patients include (1) individual psychotherapy to improve insight into the illness and help the patient cope with stress; (2) group therapy to enhance socialization skills; (3) behavioral or cognitive therapy; (4) and vocational training. Referral to community resources such as the National Alliance on Mental Illness (NAMI) may provide additional support for the patient and family.

Before initiating therapy, the treatment goals and baseline level of functioning must be established and documented. **Target symptoms** must also be identified and documented. Target symptoms are critical monitoring parameters used to assess changes in an individual's clinical status and response to medications. Examples of target symptoms include frequency and type of agitation, degree of suspiciousness, delusions, hallucinations, loose associations, grooming habits and hygiene, sleep patterns, speech patterns, social skills, and judgment. The ultimate goal is to restore behavioral, cognitive, and psychosocial processes and skills to as close to baseline levels as possible so that the patient can be reintegrated into the community. Realistically, unless the psychosis is part of another medical diagnosis such as substance abuse, most patients will have recurring symptoms of the mental disorder for most of their lives. Therefore treatment is focused on decreasing the severity of the target symptoms that most interfere with functioning. A variety of scales have been developed to assist with the objective measurement of change in target symptoms in response to psychotherapy and pharmacotherapy. These include the Brief Psychiatric Rating Scale (BPRS), the Positive and Negative Syndrome Scale for Schizophrenia (PANSS), the Clinical Global Impression (CGI) scale, and the Rating of Aggression Against People and/or Property (RAAPP) scale.

DRUG THERAPY FOR PSYCHOSIS

Pharmacologic treatment of psychosis includes several classes of drugs. The most specific are the first- and second-generation antipsychotic agents, but benzodiazepines (see Chapter 15, p. 222) are often used to control acute psychotic symptoms. Beta-adrenergic–blocking agents (beta blockers) (e.g., propranolol) (see Chapter 12, p. 180), lithium (see Chapter 16, p. 249), anticonvulsants (valproic acid) (see Chapter 18, p. 285), carbamazepine (see Chapter 18, p. 275), antiparkinsonian agents (see Chapter 14), and anticholinergic agents (see Chapters 12, 14, pp. 183 and 215) occasionally play a role in controlling the adverse effects of medications used in antipsychotic therapy.

Antipsychotic (also known as *neuroleptic*) medications can be classified in several ways. Traditionally, they have been divided into phenothiazines and nonphenothiazines. Antipsychotic medications can also be classified as low-potency or high-potency drugs. The terms *low potency* and *high potency* refer only to the milligram doses used for these medicines and not to any difference in effectiveness (e.g., 100 mg of chlorpromazine, a low-potency drug, is equivalent in antipsychotic activity to 2 mg of haloperidol, a high-potency drug). Chlorpromazine and thioridazine are low-potency drugs, whereas trifluoperazine, fluphenazine, thiothixene, haloperidol, and loxapine are high-potency drugs. Since 1990, antipsychotic medications have also been classified as **typical (first-generation) antipsychotic agents** or **atypical (second-generation) antipsychotic agents** on the basis of their mechanism of action (Table 17-1). The atypical antipsychotic agents are aripiprazole, asenapine, clozapine, iloperidone, olanzapine, quetiapine, risperidone, lurasidone, and ziprasidone. All of the remaining antipsychotic agents listed in Table 17-1 are typical antipsychotic agents.

ACTIONS

The typical antipsychotic medications block the neurotransmitter dopamine in the central nervous system (CNS). The atypical antipsychotic agents block dopamine receptors, but they also block serotonin receptors to varying degrees. However, the exact mechanisms whereby these actions prevent psychotic symptoms are unknown. There is substantially more to the development of psychotic symptoms than elevated dopamine levels. There are at least five known types of dopamine receptors and several more types of serotonin receptors in various areas of the CNS. Antipsychotic medications also stimulate or block cholinergic, histaminic, nicotinic, alpha-adrenergic, and beta-adrenergic neurotransmitter receptors to varying degrees, accounting for many of the adverse effects of therapy.

USES

All antipsychotic medications are equal in efficacy when used in **equipotent doses.** There is some unpredictable variation among patients, however, and individual patients sometimes show a better response to particular drugs. In general, medication should be selected on the basis of the need to avoid certain adverse effects when dealing with concurrent medical or psychiatric disorders. Despite practice trends, no proof exists that agitation responds best to sedating drugs or that withdrawn patients respond best to nonsedating drugs. Medication history should be a major factor in drug selection. The final important factors in drug selection are the clinically important differences in the frequency of adverse effects. No single drug is

least likely to cause all adverse effects; thus individual response should be the best determinant of which drug is to be used. The atypical antipsychotic agents tend to be more effective in relieving the negative and cognitive symptoms associated with schizophrenia and treating refractory schizophrenia, and they have a much lower incidence of **extrapyramidal symptoms (EPSs)** and hyperprolactinemia.

The initial goals of antipsychotic therapy are calming the agitated patient who may be a physical threat to himself or herself or to others and beginning the treatment of the psychosis and thought disorder. Combined therapy with benzodiazepines (often lorazepam) and antipsychotic medications allows lower dosages of the antipsychotic medication to be used, reducing the risk of serious adverse effects more commonly seen with higher-dose therapy. Some therapeutic effects, such as reduced psychomotor agitation and insomnia, are observed within 1 week of therapy, but reductions in hallucinations, delusions, and thought disorder often require 6 to 8 weeks of treatment to achieve the full therapeutic effect. Rapid increases in the dosing of antipsychotic medications will not reduce the antipsychotic response time. Patients, families, and the healthcare team must be informed about giving antipsychotic agents an adequate chance to work before unnecessarily escalating the dosage and increasing the risk of adverse effects.

 Clinical Pitfall

During episodes of acute psychosis, the patient is out of touch with reality and often does not understand the need to take medicines that will help stabilize his or her condition. The nurse must ensure that the patient has actually swallowed the medication when it is administered and not just "mouthed" or "cheeked" it. Outpatients often require that medication administration be supervised to ensure adherence to the medication regimen. In some cases, it is necessary to inject long-acting medicines to overcome a patient's nonadherence problem. After an acute psychotic episode has resolved and the patient is free from overt psychotic symptoms, a decision must be made as to whether maintenance therapy is necessary. This will depend on the diagnosed psychotic disorder and the patient's tolerance of the adverse effects of the medication. However, most psychotic disorders are treated with lower maintenance dosages to minimize the risk of recurrence of the disorder episodes (Box 17-1).

ADVERSE EFFECTS OF ANTIPSYCHOTIC DRUG THERAPY

EXTRAPYRAMIDAL SYMPTOMS

Many of the serious adverse effects of antipsychotic medications can be attributed to the pharmacologic effect of blocking dopaminergic, cholinergic, histaminic, serotonergic, and adrenergic neurotransmitter receptors. Although these agents block D_2 receptors in the mesolimbic area of the brain to stop psychotic

Table 17-1   Antipsychotic Agents

GENERIC NAME	BRAND NAME	AVAILABILITY	ADULT DOSAGE RANGE (mg)	MAJOR ADVERSE EFFECTS			
				SEDATION	EXTRAPYRAMIDAL SYMPTOMS	HYPOTENSION	ANTICHOLINERGIC EFFECTS
Typical (First-Generation) Antipsychotic Agents							
Phenothiazines							
chlorpromazine ⬆⬇ *Do not confuse chlorpromazine with chlordiazepoxide, chlorhexidine, chlorpropamide, or chlorthalidone.*	Teva-Chlorpromazine 🍁	Tablets: 10, 25, 50, 100, 200 mg Injection: 25 mg/mL	25-2000	+++	++	+++	++
fluphenazine 🍁	Modecate 🍁	Tablets: 1, 2.5, 5, 10 mg Elixir: 2.5 mg/5 mL Concentrate: 5 mg/mL Injection: 2.5 mg/mL	0.5-40	+	+++	+	+
perphenazine	—	Tablets: 2, 4, 8, 16 mg	12-64	+	+++	+	++
prochlorperazine	Compazine, Compro, PMS-Prochlorperazine 🍁	Tablets: 5, 10 mg Injection: 5 mg/mL Suppository: 25 mg	15-150	+	+++	+	+
thioridazine	—	Tablets: 10, 25, 50, 100 mg	150-800	+++	+	+++	+++
trifluoperazine	—	Tablets: 1, 2, 5, 10 mg	2-40	+	+++	+	+
Thioxanthenes							
thiothixene		Capsules: 1, 2, 5, 10, mg	6-60	+	+++	+	+
Nonphenothiazines							
haloperidol	Haldol, Apo-Haloperidol 🍁	Tablets: 0.5, 1, 2, 5, 10, 20 mg Concentrate: 2 mg/mL Injection: 5 mg/mL Injection, sustained-release: 50, 100 mg	1-100	+	+++	+	+
loxapine ⬆⬇ *Do not confuse loxapine with Lexapro.*	Loxitane, Xylac 🍁	Capsules: 5, 10, 25, 50 mg	20-250	++	+++	++	+

Atypical (Second-Generation) Antipsychotic Agents

Generic name	Brand name / Notes	Availability	Dosage range (mg)				
aripiprazole	Abilify	Tablets: 2, 5, 10, 15, 20, 30 mg; Tablets, orally disintegrating: 10, 15 mg; Solution: 1 mg/mL; Injection: 7.5 mg/mL; Injection suspension: 300, 400 mg	10-30	0	+	+	+
asenapine	Saphris	Tablet, sublingual: 5, 10 mg	5-20	+	++	++	++
clozapine	Clozaril, Gen-clozapine ⬥ *Do not confuse Clozaril with Clinoril or Colazal.*	Tablets: 25, 50, 100, 200 mg; Tablets, orally disintegrating: 12.5, 25, 100, 150, 200 mg	300-900	++	+++	+	+++
iloperidone	Fanapt	Tablets: 1, 2, 4, 6, 8, 10, 12 mg	2-24	++	++	+	++
lurasidone	Latuda	Tablets: 20, 40, 60, 80, 120 mg	20-160	++	++	++	++
olanzapine ⇅ *Do not confuse olanzapine with oxcarbazepine.*	Zyprexa ⇅ *Do not confuse Zyprexa with Celexa, Zaroxolyn, or Zyrtec.*	Tablets: 2.5, 5, 7.5, 10, 15, 20 mg; Tablets, orally disintegrating: 5, 10, 15, 20 mg; Injection: 10 mg; Injection, sustained release: 210, 300, 405 mg	PO: 5-20 mg; IM: 30 mg	+++	++	+	++
quetiapine	Seroquel, Seroquel XR ⇅ *Do not confuse Seroquel with Symmetrel or Sertraline.*	Tablets: 25, 50, 100, 200, 300, 400 mg; Tablets, extended release: 50, 150, 200, 300, 400 mg	50-800	0	++	+	++
risperidone	Risperdal ⇅ *Do not confuse Risperdal with estradiol, reserpine, Restoril, risedronate, or ropinirole.*	Tablets: 0.25, 0.5, 1, 2, 3, 4 mg; Tablets, orally disintegrating 0.25, 0.5, 1, 2, 3, 4 mg; PO solution: 1 mg/mL; IM injection, suspension: 12.5, 25, 37.5, 50 mg	2-16	+	+	++	++
ziprasidone ⇅ *Do not confuse ziprasidone with zidovudine.*	Geodon	Capsules: 20, 40, 60, 80 mg; Injection: 20 mg	40-160	++	+	++	+

+, Low; ++, moderate; +++, high.
⬥ Available in Canada.

Box 17-1	Antipsychotic Medicines

Patients who begin antipsychotic drug therapy can expect some therapeutic effects, such as reduced psychomotor agitation and insomnia, within 1 week of starting treatment. However, reduction in hallucinations, delusions, and thought disorders often requires 6 to 8 weeks for a full therapeutic response to be achieved. Rapid increases in dosages of antipsychotic medications will not reduce the antipsychotic response time, but will increase the frequency of adverse effects.

Antipsychotic medicines may produce extrapyramidal effects. Tardive dyskinesia may be reversible during its early stages, but it becomes irreversible with continued use of the antipsychotic medication. Regular assessment for tardive dyskinesia should be performed for all patients receiving antipsychotic drugs. Older adult patients should be observed for hypotension and tardive dyskinesia.

symptoms, blockade of D_2 receptors in other areas of the brain explains the occurrence of extrapyramidal symptoms (EPSs).

Extrapyramidal symptoms are the most troublesome adverse effects and the most common cause of nonadherence associated with antipsychotic therapy. There are four categories of EPSs: dystonic reactions, pseudoparkinsonism, akathisia, and tardive dyskinesia.

Acute dystonia has the earliest onset of all the EPSs. **Dystonias** are spasmodic movements (prolonged tonic contractions) of muscle groups such as tongue protrusion, rolling back of the eyes (oculogyric crisis), jaw spasm (trismus), and neck torsion (torticollis). These symptoms are often frightening and painful for the patient. Approximately 90% of all dystonic reactions occur during the first 72 hours of therapy. Dystonic reactions are most frequent in male patients, younger patients, and patients receiving high-potency medications such as haloperidol. Dystonic reactions are generally brief, and they are the EPSs most responsive to treatment. Acute dystonic reactions may be controlled by intramuscular injections of diphenhydramine, benztropine, diazepam, or lorazepam. Rating scales for assessing patients with different forms of dystonias include the Toronto Western Spasmodic Torticollis Rating Scale (TWSTRS), the Global Dystonia Scale (GDS), the Unified Dystonia Rating Scale (UDRS), and the Fahn-Marsden Scale.

Pseudoparkinsonian symptoms of tremor, muscular rigidity, masklike expression, shuffling gait, and loss or weakness of motor function typically begin after 2 to 3 weeks of antipsychotic drug therapy, but may occur up to 3 months after starting therapy. They are more commonly seen in older adults. These symptoms result from a relative deficiency of dopamine, with cholinergic excess caused by antipsychotic medica-

tions, and are well controlled by anticholinergic antiparkinsonian drugs (e.g., benztropine, diphenhydramine, trihexyphenidyl).

Akathisia is a syndrome consisting of subjective feelings of anxiety and restlessness and objective signs of pacing, rocking, and inability to sit or stand in one place for extended periods. Akathisia can increase aggression and is a frequent cause of noncompliance. It occurs more commonly when high-potency antipsychotic medications are used. The mechanism of action is unknown. Reducing the dosage of the antipsychotic medication or switching to a lower-potency drug should be considered. Treatment with anticholinergic agents, benzodiazepines (e.g., diazepam, lorazepam), beta blockers (e.g., propranolol), and clonidine has shown varying degrees of success.

Tardive dyskinesia is a syndrome of persistent and involuntary hyperkinetic abnormal movements. It develops in about 20% to 25% of patients receiving typical antipsychotic medications on a long-term basis (e.g., months to years). There appears to be a lower incidence in patients receiving atypical antipsychotic agents, but these agents are newer and it sometimes takes years for tardive dyskinesia to develop. This drug-induced, late-appearing neurologic disorder is noted for such symptoms as buccolingual masticatory (BLM) syndrome or orofacial movements. The BLM movements begin with mild forward, backward, or lateral tongue movement. As the disorder progresses, more obvious movements appear, including tongue thrusting, rolling, or fly-catching movements, as well as chewing or lateral jaw movements that produce smacking noises. Symptoms may interfere with the patient's ability to chew, speak, or swallow. Facial movements include frequent blinking, brow arching, grimacing, and upward deviation of the eyes. The severity of symptoms of tardive dyskinesia can fluctuate daily, and symptoms often will remit during sleep. The clinical manifestations of tardive dyskinesia are similar to those of dystonias, but there are some significant differences. Tardive dyskinesia typically appears after antipsychotic dosage reduction or discontinuation, it improves when the antipsychotic dosage is increased, it worsens with the administration of anticholinergic agents, and it may persist for months or years after antipsychotic medicines are discontinued. The exact cause of tardive dyskinesia is unknown. Early signs may be reversible, but, over time, they may become irreversible, even with discontinuation of the antipsychotic medicine.

The best treatment approach to tardive dyskinesia is prevention. Patients who receive maintenance antipsychotic drug therapy should be assessed for early signs of tardive dyskinesia at least semiannually and preferably quarterly. Findings should be documented in patient records to ensure continuity of care and medicolegal protection. Because of the variability in severity and presentation, rating scales have been developed to standardize assessments and diagnoses. The **Abnormal Involuntary Movement Scale (AIMS)** rates dyskinetic movements, but it is not exclusively diagnostic for tardive dyskinesia (see Evolve website). The **Dyskinesia Identification System: Condensed User Scale (DISCUS)** rates the presence and severity of abnormal movements and considers other variables when formulating a conclusion. The DISCUS evaluation specifically describes the type of tardive dyskinesia and allows diagnoses to change over time (see Evolve website).

Treatment of tardive dyskinesia is not particularly successful. The most beneficial treatments are anticholinergic withdrawal, adrenergic blocking agents (e.g., beta blockers, clonidine), and benzodiazepines. Antipsychotic dosages may be increased, but they may only mask symptoms, and they eventually will worsen tardive dyskinesia. Patients receiving typical antipsychotic therapy who have severe symptoms of tardive dyskinesia and who must be maintained on antipsychotic therapy may be candidates for atypical antipsychotic therapy.

Neuroleptic malignant syndrome (NMS) is a potentially fatal adverse effect of antipsychotic therapy in which the patient displays EPSs as part of the symptoms of the disorder. It occurs in 0.5% to 1.4% of patients receiving antipsychotic therapy and is reported most often with high-potency antipsychotic agents given intramuscularly. It typically occurs after 3 to 9 days of treatment with antipsychotic medications, and it is not related to dosage or previous drug exposure. Once NMS begins, symptoms rapidly progress over 24 to 72 hours. Symptoms usually last for 5 to 10 days after discontinuation of oral medications and 13 to 30 days with **depot antipsychotic medicine** (*depot*, injectable, slow-release dose form). Most cases of NMS occur in patients younger than 40 years old, and it occurs twice as often in men. The syndrome is characterized by the following: fever, severe EPSs (e.g., lead-pipe rigidity, trismus, choreiform movements, opisthotonos), autonomic instability (e.g., tachycardia, labile hypertension, diaphoresis, incontinence), and alterations in consciousness (e.g., stupor, mutism, coma). Mortality rates have been as high as 30%, but prompt recognition of the symptoms has reduced the mortality rate to 4% in recent years. It is hypothesized that the cause of the symptoms is excessive dopamine depletion. Treatment includes bromocriptine or amantadine as dopamine agonists and dantrolene as a muscle relaxant. Fever is treated with cooling blankets, adequate hydration, and antipyretics. After the patient's condition has stabilized, a thorough evaluation of the medications being prescribed must be made. Resumption of the antipsychotic medication may result in a recurrence of NMS; therefore the lowest dose possible of an antipsychotic agent is prescribed, and close observation of the patient's response is required.

SEIZURES

Antipsychotic agents may lower the seizure threshold in patients with seizure disorders and even in those with no previous history of seizures. The low-potency typical agents and clozapine, an atypical agent, have a higher incidence of inducing seizures.

WEIGHT GAIN

Antipsychotic drug therapy often causes substantial weight gain. There is a higher prevalence of obesity associated with schizophrenia, and the weight gain often contributes to nonadherence to therapy. Obesity leads to an increased risk of type 2 diabetes mellitus, dyslipidemia, hypertension, coronary heart disease, and stroke (see Chapter 20). The frequency and amount of weight gain are generally greater with atypical agents than with typical medications, although individual atypical agents vary in the extent to which they cause weight gain. Of the atypical agents, clozapine and olanzapine cause the most weight gain, moderate weight gain is reported with risperidone and quetiapine, and aripiprazole and ziprasidone cause the least weight gain.

HYPERGLYCEMIA

A relatively new adverse effect being reported—particularly with atypical antipsychotic agents—is hyperglycemia and the development of diabetes mellitus. The mechanism whereby this occurs is unknown, and research in this area is more difficult because patients with schizophrenia also have a two- to three-fold higher incidence of diabetes mellitus than the general population. Hyperglycemia occurs more frequently with clozapine, olanzapine, and quetiapine, but development of hyperglycemia with the other atypical agents cannot yet be ruled out because these agents are new.

DYSLIPIDEMIA

Clozapine, olanzapine, and quetiapine appear to increase serum triglyceride levels. They do not increase cholesterol levels, although they may appear to do so because serum triglycerides are a component of total serum cholesterol values. The increase in serum triglyceride levels may occur without a change in weight, although increased body weight will contribute to the hypertriglyceridemia.

DYSRHYTHMIAS

Thioridazine, ziprasidone, haloperidol, quetiapine, olanzapine, asenapine, iloperidone, lurasidone, and risperidone have rarely been associated with torsades de pointes—a ventricular dysrhythmia associated with prolongation of the QTc interval on the electrocardiogram, syncope, and sudden death. Bradycardia, electrolyte imbalance (hypokalemia, hypomagnesemia), presence of congenital prolongation of the QTc interval, and concomitant use of other medications that may significantly prolong the QTc interval (e.g., quinidine, sotalol, moxifloxacin, dofetilide) can increase the risk of torsades de pointes and sudden death in patients receiving antipsychotic agents.

OTHER ADVERSE EFFECTS

Other adverse effects of antipsychotic therapy can also be predicted on the basis of the receptor-blocking activity of the agents:

- Blocking the cholinergic (acetylcholine) receptors explains the anticholinergic effects (e.g., dry mouth, constipation, sinus tachycardia, blurred vision, inhibition or impairment of ejaculation, urinary retention) associated with antipsychotic agents.
- Blocking histamine-1 receptors causes sedation, drowsiness, and appetite stimulation, and contributes to the hypotensive effects and potentiation of CNS depressant drugs. Antipsychotic agents also block alpha-1 and alpha-2 adrenergic receptors, causing postural hypotension, sexual dysfunction, reflex tachycardia, and potentiation of antihypertensive agents. The most potent alpha-1 blockers are chlorpromazine and thioridazine, whereas haloperidol has almost no effect on alpha-1 receptors.

Antipsychotic agents may produce many adverse effects other than those already listed, including hepatotoxicity, blood dyscrasias, allergic reactions, endocrine disorders, skin pigmentation, and reversible effects in the eyes. Patients receiving clozapine are particularly susceptible to developing agranulocytosis. Regularly scheduled white blood cell (WBC) counts are mandatory.

 Clinical Pitfall

Antipsychotic medicines may have adverse effects such as seizure activity, parkinsonian symptoms, tardive dyskinesia, and hepatotoxicity that require management by the prescribing healthcare provider. The patient and those providing supervision need to understand the importance of reporting any of these symptoms promptly for appropriate interventions.

❖ NURSING IMPLICATIONS FOR ANTIPSYCHOTIC THERAPY

■ Assessment

History of Behavior

- Gather information from the patient and other individuals relating to the onset, duration, and progression of the patient's symptoms. Has the patient previously been treated for this or other mental disorders? Does the patient have any coexisting health conditions?
- Take a detailed history of all medications that the patient is taking or has taken during the past 3 months.
- Inquire about the use of substances.

Basic Mental Status

- Note the patient's general appearance and appropriateness of attire. Is the patient clean and neat? Is the posture erect, stooped, or slumped? Is the patient oriented to date, time, place, and person?
- What coping mechanisms has the patient been using to deal with the situation? How adaptive are the coping mechanisms? Initiate changes in maladaptive coping mechanisms by guiding the patient toward the use of more adaptive coping strategies.
- Has the patient been able to carry out self-care activities and social and work obligations?
- Are symptoms of depression present? Symptoms may not be evident during the acute phase of schizophrenia.

Interpersonal Relationships. Assess the quality of the relationships in which the patient is involved. Identify people in the patient's life who are supportive. Ask the family and significant others to describe the relationship they have with the patient. Has there been deterioration in their closeness and their ability to interrelate effectively?

Mood and Affect. Patients experiencing altered thinking, behavior, or feelings require careful evaluation of their verbal and nonverbal actions. Often the thoughts, feelings, and behaviors displayed are inconsistent with the so-called "normal" responses of individuals in similar circumstances.

- Is the facial expression worried, sad, angry, or blank?
- Is the patient displaying behaviors that are inappropriate or blunted? Does the patient have a flat affect?
- Is the patient apathetic to normal situations?
- Is there consistency when the patient is expressing feelings verbally and nonverbally?
- Does the patient overreact to situations at times?

Clarity of Thoughts and Perception

- Does the patient suffer from delusions, disorganized speech pattern, flight of ideas, autism, grandiose ideas, or mutism? Ask about the presence of hallucinations (auditory, visual, tactile).
- Does the patient talk about unrelated topics (loose association) as though they are connected and related?
- Is the patient self-absorbed and not in contact with reality?
- Does the patient display an interruption of thoughts?
- Does the patient display paranoid behavior?

Suicidal Ideation. If the individual is suspected of being suicidal, ask the patient whether he or she has ever had thoughts about suicide. If the response is "yes," get more details. Has a specific plan been formulated? How often do these thoughts occur? Does the patient make direct or indirect statements regarding death (e.g., "things would be better" if death occurred)?

Psychomotor Function. What is the patient's activity level? Is the individual unable to sit still and instead paces continually? Is the patient catatonic (i.e., immobile as a result of psychological functioning)?

Sleep Pattern. What is the patient's normal sleep pattern, and how has it varied since the onset of the psychotic symptoms? Ask specifically whether insomnia is present. Ask the patient to describe the perception of the amount and quality of sleep nightly. What is the level of fatigue? Are naps taken regularly?

Dietary History. Ask questions about the patient's appetite and note weight gains or losses not associated with intentional dieting.

▪ Implementation

- Nursing interventions must be individualized and based on patient assessment data.
- Provide the individual with a structured environment that is safe and that decreases external stimuli.
- Provide an environment of acceptance that focuses on the individual's strengths while minimizing weaknesses.
- Provide an opportunity for the patient to express feelings. Use active listening and therapeutic communication techniques. Allow the patient to express feelings in nonverbal ways, such as involvement in physical activities or occupational therapy.
- Allow the patient to make decisions, if capable; make those decisions that the patient is not capable of making. Provide a reward for progress when decisions are initiated appropriately.
- Involve the patient in self-care activities. Assist with personal grooming as needed. Ensure that the patient is dressed appropriately.
- Set limits for the patient to handle inappropriate behaviors, and enforce them in a kind, firm manner.
- Once the content is known, do not reinforce the patient's hallucinations or delusions.
- When the patient has altered perceptions, provide diversionary activities and minimize interactions, such as viewing television programs that may reinforce the distorted perceptions.
- Be open and direct when handling a patient who is highly suspicious. Speak distinctly to be heard; do not whisper or laugh in circumstances that the patient could misconstrue.
- If the patient is suicidal, ask for details about the plan being formulated. Follow up on details obtained with appropriate family members or significant others (e.g., have guns removed from the home if this is part of the suicide plan). Provide for patient safety and supervision, and record observations at specified intervals consistent with the severity of the suicide threat and the policies of the practice site.
- Use physical restraints within the guidelines of the clinical setting as appropriate to the behaviors being exhibited. Use the least restrictive alternative possible for the circumstances. Have sufficient staff available to assist with violent behavior to demonstrate the ability to control the situation while providing for the safety and well-being of the patient and fellow staff members.
- Provide for nutritional needs by having high-protein, high-calorie foods appropriate for the individual to eat while pacing or highly active. Have nutritious snacks that the patient is known to like available on the unit, and offer them throughout the day. Give vitamins and liquid supplemental feedings as ordered.
- Provide an opportunity for the individual to be involved in selecting foods appropriate to needs (to lose or gain weight). If the person is paranoid and suspects being poisoned, allow the individual to self-serve food, open canned food, and perform other activities, as appropriate within the setting.
- Manipulative behavior must be handled in a consistent manner by all staff members. Set limits and use consequences that are agreed to in advance by all staff members. When the patient attempts to blame others, refocus on the patient's responsibilities. Give positive reinforcement for nonmanipulative behaviors when they occur.

▪ Patient Education

- Orient the individual to the unit. Explain the rules and the process of privileges and how they are obtained or lost. (The extent of the orientation and explanations given will depend on the patient's orientation to date, time, and place, as well as his or her abilities.)
- Explain the unit rules and the therapeutic rules. Keep the explanations clear and concise.
- Base patient education on assessment data and individualize instruction to provide the patient with a structured environment in which to grow and enhance his or her self-esteem.
- Explain the activity groups available and how and when the individual will participate in them. A variety of group process activities (e.g., social skills group, self-esteem group, physical exercise group) are available in different therapeutic settings.
- Involve the patient and family in establishing outcomes, and integrate the patient into the appropriate group processes to develop positive experiences to enhance coping skills. Patients who are disruptive or withdrawn or who have impaired communication require individualized approaches to patient education.
- Before discharge, make sure the patient and the family understand the desired treatment outcomes and the entire follow-up plan (e.g., frequency of therapy sessions, prescribed medications, physician visits, return-to-work goals).

Fostering Health Maintenance

- Throughout the course of treatment, discuss medication information and how it will benefit the patient's symptoms and circumstances. Drug therapy is a major portion of antipsychotic therapy. Although symptoms may improve, they may not be totally eliminated. The onset of a drug's effectiveness varies widely, depending on the drug and the route of administration.

- Nonadherence is a major problem in this group of patients; therefore tracking the medications being taken requires careful scrutiny. On an outpatient basis, many of these patients need their medications administered by another responsible individual; the patient may find this stressful. Nonadherence is thought to be a major cause of repeat hospitalization in these patients. Long-acting injections may be used for some patients in an attempt to overcome this problem. On an inpatient basis, the nurse must always check to be sure that the patient is actually swallowing the medication because there is a high incidence of "cheeking" (i.e., hiding drugs between the teeth and gums).
- Use baseline clinical evaluation rating scales (e.g., BPRS, CGI, PANSS) and adverse effect scales (e.g., GDS, TWSTRS for dystonias, DISCUS or AIMS for EPSs) at specified intervals; record and report findings in accordance with agency policy.
- Provide the patient and significant others with important information contained in the specific drug monograph for the medicines prescribed. Additional health teaching and nursing interventions for common and serious adverse effects are described in the drug monographs that follow.
- Seek cooperation and understanding of the following points so that medication adherence is increased: name of the medication; its dosage, route, and time of administration; and its common and serious adverse effects. Encourage the patient not to discontinue or adjust the drug dosage without consulting the healthcare provider. Provide the patient and family with information about available community resources, including the NAMI.

Patient Self-Assessment. Enlist the patient's help with developing and maintaining a written record of monitoring parameters. See the Template for Developing a Written Record for Patients to Monitor Their Own Therapy on the Evolve website, and complete the Premedication Data column for an assessment of the patient's physical and mental capabilities as a baseline to track the patient's response to drug therapy. Ensure that the patient understands how to use the form, and instruct the patient to bring the completed form to follow-up visits. Because there are a number of debilitating adverse effects and others that are life threatening if they are not acted on correctly, it is important to maintain open communication with healthcare providers, nurses, therapists, and pharmacists throughout the course of therapy.

DRUG CLASS: ANTIPSYCHOTIC AGENTS

Phenothiazines, thioxanthenes, haloperidol, aripiprazole, asenapine, loxapine, clozapine, iloperidone, olanzapine, quetiapine, risperidone, ziprasidone

Typical (First-Generation) Antipsychotic Agents
phenothiazines (fēn-ō-THĪ-ă-zēnz)
thioxanthenes (thē-ō-ZĂN-thēnz)
  thiothixene
Nonphenothiazines
haloperidol (hăl-ō-PĚR-ĭ-dŏl)
  Haldol, Apo-Haloperidol (HĂL-dŏl, ă-pō-hăl-ō-PĚR-ĭ-dŏl)
loxapine (LŎKS-ă-pēn)
  ⮀ Do not confuse loxapine with Lexapro.
  Loxitane, Xylac (LŎKS-ĭ-tăn, ZĪ-lăk)

Atypical (Second-Generation) Antipsychotic Agents
aripiprazole (ăr-ĭ-PĬP-ră-zōl)
  Abilify (ă-BĬL-ĭ-fī)
asenapine (ă-SĚN-ă-pēn)
  Saphris (SĂF-rĭs)
clozapine (CLŎZ-ă-pēn)
  Clozaril, Gen-clozapine (CLŎZ-ă-rĭl, jĕn-CLŎZ-ă-pēn)
  ⮀ Do not confuse Clozaril with Clinoril or Colazal.
iloperidone (ĭ-lō-PĚR-ĭ-dōn)
  Fanapt (FĂN-ăpt)
olanzapine (ō-LĂN-ză-pēn)
  ⮀ Do not confuse olanzapine with oxcarbazepine.
  Zyprexa (zī-PRĚK-să)
  ⮀ Do not confuse Zyprexa with Celexa, Zaroxolyn, or Zyrtec.
quetiapine (kwĕt-Ī-ă-pēn)
  Seroquel, Seroquel XR (SĚR-ō-kwĕl)
  ⮀ Do not confuse Seroquel with Symmetrel or Sertraline.
risperidone (rĭs-PĚR-ĭ-dōn)
  Risperdal (RĬS-pĕr-dăl)
  ⮀ Do not confuse Risperdal with estradiol, reserpine, Restoril, risedronate, or ropinirole.
ziprasidone (zĭ-PRĂ-sĭ-dōn)
  ⮀ Do not confuse ziprasidone with zidovudine.
  Geodon (GĒ-ō-dŏn)

ACTIONS

Although the antipsychotic medications are from distinctly different chemical classes, all are similar in that they act by blocking the action of dopamine in the brain. The atypical antipsychotic agents block serotonin receptors in addition to dopamine receptors. Because all the antipsychotic agents work at different sites in the brain, adverse effects are observed in different body systems. Atypical antipsychotic agents tend to be more effective and have fewer adverse effects than typical agents.

USES

Antipsychotic agents are used to treat psychoses associated with mental illnesses such as schizophrenia, mania, psychotic depression, and psychotic organic brain syndrome. Medications used to treat these disorders are grouped into two broad categories: first-generation antipsychotic drugs (also known as *typical antipsychotic drugs,* including the phenothiazines and nonphenothiazines [e.g., thioxanthenes, haloperidol, loxapine]) and second-generation antipsychotic drugs (also known as *atypical antipsychotic drugs* (see Table 17-1) [e.g., aripiprazole, asenapine, clozapine, iloperidone, lurasidone, olanzapine, quetiapine, risperidone, ziprasidone]). Aripiprazole, olanzapine, quetiapine, risperidone, and ziprasidone are now considered to be first-line, second-generation antipsychotic drugs that provide significant relief of active psychotic symptoms such as hallucinations, delusions, and thought disorganization for approximately 70% of patients with schizophrenia. Aripiprazole is approved for treating schizophrenia in 13- to 17-year-old patients and as an adjunctive treatment to antidepressant therapy in adults with major depressive disorder. It is also approved for treating acute manic and mixed episodes associated with bipolar disorder. Quetiapine is approved for treating schizophrenia and depressive episodes associated with bipolar disorder. Clozapine is reserved for more resistant cases that do not respond adequately to the other atypical agents. All these antipsychotic medications also significantly reduce the risk of recurrence.

As clinical experience is being gained with the relatively new second-generation antipsychotic drugs, dramatic weight gain, diabetes mellitus, electrocardiographic changes (e.g., QT-interval prolongation), and dyslipidemia have been reported. The risk of these potentially serious adverse effects is not the same with all drugs, but the U.S. Food and Drug Administration has issued precautionary statements to encourage close monitoring of body weight, blood glucose, and serum lipid levels in all patients receiving these antipsychotic agents.

THERAPEUTIC OUTCOME

The primary therapeutic outcome expected from antipsychotic therapy is maintaining the individual at an optimal level of functioning, with minimal exacerbations of psychotic symptoms and minimal adverse effects from medicines.

❖ NURSING IMPLICATIONS FOR ANTIPSYCHOTIC AGENT THERAPY

▪ Premedication Assessment

1. Obtain baseline blood pressures with the patient supine, sitting, and standing; record and report significant lowering to the healthcare provider before administering the medicine. Monitor on a yearly basis thereafter.
2. Check the patient's electrolyte levels, body weight, waist circumference, height, blood glucose level, lipid profile, hepatic function, cardiac function, and thyroid function before initiating therapy and periodically throughout the course of treatment. Weight should be monitored every 4 weeks until 12 weeks after initiating therapy and then every 3 months. Monitor waist circumference and fasting plasma glucose level annually and fasting lipid levels every 5 years.
3. Use baseline clinical evaluation rating scales (e.g., BPRS, CGI, PANSS) and adverse effect scales (e.g., GDS, TWSTRS for dystonias, DISCUS or AIMS for EPSs) at specified intervals; record and report findings in accordance with agency policy.
4. Use of clozapine requires a baseline WBC count and weekly WBC counts for the first 6 months of treatment because of the high incidence of agranulocytosis. Thereafter, if WBC counts are acceptable (i.e., $\geq 3500/mm^3$) and if the absolute neutrophil count is more than $2000/mm^3$, WBC counts can be monitored every other week. White blood cell counts must be monitored weekly for at least 4 weeks after the discontinuation of clozapine.

▪ Availability, Dosage, and Administration

See Table 17-1. The dosage must be individualized according to the patient's degree of mental and emotional disturbance. It will often take several weeks for a patient to show optimal improvement and become stabilized on an adequate maintenance dosage. As a result of the cumulative effects of antipsychotic agents, the patient must be reevaluated periodically to determine the lowest effective dosage necessary to control psychiatric symptoms.

▪ Common Adverse Effects
Neurologic

Chronic fatigue, drowsiness. Chronic fatigue and drowsiness are common problems associated with medications used to treat psychoses. Sedative effects associated with antipsychotic therapy can be minimized by giving the dose of medication at bedtime. The patient should not take these medications while working with machinery, operating a motor vehicle, administering medication, or performing other duties that require mental alertness.

Cardiovascular

Orthostatic hypotension. All antipsychotic agents may cause some degree of orthostatic hypotension manifested by dizziness and weakness, particularly when therapy is initiated. Monitor the patient's blood pressure daily in the supine, sitting, and standing positions. Anticipate the development of postural hypotension, and take measures to prevent an occurrence. Teach the patient to rise slowly from a supine or sitting position, and encourage the patient to sit or lie down if feeling faint.

Sensory

Blurred vision. Caution the patient that blurred vision may occur, and make appropriate suggestions to ensure the patient's personal safety.

Genitourinary

Urinary retention. Urinary retention may occur after the administration of antipsychotic agents.

Gastrointestinal

Constipation; dryness of mucosa of the mouth, throat, nose. Mucosal dryness may be relieved by sucking hard candy or ice chips or by chewing gum. A high-fiber diet, stool softeners (e.g., docusate), or the occasional use of a stimulant laxative (e.g., bisacodyl) may be required to treat constipation.

■ Serious Adverse Effects

Neurologic

Seizure activity. Provide for patient safety during episodes of seizures; report this symptom to the healthcare provider for further evaluation. An adjustment of anticonvulsant therapy may be required, especially for seizure-prone patients.

Parkinsonian symptoms. Report the development of drooling, cogwheel rigidity, shuffling gait, mask-like expression, or tremors. Anticholinergic agents may be used to help control these symptoms.

Tardive dyskinesia. Tardive dyskinesia occurs much more commonly with the first-generation antipsychotic drugs. Report the development of fine tremors of the tongue, "fly-catching" tongue movements, and lip smacking. This is particularly important for patients who have been receiving antipsychotic drugs and anticholinergic medications for several years.

Gastrointestinal

Hepatotoxicity. The symptoms of hepatotoxicity are anorexia, nausea, vomiting, jaundice, hepatomegaly, splenomegaly, and abnormal liver function test results (e.g., elevated bilirubin, aspartate aminotransferase [AST], alanine aminotransferase [ALT], gamma-glutamyltransferase [GGT], and alkaline phosphatase levels, increased prothrombin time).

Hematologic

Blood dyscrasias. Routine laboratory studies (e.g., red blood cell [RBC], WBC, and differential counts) should be scheduled. This is particularly important for patients receiving clozapine. Monitor for sore throat, fever, purpura, jaundice, or excessive and progressive weakness.

Hypersensitivity

Hives, pruritus, rash. Report these symptoms to the healthcare provider for further evaluation.

Other

Photosensitivity. The patient should be cautioned to avoid prolonged exposure to sunlight and ultraviolet light. Suggest that the patient wear long-sleeved clothing, a hat, and sunglasses when exposed to sunlight. Advise against using artificial tanning lamps.

■ Drug Interactions

Drugs That Increase Adverse Effects. Antihistamines, alcohol, analgesics, anesthetics, tranquilizers, barbiturates, opiates, St. John's wort, and sedative-hypnotics increase the toxic effects of antipsychotic drugs. Monitor the patient for excessive sedation and reduce the dosage of the previously mentioned drugs if necessary.

 Herbal Interactions

St. John's Wort

St. John's wort increases the toxic effects of antipsychotic medications.

Drugs That Decrease Therapeutic Effects

Dopamine agonists. Dopamine agonists (i.e., levodopa, bromocriptine, pergolide, amantadine, ropinirole, pramipexole) block the dopamine antagonist effects of the antipsychotic agents. Avoid concurrent use.

Carbamazepine. Carbamazepine stimulates the metabolism of haloperidol, clozapine, aripiprazole, iloperidone, olanzapine, risperidone, and ziprasidone. Adjustment of the dosage of the antipsychotic medicine may be required.

Erythromycin, clarithromycin, fluoxetine, fluvoxamine, grapefruit juice, ketoconazole, nefazodone. All of these agents inhibit the metabolism of aripiprazole, asenapine, clozapine, iloperidone, quetiapine, and ziprasidone, causing an increase in serum levels and potential toxicity from the antipsychotic drug. Dosages of the antipsychotic drug may need to be reduced by up to 50% to avoid toxicities.

Cimetidine. Cimetidine inhibits the metabolism of quetiapine, clozapine, and risperidone. The dosage of these medicines may need to be reduced to prevent adverse effects.

Phenytoin. Phenytoin increases the metabolism of quetiapine, thioridazine, and haloperidol. Increases in dosage of the antipsychotic medication may be necessary.

Beta blockers. Beta blockers (e.g., propranolol, timolol, nadolol, pindolol) significantly enhance the hypotensive effects of antipsychotic agents. Concurrent therapy is not recommended unless it is used to treat the adverse effects of antipsychotic agents.

Barbiturates. Barbiturates may stimulate the rate of metabolism of phenothiazines. Dosage adjustments of the antipsychotic agent may be necessary.

Insulin, oral hypoglycemic agents. Patients with prediabetes or diabetes must be monitored for the development of hyperglycemia, particularly during the early weeks of therapy. Assess patients regularly for glycosuria and report it to the healthcare provider if it occurs with any frequency. Patients receiving oral hypoglycemic agents or insulin may require a dosage adjustment.

Venlafaxine. Venlafaxine significantly inhibits the metabolism of haloperidol. Doses of haloperidol may have to be given less often to prevent potential toxicity.

Get Ready for the NCLEX® Examination!

Key Points

- Psychoses are symptoms of psychotic disorders—that is, illnesses in which the patient has lost touch with reality. The underlying illness must be treated, not just the psychosis.
- A combination of nonpharmacologic and pharmacologic therapies provides the most successful therapeutic outcomes.
- The emphasis on community treatment has ensured that almost all health care settings treat patients with psychotic symptoms. Community hospitals and health maintenance organizations now provide care to many psychiatric patients, and nurses increasingly serve residential care facilities. Many patients require years of antipsychotic drug treatment to prevent exacerbations of their illness.
- Although antipsychotic medications cause many adverse effects, most can be minimized by patient education, manipulation of dosage and administration, and sometimes adjunctive drug treatments. These patients require careful monitoring of target symptoms to maximize response and minimize adverse effects.

Additional Learning Resources

SG Go to your Study Guide for additional Review Questions for the NCLEX® Examination, Critical Thinking Clinical Situations, and other learning activities to help you master this chapter content.

evolve Go to your Evolve website (http://evolve.elsevier.com/Clayton) for additional online resources.

Review Questions for the NCLEX® Examination

1. A nurse is assessing a patient who has been admitted to the psychiatric unit and who has been hearing voices that told her to lock all her doors and not answer any phone calls. The nurse should administer which scale specific for schizophrenia?
   1. AIMS
   2. TWSTRS
   3. PANSS
   4. DISCUS

2. Which premedication assessments does the nurse complete for patients who have been prescribed antipsychotic agents? *(Select all that apply.)*
   1. Baseline rating scales (e.g., BPRS, CGI)
   2. Height and waist circumference
   3. Positional blood pressure reading
   4. Sleep patterns
   5. Dietary history

3. A patient who has been taking an antipsychotic agent develops tongue protrusion, jaw spasms, and neck torsions. What are these extrapyramidal symptoms referred to as?
   1. Akathisia
   2. Dystonias
   3. Neuroleptic malignant syndrome
   4. Pseudoparkinsonian symptoms

4. What are the major adverse effects of antipsychotic medications? *(Select all that apply.)*
   1. Extrapyramidal symptoms
   2. Seizures
   3. Weight loss
   4. Hypoglycemia
   5. Dyslipidemia

5. A psychotic patient began antipsychotic medications 1 week ago. What does the nurse expect the patient to experience? *(Select all that apply.)*
   1. Reduced auditory hallucinations
   2. Reduced delusions
   3. Rapid weight gain
   4. Reduced agitation
   5. Reduced insomnia

Objectives

1. Identify the different types of seizure disorders.
2. Identify nursing interventions during the management of seizure activity.
3. Cite the desired therapeutic outcomes from antiepileptic agents used for seizure disorders.
4. Identify the drug classes used to treat seizure disorders.
5. Describe the neurologic assessment performed on patients taking antiepileptic agents to monitor for common and serious adverse effects.

Key Terms

seizures (SĒ-zhŭrz) (p. 266)
epilepsy (ĔP-ĭ-lĕp-sē) (p. 266)
generalized seizures (JĔN-ŭr-ăl-īzd) (p. 266)
partial seizures (PĂR-shŭl) (p. 266)
anticonvulsants (ăn-tī-kŏn-VŬL-sănts) (p. 266)
antiepileptic drugs (ăn-tī-ĕp-ĭ-LĔP-tĭk) (p. 266)
tonic phase (TŎN-ĭk) (p. 267)
clonic phase (KLŎN-ĭk) (p. 267)
postictal state (PŌST-ĭk-tĕl) (p. 267)
status epilepticus (STĂ-tŭs ĕp-ĭ-LĔP-tĭk-ŭs) (p. 267)

atonic seizure (ĕ-TŎN-ĭk) (p. 267)
myoclonic seizures (mī-ō-KLŎN-ĭk) (p. 267)
absence (petit mal) epilepsy (ĂB-sĕns) (p. 267)
seizure threshold (THRĔSH-hōld) (p. 267)
gamma-aminobutyric acid (GABA) (GĂM-ă ă-mēn-ō-byū-TĪR-ĭk) (p. 268)
treatment responsive (TRĒT-mĕnt rē-SPŎN-sĭv) (p. 268)
treatment resistant (TRĒT-mĕnt rē-ZĪS-tĕnt) (p. 268)
gingival hyperplasia (JĬN-jĭ-văl hī-pŭr-PLĀ-zhă) (p. 270)
nystagmus (nĭs-TĂG-mŭs) (p. 274)

SEIZURE DISORDERS

Seizures are a symptom of an abnormality in the nerve cells of the brain. A seizure is a brief period of abnormal electrical activity in these nerve centers. Seizures may be convulsive (i.e., accompanied by violent, involuntary muscle contractions) or nonconvulsive. During a seizure, there is often a change in the person's consciousness, sensory and motor systems, subjective well-being, and objective behavior. Seizures may result from fever, head injury, brain tumor, meningitis, hypoglycemia, a drug overdose or withdrawal, or poisoning. It is estimated that 8% to 10% of all people will have a seizure during their lifetimes. If the seizures are chronic and recurrent, the patient is diagnosed as having epilepsy. Epilepsy is the most common of all neurologic disorders. It is not a single disease, but rather several different disorders that have one common characteristic: a sudden discharge of excessive electrical energy from nerve cells in the brain. An estimated 2.3 million Americans have these disorders, and approximately 125,000 new cases are diagnosed annually. The cause of epilepsy may be unknown (i.e., idiopathic), or it may be the result of a head injury, a brain tumor, meningitis, or a stroke.

Epilepsy has been classified in several ways. Traditionally, the most important subdivisions have been

grand mal, petit mal, psychomotor, and *Jacksonian* types. These conditions also can be grouped based on type of seizure, cause, location in the brain involved, causal factors, and the patient's age at onset, as well as their severity, frequency, and prognosis. An international commission reclassified epilepsies into two broad categories based on their clinical and electroencephalographic (EEG) patterns: generalized and partial (localized). Generalized seizures refer to those that affect both hemispheres of the brain, are accompanied by a loss of consciousness, and may be subdivided into convulsive and nonconvulsive types. Partial seizures may be subdivided into simple and complex symptom types; a change in consciousness occurs with complex seizures. Partial seizures begin in a localized area in one hemisphere of the brain. Both simple and complex partial seizures can evolve into generalized seizures, which is a process that is referred to as *secondary generalization.* Epilepsy is treated almost exclusively with medications known as *anticonvulsants* or a term gaining more widespread use, *antiepileptic drugs*.

DESCRIPTIONS OF SEIZURES

GENERALIZED CONVULSIVE SEIZURES

The most common generalized convulsive seizures are the tonic-clonic, atonic, and myoclonic seizures.

Tonic-Clonic (Grand Mal) Seizures

Tonic-clonic (grand mal) seizures are the most common type of seizure. During the tonic phase, patients suddenly develop intense muscular contractions that cause them to fall to the ground, lose consciousness, and lie rigid. The back may arch, the arms may flex, the legs may extend, and the teeth may clench. Air is forced up the larynx, extruding saliva as foam and producing an audible sound like a cry. Respirations stop, and the patient may become cyanotic. The tonic phase usually lasts 20 to 60 seconds before diffuse trembling sets in. The clonic phase, which is manifested by bilaterally symmetric jerks alternating with the relaxation of the extremities, then begins. The clonic phase starts slightly and gradually becomes more violent, and it involves the whole body. Patients often bite their tongues and become incontinent of urine or feces. Usually, within 60 seconds, this phase proceeds to a resting, recovery phase of flaccid paralysis and sleep that lasts 2 to 3 hours (the postictal state). The patient has no recollection of the attack on awakening. The severity, frequency, and duration of attacks are highly variable; they may last from 1 to 30 minutes and occur as frequently as daily or as infrequently as every few years. Status epilepticus is a rapidly recurring generalized seizure that does not allow the individual to regain normal function between seizures. It is a medical emergency that requires prompt treatment to minimize permanent nerve damage and prevent death.

Atonic or Akinetic Seizures

A sudden loss of muscle tone is known as an *atonic seizure* or a *drop attack*. This may be described as a head drop, the dropping of a limb, or the slumping of the body to the ground. A sudden loss of muscle tone results in a dramatic fall. Seated patients may slump forward violently. Patients usually remain conscious. The attacks are short, but injury frequently occurs from the uncontrolled falls. These patients often wear protective headgear to minimize trauma.

Myoclonic Seizures

Myoclonic seizures involve lightning-like repetitive contractions of the voluntary muscles of the face, trunk, and extremities. The jerks may be isolated events, or they may be rapidly repetitive. It is not uncommon for patients to lose their balance and fall to the floor. These attacks occur most often at night as the patient enters sleep. There is no loss of consciousness with myoclonic seizures.

GENERALIZED NONCONVULSIVE SEIZURES

By far the most common generalized nonconvulsive seizure disorder is absence (petit mal) epilepsy. These seizures occur primarily in children, and they usually disappear at puberty; however, the patient may develop a second type of seizure activity. Attacks consist of paroxysmal episodes of altered consciousness lasting 5 to 20 seconds. There are no prodromal or postictal phases. Patients appear to be staring into space, and they may exhibit a few rhythmic movements of the eyes or head, lip smacking, mumbling, chewing, or swallowing movements. Falling does not occur, patients do not convulse, and they will have no memory of the events that occur during the seizures.

Partial (Localized) Seizures

Classification of **partial seizures** is subdivided into partial simple motor seizures and partial complex seizures. *Partial simple motor (Jacksonian) seizures* involve localized convulsions of voluntary muscles. A single body part such as a finger or an extremity may start jerking. Turning the head, smacking the lips, mouth movements, drooling, abnormal numbness, tingling, and crawling sensations are other indications of partial simple motor seizures. The muscle spasm may end spontaneously, or it may spread over the whole body. The patient does not lose consciousness unless the seizure develops into a generalized convulsion. *Partial seizures with complex symptoms (psychomotor seizures)* are manifested by a vast array of possible symptoms. The patient's outward appearance may be normal, or there may be aimless wandering, lip smacking, unusual and repeated chewing, or swallowing movements. The person is conscious, but may be in a confused, dreamlike state. The attacks, which may occur several times daily and last for several minutes, commonly end during sleep or with a clouded sensorium, and the patient usually has no recollection of the events of the attack.

ANTICONVULSANT THERAPY

Identifying the cause of seizure activity is important for determining the type of therapy required. Contributing factors (e.g., head injury, fever, hypoglycemia, drug overdose) must be specifically treated to correct the underlying cause before chronic anticonvulsant therapy is started. After the underlying cause is treated, it is rare that chronic antiepileptic therapy is needed. When seizure activity continues, drug therapy is the primary form of treatment. The goals of therapy are to improve the patient's quality of life, reduce the frequency of seizure activity, and minimize the adverse effects of the medication. Therapeutic outcomes must be individualized for each patient. The selection of the medication depends on the type of seizure, the age and gender of the patient, any other medical conditions present, and the potential adverse effects of the individual medications.

ACTIONS

Unfortunately, the mechanisms of seizure activity are extremely complex and not well understood. In general, anticonvulsants increase the seizure threshold and regulate neuronal firing by inhibiting excitatory processes or enhancing inhibitory processes. The medications can also prevent the seizure from spreading to adjacent neurons. Phenytoin, carbamazepine, lamotrigine, zonisamide, and valproic acid act on sodium and calcium channels to stabilize the neuronal membrane and may decrease the release of excitatory neurotransmitters. Barbiturates, benzodiazepines, tiagabine, gabapentin, and pregabalin enhance the inhibitory effect of gamma-aminobutyric acid (GABA), an inhibitory neurotransmitter that counterbalances the effect of excitatory neurotransmitters. Gamma-aminobutyric acid opens chloride channels resulting in a hyperpolarized cell membrane preventing excitation of the cell, stopping further propagation of the seizure. Seizure control medications are sometimes subdivided into broad-spectrum and narrow-spectrum agents in relation to their efficacy against different types of seizures. The broad-spectrum agents are levetiracetam, topiramate, valproic acid, zonisamide, and lamotrigine. These drugs are often used for the initial treatment of a patient with a newly diagnosed seizure disorder. The narrow-spectrum agents are phenytoin, carbamazepine, oxcarbazepine, tiagabine, gabapentin, and pregabalin (French, 2008).

In general, anticonvulsant therapy should start with the use of a single drug selected from a group of first-line agents based on the type of seizure. Table 18-1 lists the antiepileptic drugs of choice for primary seizure disorders. The agents classified as first-line therapy are fairly similar with regard to their potential to prevent seizures, but their adverse effects vary. Thus the drug chosen is selected first on its ability to control a certain form of epilepsy and then on its adverse effect profile and its likelihood to cause adverse effects in a particular patient. In general, if treatment is not successful with the first agent chosen, that agent is discontinued and another first-line agent is started. If treatment fails

with the second agent, the healthcare provider may decide to discontinue the second agent and start a third first-line agent, or combination therapy may be started by adding an alternative medication to one of the first-line therapies. Occasionally some patients will require multiple-drug therapy with a combination of agents and will still not be completely free of seizures. Those patients with newly diagnosed epilepsy who respond to treatment are referred to as "treatment responsive," and those who do not respond to first-line agents are referred to as "treatment resistant." About half of patients with newly diagnosed epilepsy become free of seizures while using the first prescribed antiepileptic drug. Almost two thirds of patients become free of seizures after receiving the second or third agent.

Nonpharmacologic treatment of refractory seizures includes surgical intervention, the use of an implantable vagus nerve stimulator for children who are 12 years old and older, and a ketogenic diet. The ketogenic diet is used for children, and it includes the restriction of carbohydrate and protein intake; fat is the primary fuel that produces acidosis and ketosis. Although the diet has been shown to reduce refractory seizures in children who have not achieved effective control with drug therapy, the adverse effects of this diet include high blood lipid levels with long-term effects that are not known.

According to a report by the U.S. Food and Drug Administration (2008), patients who were receiving antiepileptic drugs had approximately twice the risk of suicidal behavior or ideation (0.43%) compared with patients receiving placebo (0.22%). The increased risk of suicidal behavior and suicidal ideation was observed as early as 1 week after starting the antiepileptic drug, and it continued through 24 weeks of use of the medication. Healthcare professionals should closely monitor all patients currently receiving antiepileptic drugs for notable changes in behavior that could indicate the

Table 18-1 Antiepileptic Drugs of Choice Based on Type of Seizure

GENERALIZED SEIZURES			
GENERALIZED TONIC-CLONIC	ABSENCE	ATONIC OR MYOCLONIC	PARTIAL SEIZURES
Drugs of Choice			
topiramate	lamotrigine	ethosuximide lamotrigine valproate levetiracetam	carbamazepine phenytoin oxcarbazepine topiramate gabapentin valproate phenobarbital
Alternatives			
lamotrigine levetiracetam	valproate ethosuximide levetiracetam	clonazepam topiramate zonisamide	levetiracetam zonisamide clobazam lacosamide

Modified from Rogers SJ, Cavazos JE: Epilepsy. In DiPiro JT, Talbert RL, Yee GC, et al, editors: *Pharmacotherapy: A pathophysiologic approach*, ed 9, New York, 2014, McGraw-Hill, p. 861.

concurrent therapy for signs of phenytoin toxicity, including nystagmus, sedation, and lethargy. Serum levels may be ordered, and a reduced dosage of phenytoin may be required.

Ketoconazole. The concurrent administration with ketoconazole may alter the metabolism of one or both drugs. Monitoring the levels of both drugs is recommended.

 Medication Safety Alert

Phenytoin is associated with many drug interactions. Those listed earlier are the most common drug interactions recognized, but it is only a representative list. Consult a resource such as Drug Interaction Facts for a more complete description.

DRUG CLASS: SUCCINIMIDES

ACTIONS

The succinimides elevate the seizure threshold by depression of nerve transmission in the cortex by reducing the current in the T-type calcium channels found in primary afferent neurons.

USES

Succinimides (e.g., ethosuximide, methsuximide) are used to control absence (i.e., petit mal) seizures.

THERAPEUTIC OUTCOMES

The primary therapeutic outcomes expected from the succinimides are as follows:
1. Reduced frequency of seizures and reduced injury from seizure activity
2. Minimal adverse effects from therapy

❖ NURSING IMPLICATIONS FOR SUCCINIMIDES

■ **Premedication Assessment**
1. Perform a baseline assessment of the patient's speech patterns; degree of alertness; and orientation to name, place, and time before initiating therapy.
2. Monitor the patient's behavioral responses to therapy.
3. Review the patient's medical record to document the frequency of seizure activity.

■ **Availability, Dosage, and Administration**
See Table 18-2.

■ **Common Adverse Effects**
Gastrointestinal
Nausea, vomiting, indigestion. These effects are common during the initiation of therapy. Gradual increases in dosage and administration with food or milk will reduce gastric irritation.
Neurologic
Sedation, drowsiness, dizziness, fatigue, lethargy. These symptoms tend to disappear with continued therapy and possible dosage adjustment. Encourage the patient

not to discontinue therapy without first consulting the physician. The patient should be warned not to work with machinery, operate a motor vehicle, administer medication, or perform other duties that require mental alertness. Provide for patient safety during episodes of dizziness; report these changes to the healthcare provider for further evaluation.

■ **Drug Interactions**
Drugs That Enhance Toxic Effects. Antihistamines, alcohol, analgesics, anesthetics, tranquilizers, other anticonvulsants, and sedative-hypnotics enhance the toxic effects of succinimides.

DRUG CLASS: MISCELLANEOUS ANTICONVULSANTS

> **carbamazepine** (kăr-bă-MĂZ-ă-pĕn)
> **Tegretol** (TĔG-rĕ-tŏl)
> ⇄ *Do not confuse Tegretol with Toradol, Trental, or Trileptal.*

ACTIONS

Carbamazepine blocks the reuptake of norepinephrine and decreases the release of norepinephrine and the rate of dopamine and GABA turnover. Despite knowledge of these pharmacologic effects, the mechanisms of action as an anticonvulsant, selective analgesic, and antimanic agent are not fully known. Carbamazepine is structurally related to the tricyclic antidepressants.

USES

Carbamazepine is an anticonvulsant often used in combination with other anticonvulsants to control generalized tonic-clonic and partial seizures. It is not effective for controlling myoclonic or absence seizures. Carbamazepine has also been used successfully to treat the pain associated with trigeminal neuralgia (tic douloureux). It may also be used to treat manic-depressive disorders when lithium therapy has not been optimal.

In March 2008, the U.S. Food and Drug Administration issued an alert to healthcare professionals about dangerous and possibly fatal skin reactions that may occur with carbamazepine in certain patient populations. These skin reactions are significantly more common among patients with a particular human leukocyte antigen: the HLA-B*1502 allele. This allele occurs almost exclusively in persons of Asian ancestry, including South Asian Indians. Patients with this ancestry should be screened with available genetic tests for the allele before starting treatment with carbamazepine. If test results are positive, the drug should not be started unless the expected benefit clearly outweighs the risk of serious skin reactions. Patients who test positive for the allele may also be at increased risk from other antiepileptic drugs that have caused serious skin reactions. More than 90% of all serious skin reactions occur within the first few months of treatment. This means that patients who have been on the drug for longer periods without developing skin reactions have a low risk of reaction in the future, even if they have tested positive for the allele.

THERAPEUTIC OUTCOMES

The primary therapeutic outcomes expected from carbamazepine are as follows:
1. Reduced frequency of seizures and reduced injury from seizure activity
2. Minimal adverse effects from therapy

❖ NURSING IMPLICATIONS FOR CARBAMAZEPINE

▪ Premedication Assessment

1. As a result of serious adverse reactions, the manufacturer recommends that the following baseline studies be repeated at regular intervals: complete blood count (CBC), liver function tests, urinalysis, blood urea nitrogen (BUN), serum creatinine, and ophthalmologic examination.
2. Review the patient's history to exclude Asian ancestry, including South Asian Indian ancestry. If the patient does have this ancestry, bring it to the prescriber's attention so that genetic testing may be completed.
3. Perform a baseline assessment of the patient's speech patterns; degree of alertness; and orientation to name, place, and time before initiating therapy. Monitor the patient's behavioral responses to therapy.
4. Review the patient's medical record to document the frequency of seizure activity.

▪ Availability

PO: 200-mg tablets; 100-mg chewable tablets; 100-, 200-, and 400-mg extended-release tablets (12 hr); 100-, 200-, and 300-mg extended-release capsules (12 hr); 100 mg/5 mL suspension.

▪ Dosage and Administration

Adult: PO: Initial dosage is 200 mg twice daily on the first day. Dosage may be increased by 200 mg/day at weekly intervals. Max: 1000 mg/day in adolescents 12 to 15 years or 1200 mg/day in those younger than 15 years. In rare instances, doses ≥1600 mg/day in adults may be necessary. Therapeutic plasma levels for carbamazepine range from 4 to 12 mg/L.

▪ Common Adverse Effects

These effects can be reduced by slowly increasing the dosage. They are usually mild and tend to resolve with continued therapy. Encourage the patient not to discontinue therapy without first consulting the healthcare provider.

Gastrointestinal. Gastrointestinal effects include nausea and vomiting.

Neurologic

Drowsiness, dizziness. Provide for patient safety during episodes of drowsiness or dizziness. Patients must be warned not to work around machinery, operate motor vehicles, or perform other duties that require constant mental alertness until it is known how they are affected by this medication.

▪ Serious Adverse Effects

Cardiovascular

Orthostatic hypotension, hypertension. Monitor the patient's blood pressure daily in the supine and standing positions. Anticipate the development of postural hypotension, and take measures to prevent an occurrence. Teach the patient to rise slowly from a supine or sitting position, and encourage the patient to sit or lie down if feeling faint.

Dyspnea, edema. If carbamazepine is used by a patient with a history of heart failure, monitor daily weights, lung sounds, and accumulation of edema.

Neurologic

Slurred speech, sedation, confusion. Perform a baseline assessment of the patient's speech patterns; degree of alertness; and orientation to name, place, and time before initiating therapy. Make regularly scheduled subsequent evaluations of the patient's mental status, and compare findings. Report any significant alterations to the healthcare provider.

Genitourinary

Nephrotoxicity. Monitor the patient's urinalysis and kidney function tests for abnormal results. Report increasing BUN and creatinine levels, decreasing urine output or specific gravity despite the amount of fluid intake, casts or protein in the urine, frank blood or smoky-colored urine, or RBCs in excess of 0 to 3 on the urinalysis report.

Gastrointestinal

Hepatotoxicity. The symptoms of hepatotoxicity include anorexia, nausea, vomiting, jaundice, hepatomegaly, splenomegaly, and abnormal liver function tests (i.e., elevated bilirubin, AST, ALT, GGT, alkaline phosphatase levels; increased PT).

Hematologic

Blood dyscrasias. Routine laboratory studies (i.e., RBC, WBC, differential counts) should be scheduled. Monitor the patient for sore throat, fever, purpura, jaundice, or excessive and progressive weakness.

Integumentary

Dermatologic reactions. Report a rash or pruritus immediately, and withhold additional doses pending approval by the healthcare provider.

▪ Drug Interactions

Drugs That Enhance Therapeutic and Toxic Effects. Isoniazid, cimetidine, fluoxetine, fluvoxamine, ketoconazole, and macrolide antibiotics (e.g., erythromycin, clarithromycin) inhibit the metabolism of carbamazepine. Monitor the patient for signs of toxicity, such as disorientation, ataxia, lethargy, headache, drowsiness, nausea, and vomiting. Dosage reductions in carbamazepine may be necessary.

Verapamil, Diltiazem, Danazol, Lamotrigine, Nefazodone. These drugs increase serum levels of carbamazepine. Monitor the patient for signs of toxicity (e.g., disorientation, ataxia, lethargy, headache, drowsiness, nausea, vomiting). A 40% to 50% decrease in the carbamazepine dosage may be necessary.

Warfarin. Carbamazepine may diminish the anticoagulant effects of warfarin. Monitor the PT, and increase the dosage of warfarin, if necessary.

Phenobarbital, Phenytoin, Valproic Acid. Carbamazepine enhances the metabolism of these agents. Monitor the patient for an increased frequency of seizure activity. Monitoring changes in serum levels should help predict possible increased seizure activity.

Doxycycline. Carbamazepine enhances the metabolism of this antibiotic. Monitor the patient for signs of continued infection.

Oral Contraceptives. Carbamazepine enhances the metabolism of estrogens. Spotting or bleeding may be an indication of reduced contraceptive activity. The use of other forms of birth control is recommended.

---

gabapentin (găb-ă-PĔN-tĭn)
Neurontin (nyŭr-ŎN-tĭn)
⇄ *Do not confuse Neurontin with Neoral or Noroxin.*

ACTIONS

The mechanism of action of gabapentin is unknown. It does not appear to enhance GABA.

USES

Gabapentin is an anticonvulsant usually used in combination with other anticonvulsants to control partial seizures. Gabapentin is also approved for use in patients with diabetic neuropathy, fibromyalgia, and postherpetic neuralgia.

THERAPEUTIC OUTCOMES

The primary therapeutic outcomes expected from gabapentin are as follows:
1. Reduced frequency of seizures and reduced injury from seizure activity
2. Symptomatic relief from diabetic neuropathy, fibromyalgia, and postherpetic neuralgia
3. Minimal adverse effects from therapy

❖ NURSING IMPLICATIONS FOR GABAPENTIN

▪ Premedication Assessment
1. Perform a baseline assessment of the patient's speech patterns; degree of alertness; and orientation to name, place, and time before initiating therapy. Monitor the patient's behavioral responses to therapy.

2. Review the patient's medical record to document the frequency of seizure activity.
3. When gabapentin is used as an analgesic, perform a pain assessment before administering it and at appropriate intervals during therapy. Report poor pain control, and obtain a modification in the patient's orders.

▪ Availability
PO: 100-, 300-, and 400-mg capsules; 300-, 600-, and 800-mg tablets; 250 mg/5 mL oral solution.

▪ Dosage and Administration
Adult: PO: 900 to 1800 mg daily. Initially administer 300 mg at bedtime on day 1, 300 mg two times on day 2, and then 300 mg three times on day 3. May increase using 300-, 400-, 600-, or 800-mg dosage forms given three times per day. Effective dose is 900 to 1800 mg/day, but up to 2400 mg/day has been used long term. Dosages of 3600 mg/day have been given to limited patients for a relatively short duration. The maximum time between doses for the three-times-daily schedule should not exceed 12 hours. Therapeutic blood levels for gabapentin are 12 to 20 mg/L. If the patient also uses antacids, administer gabapentin at least 2 hours after the last dose of antacid, because antacids reduce the absorption of gabapentin.

▪ Common Adverse Effects
Neurologic
Sedation, drowsiness, dizziness. These symptoms tend to disappear with continued therapy and possible dosage adjustment. Encourage the patient not to discontinue therapy without first consulting the healthcare provider. Provide for patient safety during episodes of drowsiness or dizziness. Patients must be warned not to work around machinery, operate motor vehicles, or perform other duties that require constant mental alertness until it is known how they are affected by this medication.
Sensory
Blurred vision. Caution the patient that blurred vision may occur, and make appropriate suggestions for the patient's personal safety.

▪ Serious Adverse Effects
Neurologic
Slurred speech, lethargy, confusion. Perform a baseline assessment of the patient's speech patterns; degree of alertness; and orientation to name, place, and time before initiating therapy. Make regularly scheduled subsequent evaluations of the patient's mental status, and compare findings. Report any significant alterations.

▪ Drug Interactions
Enhanced Sedation. Central nervous system (CNS) depressants—including sleep aids, analgesics, tranquilizers, and alcohol—enhance the sedative effects of

gabapentin. Patients must be warned not to work around machinery, operate motor vehicles, or perform other duties that require constant mental alertness until it is known how they are affected by this medication. Provide for patient safety during episodes of drowsiness or dizziness.

Urine Protein. False-positive readings for protein in the urine have been reported by patients who are taking gabapentin who use the N-Multistix SG dipstick test. The manufacturer recommends that the more specific sulfosalicylic acid precipitation procedure be used to determine the presence of urine protein.

---

lamotrigine (lă-MŎ-trĭ-gēn)
⇄ *Do not confuse lamotrigine with Lamivudine.*
Lamictal (lă-MĬK-tăl)
⇄ *Do not confuse Lamictal with labetalol, Lamisil, Lomotil, or Ludiomil.*

ACTIONS

Lamotrigine is a newer anticonvulsant of the phenyltriazine class that is unrelated to other antiepileptic medications currently available. It is thought to act by blocking voltage-sensitive sodium and calcium channels in the neuronal membranes. This stabilizes the neuronal membranes and inhibits the release of excitatory neurotransmitters (e.g., glutamate), which may induce seizure activity.

USES

Lamotrigine is used in combination with other anticonvulsants to treat partial onset seizures and the generalized seizures of Lennox-Gastaut syndrome in pediatric and adult patients. Lamotrigine is also approved for use in combination with other standard therapies to treat bipolar disorder to delay the time to the onset of mood episodes (i.e., depression, mania, mixed episodes).

THERAPEUTIC OUTCOMES

The primary therapeutic outcomes expected from lamotrigine are as follows:
1. Reduced frequency of seizures and reduced injury from seizure activity
2. Treatment of bipolar disorder
3. Minimal adverse effects from therapy

❖ NURSING IMPLICATIONS FOR LAMOTRIGINE

▪ Premedication Assessment
1. Perform a baseline assessment of the patient's speech patterns; degree of alertness; and orientation to name, place, and time before initiating therapy. Monitor the patient's behavioral responses to therapy.
2. Review the patient's medication history to determine whether the patient is already taking valproic acid for seizure control.
3. Review the patient's medical record to document the frequency of seizure activity.

▪ Availability
PO: 25-, 50-, 100-, 150-, 200-, and 250-mg tablets; 2-, 5-, and 25-mg chewable tablets; 25-, 50-, 100-, and 200-mg orally disintegrating tablets; 25-, 50-, 100-, 200-, 250-, and 300-mg extended-release tablets.

▪ Dosage and Administration
Seizure Disorder. **Adult:** *PO:* If the patient is already taking valproic acid for seizure control, initiate lamotrigine therapy at 25 mg every other day for 2 weeks, followed by 25 mg daily for 3 to 4 weeks; then the dose may be increased by 25 to 50 mg PO daily every 1 to 2 weeks until the maintenance dosage is achieved. The usual maintenance dose is 100 to 400 mg/day PO, given in one to two divided doses. The usual maintenance dose for patients who add lamotrigine to valproic acid alone ranges from 100 to 200 mg/day.

If the patient is not already taking metabolism-inducing medications (e.g., valproic acid, carbamazepine, phenytoin, phenobarbital, rifampin) for seizure control, initiate lamotrigine therapy at 25 mg PO every day for 2 weeks, then 50 mg/day PO for weeks 3 to 4, and then the dose may be increased by 50 mg/day PO every 1 to 2 weeks until the maintenance dosage is achieved. The usual maintenance dose is 225 to 375 mg/day PO, given in two divided doses. If the patient is already receiving metabolism-inducing medications for seizure control, the dosage of lamotrigine should be approximately two times these dosages up to 400 mg daily in divided doses; see the manufacturer's recommendations. Therapeutic blood levels for lamotrigine are 3 to 14 mg/L.

Bipolar Disorder. **Adult:** *PO:* Initial dosage depends on other medications that are being taken, as described previously. Target dosage is 200 mg/daily of immediate-release medication.

▪ Common Adverse Effects
Gastrointestinal
Nausea, vomiting, indigestion. These effects are common during the initiation of therapy. Gradual increases in dosage and administration with food or milk will reduce gastric irritation.

Neurologic
Sedation, drowsiness, dizziness. These symptoms tend to disappear with continued therapy and possible dosage adjustment. Encourage the patient not to discontinue therapy without first consulting the healthcare provider. Provide for patient safety during episodes of drowsiness or dizziness. Patients must be warned not to work around machinery, operate motor

USES

Primidone is used in combination with other anticonvulsants to treat both partial-onset seizures and generalized tonic-clonic seizures.

THERAPEUTIC OUTCOMES

The primary therapeutic outcomes expected from primidone are as follows:
1. Reduced frequency of seizures and reduced injury from seizure activity
2. Minimal adverse effects from therapy

❖ NURSING IMPLICATIONS FOR PRIMIDONE

▪ Premedication Assessment
1. Review the patient's routine blood studies to detect blood dyscrasias.
2. Perform a baseline assessment of the patient's speech patterns; degree of alertness; and orientation to name, place, and time before initiating therapy. Monitor the patient's behavioral responses to therapy. In children, assess the degree of excitability present.
3. Review the patient's medical record to document the frequency of seizure activity.

▪ Availability
PO: 50- and 250-mg tablets.

▪ Dosage and Administration
Adult: PO: Initially 100 to 125 mg daily at bedtime for 3 days. On days 4 through 6, increase the dosage to 100 to 125 mg twice daily. On days 7 through 9, increase to 100 to 125 mg three times daily. Increase by 100 to 125 mg/day every 3 or 4 days until therapeutic response or intolerance develops. The typical dosage is 750 to 1500 mg/day. Do not exceed 2000 mg/day.

▪ Common Adverse Effects
These symptoms tend to disappear with continued therapy and possible dosage adjustment. Encourage the patient not to discontinue therapy without first consulting the healthcare provider.

Neurologic

Sedation, drowsiness, dizziness. People who work around machinery, operate motor vehicles, or perform other duties that require constant mental alertness should be particularly cautious until they know how this medication will affect them. Provide for patient safety during episodes of dizziness, and report these patients for further evaluation.

Sensory

Blurred vision. Caution the patient that blurred vision may occur, and make appropriate suggestions for the patient's safety.

▪ Serious Adverse Effects
Hematologic

Blood dyscrasias. Blood dyscrasias have rarely been reported with the use of primidone. Routine laboratory studies (e.g., RBC, WBC, differential counts) should be scheduled. Monitor the patient for sore throat, fever, purpura, jaundice, or excessive and progressive weakness.

Neurologic

Paradoxical excitability. Primidone may cause paradoxical excitability in children. During a period of excitement, protect patients from harm, and provide for the physical channeling of energy (e.g., walk with them). Notify the healthcare provider of the need for a possible change in medication.

▪ Drug Interactions
NOTE: See Chapter 13 for the drug interactions associated with phenobarbital, because primidone is metabolized to phenobarbital.

Oral Contraceptives. Spotting or bleeding may be an indication of reduced contraceptive activity. Recommend the patient use alternative forms of birth control while taking this medication.

Phenytoin. Phenytoin may increase phenobarbital serum levels when it is taken concurrently with primidone. Monitor patients for increased sedation.

---

tiagabine (tē-ĂG-ă-bēn)
⇄ *Do not confuse tiagabine with tizanidine.*
Gabitril (GĂB-ĭ-trĭl)
⇄ *Do not confuse Gabitril with gabapentin.*

ACTIONS

The mechanism of action of tiagabine is unknown. It appears to prevent the reuptake of GABA into presynaptic neurons, thus permitting more GABA to be available to act as an inhibitory neurotransmitter.

USES

Tiagabine is an anticonvulsant usually used in combination with other anticonvulsants to control partial seizures.

THERAPEUTIC OUTCOMES

The primary therapeutic outcomes expected from tiagabine are as follows:
1. Reduced frequency of seizures and reduced injury from seizure activity
2. Minimal adverse effects from therapy

❖ NURSING IMPLICATIONS FOR TIAGABINE

▪ Premedication Assessment
1. Perform a baseline assessment of the patient's speech patterns; degree of alertness; and orientation to name, place, and time before initiating therapy. Monitor the patient's behavioral responses to therapy.
2. Review the patient's medical record to document the frequency of seizure activity.

▪ Availability
PO: 2-, 4-, 12-, and 16-mg tablets.

■ **Dosage and Administration**

Adult: PO: Initially 4 mg once daily. Increase daily dosage by 4 to 8 mg at weekly intervals until a clinical response is achieved or until a total daily dosage of 56 mg has been reached. A total daily dosage of 32 to 56 mg may be taken in two to four divided doses. The therapeutic blood levels for this drug have not been established.

■ **Common Adverse Effects**

Neurologic

Sedation, drowsiness, dizziness. These symptoms tend to disappear with continued therapy and possible dosage adjustment. Encourage the patient not to discontinue therapy without first consulting the healthcare provider. People who work around machinery, operate motor vehicles, or perform other duties that require constant mental alertness should be particularly cautious until they know how this medication will affect them. Provide for patient safety during episodes of dizziness, and report these patients for further evaluation.

■ **Serious Adverse Effects**

Neurologic

Neurologic assessment, memory loss. Perform a baseline assessment of the patient's speech patterns and degree of alertness, as well as his or her orientation to name, place, and time before the therapy. Make regularly scheduled subsequent evaluations of mental status, and compare findings. Report any significant alterations.

■ **Drug Interactions**

Drugs That Decrease Therapeutic Effects. Phenobarbital, primidone, phenytoin, and carbamazepine may enhance the metabolism of tiagabine and thus decrease its therapeutic effect. Monitor the patient for the increased frequency of seizure activity. Monitoring changes in serum levels should help predict the potential for increased seizure activity.

Enhanced Sedation. Central nervous system depressants—including sleep aids, analgesics, tranquilizers, and alcohol—may enhance the sedative effects of tiagabine. Patients must be warned not to work around machinery, operate motor vehicles, or perform other duties that require constant mental alertness until they know how they will be affected by this medication. Provide for patient safety during episodes of drowsiness or dizziness.

---

topiramate (tō-PĬR-ă-māt)

⇄ *Do not confuse topiramate with torsemide.*

Topamax (TŌ-pă-măks)

ACTIONS

The mechanism of action of topiramate as an anticonvulsant is unknown. Three potential mechanisms may support anticonvulsant activity: (1) the prolonged blockade of sodium channels in the neuronal membrane; (2) the potentiation of the activity of the inhibitory neurotransmitter GABA; and (3) the antagonism of certain receptors of the excitatory neurotransmitter.

USES

Topiramate is an anticonvulsant used in combination with other anticonvulsants to control partial and generalized tonic-clonic seizures. It is also used for patients 2 years old and older who have seizures associated with Lennox-Gastaut syndrome.

Topiramate has also been approved for adults for the prevention (but not treatment) of migraine headaches.

THERAPEUTIC OUTCOMES

The primary therapeutic outcomes expected from topiramate are as follows:
1. Reduced frequency of seizures and reduced injury from seizure activity
2. Prevention of migraines
3. Minimal adverse effects from therapy

❖ NURSING IMPLICATIONS FOR TOPIRAMATE

■ **Premedication Assessment**

1. Perform a baseline assessment of the patient's speech patterns and degree of alertness, as well as orientation to name, place, and time before initiating therapy. Monitor the patient's behavioral responses to therapy.
2. Obtain the patient's baseline weight for future reference. Weight loss may be an adverse effect of topiramate therapy.
3. Assess the patient's baseline state of hydration. Rare cases of oligohidrosis (decreased sweating) and hyperthermia have been reported, particularly in children and in those patients who are taking other medications with anticholinergic activity. Proper hydration before and during activities such as exercise or exposure to warm temperatures is recommended.
4. Review the patient's medical record to document the frequency of seizure activity.
5. If this drug is used for migraine prevention, review the patient's medical record to document the frequency of migraine headaches.
6. Ask female patients if there is a possibility of pregnancy at this time. If so, notify the healthcare provider of this possibility before starting therapy.

■ **Availability**

PO: 25-, 50-, 100-, and 200-mg tablets; 15- and 25-mg sprinkle capsules; 25-, 50-, 100-, and 200-mg extended-release sprinkle capsules (24 hr).

■ **Dosage and Administration**

Anticonvulsant. Adult: PO: Initially 25 mg twice daily. Increase the daily dosage by 50 mg at weekly

Gastrointestinal

Nausea, vomiting, dry mouth. These effects tend to occur most often with the initial dose. Symptoms can be reduced by keeping the patient supine. Provide patient safety, assurance, and comfort.

Constipation. Continued use may cause constipation. Maintain the patient's state of hydration and obtain an order for stool softeners or bulk-forming laxatives if necessary. Encourage the inclusion of sufficient roughage, fresh fruits, vegetables, and whole-grain products in the diet.

▪ Serious Adverse Effects

Neurologic

Confusion, disorientation, hallucinations. Butorphanol and pentazocine and, to a lesser degree, nalbuphine, may produce hallucinations. Patients may complain of seeing multicolored flashing patterns or animals, with and without sound, or may have very vivid dreams. These adverse effects have been reported after only one or two doses of medication and may occur in as many as one third of patients taking butorphanol or pentazocine.

Perform a baseline assessment of the patient's degree of alertness and orientation to name, place, and time before initiating therapy. Make regularly scheduled subsequent evaluations of mental status, and report alterations from baseline. Provide for patient safety during these episodes. If recurring, seek a change in the medication order.

Respiratory

Respiratory depression. Opiate partial agonists make the respiratory centers less sensitive to carbon dioxide, causing respiratory depression. This may occur before the reduction in respiratory rate or tidal volume is noticeable. Check the respiratory rate and depth often.

Psychological

Excessive use or abuse. Repeated use may lead to tolerance and physical dependence. Evaluate the patient's response to the analgesic. Identify underlying needs and plan for more appropriate management of those needs. Discuss the case with the healthcare provider and make plans to approach gradual withdrawal of the medications being abused cooperatively. Suggest a change to a milder analgesic when indicated.

The patient does not have to experience symptoms of withdrawal to be treated for physical dependence, which is usually a gradual reduction of the daily opiate agonist dosage. If withdrawal symptoms become severe, the patient may receive methadone. Temporary administration of tranquilizers and sedatives may aid in reducing patient anxiety and craving for the opiate agonist.

Assist the patient in recognizing the abuse problem. Provide for emotional support of the individual by displaying an accepting attitude and by being kind but firm.

▪ Drug Interactions

Central Nervous System Depressants. General anesthetics, phenothiazines, tranquilizers, sedative-hypnotics, tricyclic antidepressants, antihistamines, and alcohol enhance the depressant effects of the opiate partial agonists. Respiratory depression, hypotension, and profound sedation or coma may result

Table 19-2 Opiate Partial Agonists

GENERIC NAME	BRAND NAME	AVAILABILITY	ADULT DOSAGE RANGE	DURATION (hr)	DOSAGE EQUIVALENT TO MORPHINE (10 mg)
buprenorphine	Buprenex, Subutex	Tablets, sublingual: 2, 8 mg Injection: 0.3 mg/mL in 1-mL ampules Patch (weekly): 5, 10, 15, 20 mcg/hr	0.3-0.6 mg, repeat in 5-6 hr	6	IM/IV: 0.4 mg
butorphanol	—	Injection: 1, 2 mg in 1-, 2-, 10-mL vials Nasal spray: 10 mg/mL	IM: 2 mg, repeat in 3-4 hr; maximum dosage, 4 mg IV: 1 mg, repeat in 3-4 hr Nasal: 1 spray in each nostril repeated in 3-4 hr	IM: 3-4	IM: 2 mg
nalbuphine	—	Injection: 10, 20 mg/mL in 1-, 10-mL vials	Subcut, IM, IV: 10 mg/70 kg, repeat q3-6h; maximum daily dosage, 160 mg	3-6	IM/IV/subcut: 10 mg
pentazocine	Talwin	Injection: 30 mg/mL in 1-, 10-mL vials Tablets: (with naloxone)* 50 mg	PO: 50-100 mg q3-4h; do not exceed 600 mg daily Subcut, IM, IV: 30 mg q3-4h; maximum daily dosage 360 mg	4-5	30-60 mg

*Tablets contain naloxone to prevent abuse.

from this interaction unless the dosage of the opiate partial agonist has been reduced appropriately (usually by one third to one half the normal dose).

Opiate Agonists. Opiate partial agonists have weak antagonist activity. When administered to patients who have been receiving opiate agonists such as morphine or meperidine on a regular basis, it may precipitate withdrawal symptoms.

DRUG CLASS: OPIATE ANTAGONISTS

naloxone (năl-ŎKS-ōn)
  Evzio

ACTIONS

Naloxone is a so-called pure opiate antagonist because it has no other known effect than reversal of the CNS depressant effects of opiate agonists and opiate partial agonists. When administered to patients who have not recently received opiates, there is no respiratory depression, psychomimetic effect, circulatory change, or other pharmacologic activity. If administered to a person addicted to opiate agonists or opiate partial agonists, withdrawal symptoms may be precipitated.

USES

Naloxone is a drug of choice for treatment of respiratory depression when excessive doses of opiate agonists or opiate partial agonists have been administered, or when the causative agent is unknown. Naloxone is not effective in reversing CNS depression induced by tranquilizers or sedative-hypnotics. Naloxone has been added to pentazocine formulations to reduce its abuse by blocking the euphoric high associated with pentazocine.

Many emergency services (police, fire, ambulance) across the nation now carry prefilled syringes of naloxone (Evzio) to administer to patients emergently for potential overdoses of opiates (heroin, morphine, oxycodone, hydromorphone). This is similar to EpiPen or Auvi-Q use in acute anaphylaxis by allergens (e.g., bee stings).

THERAPEUTIC OUTCOMES

The primary therapeutic outcome expected from naloxone is reversal of respiratory depression secondary to opiate overdose.

❖ NURSING IMPLICATIONS FOR NALOXONE

▪ Premedication Assessment

1. Perform baseline neurologic assessment (e.g., orientation to date, time, and place; mental alertness; bilateral hand grip; and motor functioning).
2. Monitor vital signs; blood pressure, pulse, and respirations should be taken at frequent intervals until resolution of CNS depression. Then, schedule vital signs to be taken at appropriate intervals because the duration of action of naloxone is short.
3. Check prior use or dependence on opiate agonists or opiate partial agonists. Diagnostic testing for narcotic dependence may be performed in accordance with policies of the clinical site. Inform patient of risks involved.
4. Have supportive equipment available in immediate area to maintain respirations.
5. Check bowel sounds. Review voiding pattern and urine output.

▪ Availability

Injection: 0.4 mg/mL in 1-mL prefilled syringes; 1 mg/mL in 2-mL prefilled syringes and 1- and 10-mL vials; 0.4 mg in 0.4-mL prefilled autoinjector.

▪ Dosage and Administration

Adult: IV: Postoperative opiate depression, 0.1 to 0.2 mg every 2 to 3 minutes until the desired response is achieved. Opiate overdose, 0.4 to 2 mg every 2 to 3 minutes. If no response is seen after 10 minutes, the depressive condition may be caused by a drug or disease process not responsive to naloxone.

▪ Common Adverse Effects

Naloxone rarely manifests any adverse effects. In rare cases when extremely high doses have been used, mental depression, apathy, inability to concentrate, sleepiness, irritability, anorexia, nausea, and vomiting have been reported. These adverse effects usually occurred in the first few days of treatment and dissipated rapidly with continued therapy.

Cardiovascular. Use with caution in patients with cardiovascular disease or in patients taking cardiovascular medicines (e.g., antihypertensives, antiarrhythmics). Abrupt reversal of opiate overdose by opioid antagonists may cause arrhythmias, pulmonary edema, and ventricular fibrillation.

Neurologic

Mental depression, apathy. Be aware of the potential for suicidal thoughts or suicide. Inform the healthcare provider immediately if the patient has any new or worsening symptoms of depression.

Gastrointestinal

Nausea, vomiting. Naloxone should be used with caution following the use of opiates during surgery because it may result in excitement, increased blood pressure, and a clinically important reversal of analgesia. The early reversal of opiate effects may induce nausea, vomiting, sweating, and tachycardia.

Naloxone should be given with caution to patients known or suspected to be physically dependent on opiates, including neonates born to women who are opiate dependent, because the drug may precipitate severe withdrawal symptoms. The severity of the symptoms depends on the dose of naloxone and the degree of dependence.

▪ Drug Interactions

There are no drug interactions other than that of the antagonist activity toward opiate agonists and opiate partial agonists.

---

naltrexone (năl-TRĔKS-ōn)
   Revia (rē-VĒ-ă)

ACTIONS

Naltrexone is a pure opioid antagonist closely related to naloxone. It differs, however, in that it is active after oral administration and has a considerably longer duration of action. Naltrexone blocks the effects of opioids by competing for binding sites at opioid receptors. The mechanism of action of naltrexone in patients with alcoholism is not known.

USES

Naltrexone is used clinically to block the pharmacologic effects of exogenously administered opiates in patients who are enrolled in drug abuse treatment programs. Naltrexone may diminish or eliminate opiate-seeking behavior by blocking the euphoric reinforcement produced by self-administration of opiates and by preventing the conditioned abstinence syndrome (i.e., opiate craving) that occurs after opiate withdrawal.

Naltrexone is also used as an adjunct in the treatment of alcoholism to support abstinence and reduce relapse rates and alcohol consumption. It must be used with other treatment forms such as group and behavior therapy; the expected effect of the drug treatment is a modest improvement in the outcome of conventional treatment.

THERAPEUTIC OUTCOMES

The primary therapeutic outcomes expected from naltrexone are as follows:
1. Improved adherence with a substance abuse treatment program by reducing the craving for opioids
2. Improved adherence with an alcohol abuse treatment program by diminishing the craving for alcohol

❖ NURSING IMPLICATIONS FOR NALTREXONE

▪ Premedication Assessment
1. Perform baseline neurologic assessment (e.g., orientation to date, time, and place; mental alertness; bilateral hand grip; and motor functioning).
2. Monitor vital signs: temperature, blood pressure, pulse, and respirations.
3. Check laboratory values for hepatotoxicity; urine screen for opiate use.
4. Monitor for GI symptoms before and during therapy.
5. The manufacturer recommends that baseline determinations of liver function should be obtained in all patients before initiating therapy and repeated monthly for the next 6 months.
6. The manufacturer recommends a minimum of 7 to 10 days of abstinence from all opiates, a urinalysis to confirm the absence of opiates, and the use of a naloxone challenge test to ensure that the patient will not develop withdrawal symptoms.

▪ Availability
PO: 50-mg tablets; *IM:* 380 mg/vial suspension, extended-release injection

▪ Dosage and Administration
Behavior Modification. Naltrexone therapy in combination with behavioral therapy is more effective than naltrexone or behavioral therapy alone in prolonging opiate or alcohol cessation in patients formerly physically dependent on opiates or alcohol.

Treatment of Opiate Agonist Dependence. PO: Induction regimen of 25 mg. Observe for development of withdrawal symptoms. If none occur, administer 50 mg the next day. The maintenance regimen is 50 mg daily. Alternative regimens of 100 mg every other day or 150 mg every third day have been used to improve adherence during a behavior modification program (see Chapter 48).

Withdrawal Symptoms. Naltrexone may precipitate acute and severe withdrawal symptoms in patients who are physically dependent on opioids. Addicts must be completely detoxified and opioid free before taking naltrexone. The manufacturer recommends a minimum of 7 to 10 days of abstinence from all opiates, a urinalysis to confirm the absence of opiates, and the use of a naloxone challenge test to ensure that the patient will not develop withdrawal symptoms.

Patients undergoing naltrexone therapy must be carefully instructed about the expectations of behavioral modification associated with therapy. They should also be advised that self-administration of small doses of opiates (e.g., heroin) during naltrexone therapy will not result in any euphoric effect and that large doses may result in serious adverse effects, including coma and death. Patients should also be given identification to notify medical personnel that they are taking a long-acting opiate antagonist.

Treatment of Alcoholism. PO: 50 mg once daily (see also Chapter 48).

IM: 380 mg IM every 4 weeks as a gluteal injection, alternating buttocks.

▪ Common Adverse Effects
Many adverse effects have been associated with naltrexone therapy, but it is difficult to know exactly which ones are secondary to naltrexone alone because some patients may experience mild opiate withdrawal symptoms as well. The adverse effects of drug and alcohol abuse and poor nutritional states may contribute to the patient's discomfort.

Gastrointestinal

Nausea, vomiting, anorexia. Adverse effects are usually mild and tend to resolve with continued therapy. Encourage the patient not to discontinue therapy without first consulting the healthcare provider and treatment program.

Neurologic

Headache. Adverse effects are usually mild and tend to resolve with continued therapy. Encourage the patient not to discontinue therapy without first consulting the healthcare provider and treatment program.

■ **Serious Adverse Effects**

Gastrointestinal

Hepatotoxicity. Hepatotoxicity has been reported after doses of 300 mg daily for 3 to 8 weeks. The symptoms of hepatotoxicity are jaundice, nausea, vomiting, anorexia, hepatomegaly, splenomegaly, and abnormal liver function test results (e.g., elevated bilirubin, aspartate aminotransferase [AST], alanine aminotransferase [ALT], alkaline phosphatase levels; increased prothrombin time). Because many of these patients do not develop clinical symptoms but do develop abnormal liver function, strongly encourage patients to report for blood tests as scheduled. Report abnormal values to the appropriate healthcare provider.

■ **Drug Interactions**

Opiate-Containing Products. Patients taking naltrexone will probably not benefit from opioid-containing medicines such as analgesics, cough and cold preparations, and antidiarrheal preparations. These products should be avoided during naltrexone therapy when nonopiate therapy is available.

Clonidine. Clonidine may be administered in patients to reduce the severity of withdrawal symptoms precipitated or exacerbated by naltrexone.

DRUG CLASS: PROSTAGLANDIN INHIBITORS

acetaminophen (ă-sēt-ă-MĬN-ō-fĕn)
  Tylenol (TĬ-lĕ-nŏl)

ACTIONS

Acetaminophen is a synthetic nonopiate analgesic that works by prostaglandin inhibition in the CNS and blocks generation of pain impulses in the peripheral tissue. Control of elevated body temperature (antipyresis) results from inhibition of the heat-regulating center in the hypothalamus. Antipyretic effectiveness and analgesic potency are similar to those of aspirin in equal doses.

USES

Acetaminophen is an effective analgesic-antipyretic for discomfort associated with bacterial and viral infections, headache, and musculoskeletal pain. It is a good substitute for patients who cannot take products containing aspirin because of allergic reactions; hypersensitivities; anticoagulant therapy; or possible bleeding problems from gastric or duodenal ulcers, gastritis, and hiatus hernia. This drug has no antiinflammatory activity and is therefore ineffective (other than as an analgesic) for the relief of symptoms of rheumatoid arthritis or other inflammation.

THERAPEUTIC OUTCOMES

The primary therapeutic outcomes expected from acetaminophen are reduced pain and fever.

❖ **NURSING IMPLICATIONS FOR ACETAMINOPHEN**

■ **Premedication Assessment**

1. Take vital signs: temperature, blood pressure, pulse, and respirations.
2. Check laboratory data for hepatotoxicity or nephrotoxicity.
3. Monitor for GI symptoms before and during therapy.
4. Check bowel sounds and review voiding pattern and urine output.
5. When used as an analgesic, perform pain assessment before administering acetaminophen and at appropriate intervals during therapy. Report poor pain control promptly and obtain modification in orders.
6. When used as an antipyretic, take baseline temperature and continue monitoring temperature at appropriate intervals (e.g., every 2 to 4 hours, depending on severity of temperature elevation).

■ **Availability**

PO: 160-, 325-, 500-, and 650-mg tablets; 80- and 500-mg chewable tablets; 650-mg extended-release tablets; 80- and 500-mg dispersible tablets; 80 mg/0.8 mL drops; 80 mg/2.5 mL elixir; 80, 120, 160 mg/5 mL elixir; 160 mg/5 mL and 500 mg/15 mL liquid; 80 mg/1.66 mL and 100 mg/mL solution.

Rectal: 80-, 120-, 325-, or 650-mg suppositories.

IV: 10 mg/mL solution in 100-mL vial.

To avoid toxicity, it is recommended that the adult receive no more than 4 g of acetaminophen daily. Patients who are chronic alcoholics should take no more than 2 g per day.

■ **Dosage and Administration**

Adult: PO: 325 to 650 mg every 4 to 6 hours. Doses up to 1000 mg may be given four times daily for short-term therapy. Do not exceed 4 g daily. *IV:* Greater than 50 kg: 1 g every 6 hours. Do not exceed 4 g in 24 hours. Less than 50 kg: 15 mg/kg (up to 750 mg) as a single dose and 75 mg/kg (up to 3750 mg) in 24 hours.

Pediatric: PO: 0 to 3 months, 40 mg; 4 to 11 months, 80 mg; 12 to 24 months, 120 mg; 2 to 3 years, 160 mg;

4 to 5 years, 240 mg; 6 to 8 years, 320 mg; 9 to 10 years, 400 mg; 11 to 12 years, 480 mg; older than 14 years, 650 mg. *Rectal:* Same as for oral doses. Administer every 4 hours with no more than five doses per day. **2 to 12 years of age:** *IV:* 15 mg/kg as a single dose and 75 mg/kg in 24 hours. **13 years of age and older; 50 kg or more:** *IV:* 1000 mg every 6 hours or 650 mg every 4 hours. Do not exceed 1000 mg as a single dose and 4000 mg in 24 hours. **13 years and older; less than 50 kg:** *IV:* 15 mg/kg every 6 hours or 12.5 mg/kg every 4 hours. Do not exceed 15 mg/kg (up to 750 mg) as a single dose and 75 mg/kg (up to 3750 mg) in 24 hours. *Antidote.* The antidote is acetylcysteine.

▪ Common Adverse Effects

When used as directed, acetaminophen is extremely well tolerated.

Gastrointestinal

Gastric irritation. If gastric irritation occurs, administer medication with food, milk, antacids, or large amounts of water. If symptoms persist or increase in severity, report for healthcare provider evaluation.

▪ Serious Adverse Effects

Gastrointestinal

Hepatotoxicity. Overdosage caused by acute and chronic ingestion has risen dramatically in the past few years. Severe life-threatening hepatotoxicity has been reported in patients who ingest 5 to 8 g daily for several weeks or attempt suicide by consuming large quantities at one time. Hepatotoxicity is also more frequent with heavy alcohol use and ingestion of acetaminophen.

Early indications of toxicity include anorexia, nausea, vomiting, low blood pressure, drowsiness, confusion, and abdominal pain—symptoms often attributed to other causes. Within 2 to 4 days, symptoms of hepatotoxicity develop (jaundice and a rise in the AST and ALT levels and prothrombin time). If acetaminophen toxicity is suspected, consult the manufacturer, a university drug information center, or a poison control center for the most current recommendations for therapy.

▪ Drug Interactions

Barbiturates, Carbamazepine, Phenytoin, Sulfinpyrazone. If acetaminophen is taken in large doses or over the long term, these agents may enhance hepatotoxicity.

Alcohol. Chronic excessive ingestion of alcohol may increase the potential for hepatotoxicity with therapeutic doses or overdoses of acetaminophen.

---

salicylates (săl-ĭ-SĬL-āts)

ACTIONS

Salicylates are the most common analgesics used for the relief of slight to moderate pain. Salicylates were introduced into medicine in the late nineteenth century because of their three primary pharmacologic effects as analgesic, antipyretic, and antiinflammatory agents. Although the mechanisms of action are not fully known, most of the activity of salicylates comes from inhibiting prostaglandin synthesis. Salicylates inhibit the formation of prostaglandins that sensitize pain receptors to stimulation causing pain (analgesia), they inhibit the prostaglandins that produce the signs and symptoms of inflammation (e.g., redness, swelling, warmth), and they inhibit the synthesis and release of prostaglandins in the brain that cause the elevation of body temperature (antipyresis). A major benefit of salicylates is that they do not dull the consciousness level and do not cause mental sluggishness, memory disturbances, hallucinations, euphoria, or sedation.

A unique property of aspirin, compared with other salicylates, is inhibition of platelet aggregation and enhancement of bleeding time. The platelet loses its ability to aggregate and form clots for the duration of its lifetime (7 to 10 days). The mechanism of action is inhibition of the synthesis of thromboxane A2, a potent vasoconstrictor and inducer of platelet aggregation.

USES

The combination of pharmacologic effects makes salicylates the drug of choice for symptomatic relief of discomfort, pain, inflammation, or fever associated with bacterial and viral infections, headache, muscle aches, and rheumatoid arthritis. Salicylates can be taken to relieve pain on a long-term basis without causing drug dependence. The use of salicylates in children is not recommended because of the associated risk of Reye's syndrome.

Because of its antiplatelet activity, aspirin is also indicated for reducing the risk of recurrent transient ischemic attacks (TIAs) or stroke. Aspirin is also used to reduce the risk of MI in patients with previous MI or unstable angina pectoris. Aspirin is administered on arrival to the emergency room to those patients experiencing an acute MI.

THERAPEUTIC OUTCOMES

The primary therapeutic outcomes expected from salicylates are reduced pain, reduced inflammation, and elimination of fever. The primary therapeutic outcomes expected from aspirin when used for antiplatelet therapy are reduced frequency of TIA, stroke, or MI.

❖ NURSING IMPLICATIONS FOR SALICYLATES

▪ Premedication Assessment

1. Perform baseline neurologic assessment (e.g., orientation to date, time, and place; mental alertness; bilateral hand grip; motor functioning).
2. Monitor vital signs (i.e., temperature, blood pressure, pulse, respirations).
3. Check laboratory values for hepatotoxicity, renal impairment, and clotting time.

4. Monitor for GI symptoms before and during therapy; conduct stool guaiac test if GI tract bleeding is suspected.
5. Check for concurrent use of anticoagulant agents.
6. If the patient is taking oral hypoglycemics, review baseline serum glucose level.
7. When used as an analgesic, perform pain assessment before administering salicylates and at appropriate intervals during therapy. Report poor pain control promptly and obtain modification in orders.

■ **Availability**

See Tables 19-3 and 19-4.

■ **Dosage and Administration**

Treatment of Pain, Arthritis, Acute Rheumatic Fever, and Myocardial Infarction Prophylaxis. See Table 19-3.

Stroke Prevention. See Table 19-3.

■ **Common Adverse Effects**

As beneficial as salicylates are, they are not without adverse effects. In normal therapeutic dosages, they may produce GI irritation, occasional nausea, and gastric hemorrhage. Extreme caution should be used with administration to patients with a history of peptic ulcer, liver disease, or coagulation disorders.

Gastrointestinal

Gastric irritation. If gastric irritation occurs, give medication with food, milk, or antacids (1 hour later) or with large amounts of water. If symptoms persist or increase in severity, notify the healthcare provider. Aspirin is available in an enteric-coated form to reduce gastric irritation.

■ **Serious Adverse Effects**

Gastrointestinal

Gastrointestinal bleeding. Dark, tarry stools and bright red or coffee-ground emesis may occur. Test any suspect stools or emesis for presence of occult blood.

Toxicity

Salicylism. Patients receiving higher doses on a continuing basis are susceptible to developing salicylate intoxication (salicylism). Symptoms include tinnitus (ringing in the ears), impaired hearing, dimming of vision, sweating, fever, lethargy, dizziness, mental confusion, nausea, and vomiting. This condition is reversible on dosage reduction. Massive overdosage may lead to respiratory depression and coma. There is no antidote; primary treatment is discontinuing the drug, gastric lavage, forcing IV fluids, and alkalizing the urine with IV sodium bicarbonate.

Patients who develop signs of salicylate toxicity should be reevaluated for other underlying diseases and the possibility that other medications would be more effective.

■ **Drug Interactions**

Nonsteroidal Antiinflammatory Drugs. It is possible that cyclooxygenase-1 (COX-1) inhibitors reduce the platelet-inhibiting effects of aspirin when administered at about the same time. The NSAID may block the receptor on platelets that aspirin would normally bind to, preventing the platelet inhibition caused by aspirin. One approach to avoid this interaction is to take aspirin several hours before the COX-1 NSAID. This might not be possible for a patient with severe rheumatoid arthritis who needs the analgesic effects around the clock.

Sulfinpyrazone, Probenecid. Salicylates inhibit the excretion of uric acid by these agents. Although an occasional aspirin will not interfere with their effectiveness, regular use of salicylates or products containing salicylate should be discouraged. If analgesia is required, suggest acetaminophen.

Warfarin. Salicylates may enhance the anticoagulant effects of warfarin. Observe for petechiae; ecchymoses; nosebleeds; bleeding gums; dark, tarry stools; and bright red or coffee-ground emesis. Monitor prothrombin time and reduce the dosage of warfarin if necessary.

Valproic Acid. Monitor the patient with concurrent therapy for signs of valproic acid toxicity, such as sedation or lethargy. Serum levels may be ordered, and the dosage of valproic acid may need to be reduced.

Oral Hypoglycemic Agents. Salicylates may enhance the hypoglycemic effects of these agents. Monitor for hypoglycemia, headache, weakness, decreased coordination, general apprehension, diaphoresis, hunger, or blurred or double vision. The dosage of the hypoglycemic agent may need to be reduced. Notify the healthcare provider if any of the previous symptoms appear.

Methotrexate. Monitor for signs of methotrexate toxicity: bone marrow suppression, decreased white blood cell (WBC) count, decreased red blood cell (RBC) count, sore throat, fever, or lethargy.

Corticosteroids. Although often used together, salicylates and corticosteroids may produce GI ulceration. Monitor for signs of GI bleeding; observe for the development of dark, tarry stools and bright red or coffee-ground emesis.

Ethanol. The patient should avoid aspirin within 8 to 10 hours of heavy alcohol use. Small amounts of GI bleeding often occur. If aspirin therapy is absolutely necessary, an enteric-coated product should be used.

DRUG CLASS: NONSTEROIDAL ANTIINFLAMMATORY DRUGS

ACTIONS

Nonsteroidal antiinflammatory drugs (NSAIDs) are also known as *aspirin-like drugs.* They are chemically unrelated to salicylates but are prostaglandin inhibitors

Table 19-3 Nonsteroidal Antiinflammatory Drugs

GENERIC NAME	BRAND NAME	AVAILABILITY	USES AND DOSAGES	MAXIMUM DAILY DOSAGE (mg)
Salicylates				
aspirin	Ecotrin, St. Joseph	Tablets: 81, 325, 500 mg Tablets, sustained release: 81, 162, 325, 500 mg Tablets, dispersible: 81 mg Tablets, chewable: 81 mg Suppositories: 60, 120, 200, 300, 600 mg	Minor aches and pains: 325-600 mg q4h Arthritis: 2.6-5.2 g/day in divided doses Acute rheumatic fever: 7.8 g/day Myocardial infarction prophylaxis: 75-325 mg daily Ischemic stroke and TIA: 50-325 mg daily	—
diflunisal	Dolobid	Tablets: 500 mg	Mild to moderate pain: Initially, 1000 mg, then 500 mg q8h Osteoarthritis and rheumatoid arthritis: 250-500 mg twice daily	1500
magnesium salicylate	Doan's	Tablets: 325, 580, 600 mg	Mild aches and pains: 500-650 mg three or four times daily	9600
salsalate	—	Tablets: 500, 750 mg	Mild pain: 500-700 mg four to six times daily	3000
Nonsteroidal Antiinflammatory Drugs				
Cyclooxygenase-1 (COX-1) Inhibitors				
diclofenac	Cataflam, Voltaren, Teva-Diclophenac ❦ Flector Solaraze Voltaren	Tablets: 50 mg Tablets, delayed release (24 hr): 25, 50, 75, 100 mg Capsules: 18, 25, 35 mg Patch, transdermal: 1.3% Gel, transdermal: 3% Gel, transdermal: 1%	Rheumatoid and osteoarthritis, ankylosing spondylitis: 25-50 mg two or three times daily Primary dysmenorrhea: 50 mg three times daily Apply to pain site twice daily. Do not apply to broken skin. For actinic keratoses: Apply twice daily. Avoid direct sun exposure. Osteoarthritis: Apply to affected arm, hand, foot, and knee joints four times daily. Do not apply to spine, hips, or shoulders.	200
etodolac	—	Capsules: 200, 300 mg Tablets: 400, 500 mg Tablets, extended release: 400, 500, 600 mg	Osteoarthritis, pain: 300-400 mg three or four times daily	1200
fenoprofen	Nalfon	Capsules: 400 mg Tablets: 600 mg	Rheumatoid and osteoarthritis: 300-600 mg three or four times daily Mild to moderate pain: 200 mg q4-6h	3200
flurbiprofen	—	Tablets: 50, 100 mg	Rheumatoid and osteoarthritis: 50-100 mg two or three times daily	300
ibuprofen	Motrin, Advil, Apo-Ibuprofen ❦	Tablets: 100, 200, 400, 600, 800 mg Tablets, chewable: 50, 100, 200 mg Capsules: 200 mg Suspension: 40 mg/mL, 50 mg/1.25 mL; 100 mg/5 mL Oral drops: 40 mg/mL	Rheumatoid and osteoarthritis: 300-600 mg three or four times daily Mild to moderate pain: 400 mg q4-6h Primary dysmenorrhea: 400 mg q4h Fever: Pediatric: 5-10 mg/kg three or four times daily	2400

Continued

Table 19-3 Nonsteroidal Antiinflammatory Drugs—cont'd

GENERIC NAME	BRAND NAME	AVAILABILITY	USES AND DOSAGES	MAXIMUM DAILY DOSAGE (mg)
indomethacin	Indocin, Tevo-Indomethacin ♣	Capsules: 25, 50 mg Capsules, sustained release: 75 mg Oral suspension: 25 mg/5 mL Suppository: 50 mg	Rheumatoid and osteoarthritis, ankylosing spondylitis: 25-50 mg three or four times daily Acute painful shoulder: 25-50 mg two or three times daily Acute gouty arthritis: 50 mg three times daily Closure of patent ductus arteriosus: IV, one to three doses at 12- to 24-hr intervals	—
ketoprofen	Apo-Keto ♣	Capsules: 50, 75 mg Capsules, extended release (24 hr): 200 mg	Rheumatoid and osteoarthritis: Initially, 75 mg three times daily or 50 mg four times daily; reduce initial dose by $\frac{1}{2}$ to $\frac{1}{3}$ in older patients or those with impaired renal function Mild pain, primary dysmenorrhea: 25-50 mg three or four times daily	300
ketorolac ❶	Apo-Ketorolac ♣	Tablets: 10 mg Injection: 15, 30, 60 mg/mL in 1-, 2-mL prefilled syringes; 300 mg/10 mL in 10-mL vials Nasal solution: 15.75 mg/spray	Injectable analgesic, anti-inflammatory, antipyretic used for acute, short-term pain management; 30-60 mg IM, initially, 15-30 mg q6h PRN pain; then PO, up to 40 mg/24 hr; do not exceed 5 days of therapy	120-150
meclofenamate	—	Capsules: 50, 100 mg	Rheumatoid and osteoarthritis: 200-400 mg daily in three or four equal doses Mild to moderate pain: 50-100 mg three or four times daily Primary dysmenorrhea: 100 mg three times daily	400
mefenamic acid	Ponstel, Apo-mefenamic ♣	Capsules: 250 mg	Moderate pain or primary dysmenorrhea: Initially, 500 mg, then 250 mg q6h; do not exceed 7 days of therapy	1000
meloxicam	Mobic	Tablets: 7.5, 15 mg Liquid: 7.5 mg/5 mL	Osteoarthritis: 7.5-15 mg daily	15
nabumetone	—	Tablets: 500, 750 mg	Rheumatoid and osteoarthritis: 1000-1500 mg daily in one or two doses	2000
naproxen	Naprosyn, Aleve, Anaprox, Anaprox DS	Tablets: 220, 250, 275, 375, 500, 550 mg Tablets, extended release (24 hr): 375, 500, 750 mg Oral suspension: 125 mg/5 mL	Rheumatoid arthritis, osteoarthritis, ankylosing spondylitis: 250-375 mg twice daily Acute gout: 750-825 mg initially, followed by 250-275 mg q8h Moderate pain, primary dysmenorrhea, acute tendonitis, bursitis: 500-550 mg followed by 250-275 mg	1000
oxaprozin	Daypro	Caplets: 600 mg	Rheumatoid arthritis, osteoarthritis: 1200 mg once daily	1800
piroxicam	Feldene, Teva-Piroxicam ♣	Capsules: 10, 20 mg	Rheumatoid arthritis osteoarthritis: 20 mg once daily	200

Table 19-3   Nonsteroidal Antiinflammatory Drugs—cont'd

GENERIC NAME	BRAND NAME	AVAILABILITY	USES AND DOSAGES	MAXIMUM DAILY DOSAGE (mg)
sulindac	Apo-Sulin ♣	Tablets: 150, 200 mg	Rheumatoid arthritis, osteoarthritis, ankylosing spondylitis: 150 mg twice daily Acute painful shoulder: 200 mg twice daily	400
tolmetin	—	Tablets: 200, 600 mg Capsules: 400 mg	Rheumatoid arthritis, osteoarthritis: 400-600 mg three times daily	2000
Cyclooxygenase-2 (COX-2) Inhibitors				
celecoxib	Celebrex	Capsules: 50, 100, 200, 400 mg	Rheumatoid arthritis, osteoarthritis: 100-200 mg twice daily Ankylosing spondylitis: 200-400 mg daily Acute pain and primary dysmenorrhea: 400 mg initially, followed by 200 mg on the first day, then 200 mg twice daily Familial adenomatous polyposis (FAP): 400 mg twice daily taken with food	—

♣ Available in Canada.   ❶ High-alert medication.
TIA, transient ischemic attack.

Table 19-4   Ingredients of Selected Analgesic Combination Products

PRODUCT	NONCONTROLLED SUBSTANCE			CONTROLLED SUBSTANCE	
	ASPIRIN (mg)	ACETAMINOPHEN* (mg)	OTHER (mg)	CODEINE (mg)	OTHER (mg)
Anacin caplets and tablets	400	—	Caffeine, 32	—	—
Anacin Maximum Strength	500	—	Caffeine, 32	—	—
BC Powder Arthritis Strength	742	—	Caffeine, 38 Salicylamide, 222	—	—
Excedrin Extra Strength	250	250	Caffeine, 65	—	—
Fioricet		325	Caffeine, 40	—	Butalbital, 50
Fiorinal	325	—	Caffeine, 40	—	Butalbital, 50
Fiorinal with Codeine	325	—	Caffeine, 40	30	Butalbital, 50
Lortab 10/325	—	325	—	—	Hydrocodone, 10
Norco	—	325	—	—	Hydrocodone, 10
Percocet 7.5	—	325	—	—	Oxycodone, 7.5
Percodan	325	—	—	—	Oxycodone, 4.5
Percogesic	—	325	Diphenhydramine 12.5	—	—
Talwin Compound caplets	325	—	—	—	Pentazocine, 12.5
Tylenol	—	325	—	—	—

Tylenol with
  Codeine No. 3
  Codeine No. 4
	—
	—
		300
		300
			—
			—
				30
				60
					—
					—

Vicodin	—	300	—	—	Hydrocodone, 5
Vicodin ES	—	300	—	—	Hydrocodone, 7.5
Vicodin HP	—	300	—	—	Hydrocodone, 10 mg
Vicoprofen	—	—	—	—	Hydrocodone, 7.5 Ibuprofen, 200

*As of January 2014, acetaminophen content in combination products is limited to a maximum of 325 mg per tablet or capsule.

and share many of the same therapeutic actions and adverse effects. NSAIDs block cyclooxygenase (COX-1 and COX-2). They all have varying degrees of analgesic, antipyretic, and antiinflammatory activity. Celecoxib is a COX-2 selective inhibitor, whereas all other NSAIDs are nonselective COX-1 and COX-2 inhibitors.

USES

In clinical studies, all of these agents (see Table 19-3) are superior to placebos. Depending on the agent used, the dosage, and the patient, the adverse effects of therapy tend to be somewhat less than those associated with salicylate therapy. There is little difference between them in effectiveness or tolerance, but there is a difference in response among individuals, and switching to another NSAID for better therapeutic effect is appropriate. Longer-acting NSAIDs may be useful for patients who have difficulty remembering to take frequent doses. There is also substantial cost difference among NSAIDs, so it makes sense to try the lower-cost agents before moving to the more expensive agents. Many of these products are also available in generic form that will further reduce expense of therapy.

These agents are used to relieve the pain and inflammation of rheumatoid arthritis, osteoarthritis, ankylosing spondylitis, and gout. Certain agents (e.g., ibuprofen, ketoprofen, naproxen, diclofenac, celecoxib) are also approved for use to control the discomfort of primary dysmenorrhea. Ibuprofen, naproxen, and ketoprofen are available over the counter (OTC) to be used for the temporary relief of minor aches and pains associated with the common cold, headache, toothache, muscle aches, backaches, arthritis, and menstrual cramps, as well as to reduce fever. COX-2 inhibitors appear to have the advantage of causing fewer GI adverse effects, such as upper GI bleeding. This is significant because 7% to 8% of patients experience GI bleeding while using NSAIDs, and it is a primary cause of hospitalizations caused by adverse effects of medications.

In April 2005, the U.S. Food and Drug Administration (FDA) issued a warning about an increased risk of potentially fatal cardiovascular adverse effects (heart attack, stroke) that could be a class effect of NSAIDs. The FDA also reiterated the well-described risk of serious and potentially life-threatening GI bleeding associated with NSAIDs. Nonsteroidal antiinflammatory drugs have also been associated with allergic reactions, including severe skin reactions and anaphylaxis, some of which occurred in patients without known prior exposure. If an NSAID is prescribed for chronic use, the lowest effective dose for the shortest duration should be used. Nonsteroidal antiinflammatory drugs should not be used in patients immediately after coronary artery bypass graft (CABG) surgery.

THERAPEUTIC OUTCOMES

The primary therapeutic outcomes expected from NSAIDs are reduced pain, reduced inflammation, and elimination of fever.

❖ NURSING IMPLICATIONS FOR NSAIDs

▪ Premedication Assessment
1. Perform baseline neurologic assessment (e.g., orientation to date, time, and place; mental alertness; bilateral hand grip; motor functioning; peripheral sensations; and vision and hearing).
2. Monitor vital signs (i.e., temperature, blood pressure, pulse, and respirations).
3. Check laboratory data for hepatotoxicity, nephrotoxicity, bleeding time, and blood dyscrasias.
4. Monitor for GI symptoms before and during therapy; conduct a stool guaiac test if GI tract bleeding is suspected.
5. Check bowel sounds and note stool consistency. Review voiding pattern and urine output.
6. Check for concurrent use of anticoagulant agents.
7. When used as an analgesic, perform pain assessment before administering NSAIDs and at appropriate intervals during therapy. Report poor pain control promptly and obtain modification in orders.

▪ Availability, Dosage, and Administration
See Table 19-3.

 Medication Safety Alert

Do not administer NSAIDs to patients who are allergic to aspirin.

▪ Common Adverse Effects
Gastrointestinal
Gastric irritation, constipation. If gastric irritation occurs, give medication with food, milk, antacids, or large amounts of water. If symptoms persist or increase in severity, notify the healthcare provider. The use of stool softeners or bulk-forming laxatives may be necessary. Maintain the patient's state of hydration. Encourage the patient to include sufficient roughage, fresh fruits, vegetables, and whole-grain products in the diet.

▪ Serious Adverse Effects
Gastrointestinal
Gastrointestinal bleeding. Observe for the development of dark, tarry stools and bright red or coffee-ground emesis. Other factors for increased risk of bleeding include concurrent use of oral corticosteroids, anticoagulants, smoking, consuming more than three alcoholic drinks per day, age older than 60 years, and poor general health status. Special care should be taken in elderly or debilitated patients.

Hepatotoxicity. The symptoms of hepatotoxicity are anorexia, nausea, vomiting, jaundice, hepatomegaly, splenomegaly, and abnormal liver function tests (e.g., elevated bilirubin, AST, ALT, alkaline phosphatase levels; increased prothrombin time).

Hypersensitivity

Hives, pruritus, rash, facial swelling. Report symptoms for further evaluation by the healthcare provider as soon as possible. This could become a medical emergency.

Genitourinary

Nephrotoxicity. Monitor urinalysis and kidney function tests for abnormal results. Report increasing blood urea nitrogen (BUN) and creatinine levels, decreasing urine output or urine specific gravity despite amount of fluid intake, casts or protein in the urine, frank blood- or smoky-colored urine, or RBCs in excess of 0 to 3 on the urinalysis report.

Hematologic

Blood dyscrasias. Routine laboratory studies (e.g., RBC, WBC, differential counts) should be scheduled. Monitor for sore throat, fever, purpura, jaundice, or excessive and progressive weakness.

■ **Drug Interactions**

Warfarin. Nonsteroidal antiinflammatory drugs increase bleeding risk through platelet inhibition. When used concurrently with warfarin, the patient may be at greater risk of bleeding even though the PT and INR are within therapeutic range. Observe for petechiae; ecchymoses; nosebleeds; bleeding gums; dark, tarry stools; and bright red or coffee-ground emesis. The dosage of warfarin may need to be reduced.

Phenytoin. Monitor the patient with concurrent therapy for signs of phenytoin toxicity, such as nystagmus, sedation, or lethargy. Serum levels may be ordered, and the dosage of phenytoin may need to be reduced.

Valproic Acid. Aspirin inhibits valproic acid metabolism, increasing valproic acid blood levels. Monitor for valproic acid toxicity: sedation, drowsiness, dizziness, or blurred vision. Serum levels may be ordered, and the dosage of valproic acid may need to be reduced.

Oral Hypoglycemic Agents. Monitor for hypoglycemia: headache, weakness, decreased coordination, general apprehension, diaphoresis, hunger, blurred or double vision. The dosage of the hypoglycemic agent may need to be reduced. Notify the healthcare provider if any of these symptoms appear.

Furosemide, Thiazide Diuretics. Nonsteroidal antiinflammatory drugs inhibit the diuretic activity of these agents. The dosage of the diuretic agents may need to be increased or NSAIDs discontinued. Maintain accurate intake and output and blood pressure records, and monitor for a decrease in diuretic and antihypertensive activity.

Probenecid. Probenecid inhibits the excretion of NSAIDs. Monitor for signs of toxicity: headache, drowsiness, and mental confusion.

Lithium. Nonsteroidal antiinflammatory drugs (except possibly sulindac and aspirin) may induce lithium toxicity. Monitor for lithium toxicity: nausea, anorexia, fine tremors, persistent vomiting, profuse diarrhea, hyperreflexia, lethargy, and weakness.

Aspirin. COX-1 inhibitors may reduce the platelet-inhibiting effects of aspirin when administered at about the same time. An NSAID may block the receptor on platelets that aspirin would normally bind to, preventing the platelet inhibition caused by aspirin. To avoid this interaction, take the aspirin several hours before the COX-1 NSAID. This might not be possible for the person with severe rheumatoid arthritis who needs the analgesic effects around the clock.

Cholestyramine. Cholestyramine resins bind to NSAIDs in the gut, inhibiting absorption. Separate dosage administration by 2 hours. The NSAID dosage may need to be increased.

Get Ready for the NCLEX® Examination!

Key Points

- The pain experience is highly subjective and influenced by behavioral, physiologic, sensory, emotional (e.g., attention, anxiety, fatigue, suggestion, prior conditioning), and cultural factors for a particular person under a certain set of circumstances.
- Pain is usually described as acute or short term and as chronic or long term.
- Analgesics are drugs that relieve pain without producing loss of consciousness or reflex activity.
- Analgesic medications have been divided into opiate agonists, opiate partial agonists, opiate antagonists, and prostaglandin inhibitors (acetaminophen, salicylates, and nonsteroidal antiinflammatory drugs [NSAIDs]).
- Pain management has made significant progress, primarily because of better understanding of the pain experience; however, there is still a great deal to do in educating patients, family, and some healthcare providers about appropriate pain management.
- Nurses can play an important role in providing counseling and guidance to these groups in understanding pain and how to maintain an appropriate balance between daily activities and timing of analgesics to optimize quality of life.

Additional Learning Resources

SG Go to your Study Guide for additional Review Questions for the NCLEX® Examination, Critical Thinking Clinical Situations, and other learning activities to help you master this chapter content.

evolve Go to your Evolve website (http://evolve .elsevier.com/Clayton) for additional online resources.

Review Questions for the NCLEX® Examination

1. Nurses working with patients in pain must recognize and avoid common misconceptions about pain. With regard to the pain experience, which statement is correct?
   1. The patient is the best authority on the pain experience.
   2. Chronic pain is mostly psychological in nature.
   3. Regular use of analgesics leads to drug dependence.
   4. The amount of tissue damage does not affect the perception of pain.

2. The nurse was reviewing an order for the pain medication tramadol (Ultram) for a postop patient and realized the drug is classified as a(an):
   1. opiate partial agonist.
   2. opiate agonist.
   3. opiate antagonist.
   4. prostaglandin inhibitor.

3. Nurses frequently assess a patient who is in pain. When assessing the pain, the nurse will do the following? *(Select all that apply.)*
   1. Request that the patient wait until the proper time to take pain medication
   2. Question the patient about the location of the pain
   3. Offer the patient a pain scale to quantify the pain
   4. Use open-ended questions to find out about the pain
   5. Ask about what has worked in the past to control the pain

4. A patient will be receiving pain medication administered through a PCA system. To help family members understand how this therapy works, what does the nurse explain to the family?
   1. "It is important to allow the patient to have control over the frequency of administration of the pain medication."
   2. "This system of pain medication allows the patient to control the dose of the medication."
   3. "The patient is supposed to control the delivery of the medication, but you can push the button too if you see the patient in pain."
   4. "The types of medications that are commonly used in this PCA system are the nonsteroidal anti-inflammatory drugs."

5. While preparing aspirin for the patient, the nurse reviewed the pharmacologic effects of salicylates: *(Select all that apply.)*
   1. analgesic.
   2. antiepileptic.
   3. antipyretic.
   4. antiinflammatory.
   5. antiemetic.

6. The patient who was taking aspirin for arthritis stated to the nurse that it was not working anymore and planned to stop taking it. The best response by the nurse would be:
   1. "I can see why you would want to stop taking it; you might be showing signs of physical dependence."
   2. "Okay, you have that right to refuse these drugs."
   3. "What prompted that? I'm sure the medication is working just fine."
   4. "I understand your frustration, but I think you need to talk this over with your healthcare provider first before making any decisions."

7. The nurse was explaining to the patient the many properties of diflunisal (Dolobid) to the patient with osteoarthritis: *(Select all that apply.)*
   1. "This drug is classified as a prostaglandin inhibitor."
   2. "The adverse effects that need to be monitored include GI bleeding and liver function tests."
   3. "When taking salicylate therapy you need to be careful with diuretic agents, as the Dolobid may increase the effectiveness of the diuretic."
   4. "This drug may require the monitoring of your kidney function so that adverse effects are identified."
   5. "If you need to take this long term, we will generally have you take the lowest effective dose to minimize adverse effects."

Introduction to Cardiovascular Disease and Metabolic Syndrome

Objectives

1. Identify the major risk factors for the development of metabolic syndrome.
2. Discuss the importance of lifestyle modification in the management of metabolic syndrome.
3. Explain the treatment goals for type 2 diabetes management, lipid management, and hypertension management.
4. Discuss the drug management of the underlying diseases used by patients with metabolic syndrome.

Key Terms

cardiovascular disease (kăr-dē-ō-VĂS-kyū-lăr) (p. 317)
atherosclerotic cardiovascular disease (ASCVD) (ăth-ĕr-ō-sklĕ-RŎ-tĭk) (p. 317)
coronary artery disease (CAD) (KŎR-ō-năr-ē ĂR-tĕr-ē) (p. 317)
angina pectoris (ăn-JĪ-nă PĔK-tŏr-ĭs) (p. 317)
myocardial infarction (MI) (mī-ō-KĂR-dē-ăl ĭn-FĂRK-shŭn) (p. 317)
stroke (STRŌK) (p. 317)
hypertension (hī-pĕr-TĔN-shŭn) (p. 317)

dysrhythmias (dĭs-RĬTH-mē-ăz) (p. 317)
peripheral vascular disease (pĕ-RĬF-ĕr-ăl VĂS-kū-lăr) (p. 317)
peripheral arterial disease (pĕ-RĬF-ĕr-ăl ăr-TĒR-ē-ŭl) (p. 317)
heart failure (HĂRT FĀL-yŭr) (p. 317)
insulin resistance syndrome (ĬN-sŭl-ĭn rē-ZĬS-tĕns) (p. 318)
metabolic syndrome (MĔT-ah-BŎL-ĭk) (p. 318)
body mass index (BMI) (BŎ-dē MĂS ĬN-dĕks) (p. 319)

CARDIOVASCULAR DISEASES

Cardiovascular disease (CVD) is a collective term used to refer to disorders of the circulatory system (heart, arteries, veins) of the body. The total direct and indirect cost of CVD for 2010 is estimated to be $315 billion. This includes direct costs (e.g., professional personnel, hospital services, prescribed medications, home health care, and other medical durables) and lost productivity from indirect costs of premature death. By comparison, the direct and indirect costs for cancer and benign neoplasms was $201.5 billion (Go, 2013).

These diseases have been subdivided into the areas or organs of the body in which the pathology is most obvious, such as **atherosclerotic cardiovascular disease (ASCVD),** which refers to narrowing of arteries by atherosclerotic plaques caused by hypercholesterolemia, and **coronary artery disease (CAD)** (see Chapter 21), which refers to narrowing or obstruction of the arteries of the heart, leading to **angina pectoris** and **myocardial infarction (MI)** (Chapter 24). **Stroke** (see Chapter 26) refers to either an obstruction (ischemic stroke) or rupture (hemorrhagic stroke) of blood vessels in the brain. An increase in the pressure with which blood circulates through the arteries and veins is referred to as **hypertension** (see Chapter 22). **Dysrhythmias** (see Chapter 23) are abnormalities in the electrical conduction pathways of the heart that lead to inefficient pumping of blood through the circulatory system. **Peripheral vascular disease** involves disorders of the blood vessels of the arms and legs. It can be subdivided into two types, depending on whether it is arterial or venous in origin: **peripheral arterial disease** (see Chapter 25), such as obstructive arterial disease, or venous disorders, such as acute deep vein thrombosis (see Chapter 26). The long-term pathology of any one or a combination of these diseases affecting the circulatory system leads to **heart failure** (see Chapter 27) and eventual death.

METABOLIC SYNDROME

Many causative factors lead to cardiovascular disorders (Box 20-1). Lifestyle is recognized as the greatest

Box **20-1**	Cardiovascular Disorders

- Coronary artery disease
- Angina pectoris
- Acute myocardial infarction
- Congenital heart disease
- Pulmonary stenosis
- Coarctation of the aorta
- Atrial septal defect
- Ventricular septal defect
- Valvular heart disease
- Mitral stenosis and regurgitation
- Aortic stenosis and regurgitation
- Tricuspid stenosis and regurgitation
- Disorders of heart rate and rhythm (dysrhythmias)
- Cardiomyopathies
- Pericarditis
- Rheumatic heart disease
- Cancers of the heart
- Heart failure

Table **20-1**	Definitions and Characteristics of Metabolic Syndrome*

RISK FACTOR DEFINING LIMIT	NATIONAL CHOLESTEROL EDUCATION PROGRAM (UNITED STATES)	
	MEN	WOMEN
Waist circumference (inches)†	>40	>35
High-density lipoprotein cholesterol (mg/dL)	<40	<50
Triglycerides (mg/dL)‡	>150	>150
Blood pressure (mm Hg)	>130/85	>130/85
Fasting glucose (mg/dL)	>100	>100

Data from Alberti KG, Eckel RH, Grundy SM, et al: International Diabetes Federation Task Force on Epidemiology and Prevention; National Heart, Lung, and Blood Institute; American Heart Association; World Heart Federation; International Atherosclerosis Society; International Association for the Study of Obesity: Harmonizing the metabolic syndrome: a joint interim statement of the International Diabetes Federation Task Force on Epidemiology and Prevention; National Heart, Lung, and Blood Institute; American Heart Association; World Heart Federation; International Atherosclerosis Society; and www.idf.org/. The IDF consensus worldwide definition of the metabolic syndrome. Brussels, Belgium. International Diabetes Federation (2014).
*People with central obesity and at least two of the remaining four factors are considered to have metabolic syndrome.
†There are specific circumferences for different ethnicities in the citation accompanying the table.
‡This also applies to those with previously diagnosed type 2 diabetes.

contributor to a variety of diseases that reduce the quality of life and end lives prematurely. These diseases also cost the American economy billions of dollars that could be used in many more positive, beneficial ways. Since the 1920s, investigators have hypothesized about various factors that lead to cardiovascular disease. Research during the 1960s indicated that persons with hypertension, diabetes mellitus, dyslipidemia, and obesity—alone or in combination—were at greater risk for progressive cardiovascular disease.

In 1988 a unifying pathway of insulin resistance, called *syndrome X,* was described. In 1998 the World Health Organization provided a working definition for this syndrome and renamed it *metabolic syndrome.* Insulin resistance leads to type 2 diabetes and induces atherosclerosis, which leads to coronary artery disease. Over the past 20 years, the hypothesis of insulin resistance has been studied in great depth, and the syndrome has been renamed to be more descriptive of the underlying causes. Other terms include *diabesity* and, more recently, **insulin resistance syndrome.**

Metabolic syndrome is still the most commonly used term worldwide. The key characteristics of metabolic syndrome are the presence of type 2 diabetes mellitus, abdominal obesity, hypertriglyceridemia, low levels of high-density lipoproteins (HDLs), and hypertension. Although metabolic syndrome occurs worldwide, an estimated 34% of adults (i.e., one in three) in the United States have metabolic syndrome. More than 4% of adolescents between the ages of 12 and 19 years also have metabolic syndrome. Within ethnic groups, African American males have the lowest rate (14%), whereas Hispanic American women have the highest rate (27%).

Table 20-1 gives the definition of metabolic syndrome provided in a consensus statement by several international organizations that study atherosclerosis, obesity, cardiovascular disease, and diabetes (Alberti, 2009). People with central obesity and two of the four other criteria are defined as having metabolic syndrome.

RESULTING CONDITIONS

People with metabolic syndrome are three times more likely to have (and twice as likely to die of) a heart attack or stroke than people without the syndrome. People with metabolic syndrome have a fivefold greater risk of developing type 2 diabetes. On a global scale, up to 80% of the 200 million people with diabetes will die as a result of cardiovascular disease. This puts the prevalence of metabolic syndrome and diabetes substantially ahead of HIV/AIDS in terms of morbidity and mortality, yet the problem is not as well recognized (International Diabetes Federation, 2014). In addition to type 2 diabetes and heart disease, other factors associated with metabolic syndrome include renal disease, obstructive sleep apnea, polycystic ovary syndrome, cognitive decline in older adults, and dementia in older adults.

RISK FACTORS

Obesity and Sedentary Lifestyle

Risk factors for the development of metabolic syndrome include poor diet, sedentary lifestyle (lack of exercise), and genetic predisposition. The dietary habits of most Americans have changed significantly over the past 20 years, causing a dramatic increase in weight gain in the United States. Simply put, weight gain occurs when energy intake (food calories) exceeds energy expenditure (burning calories). The 1998 National Heart, Lung, and Blood Institute expert report titled "Clinical Guidelines on the Identification, Evaluation and Treatment of Overweight and Obesity in Adults" describes weight in proportion to height as the **body mass index (BMI).** BMI is calculated the same way for both adults and children. The calculation is based on the following formulas:

Kilograms and Meters (or Centimeters)

$$BMI = \frac{\text{Weight in kilograms (kg)}}{(\text{Height in meters [m]})^2}$$

With the metric system, the formula for BMI is weight in kilograms divided by height in meters squared. Because height is commonly measured in centimeters, divide the height in centimeters by 100 to obtain the height in meters.
Example: Weight = 68 kg, Height = 165 cm (1.65 m)
Calculation: $68 \div (1.65)^2 = 24.98$

Pounds and Inches

$$BMI = \frac{\text{Weight in pounds (lb)}}{(\text{Height in inches [in]})^2} \times 703$$

Calculate the BMI by dividing the weight in pounds (lb) by the height in inches (in) squared and multiplying by a conversion factor of 703.
Example: Weight = 150 lb, Height = 5'5" (65")
Calculation: $(150 \div 65^2) \times 703 = 24.96$

The National Heart, Blood, and Lung Institute guidelines also describe overweight and obesity in terms of the BMI. See Table 20-2 for the relationship between BMI and weight (healthy weight, overweight, or obesity).

In 1991 four U.S. states had obesity prevalence rates of 15% to 19%, and none had rates of 20% or more. In 2006 only 4 states had prevalence rates of less than 20%, 20 states had rates of 20% to 24%, 22 states had rates of more than 25%, and 2 states had an obesity prevalence of 30% or more. In 2010 no state had a prevalence of obesity less than 20%; 36 states had a prevalence of 25% or more, and 12 of these states had a prevalence of 30% or more (CDC, 2013—most recent comparison data). See Figure 20-1 for comparison of obesity rates by race/ethnicity and state.

A sedentary lifestyle contributes to overweight and obesity. New technologies such as labor-saving devices and remote-control devices, as well as the availability of entertainment through television and computers, have significantly reduced daily caloric expenditure. Today, despite common knowledge that regular exercise promotes health, more than 60% of Americans are

Table 20-2	Relationship Between Body Mass Index and Categories of Obesity
BODY MASS INDEX (kg/m²)	**RELATIONSHIP TO WEIGHT**
<18.5	Underweight
18.5 to 24.9	Normal weight
25 to 29.9	Overweight
30 to 34.9	Obesity, class I
35 to 39.9	Obesity, class II
>40	Obesity, class III (extreme obesity)

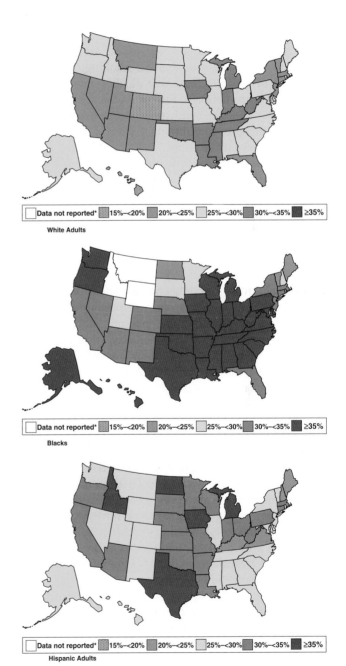

FIGURE 20-1 Prevalence of self-reported obesity among U.S. adults by race, ethnicity, and state, 2011-2013. (From Behavioral Risk Factor Surveillance System, National Center for Chronic Disease Prevention and Health Promotion, Division of Population Health, Centers for Disease Control and Prevention, retrieved from http://www.cdc.gov/obesity/data/prevalence-maps.html.)

not regularly physically active, and 32% do not engage in aerobic, leisure-time physical activity (Go, 2014).

Longer working hours that lead to less time to prepare food at home and larger portions of commercially prepared food aggravate the problem. The ease and convenience of food preparation (e.g., fast-food restaurants, drive-thrus, the use of a microwave versus a convection oven) and increases in portion sizes (e.g., "Supersize it, please!") have placed too many easily consumed calories on the table. Consequently, reduced physical activity and increased caloric intake have resulted in a national epidemic of obesity.

Alcohol and Smoking

Other negative lifestyle choices, such as excessive consumption of alcohol and cigarette smoking, aggravate metabolic syndrome. Excessive alcohol consumption causes fat accumulation in the liver, which is also associated with metabolic syndrome. Cigarette smoking is a major contributor to pulmonary disease (see Chapter 30) and hypertension (see Chapter 22). One study showed that employees with chronic work stress were more than twice as likely to have metabolic syndrome than those without work-related stress. Another study demonstrated that patients with job-related stress had a twofold increase in the risk of recurrent unstable angina and myocardial infarction.

Genetic Factors

Genetic factors influence each component of the syndrome as well as the syndrome itself. A family history of first-degree relatives (e.g., parents, siblings) that includes type 2 diabetes, hypertension, and early heart disease (e.g., angina, "heart attack") greatly increases the likelihood that an individual will develop metabolic syndrome (Figure 20-2).

TREATMENT

The variety of factors associated with the presence of metabolic syndrome requires that an individualized approach to treatment is necessary based on a person's specific risk factors and diseases present. Lifestyle management is critical to prevent and treat the comorbidities that make up the metabolic syndrome. Research indicates that lifestyle changes alone may delay the onset of type 2 diabetes mellitus by more than 50%. The overall treatment goals for metabolic syndrome are listed in Box 20-2.

Weight loss and increased physical activity are usually the first steps of treatment. Reducing the number of calories consumed—while at the same time burning more calories—can have very positive effects in treating metabolic syndrome. Even a 10- to 15-pound weight loss can improve hypertension and hyperglycemia. Initial therapeutic goals are a 7% to 10% weight reduction during the first year of treatment, with an ongoing goal of a BMI less than 25 kg/m². Several dietary approaches can be used to lose weight.

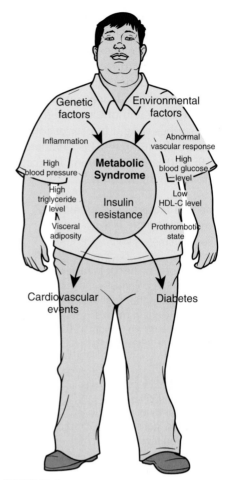

FIGURE 20-2 Mechanisms of metabolic syndrome.

Box 20-2 | **General Treatment Goals for Patients With Metabolic Syndrome**

BLOOD PRESSURE GOALS
- <150/90 mm Hg
- Blood pressure should be measured at every visit

LIPID GOALS
- Low-density lipoproteins (LDL)—individualized for each patient

BLOOD GLUCOSE GOALS
- Hemoglobin A1c <7%
- Fasting plasma glucose <120 mg/dL
- Postprandial plasma glucose <180 mg/dL

Adopting the DASH (*D*ietary *A*pproaches to *S*top *H*ypertension) diet may help patients who also have hypertension (see Chapter 22). The Mediterranean diet—one rich in "good" fats (e.g., olive oil), containing a reasonable amount of carbohydrates, and with protein from fish and chicken—is frequently recommended. The diet should reduce intake of saturated fat (<7% of total calories), lower cholesterol levels (<200 mg/day), and lower total fat intake (25% to 35% of total calories). Most dietary fat should be unsaturated, and the intake of simple sugars should be reduced. Nonpharmacologic therapy must include eliminating cigarette smoking, restricting alcohol intake, reducing stress, and controlling sodium (see Chapter 22). Other appropriate diet plans are the U.S. Department of Agriculture (USDA) Food Pattern or the American Heart Association (AHA) Diet (Eckel, 2013).

The latest report from the National Academy of Sciences/Institute of Medicine (2014) stresses the importance of balancing diet with physical activity to improve circulation, increase HDL levels, and burn calories. Muscles are the primary storage and uptake site for glucose, and because exercise leads to more muscle and less fat, blood glucose levels tend to return to normal levels. The report makes recommendations regarding the daily maximum caloric intake of food to be consumed based on height, weight, and gender for four different levels of physical activity (sedentary, low active, active, and very active). The report also illustrates how difficult it is to lose weight by reduction of calories alone and how important it is to maintain a level of physical activity to prevent a reduction in lean body mass (protein wasting). The report recommends 60 minutes of moderate-intensity physical activity (e.g., walking at a rate of 4 to 5 miles per hour) or high-intensity activity (e.g., jogging at a rate of 4 to 5 miles in 20 to 30 minutes) four to seven times weekly—in addition to the activities of daily living—to maintain the body weight of adults within the recommended body mass index range (18 to 25 kg/m^2). The exercise does not have to be completed at the same time; rather, it can be worked into a person's daily activities. More recent guidelines to reduce low-density lipoprotein (LDL) cholesterol and non-HDL cholesterol (see Chapter 21) and blood pressure (see Chapter 22) recommend at least three to four exercise sessions per week, in addition to activities of daily living, lasting an average of 40 minutes per session, involving moderate- to vigorous-intensity physical activity (Eckel, 2013).

If, after lifestyle modifications and diet and exercise, the patient is not able to meet the therapeutic goals for treating metabolic syndrome, then drug therapy may be necessary. Patient education is vitally important to make patients aware of and treat metabolic syndrome. This education should be emphasized and reiterated frequently by the physician, the pharmacist, and the nurse.

The primary prevention of metabolic syndrome is becoming a common thread in the curriculum of children in the primary grades. This education focuses on the importance of moderate activity, dietary choices, and the prevention of alcohol consumption and smoking. Resources from the National Institutes of Health, such as the MyPlate Food Guide (see Chapter 46), are often used as guidelines for this education; age- and gender-related activity and dietary information are also described.

Drug Therapy to Treat Underlying Conditions for Metabolic Syndrome

Hypertension. A combination of a thiazide diuretic plus an angiotensin-converting enzyme inhibitor, calcium channel blocker, or angiotensin receptor blocker will be necessary to treat hypertension in nonblack patients. In the general black population, including those with diabetes, initial treatment should include a thiazide-type diuretic or calcium channel blocker. Other combinations of therapy may be used, depending on the person's race and the presence of other diseases. (See Chapter 22 for a discussion of the treatment of hypertension.)

Dyslipidemia. The treatment of dyslipidemia is generally to lower triglyceride and LDL cholesterol levels and to raise the HDL cholesterol level. After lifestyle changes, the medicines most commonly used are 3-hydroxymethylglutaryl coenzyme A reductase inhibitors (also known as statins) and fibric acid derivatives. (See Chapter 21 for a discussion of the treatment of dyslipidemias.)

Type 2 Diabetes Mellitus. Several different classes of medicines may be used to treat insulin resistance and type 2 diabetes. The thiazolidinediones reduce insulin resistance in the peripheral tissues. Metformin decreases the production of glucose by the liver; to a lesser extent it also reduces insulin resistance in the peripheral tissues. Alpha-glycosidase inhibitors reduce the absorption of glucose from the intestine, reducing postprandial hyperglycemia. Sulfonylureas and meglitinides stimulate the beta cells of the pancreas to release more insulin. Insulin injections also benefit patients who do not secrete adequate amounts of insulin. (See Chapter 35 for a discussion of the treatment of type 2 diabetes mellitus.)

Get Ready for the NCLEX® Examination!

Key Points

- Cardiovascular diseases are a major cause of premature death in the United States.
- More than 34% of the U.S. adult population has metabolic syndrome; these individuals are at much greater risk for cardiovascular diseases. The key characteristics of metabolic syndrome, are type 2 diabetes mellitus, abdominal obesity, hypertriglyceridemia, a low HDL cholesterol level, and hypertension.
- The most cost-effective and successful forms of treatment are smoking cessation, weight reduction, exercise, stress reduction, and dietary modifications. If changes in diet and exercise do not produce an acceptable decrease in blood lipid levels, blood glucose levels, and hypertension, then antilipemic agents, antihyperglycemic agents, and antihypertensive agents may be added to the patient's regimen.

Additional Learning Resources

SG Go to your Study Guide for additional Review Questions for the NCLEX® Examination, Critical Thinking Clinical Situations, and other learning activities to help you master this chapter content.

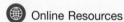 Go to your Evolve website (http://evolve .elsevier.com/Clayton) for additional online resources.

🌐 Online Resources
Centers for Disease Control and Prevention, updated 2013 trend map and other illustrations and information: http:// www.cdc.gov/obesity/data/prevalence-maps.html

Review Questions for the NCLEX® Examination

1. Which risk factors for metabolic syndrome should the nurse include when assessing a patient who came into the clinic for a yearly checkup? *(Select all that apply.)*
   1. Regular exercise
   2. Being overweight
   3. Smoking
   4. Genetic predisposition
   5. Having high blood pressure

2. A nurse tells a 45-year-old male patient whose BMI was calculated to be 29 that this number means:
   1. "This BMI indicates that you are underweight."
   2. "This means that you are within the expected normal weight."
   3. "A BMI over 25 indicates that you are considered overweight and close to obese."
   4. "According to the chart this BMI indicates that you are considered obese, class I."

3. A patient in the clinic asked the nurse for ways to reduce the risk of developing metabolic syndrome. The nurse replied:
   1. "You can't do anything to prevent metabolic syndrome because it is in your genes."
   2. "The best thing you can do to prevent metabolic syndrome is to not get diabetes."
   3. "Lifestyle modifications, including a heart-healthy diet and exercise, are important to practice to prevent the development of metabolic syndrome."
   4. "If you routinely get your blood checked for high cholesterol and eat a low-fat diet, you will not get metabolic syndrome."

4. Patients evaluated for metabolic syndrome should have which laboratory test(s) done? *(Select all that apply.)*
   1. Blood glucose
   2. Liver enzymes
   3. Thyroid hormone
   4. Lipid profile
   5. Hemoglobin A1c

5. Recommendations for patients on how to manage their diabetes to prevent metabolic syndrome include(s): *(Select all that apply.)*
   1. eating a balanced meal.
   2. maintaining an A1c of less than 8%.
   3. keeping the blood sugar less than 180 after meals.
   4. being physically active.
   5. having a BMI less than 25.

6. A patient with metabolic syndrome who requires drug therapy after lifestyle changes were not effective was told by the nurse that these drugs may be used to manage the underlying diseases (hypertension, hyperlipidemia) causing the metabolic syndrome. *(Select all that apply.)*
   1. Thiazide diuretics
   2. Testosterone
   3. Statins
   4. Analgesics
   5. Angiotensin-converting enzyme inhibitors

Drugs Used to Treat Dyslipidemias

Objectives

1. Describe atherosclerosis and identify the four major types of lipoproteins.
2. Describe the primary approaches to treat lipid disorders.
3. Determine which antilipid medications are used for cholesterol control and which can be used for triglyceride control.
4. Differentiate between how statins work to control lipid levels and how the bile acid resins work to control lipid levels.

Key Terms

atherosclerotic cardiovascular disease (ASCVD)
(ăth-ĕr-ō-sklĕ-RŌ-tĭk) (p. 323)
atherosclerosis (ăth-ĕr-ō-sklĕ-RŌ-sĭs) (p. 323)
hyperlipidemia (hī-pĕr-lĭp-ĭ-DĒ-mē-ă) (p. 323)
dyslipidemias (dĭs-lĭp-ĭ-DĒ-mē-ăz) (p. 323)

cholesterol (kō-LĔS-tĕ-rŏl) (p. 323)
triglycerides (trī-GLĬ-sĕ-rīdz) (p. 323)
lipoproteins (lī-pō-PRŌ-tēnz) (p. 323)
chylomicrons (kī-lō-MĬ-krŏnz) (p. 323)
metabolic syndrome (mĕt-ă-BŎL-ĭk SĬN-drōm) (p. 324)

ATHEROSCLEROTIC CARDIOVASCULAR DISEASE

For an introduction to cardiovascular diseases, see Chapter 20. Coronary artery disease (CAD), (also called *coronary heart disease*) is a major cause of premature death in the United States and most other industrialized nations. Almost one third (31.9%) of the U.S. population will die of a heart attack or stroke associated with **atherosclerotic cardiovascular disease (ASCVD)**, one of every six deaths in the United States. Major treatable causes of ASCVD are cigarette smoking, sedentary lifestyle, and poor eating habits leading to obesity, hypertension, type 2 diabetes mellitus and atherosclerosis (Go, 2013). **Atherosclerosis** is characterized by the accumulation of fatty deposits on the inner walls of the arteries and arterioles throughout the body that reduces the blood supply to vital organs, resulting in strokes, angina pectoris, myocardial infarction, and peripheral vascular disease. A primary cause of atherosclerosis is the abnormal elevation of cholesterol and triglyceride levels in the blood. **Hyperlipidemia** is the broad term used to classify patients with high levels of blood fats (lipids). **Dyslipidemias** are further defined under hyperlipidemia as abnormalities that involve one or more of the blood lipids. Dyslipidemias can be the result of genetic abnormalities, secondary causes (e.g., lifestyle, drugs, underlying diseases), or both. A diet that is high in saturated fats, cholesterol, carbohydrates, total calories, and alcohol and a sedentary lifestyle contribute significantly to dyslipidemias.

TYPES OF LIPOPROTEINS

Cholesterol is a naturally occurring substance that is essential for synthesizing the body steroids that are used by the endocrine system, for synthesizing the bile acids that are needed for food absorption, and for cell membrane synthesis. The body is able to manufacture enough cholesterol to meet its metabolic needs. However, the body also converts excess dietary carbohydrates into **triglycerides** (a precursor of cholesterol), and it converts dietary fat into cholesterol. After being absorbed from the gastrointestinal (GI) tract, fats (lipids), triglycerides, and cholesterol are bound to circulating proteins called **lipoproteins** for transport through the body.

Lipoproteins are subdivided into five categories on the basis of their composition: chylomicrons, very low-density lipoproteins (VLDLs), intermediate-density lipoproteins (IDLs), low-density lipoproteins (LDLs), and high-density lipoproteins (HDLs). The five types differ in relative concentrations of triglycerides, cholesterol, and proteins. Clinically, the IDL is included in the LDL measurement. **Chylomicrons** consist of about 90% triglycerides and 5% cholesterol; VLDLs represent about 15% to 20% of total serum cholesterol and most of the total blood triglyceride concentration, whereas HDLs contain about 20% to 30% cholesterol and 1% to 7% triglycerides.

The purpose of HDLs appears to be to transport cholesterol from peripheral cells to the liver for metabolism. HDLs are sometimes referred to as the "good" lipoproteins because high levels indicate that cholesterol is being removed from vascular tissue, where it may participate in the development of CAD. Low HDL levels are considered a positive risk factor for the development of CAD; high HDL levels are a negative risk factor for CAD.

LDLs account for 60% to 70% of total serum cholesterol, and are the major contributor to atherosclerosis. The probability that atherosclerosis will develop is related directly to the concentration of LDL cholesterol (LDL-C) in the blood circulation. LDL is the primary target of cholesterol-lowering therapy.

High triglyceride levels are also associated with an increased risk of CAD. Consequently, patient assessment and cholesterol-lowering treatment are based on the total cholesterol, LDL-C, HDL cholesterol (HDL-C), and triglyceride levels for individual patients. Other markers being tested to see whether they are better predictors of the risk for impending heart disease are the concentration of apolipoprotein A-1 (the major protein component of HDL); apolipoprotein B (a measure of the total number of atherogenic particles); C-reactive protein (an indicator of inflammation); and non-HDL cholesterol, the sum of the cholesterol in both LDL-C and triglyceride-rich lipoproteins.

TREATMENT OF HYPERLIPIDEMIAS

An estimated 105 million American adults have total blood cholesterol levels of 200 mg/dL or more. Of these, about 32 million American adults have levels of 240 mg/dL or more (Go, 2014). Some of the most common hyperlipidemias of genetic origin are treatable with medicines. However, it is now recognized that lifestyle is the greatest contributor to the development of hyperlipidemia. A cluster of risk factors that relate directly to excesses in lifestyle is now recognized as **metabolic syndrome** (see Chapter 20).

In November 2013 the American College of Cardiology and the American Heart Association (ACC/AHA) published new guidelines to reduce the overall risk of ASCVD (Stone, 2014). Risk reduction is the cornerstone of the guidelines: maintaining a heart-healthy diet (see Chapter 46) for a healthy weight, regular exercise, and avoidance of tobacco products. The major changes in the 2013 guidelines are the elimination of LDL and non-LDL treatment goals and the listing of four benefit groups (Table 21-1) with recommendations for the intensity of statin therapy (Table 21-2). Accompanying the guidelines is a new cardiovascular risk assessment calculator to estimate 10-year ASCVD

risk and safety recommendations on the use of statin drugs.

DRUG THERAPY FOR HYPERLIPIDEMIAS

ACTIONS

Antilipemic agents may be used to treat hyperlipidemias only if diet, exercise, and weight reduction are not successful for adequately lowering LDL-C levels. (See the individual drug monographs for information about the mechanisms of action of different antilipemic agents.) The new ACC/AHA guidelines to reduce the overall risk of ASCVD (Stone, 2013) described earlier focus on the use of statins for treatment of hypercholesterolemia because the Expert Panel making the recommendations used only evidence from randomized controlled trials published between 1995 and 2013. Although this is sound judgment, it eliminated other classes of antilipemic agents that must also be considered for use when statin therapy cannot be tolerated or when drug interactions with other medicines put the patient at risk of injury. It is also thought that the statins have antiinflammatory properties unrelated to lowering LDL that provide protection against ASCVD.

USES

Other antilipemic classes that lower LDL are the bile acid–binding resins (e.g., cholestyramine, colestipol, colesevelam) and niacin. The fibric acids (e.g., gemfibrozil, fenofibrate) are effective triglyceride-lowering agents, but are not first-line drugs for the treatment of hyperlipidemias because they do not usually produce substantial reductions in LDL-C. Omega-3 fatty acids have been approved by the U.S. Food and Drug Administration for treatment of very high triglyceride levels (>500 mg/dL) in adults. Niacin is the most effective therapy for raising HDL-C levels (20% to 35% increase). The fibrates raise HDL by 10% to 25%, and the statins raise HDL by 2% to 15%.

Selection of initial antilipemic therapy depends on the type of dyslipidemia present. Pharmacologic antilipemic therapy is often started with a statin because of their safety record and success in lowering cholesterol levels and reducing morbidity and mortality in ASCVD. The statins are the most potent and highly effective drugs for lowering LDL-C levels, and they appear to be relatively safe. However, they are substantially more expensive than other treatments. Prescription-strength niacin is effective for lowering total cholesterol and triglyceride levels and for raising HDL-C levels, but has serious adverse effects (vasomotor flushing, hepatotoxicity) in the higher doses needed for these antilipemic effects.

Before starting therapy, a lipid panel should be drawn and then repeated in 4 to 12 weeks after therapy is initiated. If the response to initial drug therapy is inadequate, it might be an indication that the patient

Table 21-1 | **Statin Benefit Groups and Recommended Treatment**

GROUP	DEFINITION	RECOMMENDATIONS
1	Patients who have already suffered a myocardial infarction, stable or unstable angina, stroke, transient ischemic attack, peripheral arterial disease, or had a revascularization procedure. Even though these patients have had serious cardiovascular events, there is strong evidence that statins reduce mortality in patients with a history of ASCVD disease.	For adults age 75 yr or younger, high-intensity statins are first-line therapy unless contraindicated. Moderate-intensity statins are a second-line choice. For adults age >75 yr, first-line therapy with moderate-intensity dosage should be considered on a case-by-case basis. Nonstatin cholesterol-lowering agents may be prescribed on a risk-to-benefit basis.
2	Adults age 21 or older with no clinical ASCVD, but with LDL-C >190 mg/dL or triglycerides of 500 mg/dL.	Evaluate for secondary causes of hyperlipidemia (e.g., high-fat diet; hypothyroidism; obstructive liver disease; medicines such as diuretics, glucocorticoids, cyclosporine, amiodarone). Primary hypercholesterolemia should be treated with high-intensity statins unless contraindicated. Treat with highest dose tolerated. Once maximum statin dosage is achieved, addition of a nonstatin to further reduce LDL-C is indicated based on tolerance.
3	Adults age 40-75 yr with diabetes and LDL-C 70-189 mg/dL but no clinical ASCVD. ASCVD is the main cause of illness and death in patients with diabetes.	Moderate-intensity statins should be started for patients with type 1 or type 2 diabetes. High-intensity statins are indicated in those with diabetes and an estimated 10-year ASCVD risk of 7.5% or greater. For adults age <40 or >75 yr, statins may be initiated taking into consideration risks, benefits, and drug interactions.
4	Adults without diabetes who have LDL 70-189 mg/dL and an estimated 10-yr ASCVD risk of 7.5% or greater. The risk calculator is for men and women, who are non-Hispanic Caucasian or African American, age 40-75 yr with or without diabetes with LDL levels of 70-189 mg/dL.	Start moderate- to high-intensity statin therapy in adults aged 40-75, with no clinical ASCVD or diabetes, with an ASCVD risk of 7.5%. Start with moderate-intensity statin therapy for those with an ASCVD 5-7.5%. Before starting therapy with the previous groups, clinicians should discuss risks/benefits and patient's preference.

Table 21-2 | **Fixed Statin Dosage Recommendations Based on Intensity***

HIGH-INTENSITY (LOWERS LDL BY >50%)	MODERATE INTENSITY (LOWERS LDL BY 30%-49%)	LOW INTENSITY (LOWERS LDL BY <30%)
Atorvastatin 40-80 mg	Atorvastatin 10-20 mg	Simvastatin 10 mg
Rosuvastatin 20-40 mg	Rosuvastatin 5-10 mg	Pravastatin 10-20 mg
	Simvastatin 20-40 mg	Lovastatin 20 mg
	Pravastatin 40-80 mg	Fluvastatin 20-40 mg
	Lovastatin 40 mg	Pitavastatin 1 mg
	Fluvastatin 80 mg	
	Pitavastatin 2-4 mg	

From Smith SC, Grundy SM: 2013 ACC/AHA Guideline recommends fixed-dose strategies instead of targeted-dose strategies instead of targeted goals to lower blood cholesterol, *J Am Coll Cardiol* 64:601-612, 2014.
*See the drug monograph on statins for monitoring drug therapy (p. 329).

is not compliant with therapy or that lifestyle changes are not being made. Have a discussion with the patient to assure that side effects are not limiting therapy. If compliant, the dosage of the statin should be increased or another drug should be added to the treatment regimen. The combination of a bile acid–binding resin with a statin can potentially lower LDL-C levels by greater than 50%. In rare cases of particularly high cholesterol levels, triple therapy with a statin, a bile acid–binding resin, *and* niacin may be required. Drug therapy is likely to continue for many years or the patient's lifetime; plasma lipid levels return to pretreatment levels after 2 to 3 weeks if therapy is discontinued.

❖ NURSING IMPLICATIONS FOR HYPERLIPIDEMIA THERAPY

▪ Assessment

History of Risk Factors. Obtain the patient's age, note gender and race, and take a family history of the incidence of elevated cholesterol and lipid levels. Ask whether any first-generation family members have a history of or have died from ASCVD. Obtain the ages and details of individuals with a history of ASCVD. Are there any living relatives with elevated cholesterol or elevated triglyceride levels?

Hypertension. Ask whether the patient has ever been told that he or she has elevated blood pressure. If yes, obtain details. Ask about medications that have been prescribed. Are the medications being taken regularly? If not, why not? Take the patient's blood pressure in lying, sitting, and standing positions.

Smoking. Obtain a history of the number of cigarettes or cigars smoked daily. How long has the patient smoked? Has the patient ever tried to stop smoking? Determine the patient's knowledge of the effects of smoking on the vascular system. How does the individual feel about modifying his or her smoking habit?

Dietary Habits

- Obtain a dietary history. Ask specific questions to obtain data related to foods eaten that are high in fat, cholesterol, refined carbohydrates, and sodium. Discuss the amount of fast foods and snack foods consumed, as well as the frequency of restaurant dining. Any of these factors tend to increase fat intake. Using a calorie counter, ask the person to estimate the number of calories eaten daily. How much meat, fish, and poultry is eaten daily (size and number of servings)? Estimate the percentage of total daily calories provided by fat.

- Discuss food preparation (e.g., baking, broiling, frying). How many servings of fruits and vegetables are eaten daily? What types of oils or fats are used in food preparation? See a nutrition text for additional dietary history questions.

- What are the frequency and volume of alcoholic beverages that are consumed?

Glucose Intolerance. Ask specific questions regarding whether the individual has now or has ever had an elevated serum glucose (blood sugar) level. If yes, what dietary modifications have been made? How successful are they? What medications are being taken for the elevated serum glucose level (e.g., oral hypoglycemic agents, insulin)?

Elevated Serum Lipid Levels. Find out whether the patient is aware of having elevated lipid, triglyceride, or cholesterol levels. If so, what measures has the patient tried for reduction, and what effect have the interventions had on the blood levels at subsequent examinations? Review available laboratory data (e.g., LDL, VLDL). A fasting lipoprotein profile that includes total cholesterol, LDL-C, HDL-C, and triglyceride levels is recommended for all adults 20 years old or older at least once every 5 years.

Obesity. Weigh the patient. Ask about any recent weight gain or loss and whether it was intentional or unintentional. Using the person's height and weight, determine the person's body mass index (see Chapter 20). If obesity is present, what strategies for weight reduction have been tried?

Psychomotor Functions

- Type of lifestyle: Ask the patient to describe his or her exercise level in terms of amount (e.g., walking 3 miles), intensity (e.g., walking 3 mph), and frequency (e.g., walking every other day). Is the patient's job physically demanding or of a sedentary nature?

- Psychological stress: How much stress does the individual estimate having in his or her life? How does the patient cope with stressful situations at home and in the work setting?

■ **Patient Education**

Nutrition. Patients who take bile acid–sequestering resins may require supplemental vitamins. (The fat-soluble vitamins—D, E, A, and K—may become deficient with long-term resin therapy.)

- Encourage the intake of high-bulk foods (e.g., whole grains, raw fruits and vegetables), as well as the intake of eight to ten 8-ounce glasses of water daily, to minimize the constipating effects of these resins.

- Arrange a dietary consultation with a nutritionist to address any dietary modifications needed (e.g., low fat, low cholesterol). Nurses should enhance and reinforce this teaching on a continuum. Stress the importance of attaining a normal weight as a major treatment goal of hyperlipidemia. See information about steps 1 and 2 of the AHA's diet recommendations for treating ASCVD.

Vitamin K Deficiency. If the patient is receiving a prescription for a bile acid–sequestering resin, teach the patient about the signs and symptoms of vitamin K deficiency, including bleeding gums, bruising, dark tarry stools, and coffee-ground emesis. This interaction is rare, but if symptoms occur they should be reported immediately to the healthcare provider.

Follow-Up Care. Stress the need for long-term regular assessment of the required serum levels (e.g., lipid profile values, liver studies, bleeding times) to track progress, identify the need for modifications in therapeutic interventions, and detect possible adverse effects of the medications. To obtain this information, blood studies and regular visits to the healthcare provider are necessary.

Relating to Medication Regimen. Examine the individual drug monographs for details about mixing drugs, scheduling medication administration, and techniques for improving compliance of patients taking these medications.

Fostering Health Maintenance

- Throughout the course of treatment, discuss medication information and how it will benefit the patient.

- Drug therapy is one component in the management of hyperlipidemia. Therapeutic lifestyle changes are as important as drug therapy; therefore the need to modify dietary habits and to control obesity, glucose levels, serum cholesterol, lipids, and hypertension must be strongly emphasized. Teach the patient about which high-cholesterol and high-fat foods to avoid (e.g., liver, egg yolks, meats, fried foods, fatty desserts, nuts [cashews, macadamia, Brazil]). Cholesterol is an animal product and not found in plants. Encourage switching to skim or 1% fat milk, substituting egg whites, and increasing consumption of fruits (especially grapefruit) and vegetables. Discuss the use of unsaturated vegetable oils, such as corn, olive, and soybean. Cessation of smoking and an increase in daily exercise (30 minutes of moderate-intensity exercise most days of the week) are strongly recommended. People with metabolic syndrome must recognize the importance of weight reduction and increased exercise to modify the insulin resistance that can dramatically affect the management of the disorder.

- Provide the patient and significant others with the important information contained in the specific drug monographs for the drugs prescribed. Additional health teaching and nursing interventions for adverse effects are described in the drug monographs that follow.
- Seek the patient's cooperation and understanding of the following points so that medication compliance is increased: the name of the medication; its dosage, route, and times of administration; and its common and serious adverse effects.

Patient Self-Assessment. Enlist the patient's help with developing and maintaining a written record of monitoring parameters (e.g., daily serum glucose levels, blood pressure, weight) (see the Patient Self-Assessment Form for Cardiovascular Agents on the Evolve website.) An individualized nutritional diary should also be kept while instituting and learning about diet modifications (e.g., a reduction in fats and refined carbohydrates, an increase in low-cholesterol foods). Complete the Premedication Data column for use as a baseline to track the patient's response to drug therapy. Ensure that the patient understands how to use the form, and instruct the patient to bring the completed form to follow-up visits. During follow-up visits, focus on issues that will foster adherence with the therapeutic interventions prescribed.

DRUG CLASS: BILE ACID–BINDING RESINS

ACTIONS

Cholestyramine, colestipol, and colesevelam are resins that bind bile acids in the intestine. After oral administration, the resin forms a nonabsorbable complex with bile acids, preventing the enterohepatic recirculation of the bile acids. Removal of bile acids causes liver cells to compensate by increasing the metabolism of cholesterol to produce more bile acids, which results in a net reduction in the total cholesterol level. Bile acid–binding resins can reduce LDL-C by 15% to 30% and increase HDL by up to 5%. Some patients also have a 5% to 10% increase in their triglyceride levels.

USES

Cholestyramine, colestipol, and colesevelam are used in conjunction with dietary therapy to decrease elevated cholesterol concentrations in patients with hyperlipidemia and to reduce the risks of atherosclerosis leading to ASCVD. These agents may also be used with statins to lower the LDL-C level even further. They are generally not used for patients who already have elevated triglyceride levels.

Other uses of the bile acid–binding resins include the treatment of pruritus secondary to partial biliary stasis, diarrhea secondary to excess fecal bile acids or pseudomembranous colitis, and digitalis glycoside toxicity.

Colesevelam has also received U.S. Food and Drug Administration approval for reducing blood glucose and hemoglobin A_1C in adult patients with type 2 diabetes. It may be used alone or in combination with metformin, sulfonylureas, or insulin. Do not use this drug in patients with type 1 diabetes.

THERAPEUTIC OUTCOMES

The primary therapeutic outcomes expected from bile acid–binding resin therapy are the reduction of the LDL and total cholesterol levels.

❖ NURSING IMPLICATIONS FOR BILE ACID–BINDING RESINS

▪ Premedication Assessment

1. Serum triglyceride, lipoprotein and cholesterol levels should be determined before the initiation of therapy and periodically thereafter.
2. Obtain patient data related to any GI alterations before the initiation of therapy (e.g., the presence of abdominal pain, nausea, flatus).

▪ Availability

Cholestyramine: *PO:* 4-g powder packets.
Colestipol: *PO:* 1-g tablets; granules in 5-g packets.
Colesevelam: *PO:* 3.75-mg packets; 625-mg tablets.

▪ Dosage and Administration

Cholestyramine: *PO:* 4 g one to six times daily. Initial dosage is 4 g daily. Maintenance dosage is 8 to 16 g/day. Maximum daily dosage is 24 g.
Colestipol: *PO:* Granules: 5 to 30 g/day in divided doses. Initial dosage is 5 g once or twice daily. Tablets: 2 to 16 g/day. Initial dosage is 2 g once or twice daily.
Colesevelam: *PO:* 6 tablets once daily or in two divided doses with liquid at meals.
Note:

- The powder resin (cholestyramine) must be mixed with 2 to 6 ounces of water, juice, soup, applesauce, or crushed pineapple, and should stand for a few minutes to allow absorption and dispersion. Do not attempt to swallow the dry powder. Follow administration with an additional glass of water.

- The recommended time of administration is with meals, but this may be modified to avoid interference with the absorption of other medications.
- Tablets should be swallowed whole; do not crush, chew, or cut them. Tablets should be taken with liquids.
- Taste may become a reason for noncompliance. Place the powder in a favorite beverage, or opt for tablets to minimize the medication's objectionable taste.

■ Common Adverse Effects

Gastrointestinal

Constipation, bloating, fullness, nausea, flatulence. These adverse effects can be minimized by starting with a low dose; mixing the drug with noncarbonated, pulpy juices or sauces; and swallowing it without gulping air. Maintain adequate fiber in the diet, and drink sufficient water.

■ Drug Interactions

Digoxin, Warfarin, Thyroid Hormones, Thiazide Diuretics, Phenobarbital, Nonsteroidal Anti-inflammatory Agents, Tetracycline, Beta-Blocking Agents, Gemfibrozil, Glipizide, Glyburide, Oral Contraceptives, Phenytoin. The resins may bind with these medicines, which reduces absorption. The interaction can usually be minimized by administering these medicines 1 hour before or 4 hours after administration of resins.

Amiodarone. The resins significantly decrease the absorption of amiodarone. The resins also block the enterohepatic recirculation of amiodarone. Consequently, amiodarone and the resins should not be used concurrently.

Fat-Soluble Vitamins (D, E, A, and K), Folic Acid. High doses of resins may reduce the absorption of these agents, but this interaction is not usually significant in normally nourished patients.

DRUG CLASS: NIACIN

> ⇌ *Do not confuse niacin with Niaspan or Naprosyn.*

ACTIONS

Niacin, also known as *nicotinic acid,* is a water-soluble B vitamin (also known as *vitamin B₃*). Its mechanisms of action as an antilipemic agent are not completely known, but they are not related to its effects as a vitamin. Niacin inhibits VLDL synthesis by liver cells, which causes a decrease in LDL and triglyceride production. Triglyceride levels are reduced by 20% to 50%, and total cholesterol and LDL-C levels can be reduced by 5% to 25%. Niacin may also reduce the metabolism

of HDL, thereby causing a 15% to 35% increase in HDL levels. Niacin also causes the release of histamine, causing peripheral vasodilation and increased blood flow (flushing of the skin).

USES

Nicotinic acid is the only form of vitamin B₃ approved by the U.S. Food and Drug Administration for the treatment of dyslipidemias. Niacin is used in conjunction with dietary therapy to decrease elevated cholesterol concentrations in patients with dyslipidemias and to reduce the risks of atherosclerosis leading to ASCVD. It can be used in combination with bile acid–binding resins or with the statins (Advicor [niacin plus lovastatin]) for greater combined lowering of cholesterol levels. Another benefit of niacin therapy is its significantly lower cost compared with the other antilipemic agents. Niacin should be used with caution in patients with diabetes because of their glucose intolerance.

Different forms of vitamin B₃ cannot be used interchangeably. Other forms of vitamin B₃ are niacinamide and inositol hexaniacinate, which do not lower elevated cholesterol levels. Immediate-release niacin products cause more facial and skin flushing, and the sustained-release products have a higher possibility of causing hepatotoxicity than the immediate-release products. Dietary supplements of niacin should not be used to treat dyslipidemia. The recommended Dietary Reference Intake for nutritional supplementation is less than 20 mg/day. The dosage of niacin required to treat dyslipidemia is 1 to 6 g/day.

THERAPEUTIC OUTCOMES

The primary therapeutic outcomes expected from niacin are reduction in LDL (5% to 25%) and total cholesterol levels, reduction in triglyceride levels (20% to 50%), and an increase in HDL levels (15% to 35%).

❖ NURSING IMPLICATIONS FOR NIACIN

■ Premedication Assessment

1. Serum triglyceride and cholesterol levels should be determined before initiation of therapy and periodically thereafter.
2. Liver function tests (bilirubin, aspartate aminotransferase [AST], alanine aminotransferase [ALT], gamma-glutamyl transferase [GGT], alkaline phosphatase levels, and prothrombin time) should be determined before initiating therapy and every 6 to 8 weeks during the first year of therapy.
3. Baseline uric acid and blood glucose levels should be determined before initiating therapy. Niacin therapy may induce hyperuricemia, gout, and hyperglycemia in susceptible patients.
4. Baseline blood pressure and heart rate should be determined before initiating therapy.
5. Obtain patient data related to any GI alterations before initiating therapy (e.g., the presence of abdominal pain, nausea, or flatus).

■ **Availability**

PO: 50-, 100-, 250-, or 500-mg tablets; 500-, 590- or 750-mg capsules; 250-, or 500-mg timed-release capsules; 250- 500-, 750-, or 1000-mg timed-release tablets.

■ **Dosage and Administration**

PO: Weeks 1 to 4: 500 mg PO at bedtime. Weeks 5 to 8: 1000 mg PO at bedtime. After week 8, titrate to patient response and tolerance. If response to 1000 mg/day is inadequate, increase dose to 1500 mg/day PO at bedtime. If response to 1500 mg/day is inadequate, may subsequently increase dose to 2000 mg/day.

■ **Common Adverse Effects**

Integumentary. Flushing, itching, and rash are common. Patients can reduce their symptoms by taking aspirin (325 mg) or ibuprofen (200 mg) 30 minutes before each dose of niacin.

Neurologic. Tingling and headache are frequently seen with these drugs.

Gastrointestinal

Nausea, gas, abdominal discomfort and pain. Gastrointestinal upset can be minimized by starting with low doses of these drugs and administering all doses with food.

The common adverse effects listed here usually occur at the beginning of therapy, especially with the immediate-release products. Tolerance develops quickly. Administer niacin with food.

Cardiovascular

Dizziness, faintness, hypotension. Niacin is a vasodilator, and it may cause hypotension, especially if a patient is receiving other antihypertensive agents. Anticipate the development of hypotension, and take measures to prevent such an occurrence. Teach the patient to rise slowly from a supine or sitting position and to sit or lie down if he or she is feeling faint. Monitor blood pressure with the patient in both the supine and sitting positions.

■ **Serious Adverse Effects**

Gastrointestinal

Hepatotoxicity. There appears to be a higher incidence of hepatotoxicity associated with the timed-release products. Some clinicians recommend limiting the timed-release products to 1500 mg daily to reduce the risk.

Fatigue, anorexia, nausea, malaise, jaundice. These are the early symptoms that are associated with hepatotoxicity. Report these to the healthcare provider for further evaluation.

Musculoskeletal

Myopathy. Symptoms of muscle aches, soreness, and weakness may be early signs of myopathy. Serum creatine phosphokinase levels that are more than 10 times the upper limit of normal confirm the diagnosis.

■ **Drug Interactions**

HMG-CoA Reductase Inhibitors. The potential of developing myopathy is increased when niacin is added to the treatment regimen. The incidence of this condition is less than 1%.

DRUG CLASS: HMG-COA REDUCTASE INHIBITORS

ACTIONS

HMG-CoA reductase enzyme inhibitors (Table 21-3) are the most potent antilipemic agents available; they are also known as *statins.* The statins competitively inhibit the enzyme that is responsible for converting HMG-CoA to mevalonate in the biosynthetic pathway to cholesterol in the liver. The reduction in liver cholesterol increases the removal of LDLs from the circulating blood. Levels of LDL-C may be reduced by as much as 50%. The statins also cause reductions in VLDL and triglyceride levels (20% to 30%) and mild increases (5% to 15%) in HDL levels. These agents are more effective if administered at night because peak production of cholesterol occurs at this time. Statins also have other beneficial effects unrelated to their lipid-lowering capacity: they reduce inflammation, platelet aggregation, thrombin formation, and plasma viscosity, thereby reducing the factors that contribute to heart attacks and strokes.

USES

Statins are used in conjunction with dietary therapy to decrease elevated cholesterol concentrations in patients with hyperlipidemia and to reduce the risks of atherosclerosis leading to ASCVD. The statins listed are similar in effectiveness at recommended starting doses and times, but they differ with regard to their potential for drug interactions. Other medicines also being taken by the patient may determine the most appropriate statin to be prescribed; this should be based on the avoidance of drug interactions.

THERAPEUTIC OUTCOMES

The primary therapeutic outcomes expected from HMG-CoA reductase inhibitors are reduction of LDL and total cholesterol levels.

❖ **NURSING IMPLICATIONS FOR HMG-COA REDUCTASE INHIBITORS**

■ **Premedication Assessment**

1. Serum triglyceride, lipoprotein and cholesterol levels should be determined before initiating therapy, then at 4 to 12 weeks, and then annually after that.

2. Liver function tests (AST, ALT) should be obtained before initiating therapy and should be measured during therapy if symptoms suggestive of hepatotoxicity develop, but do not need to be measured routinely. Obtain data related to any GI alterations before initiating therapy (e.g., presence of abdominal pain, nausea, or flatus).

3. Confirm that the patient is not pregnant before initiating a statin. Instruct the female patient to notify

Table 21-3 HMG-CoA Reductase Inhibitors (Statins)

GENERIC NAME	BRAND NAME	AVAILABILITY	DAILY DOSAGE RANGE	MAXIMUM DAILY DOSAGE RANGE
atorvastatin	Lipitor	Tablets: 10, 20, 40, 80 mg	10-40 mg daily at any time	Up to 80 mg daily
fluvastatin ⇄ Do not confuse fluvastatin with fluoxetine.	Lescol, Lescol XL	Capsules: 20, 40 mg Tablets, extended release: 80 mg	20-80 mg at bedtime	Up to 80 mg at bedtime
lovastatin ⇄ Do not confuse lovastatin with Lotensin or Lovenox.	Mevacor, Altoprev, Apo-Lovastatin ♣	Tablets: 10, 20, 40 mg Tablets, extended release: 20, 40, 60 mg	20-40 mg with evening meal or 10-60 mg daily at bedtime	80 mg daily (immediate release) or 60 mg daily at bedtime (extended release)
pitavastatin	Livalo	Tablets: 1, 2, 4 mg	2 mg once daily at any time, with or without food	Up to 4 mg daily
pravastatin	Pravachol, Nu-Pravastatin ♣ ⇄ Do not confuse Pravachol with Prevacid, Prinivil, or propranolol.	Tablets: 10, 20, 40, 80 mg	40 mg daily at any time	Up to 80 mg daily
rosuvastatin	Crestor	Tablets: 5, 10, 20, 40 mg	5-40 mg daily at any time	Up to 40 mg daily
simvastatin	Zocor ⇄ Do not confuse Zocor with Cozaar, Yocon, Zestril, Ziac, or Zoloft.	Tablets: 5, 10, 20, 40, 80 mg	5-40 mg daily at bedtime	Up to 40 mg at bedtime

♣ Available in Canada.

her healthcare provider should she contemplate conception or become pregnant while receiving statin therapy.

■ **Availability, Dosage, and Administration**
See Tables 21-3 and 21-4. Lovastatin should be administered with food at the evening meal to enhance absorption. The other statins may be administered without food.

■ **Common Adverse Effects**
Neurologic
Headaches. This symptom is usually mild and disappears with continued therapy.
Gastrointestinal
Nausea, abdominal bloating, gas. These symptoms are usually mild and disappear with continued therapy.

■ **Serious Adverse Effects**
Gastrointestinal
Hepatotoxicity. Liver function should be monitored as described previously. If the transaminases (AST, ALT) rise to three times the upper limit of normal and are persistent, then the medication should be discontinued.
Musculoskeletal
Myopathy, rhabdomyolysis. Symptoms of muscle aches, soreness, and weakness may be early signs of

myopathy. Serum creatine phosphokinase levels more than 10 times the upper limit of normal confirm the diagnosis. Myopathy is most common with lovastatin (at <1%). Myopathy is more common (5%) if statins are used in combination with niacin, gemfibrozil, or cyclosporine. Rhabdomyolysis is a very serious condition in which kidney damage results from progressing myopathy. An early indication of rhabdomyolysis is pinkish or red-tinged urine secondary to myoglobin (muscle protein) passing through damaged glomeruli into the urine (myoglobinuria).

🌐 Cultural Considerations

Chinese patients and those with a Chinese ancestry should not be treated with doses of simvastatin greater than 20 mg when also taking niacin. These patients are more susceptible to developing myopathy. The cause of the increased frequency of myopathy is unknown.

■ **Drug Interactions**
Cyclosporine, Itraconazole, Ketoconazole, Diltiazem, Fluconazole, Fibrates, Niacin, Nefazodone, Verapamil, Erythromycin, Clarithromycin, Ranolazine. The incidence of myopathy is increased when lovastatin, simvastatin, or atorvastatin is prescribed in conjunction with these medicines. These medicines

Table 21-4   HMG-CoA Reductase Inhibitor Combination Products

GENERIC NAME	BRAND NAME	AVAILABILITY	MAXIMUM DAILY DOSAGE RANGE
atorvastatin-amlodipine	Caduet	Tablets: 10 mg atorvastatin and 2.5 mg amlodipine 20 mg atorvastatin and 2.5 mg amlodipine 40 mg atorvastatin and 2.5 mg amlodipine 10 mg atorvastatin and 5 mg amlodipine 20 mg atorvastatin and 5 mg amlodipine 40 mg atorvastatin and 5 mg amlodipine 80 mg atorvastatin and 5 mg amlodipine 10 mg atorvastatin and 10 mg amlodipine 20 mg atorvastatin and 10 mg amlodipine 40 mg atorvastatin and 10 mg amlodipine 80 mg atorvastatin and 10 mg amlodipine	atorvastatin 80 mg amlodipine 10 mg
atorvastatin-ezetimibe	Liptruzet	Tablets: 10 mg atorvastatin and 10 mg ezetimibe 20 mg atorvastatin and 10 mg ezetimibe 30 mg atorvastatin and 10 mg ezetimibe 40 mg atorvastatin and 10 mg ezetimibe	atorvastatin 40 mg ezetimibe 10 mg
lovastatin-niacin (extended release)	Advicor	Tablets: 20 mg lovastatin and 500 mg niacin 20 mg lovastatin and 750 mg niacin 20 mg lovastatin and 1000 mg niacin 40 mg lovastatin and 1000 mg niacin	lovastatin 40 mg niacin 2000 mg extended release
simvastatin-ezetimibe	Vytorin	Tablets: 10 mg simvastatin and 10 mg ezetimibe 20 mg simvastatin and 10 mg ezetimibe 40 mg simvastatin and 10 mg ezetimibe 80 mg simvastatin and 10 mg ezetimibe	simvastatin 80 mg ezetimibe, 10 mg
simvastatin-niacin (extended release)	Simcor	Tablets: 20 mg simvastatin and 750 mg niacin 20 mg simvastatin and 1000 mg niacin 40 mg simvastatin and 500 mg niacin 40 mg simvastatin and 1000 mg niacin	simvastatin 40 mg niacin 2000 mg extended release

inhibit the metabolism of the statins, inducing toxicity.

Cimetidine, Ranitidine, Omeprazole. Coadministration of these drugs with fluvastatin results in significantly increased fluvastatin levels. Dosage reductions of fluvastatin may be necessary.

Propranolol. Concurrent administration of propranolol and simvastatin results in a significantly lower serum level of simvastatin. Either increase the dosage of simvastatin or switch to another statin.

Rifampin. Concurrent administration of rifampin and fluvastatin, atorvastatin, or simvastatin results in significantly lower levels of fluvastatin, atorvastatin, or simvastatin. Either increase the dosage of fluvastatin or switch to another statin.

Warfarin. When lovastatin, simvastatin, rosuvastatin, or fluvastatin and warfarin are prescribed together, the prothrombin time (international normalized ratio [INR]) may be prolonged. Observe the patient for possible overanticoagulation and bleeding.

Grapefruit Juice. Grapefruit juice inhibits the metabolism of atorvastatin, lovastatin, and simvastatin, thus increasing their plasma concentrations and resulting in a greater potential for myopathy. People who are taking these medications should avoid grapefruit juice.

DRUG CLASS: FIBRIC ACIDS

ACTIONS

The mechanism of action of the fibric acids (e.g., gemfibrozil, fenofibrate) is unknown; however, they do lower triglyceride levels by 20% to 40%. In patients with hypertriglyceridemia, these drugs raise HDL levels by 20% to 25%. They also reduce LDL-C by 10% to 15% in patients with elevated cholesterol. Fenofibrate may lower LDL-C levels more effectively than gemfibrozil. However, in patients with concurrent hypertriglyceridemia, gemfibrozil may have no effect, or it may slightly increase LDL-C levels.

USES

The fibrates are the most effective triglyceride-lowering agents. Gemfibrozil and fenofibrate are used in conjunction with dietary therapy to decrease elevated triglyceride levels in patients who are at risk for pancreatitis. Fibric acids must be used with caution in combination with statins because of the risk of myopathy and rhabdomyolysis.

THERAPEUTIC OUTCOMES

The primary therapeutic outcomes expected from fibric acid therapy are a 20% to 40% reduction in triglyceride levels and a 20% to 25% increase in HDL levels.

❖ NURSING IMPLICATIONS FOR FIBRIC ACIDS

■ Premedication Assessment

1. Serum triglyceride, lipoprotein and cholesterol levels should be measured before initiating therapy and periodically thereafter.
2. Liver function tests should be run before initiating therapy and then every 6 months thereafter.
3. Baseline blood glucose levels should be determined before gemfibrozil therapy. Gemfibrozil may cause moderate hyperglycemia.
4. Obtain patient data related to any GI alterations before initiating therapy (e.g., presence of abdominal pain, nausea, flatus).

■ Availability

Gemfibrozil (Lopid): *PO:* 600-mg tablets.
Fenofibrate: *PO:* 35-, 40-, 48-, 50-, 54-, 105-, 120-, 145-, and 160-mg tablets; 30-, 43-, 50-, 67-, 90-, 130-, 134-, 150-, and 200-mg capsules; 45- and 135-mg delayed-release capsules.

■ Dosage and Administration

Gemfibrozil: *PO:* 1200 mg/day in two divided doses, 30 minutes before the morning and evening meals.
Fenofibrate: *PO:* Initially, 45 to 160 mg/day, given with meals. Increase dosage every 4 to 8 weeks up to 160 mg daily with a meal. Dosages of fenofibrate need to be reduced in older adult patients and in patients with renal insufficiency. See the manufacturer's recommendations.

■ Common Adverse Effects

Gastrointestinal

Nausea, diarrhea, flatulence, bloating, abdominal distress. These are relatively common adverse effects. Starting with a lower dosage taken between meals can help to minimize these effects. If symptoms persist, notify the healthcare provider because potentially more serious complications may be developing.

■ Serious Adverse Effects

Gastrointestinal

Fatigue, anorexia, nausea, malaise, jaundice. These are the early symptoms associated with gallbladder disease and hepatotoxicity. Report these symptoms to the healthcare provider for further evaluation.

Musculoskeletal

Myopathy. Symptoms of muscle aches, soreness, and weakness may be early signs of myopathy. Serum creatine phosphokinase levels of more than 10 times the upper limit of normal confirm the diagnosis. Myopathy is most common with lovastatin and gemfibrozil. Myopathy is more common (5%) if statins are used in combination with niacin, gemfibrozil, or cyclosporine.

■ Drug Interactions

Warfarin. The fibric acids may enhance the pharmacologic effects of warfarin. Reduce the dosage of warfarin using the prothrombin time (INR) as an indicator to prevent bleeding.

Sulfonylureas, Insulin. Gemfibrozil may increase the pharmacologic effects of these agents. Monitor the patient for signs of hypoglycemia, and reduce the dosage of the insulin or sulfonylurea as needed.

Bile Acid–Binding Resins. These resins may bind to fenofibrate, reducing absorption. The interaction can usually be minimized by administering fenofibrate 1 hour before or 4 hours after administration of the resins.

HMG-CoA Reductase Inhibitors. The potential for developing myopathy is increased when fibric acids are added to the treatment regimen. The incidence is less than 5%.

DRUG CLASS: MISCELLANEOUS ANTILIPEMIC AGENTS

---

ezetimibe (ĕ-ZĔT-ĭ-mēb)
Zetia (ZĔ-tē-ă)

ACTIONS

Ezetimibe is the first of a new class of agents used to reduce atherosclerosis. Ezetimibe acts by blocking the absorption of cholesterol from the small intestine. Unlike bile acid–binding resins, ezetimibe does not bind to cholesterol and reduce absorption. Instead, it acts on the small intestine to inhibit absorption of cholesterol derived from the cholesterol secreted in the bile and from the diet. Studies indicate that ezetimibe reduces total cholesterol by about 12%, LDL-C by 18%, and triglycerides by 7%, and has a minimal effect on raising HDL levels.

USES

Ezetimibe is used in conjunction with dietary therapy to decrease elevated cholesterol concentrations in patients with hyperlipidemia and to reduce the risks of atherosclerosis leading to ASCVD. This agent may also be used with the statins to lower cholesterol further (Vytorin, Liptruzet). Combined therapy with fibric acid derivatives is not recommended. Ezetimibe may have an advantage over the bile acid resins because it does not elevate triglyceride levels.

THERAPEUTIC OUTCOMES

The primary therapeutic outcomes expected from ezetimibe therapy are reduction of LDL and total cholesterol levels.

❖ NURSING IMPLICATIONS FOR EZETIMIBE

▪ Premedication Assessment

1. Serum triglyceride, lipoproteins and cholesterol levels should be determined before initiating therapy and periodically thereafter.
2. Obtain patient data related to any GI alterations before initiating therapy (e.g., presence of abdominal pain, nausea, flatus).

▪ Availability

PO: 10-mg tablets.

▪ Dosage and Administration

Adult: PO: 10 mg once daily; may be taken with or without meals.

▪ Common Adverse Effects

Gastrointestinal

Abdominal pain, diarrhea. These adverse effects are mild and generally do not require discontinuation of therapy.

▪ Drug Interactions

Bile Acid–Binding Resins. These resins may bind to ezetimibe, reducing absorption. The interaction can usually be minimized by administering ezetimibe 1 hour before or 4 hours after administering the resins.

---

omega-3 fatty acids
Lovaza (lō-VĂ-ză)

ACTIONS

Lovaza was the first of a new class of agents used to reduce atherosclerosis. Lovaza is a combination product that contains two omega-3 fatty acids: eicosapentaenoic acid (EPA) and docosahexaenoic acid (DHA). Omega-3 fatty acids are sometimes referred to as *fish oils* because higher concentrations of these fatty acids are found in such oils. The mechanism of action is unknown, but the end result is that the omega-3 fatty acids reduce synthesis of triglycerides in the liver. Early studies indicate that Lovaza reduces triglyceride levels by 20% to 50%, with small increases in HDL-C levels also seen. In some cases, LDL-C levels are also increased.

USES

Lovaza is used in conjunction with dietary therapy to decrease very elevated triglyceride levels (>500 mg/dL) in adult patients. This agent may also be used with statins to lower the cholesterol level even further. Lovaza may have an advantage over fibrates and niacin because it does not cause myositis or rhabdomyolysis, particularly when combined with statins. Lovaza should be used with caution in patients who are sensitive or allergic to fish. It should be discontinued in patients who have not shown an adequate response after 2 months of treatment.

THERAPEUTIC OUTCOME

The primary therapeutic outcome expected from Lovaza therapy is the reduction of an elevated triglyceride level.

❖ NURSING IMPLICATIONS FOR OMEGA-3 FATTY ACIDS

▪ Premedication Assessment

1. Serum triglyceride, total cholesterol, HDL-C, and LDL-C levels should be determined before initiating therapy and periodically thereafter.
2. Liver function tests (AST, ALT) should be completed before initiating therapy and periodically for the first year of therapy.
3. Obtain patient data related to any GI alterations before initiating therapy (e.g., presence of abdominal pain, nausea, flatus).

▪ Availability

PO: 1-g capsules.

▪ Dosage and Administration

Adult: PO: 4 g once daily or 2 g twice daily.

▪ Common and Serious Adverse Effects

If any of the following adverse effects occur, report them to the healthcare provider immediately: arm, back, or jaw pain; chest pain or discomfort; chest tightness or heaviness; difficult or labored breathing; fast or irregular heartbeat; nausea; shortness of breath; sweating; tightness in the chest; or wheezing.

Other minor adverse effects reported during clinical studies include back pain, unusual or unpleasant aftertaste, belching, a bloated and full feeling, a change in taste, chills, cough, diarrhea, excess air or gas in stomach, fever, a general feeling of discomfort or illness, headache, hoarseness, joint pain, loss of appetite, lower back or side pain, muscle aches and pains, pain, painful or difficult urination, rash, runny nose, shivering, sore throat, sweating, trouble sleeping, unusual tiredness or weakness, or vomiting. These symptoms should be reported to the healthcare provider if they persist.

▪ Drug Interactions

No drug interactions have been reported to date.

Get Ready for the NCLEX® Examination!

Key Points

- Coronary artery disease is a major cause of premature death in the United States.
- Major treatable causes of ASCVD are hypertension, cigarette smoking, and atherosclerosis.
- A primary cause of atherosclerosis is the abnormal elevation of cholesterol and triglyceride levels in the blood in a disease known as *hyperlipidemia*. A diet high in saturated fats, cholesterol, carbohydrates, total calories, and alcohol—in combination with a sedentary lifestyle—comprise the most common and treatable causes of hyperlipidemia.
- The most cost-effective and successful forms of treatment are smoking cessation, weight reduction, exercise, and dietary modification. If changes in diet and exercise habits do not produce an acceptable decrease in blood lipid levels, an antilipemic agent may be added to the patient's regimen.
- Patients should be fully informed of the significance of hyperlipidemias, the potential complications involved with not modifying their lifestyles, and drug therapy. Drug therapy is likely to continue for many years or a lifetime.
- The primary medicines that are used to lower elevated cholesterol levels are the bile acid–binding resins, niacin, ezetimibe, and the statins. The fibric acid derivatives and omega-3 fatty acids lower triglyceride levels.

Additional Learning Resources

SG Go to your Study Guide for additional Review Questions for the NCLEX® Examination, Critical Thinking Clinical Situations, and other learning activities to help you master this chapter content.

evolve Go to your Evolve website (http://evolve .elsevier.com/Clayton) for additional online resources.

Review Questions for the NCLEX® Examination

1. The nurse teaching a patient about lipoproteins realized further education was needed when the patient made the following statement:
   1. "I understand that our body manufactures cholesterol and it is needed for normal functioning."
   2. "I need to watch my level of HDL and keep it low, while making sure my LDL level is higher."
   3. "If I overeat, my body converts the excess carbohydrates into triglycerides."
   4. "I need to watch my level of LDL and keep it low, while making sure my HDL level is higher."

2. Lifestyle modifications that can be implemented to reduce the risk of developing hyperlipidemia include: *(Select all that apply.)*
   1. maintaining a heart-healthy diet.
   2. daily dental hygiene.
   3. avoiding tobacco products.
   4. maintaining a healthy weight.
   5. regular exercise.

3. A patient taking the fibric acid gemfibrozil asks the nurse how this drug works. The best response would be:
   1. "The drug gemfibrozil is used to lower your triglyceride level."
   2. "Fibric acids are used to help lower your cholesterol level."
   3. "The doctor prescribed this drug to help lower the HDLs in your system."
   4. "This drug is useful for preventing insulin resistance."

4. A nurse teaching a patient who was prescribed niacin includes the avoidable adverse effects of: *(Select all that apply.)*
   1. headache.
   2. nausea.
   3. diarrhea.
   4. flatulence.
   5. abdominal discomfort.

5. A patient prescribed omega-3 fatty acids (Lovaza) asked the nurse what he should know about the drug. The best response would include: *(Select all that apply.)*
   1. "Lovaza is used to decrease very elevated triglyceride levels."
   2. "Lovaza is often used with statins to further lower cholesterol levels."
   3. "Lovaza may cause myositis or rhabdomyolysis."
   4. "Lovaza should be used with caution in patients who are allergic to fish."
   5. "Lovaza should be discontinued after 2 months of therapy if there is not an adequate response."

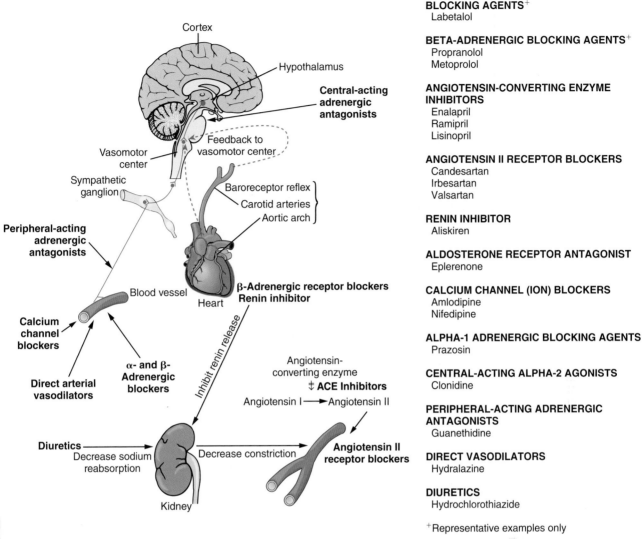

ALPHA-AND BETA-ADRENERGIC BLOCKING AGENTS[+]
Labetalol

BETA-ADRENERGIC BLOCKING AGENTS[+]
Propranolol
Metoprolol

ANGIOTENSIN-CONVERTING ENZYME INHIBITORS
Enalapril
Ramipril
Lisinopril

ANGIOTENSIN II RECEPTOR BLOCKERS
Candesartan
Irbesartan
Valsartan

RENIN INHIBITOR
Aliskiren

ALDOSTERONE RECEPTOR ANTAGONIST
Eplerenone

CALCIUM CHANNEL (ION) BLOCKERS
Amlodipine
Nifedipine

ALPHA-1 ADRENERGIC BLOCKING AGENTS
Prazosin

CENTRAL-ACTING ALPHA-2 AGONISTS
Clonidine

PERIPHERAL-ACTING ADRENERGIC ANTAGONISTS
Guanethidine

DIRECT VASODILATORS
Hydralazine

DIURETICS
Hydrochlorothiazide

[+]Representative examples only

FIGURE 22-1 Sites of action of antihypertensive agents. *ACE,* angiotensin-converting enzyme. (Modified from U.S. Department of Health and Human Services: *The sixth report of the Joint National Committee on Detection, Evaluation, and Treatment of High Blood Pressure [JNC-VI]*, Washington D.C., 1997, National Institutes of Health.)

relatively short time. Patients with an average diastolic blood pressure higher than 120 mm Hg require immediate therapy and, if significant organ damage is present, may require hospitalization for initial control.

The guidelines also provide recommendations for specific groups of patients. For example, older patients with isolated systolic hypertension should first be treated with diuretics, with or without a beta blocker, or a dihydropyridine calcium channel blocker alone. Patients with high blood pressure, diabetes, hyperlipidemia, and/or chronic kidney disease should be treated with the ACE inhibitors or ARBs. Patients who have hypertension and have suffered a myocardial infarction should be treated with a beta-adrenergic blocking agent and, in most cases, an ACE inhibitor. Other studies have demonstrated that if a patient has heart failure, a diuretic, an ACE inhibitor, and an aldosterone receptor antagonist (e.g., spironolactone, eplerenone) may be beneficial. If a patient has angina

pectoris, dihydropyridine calcium channel blockers (e.g., amlodipine, nifedipine) may be added to other therapy because they have been proven to relieve chest pain and reduce the incidence of stroke. Other combinations of therapy found to be particularly effective are an ACE inhibitor plus a diuretic or calcium channel blocker or an ARB plus a diuretic. See individual drug monographs for mechanisms of action of each class of antihypertensive agent. Do not use an ACE inhibitor and ARB together in the same patient. There is generally little therapeutic gain compared with potential adverse effects that may develop.

Patients who have modified their lifestyles with appropriate exercise, diet, weight reduction, and control of hypertension for at least 1 year may be candidates for step-down therapy. The dosage of antihypertensive medications may be gradually reduced in a slow, deliberate manner. Most patients may still require some therapy, but occasionally the medicine can be

FIGURE 22-2 Treatment algorithm for hypertension. (Modified from James PA, Oparil S, Carter BL, et al: 2014 Evidence-based Guideline for the Management of High Blood Pressure in Adults: Report from the Panel Members Appointed to the Eighth Joint National Committee [JNC 8], *JAMA*, 311(5):507-520, 2014.)

FIGURE 22-3 Effects of antihypertensive agents.

Table 22-4   Combination Drugs for Hypertension

COMBINATION TYPE	FIXED-DOSE COMBINATION (mg)*	BRAND NAME
ACEIs and CCBs	amlodipine/benazepril (2.5/10, 5/10, 5/20, 5/40, 10/20, 10/40) enalapril /felodipine (5/2.5, 5/5) trandolapril/verapamil (2/180, 1/240, 2/240, 4/240)	Lotrel Lexxel Tarka
CCBs and statin	amlodipine/atorvastatin (2.5/10 to 10/80)	Caduet
CCBs and ARBs	amlodipine/valsartan (5/160 to 10/320) amlodipine/olmesartan (5/20 to 10/40) amlodipine/telmisartan (5/40, 5/80, 10/40, 10/80)	Exforge Azor Twynsta
CCBs/diuretic/ ARBs	amlodipine/hydrochlorothiazide/valsartan (5/12.5/160 to 10/25/320) amlodipine/hydrochlorothiazide/olmesartan (5/12.5/20 to 10/25/40)	Exforge HCT Tribenzor
ACEIs and diuretics	benazepril/hydrochlorothiazide (5/6.25, 10/12.5, 20/12.5, 20/25) captopril/hydrochlorothiazide (25/15, 25/25, 50/15, 50/25) enalapril /hydrochlorothiazide (5/12.5, 10/25) fosinopril/hydrochlorothiazide (10/12.5, 20/12.5) lisinopril/hydrochlorothiazide (10/12.5, 20/12.5, 20/25) moexipril /hydrochlorothiazide (7.5/12.5, 15/12.5, 15/25) quinapril /hydrochlorothiazide (10/12.5, 20/12.5, 20/25)	Lotensin HCT Vaseretic Prinzide ⇄ *Do not confuse* *Prinzide with Prinivil.* Uniretic Accuretic

ARBs and
diuretics
	azilsartan/chlorthalidone (40/12.5 to 40/25)
	candesartan /hydrochlorothiazide (16/12.5, 32/12.5, 32/25)
	eprosartan /hydrochlorothiazide (600/12.5, 600/25)
	irbesartan/hydrochlorothiazide (150/12.5, 300/12.5)
	losartan/potassium/hydrochlorothiazide (50/12.5, 100/12.5,
	  100/25)
	
	olmesartan/hydrochlorothiazide (20/12.5, 40/12.5, 40/25)
	telmisartan/hydrochlorothiazide (40/12.5, 80/12.5, 80/25)
	valsartan/hydrochlorothiazide (80/12.5, 160/12.5, 320/12.5,
	  160/25, 320/25)
		Edarbyclor
		Atacand HCT
		Teveten/HCT
		Avalide
		Hyzaar
		⇄ *Do not confuse*
		  Hyzaar with Cozaar.
		Benicar HCT
		Micardis/HCT
		Diovan/HCT

BBs and diuretics	atenolol/chlorthalidone (50/25, 100/25)
	bisoprolol /hydrochlorothiazide (2.5/6.25, 5/6.25, 10/6.25)
	
	propranolol /hydrochlorothiazide (40/25, 80/25)
	metoprolol /hydrochlorothiazide (25/12.5, 50/12.5, 100/12.5,
	  50/25, 100/25, 100/50)
	nadolol/bendroflumethiazide (40/5, 80/5)
		Tenoretic
		Ziac
		⇄ *Do not confuse*
		  Ziac with Zocor or
		  Tiazac.
		
		Lopressor HCT
		
		Corzide

Direct renin inhibitor combination products	aliskiren/amlodipine (150/5, 150/10, 300/5, 300/10) aliskiren/amlodipine/hydrochlorothiazide (150/5/12.5, 300/5/12.5, 300/5/25, 300/10/12.5, 300/10/25) aliskiren/hydrochlorothiazide (150/12.5, 150/25, 300/12.5, 300/25)	Tekamlo Amturnide Tekturna
Diuretic and diuretic combination	amiloride HCl/hydrochlorothiazide (5/50) spironolactone/hydrochlorothiazide (25/25, 50/50) triamterene/hydrochlorothiazide (37.5/25, 50/25, 75/50)	Moduretic Aldactazide Dyazide, Maxzide

ACEI, angiotensin-converting enzyme inhibitor; *ARB,* angiotensin-receptor blocker; *BB,* beta blocker; *CCB,* calcium channel blocker.
*Some drug combinations are available in multiple fixed doses. Each drug dose is reported in milligrams.

discontinued. Patients whose drugs have been discontinued should have regular follow-up examinations because blood pressure often rises again to hypertensive levels, sometimes months or years later, especially if lifestyle modifications are not continued.

❖ NURSING IMPLICATIONS FOR HYPERTENSIVE THERAPY

▪ Assessment

History of Risk Factors

- Make note of the patient's gender, age, and race. People who are older, male, and/or African American have a higher incidence of hypertension.
- Has the patient been told previously about the elevated blood pressure readings? If so, under what circumstances were the blood pressure readings taken?
- Is there a family history of hypertension, coronary heart disease, stroke, diabetes mellitus, or dyslipidemia?

Smoking. Obtain a history of the number of cigarettes or cigars smoked daily. How long has the person smoked? Has the person ever tried to stop smoking? Ask whether the person knows what effect smoking has on the vascular system. How does the individual feel about modifying the smoking habit?

Dietary Habits. Obtain a dietary history. Ask specific questions to obtain data relating to the amount of salt used in cooking and at the table, as well as foods eaten that are high in fat, cholesterol, refined carbohydrates, and sodium. Using a calorie counter, ask the person to estimate the number of calories eaten daily. How much meat, fish, and poultry are eaten daily (size and number of servings)? Estimate the percentage of total daily calories provided by fats. Discuss food preparation (e.g., baked, broiled, fried foods). How many servings of fruits and vegetables are eaten daily? What types of oils or fats are used in food preparation? See a nutrition text for further dietary history questions. What is the frequency and volume of alcoholic beverages consumed?

Elevated Serum Lipids. Ask whether the patient is aware of having elevated lipid, triglyceride, or cholesterol levels. If elevated, what measures has the person tried for reduction and what effect have the interventions had on the blood levels at subsequent examinations? Review laboratory data available (e.g., cholesterol, triglyceride, low-density lipoprotein [LDL], very low-density lipoprotein [VLDL] levels).

Renal Function. Has the patient had any laboratory tests to evaluate renal function (e.g., urinalysis—microalbuminuria, proteinuria, microscopic hematuria) or had a blood analysis showing an elevated blood urea nitrogen (BUN) or serum creatinine level? Does the patient have nocturia?

Obesity. Ask about any recent weight gains or losses and whether intentional or unintentional. Note abnormal waist-to-hip ratio. Patients with more weight around their waist have a higher incidence of developing heart disease, hypertension, and diabetes (see Chapter 20).

Psychomotor Functions

- Determine the patient's type of lifestyle. Have the patient describe exercise level in terms of amount (e.g., walking 3 miles), intensity (e.g., walking 3 mph), and frequency (e.g., walking every other day). Is the patient's job physically demanding or of a sedentary nature?
- Determine the patient's level of psychological stress. Ask the individual to estimate the amount of stress in his or her life. How does the person cope with stressful situations at home and in the workplace?
- Has the patient experienced any fatigue or reduction in activity level caused by intolerance or palpitations, angina, or dyspnea? When walking, do severe leg cramps (claudication) force him or her to stop and rest or severely limit ambulation?

Medication History

- Has the patient ever taken or is currently taking any medications for the treatment of high blood pressure? If blood pressure medications have been prescribed but are not being taken, why was the medicine discontinued? Were any adverse effects noticed while taking the medications, and how did the patient manage them?
- Obtain a listing of all medications being taken, including prescribed, over-the-counter, herbal preparations, and street drugs. Research these medications in the drug monographs to determine potential drug-drug interactions that may affect the individual's blood pressure or the effectiveness of the medicines prescribed.
- If the patient is female, ask whether she is now or has been taking oral contraceptives or is receiving hormone replacement therapy (HRT).

Physical Assessments

Blood pressure. Obtain two or more blood pressure measurements.

- The individual should be seated quietly for at least 5 minutes in a chair with a back support (rather than an examination table), with feet on the floor and arm supported at heart level.
- An appropriately sized cuff (cuff bladder encircling at least 80% of the arm) should be used for accuracy.
- When measuring blood pressure, the cuff should be inflated to 30 mm Hg above the point at which the radial pulse disappears. The sphygmomanometer pressure should then be reduced at 2 to 3 mm/second. Two readings should be taken at least 1 minute apart.
- Verify the readings in the opposite arm. A difference in blood pressure between the two arms can be expected in about 20% of patients. The higher value should be the one used in treatment decisions.

Table 22-5   Angiotensin-Converting Enzyme (ACE) Inhibitors

GENERIC NAME	BRAND NAME	AVAILABILITY	APPROVED USES	DOSAGE RANGE
benazepril ⇄ Do not confuse benazepril with Benadryl, Benzonatate, or donepezil.	Lotensin ⇄ Do not confuse Lotensin with Lioresal, Loniten, or Lovastatin.	Tablets: 5, 10, 20, 40 mg	Hypertension	PO: Initial: 10 mg once daily Maintenance: 20-40 mg daily Maximum: 80 mg/day
captopril ⇄ Do not confuse captopril with carvedilol.	—	Tablets: 12.5, 25, 50, 100 mg	Hypertension, heart failure, diabetic nephropathy	PO: Initial: 12.5-25 mg two or three times daily 1 hr before meals Maintenance: 50-450 mg daily 1 hr before meals in two or three divided doses
enalapril ⇄ Do not confuse enalapril with Eldepryl.	Vasotec ⇄ Do not confuse Vasotec with Norvasc.	Tablets: 2.5, 5, 10, 20 mg	Hypertension, heart failure	PO: Initial: 2.5-5 mg once daily Maintenance: 10-40 mg daily
enalaprilat	Vasotec IV	Injection: 1.25 mg/mL	Hypertension	IV: 0.625-1.25 mg over 5 min every 6 hr
fosinopril ⇄ Do not confuse fosinopril with bisoprolol, furosemide	Monopril ⇄ Do not confuse Monopril with Accupril, or Monoket.	Tablets: 10, 20, 40 mg	Hypertension, heart failure	PO: Initial: 10 mg once daily Maintenance: 20-40 mg daily Maximum: 80 mg/day
lisinopril	Prinivil ⇄ Do not confuse Prinivil with Plendil, Pravachol, Prevacid, Prilosec, or Prinzide. Zestril ⇄ Do not confuse Zestril with Vistaril, Zerit, Zocor, or Zyrtec.	Tablets: 2.5, 5, 10, 20, 30, 40 mg	Hypertension, heart failure, post–myocardial infarction	PO: Initial: 5-10 mg once daily Maintenance: 20-40 mg daily Maximum: 80 mg/day
moexipril	Univasc ⇄ Do not confuse Univasc with Uniretic or Urispas.	Tablets: 7.5, 15 mg	Hypertension	PO: Initial: with diuretic, 3.75 mg; without diuretic, 7.5 mg Maintenance: 7.5-30 mg in one or two divided doses 1 hr before meals
perindopril	Aceon	Tablets: 2, 4, 8 mg	Hypertension	PO: Initial: 4 mg daily Maintenance: 4-8 mg daily Maximum: 16 mg/day
quinapril	Accupril ⇄ Do not confuse Accupril with AcipHex, Accolate, Accutane, Altace, or Aricept.	Tablets: 5, 10, 20, 40 mg	Hypertension, heart failure	PO: Initial: 10-20 mg daily without diuretic; 5 mg daily with diuretic Maintenance: 20-80 mg daily
ramipril ⇄ Do not confuse ramipril with rifampin.	Altace ⇄ Do not confuse Altace with Accupril, Amaryl, Artane, or Norvasc.	Capsules: 1.25, 2.5, 5, 10 mg	Hypertension, heart failure	PO: Initial: 1.25-2.5 mg daily Maintenance: 2.5-20 mg daily
trandolapril ⇄ Do not confuse trandolapril with tramadol.	Mavik	Tablets: 1, 2, 4 mg	Hypertension, heart failure	PO: Initial: 1 mg daily Maintenance: 2-4 mg daily

4. Ask whether the patient is pregnant or likely to become pregnant. If so, discuss with a healthcare provider before initiating ACE inhibitor therapy.
5. Ask if the patient has a persistent cough.

■ Availability, Dosage, and Administration

See Table 22-5. Captopril should be administered without food and requires two- to three-times-daily dosing. All the other agents may be administered one or two times daily.

NOTE: The initial doses of ACE inhibitors may cause hypotension with dizziness, tachycardia, and fainting; these adverse effects occur more commonly in patients also receiving diuretics. Symptoms occur within 3 hours after the first several doses. This effect may be minimized by discontinuing the diuretic 1 week before initiating ACE inhibitor therapy. Patients should be warned that this adverse effect may occur, that it is transient, and that they should lie down immediately if symptoms develop.

■ Common Adverse Effects

Gastrointestinal

Nausea, diarrhea. These adverse effects are usually mild and tend to resolve with continued therapy. Encourage the patient not to discontinue therapy without first consulting a healthcare provider.

Neurologic

Fatigue, headache. These adverse effects are usually mild and tend to resolve with continued therapy. Encourage the patient not to discontinue therapy without first consulting a healthcare provider.

Cardiovascular

Orthostatic hypotension (dizziness, weakness, faintness). Although these adverse effects are infrequent and usually mild, certain patients, particularly those also receiving diuretics, may suffer some degree of orthostatic hypotension, especially when therapy is initiated. Observe the patient closely for at least 2 hours after the initial dose is given and for at least an additional hour until blood pressure has stabilized. Monitor the blood pressure in both the supine and standing positions. Anticipate the development of postural hypotension and take measures to prevent an occurrence. Teach the patient to rise slowly from a supine or sitting position and to sit or lie down if feeling faint.

Immunologic, Inflammatory

Chronic cough. As many as one third of patients receiving ACE inhibitors may develop a chronic, dry, nonproductive, persistent cough. This is thought to be caused by an accumulation of bradykinin. It may appear from 1 week to 6 months after initiation of ACE inhibitor therapy. Women appear to be more susceptible than men. Patients should be told to contact their healthcare provider if the cough becomes troublesome. The cough resolves within 1 to 30 days after discontinuation of therapy. An ARB agent may be substituted

for the ACE inhibitor if the frequency of cough is excessive.

■ Serious Adverse Effects

Pregnancy. Medications that act directly on the renin-angiotensin system can cause fetal and neonatal harm. There is concern about the potential for birth defects in neonates whose mothers received ACE inhibitors, especially during the second and third trimesters of pregnancy. Women who wish to become pregnant or who become pregnant while receiving ACE inhibitors should discuss alternative therapies with their healthcare provider as soon as possible.

Hypersensitivity

Swelling of the face, eyes, lips, tongue; difficulty breathing. Angioedema has been reported to occur in a small number of patients, especially after the first dose. The patient should be cautioned to discontinue further therapy and seek medical attention immediately.

Life Span Considerations

Antihypertensive Therapy

Older adults are more likely to develop orthostatic hypotension with antihypertensive therapy. The patient's blood pressure should be monitored in the supine and sitting positions during the initiation of antihypertensive therapy or when the drug dosage is adjusted. Safety precautions should be initiated to prevent accidental injury. Teach the patient to rise slowly from a supine to a sitting and then a standing position.

Medication Safety Alert

Hypotension With ACE Inhibitors

The initial doses of ACE inhibitors may cause hypotension with dizziness, tachycardia, and fainting; these adverse effects occur more commonly in patients also receiving diuretics. Symptoms occur within 3 hours after the first several doses. This effect may be minimized by discontinuing the diuretic 1 week before initiating ACE inhibitor therapy. Patients should be warned that this adverse effect may occur, that it is transient, and that they should lie down immediately if symptoms develop.

Hematologic

Neutropenia. Neutropenia (300 neutrophils/mm³) and agranulocytosis (drug-induced bone marrow suppression) have rarely been observed in patients receiving ACE inhibitors. The neutropenia appears within the first 3 to 12 weeks of therapy and develops slowly; the white blood cell count falls to its nadir in 10 to 30 days. The white blood cell count returns to normal about 2 weeks after discontinuation of ACE inhibitor therapy.

The patients most susceptible are those receiving captopril who also have impaired renal function or serious autoimmune diseases, such as lupus erythematosus, or who are exposed to drugs known to affect the white cells or immune response, such as corticosteroids.

Patients at risk should have differential and total white blood cell counts determined before initiation of therapy and then every 2 weeks thereafter for the first 3 months of therapy. Stress the importance of returning for this laboratory work. Patients should be told to notify their healthcare provider promptly if any evidence of infection such as sore throat or fever, which may be an indicator of neutropenia, develops.

Renal

Hyperkalemia. Because ACE inhibitors inhibit aldosterone, patients may develop slight increases in serum potassium levels. Approximately 1% of patients may develop hyperkalemia (higher than 5.7 mEq/L). Most cases resolve without discontinuation of therapy. Patients most susceptible to the development of hyperkalemia are those with renal impairment or diabetes mellitus and those already receiving a potassium supplement or a potassium-sparing diuretic. Many symptoms associated with altered fluid and electrolyte balance are subtle and interspersed with general symptoms of drug toxicity or the disease process itself.

Gather data relative to changes in the patient's mental status (e.g., alertness, orientation, and confusion), muscle strength, muscle cramps, tremors, nausea, and general appearance (e.g., drowsy, anxious, or lethargic). Always check the electrolyte reports for early indications of electrolyte imbalance. Keep accurate records of intake and output, daily weights, and vital signs.

Nephrotoxicity. A small number of hypertensive patients who are receiving ACE inhibitors, particularly those with preexisting renal impairment and those also taking NSAIDs, have developed increased BUN and serum creatinine levels. These elevations have usually been minor and transient, especially when the ACE inhibitor was administered concomitantly with a diuretic. Renal function should be monitored during the first few weeks of therapy. Report increasing BUN and creatinine levels. Dosage reduction of the ACE inhibitor or possible discontinuation of the NSAID or diuretic may be required.

■ Drug Interactions

Drugs That Enhance Therapeutic and Toxic Effects. These include diuretics, phenothiazines, alcohol, beta-adrenergic blocking agents (e.g., metoprolol, carvedilol), and other antihypertensive agents. Monitor the blood pressure response to the cumulative effects of antihypertensive agents. Take the blood pressure in supine and standing positions.

Drugs That Reduce Therapeutic Effects. Antacids may diminish absorption of ACE inhibitors. Separate the administration times by 2 hours. Nonsteroidal antiinflammatory drugs may reduce the antihypertensive effects of the ACE inhibitors. Rifampin may decrease the antihypertensive effects of enalapril. Monitor carefully for poor blood pressure control or a gradually increasing blood pressure.

Digoxin. ACE inhibitors may increase or decrease the serum levels of digoxin. Monitor for symptoms of anorexia, nausea, vomiting, headaches, blurred or colored vision, bradycardia, heart failure, or arrhythmias. A digoxin serum level may be ordered by a healthcare provider.

Lithium. ACE inhibitors may induce lithium toxicity. Monitor for lithium toxicity manifested by nausea, anorexia, fine tremors, persistent vomiting, profuse diarrhea, hyperreflexia, lethargy, and weakness.

Hyperkalemia. ACE inhibitors may cause small increases in potassium levels by inhibiting aldosterone secretion. Patients should not take dietary supplements of potassium or potassium-sparing diuretics (e.g., triamterene, spironolactone, amiloride) without specific approval from the healthcare provider. If a patient has received spironolactone or eplerenone up to several months before ACE inhibitor therapy, the serum potassium level should be monitored closely because the potassium-sparing effect of spironolactone or eplerenone may persist.

Capsaicin. Capsaicin may cause or aggravate coughing associated with ACE inhibitor therapy. Monitor for increased frequency of dry, persistent cough. Report to the healthcare provider.

DRUG CLASS: ANGIOTENSIN II RECEPTOR BLOCKERS

ACTIONS

Angiotensin II receptor blockers (also known as ARBs; Table 22-6) are a class of antihypertensive agents that act by binding to angiotensin II receptor sites, blocking the very potent vasoconstrictor from binding to the receptor (also called AT_1 receptor) sites in the vascular smooth muscle, brain, heart, kidneys, and adrenal glands. The blood pressure–elevating and sodium-retaining effects of angiotensin II are thus blocked. The angiotensin II receptor blockers have no effect on renal function, prostaglandin levels, triglycerides, cholesterol, or blood glucose levels. These agents do not affect bradykinin and therefore do not cause a dry cough.

USES

Angiotensin II receptor blockers are as effective in lowering blood pressure as ACE inhibitors and beta blockers. Men and women usually have similar responses; however, African American patients do not respond as well to monotherapy. Angiotensin II receptor blockers are indicated for the treatment of hypertension and may be used alone or in combination with other antihypertensive agents, particularly thiazide-like diuretics. The blood pressure–lowering effect is seen within

Table 22-6   Angiotensin II Receptor Blockers (ARBs)

GENERIC NAME	BRAND NAME	AVAILABILITY	DOSAGE RANGE
azilsartan	Edarbi	Tablets: 40, 80 mg	PO: 80 mg once daily; 40 mg once daily with high-dose diuretic therapy
candesartan	Atacand ⇄ Do not confuse Atacand with antacid or Avandia.	Tablets: 4, 8, 16, 32 mg	PO: Initial: 16 mg once daily; adjust over 4-6 wk with total daily dosage from 8-32 mg Dose may be administered once or twice daily for optimal control
eprosartan	Teveten	Tablets: 400, 600 mg	PO: Initial: 600 mg once daily; adjust over 2-3 wk with total daily dosage of 400-800 mg daily Maximum: 900 mg/day Dose may be administered once or twice daily for optimal control
irbesartan	Avapro ⇄ Do not confuse Avapro with Anaprox or Avelox.	Tablets: 75, 150, 300 mg	PO: Initial: 150 mg once daily; adjust over 3-4 wk with a total daily dosage of 300 mg daily
losartan ⇄ Do not confuse losartan with loratadine.	Cozaar ⇄ Do not confuse Cozaar with Corgard, Hyzaar, or Zocor.	Tablets: 25, 50, 100 mg	PO: 50 mg once daily; adjust over 4-6 wk with a total daily dosage from 25-100 mg administered once or twice daily for optimal control
olmesartan	Benicar	Tablets: 5, 20, 40 mg	PO: Initial: 20 mg once daily; adjust over 2 wk with total daily dosage of 20-40 mg daily Twice-daily dosing offers no benefit
telmisartan	Micardis	Tablets: 20, 40, 80 mg	PO: Initial: 40 mg once daily; adjust over 4-6 wk with total daily dosage from 20-80 mg
valsartan	Diovan ⇄ Do not confuse Diovan with Darvon or Zyban.	Capsules: 40, 80, 160, 320 mg	PO: Initial: 80 mg once daily; adjust over 4-6 wk with total daily dosage from 80-320 mg

1 week, but it may take 3 to 6 weeks to achieve the full therapeutic effect. If the antihypertensive effect is not controlled by angiotensin II receptor blockers alone, a low dosage of a diuretic, usually hydrochlorothiazide, may be added. ARBs should not be administered as cotherapy with ACE inhibitors.

THERAPEUTIC OUTCOME

The primary therapeutic outcome expected from ARBs is reduction in blood pressure.

❖ NURSING IMPLICATIONS FOR ANGIOTENSIN II RECEPTOR BLOCKERS

▪ Premedication Assessment

1. Obtain baseline blood pressure readings in supine and standing positions and apical pulse. Hold medication if systolic blood pressure is less than 100 mm Hg or the heart rate is less than 50 beats per minute. Contact the prescriber.
2. Initiate laboratory studies as requested by the healthcare provider (e.g., renal function tests such as BUN, serum creatinine, electrolyte levels, and CBC) to serve as a baseline for future comparison.
3. Ask whether the patient is pregnant or likely to become pregnant. If so, discuss with the healthcare provider before initiating ARB therapy.

4. Obtain a history of bowel elimination patterns and any gastrointestinal (GI) symptoms.

▪ Availability, Dosage, and Administration
See Table 22-6.

▪ Common Adverse Effects
Gastrointestinal

Dyspepsia, cramps, diarrhea. These adverse effects are usually mild and tend to resolve with continued therapy. Encourage the patient not to discontinue therapy without first consulting the healthcare provider.

Neurologic

Headache. These adverse effects are usually mild and tend to resolve with continued therapy. Encourage the patient not to discontinue therapy without first consulting the healthcare provider.

Cardiovascular

Orthostatic hypotension (dizziness, weakness, faintness). Although these adverse effects are infrequent and usually mild, certain patients, particularly those also receiving diuretics, may suffer some degree of orthostatic hypotension, especially when therapy is initiated. Observe the patient closely for at least 2 hours after the initial dose and for at least 1 additional hour until blood pressure has stabilized.

Monitor the blood pressure in both the supine and standing positions. Anticipate the development of postural hypotension and take measures to prevent an occurrence. Teach the patient to rise slowly from a supine or sitting position and to sit or lie down if feeling faint.

■ Serious Adverse Effects

Pregnancy. Medications that act directly on the renin-angiotensin system can cause fetal and neonatal harm. There is potential for birth defects in neonates whose mothers have received ARBs, especially during the second and third trimesters of pregnancy. Women who wish to become pregnant or who become pregnant while receiving ARBs should discuss alternative therapies with their healthcare provider as soon as possible.

Renal

Hyperkalemia. Because ARBs inhibit aldosterone secretion, patients may develop slight increases in serum potassium levels. Most cases resolve without discontinuation of therapy. Patients most susceptible to the development of hyperkalemia are those with renal impairment or diabetes mellitus and those already receiving a potassium supplement, eplerenone, or potassium-sparing diuretic. Many symptoms associated with altered fluid and electrolyte balance are subtle and interspersed with general symptoms of drug toxicity or the disease process itself.

Gather data relative to changes in the patient's mental status (e.g., alertness, orientation, confusion), muscle strength, muscle cramps, tremors, nausea, and general appearance (e.g., being drowsy, anxious, lethargic). Always check the electrolyte reports for early indications of electrolyte imbalance. Keep accurate records of intake and output, daily weights, and vital signs.

■ Drug Interactions

Drugs That Enhance Therapeutic and Toxic Effects. These include diuretics, phenothiazines, alcohol, beta-adrenergic blocking agents (e.g., metoprolol, carvedilol), and other antihypertensive agents. Cimetidine and fluconazole inhibit the metabolism of losartan, causing an increased antihypertensive effect. Monitor the blood pressure response to the cumulative effects of antihypertensive agents. Take the blood pressure readings in supine and standing positions.

Drugs That Reduce Therapeutic Effects. Rifampin increases the metabolism of losartan, reducing its antihypertensive effects. The dosage of losartan may need to be increased, or the patient may be switched to another ARB.

Hyperkalemia. Angiotensin II receptor blockers may cause small increases in potassium levels by reducing aldosterone secretion. Patients should not take dietary supplements of potassium or potassium-sparing diuretics (e.g., triamterene, spironolactone,

amiloride) without specific approval from the healthcare provider. If a patient has received spironolactone or eplerenone up to several months before ARB therapy, the serum potassium level should be monitored closely because the potassium-sparing effect of spironolactone and eplerenone may persist.

DRUG CLASS: DIRECT RENIN INHIBITOR

---

aliskiren (ŏ-lĭs-KĬR-ĕn)
⇄ *Do not confuse aliskiren with Azilect.*
Tekturna (TĔK-tŭrn-ă)

ACTIONS

Renin is secreted by the kidneys in response to decreases in blood volume and renal perfusion. It is the first step in the renin-angiotensin-aldosterone system (RAAS). By regulating electrolyte and fluid balance in the body, this system plays an important role in the development of hypertension and atherosclerosis. Renin is responsible for the eventual conversion of angiotensinogen to the potent vasoconstrictor angiotensin II. Aliskiren, a direct renin inhibitor, blocks the first step in the RAAS cascade, preventing angiotensin II from activating its receptors, thus preventing the release of catecholamines, aldosterone secretion, and sodium reabsorption that would otherwise result in hypertension.

USES

Aliskiren, a direct renin inhibitor, lowers blood pressure similar to the ACE inhibitors and ARBs. It does not cause reflex tachycardia as direct vasodilator antihypertensive agents (e.g., hydralazine) do. Men and women usually have similar responses. African American patients and older patients do not respond as well to monotherapy as do younger patients. Aliskiren is indicated for the treatment of hypertension and may be used alone or in combination with other antihypertensive agents. The blood pressure–lowering effect is seen within 2 weeks, but it may take 3 to 6 weeks to achieve the full therapeutic effect. Aliskiren should be reserved for those patients who do not respond adequately to ACE inhibitors or ARBs because they have been proved to be effective antihypertensive agents and should be tried first.

THERAPEUTIC OUTCOME

The primary therapeutic outcome expected from renin inhibitors is reduction in blood pressure.

❖ NURSING IMPLICATIONS FOR ALISKIREN

■ Premedication Assessment

1. Obtain baseline blood pressure readings in supine and standing positions and apical pulse. Hold medication if systolic blood pressure is less than

100 mm Hg or the heart rate is less than 50 beats per minute, and contact the prescriber.

2. Initiate laboratory studies as requested by the healthcare provider (e.g., renal function tests such as BUN, serum creatinine, and electrolyte levels and CBC) to serve as a baseline for future comparison.

3. Ask whether the patient is pregnant or likely to become pregnant. If so, discuss with the healthcare provider before initiating renin inhibitor therapy.

4. Obtain a history of bowel elimination patterns and any GI symptoms, frequency of headaches, dizziness, and fatigue.

▪ Availability

PO: 150- and 300-mg tablets.

▪ Dosage and Administration

PO: Initially, 150 mg once daily. After a few weeks, if the blood pressure is not adequately controlled, increase to 300 mg once daily.

▪ Common Adverse Effects

Gastrointestinal

Dyspepsia, cramps, diarrhea. These adverse effects are usually mild and tend to resolve with continued therapy. Encourage the patient not to discontinue therapy without first consulting the healthcare provider.

Neurologic

Headache. These adverse effects are usually mild and tend to resolve with continued therapy. Encourage the patient not to discontinue therapy without first consulting the healthcare provider.

Cardiovascular

Orthostatic hypotension (dizziness, fatigue, faintness). Although these adverse effects are infrequent and usually mild, certain patients, particularly those also receiving diuretics, may suffer some degree of orthostatic hypotension, especially when therapy is initiated. Observe the patient closely for at least 2 hours after the initial dose and for at least 1 additional hour until blood pressure has stabilized.

Monitor the blood pressure in both the supine and standing positions. Anticipate the development of postural hypotension and take measures to prevent an occurrence. Teach the patient to rise slowly from a supine or sitting position and to sit or lie down if feeling faint.

▪ Serious Adverse Effects

Pregnancy. Medications that act directly on the renin-angiotensin system can cause fetal and neonatal harm. There is potential for birth defects in neonates whose mothers have received renin inhibitors, especially during the second and third trimesters of pregnancy. Women who wish to become pregnant or who become pregnant while receiving renin inhibitors should discuss alternative therapies with their healthcare provider as soon as possible.

Renal

Serum electrolytes. Renin inhibitors block aldosterone secretion, and patients may develop slight increases in serum potassium. Most cases resolve without discontinuation of therapy. Patients most susceptible to the development of hyperkalemia are those with renal impairment or diabetes mellitus and those already receiving a potassium supplement, eplerenone, or a potassium-sparing diuretic. Many symptoms associated with altered fluid and electrolyte balance are subtle and interspersed with general symptoms of drug toxicity or the disease process itself. Gather data relative to changes in the patient's mental status (e.g., alertness, orientation, confusion), muscle strength, muscle cramps, tremors, nausea, and general appearance (e.g., being drowsy, anxious, lethargic). Check the electrolyte reports for early indications of electrolyte imbalance. Keep accurate records of intake and output, daily weights, and vital signs.

▪ Drug Interactions

Drugs That Enhance Therapeutic and Toxic Effects. These include diuretics, phenothiazines, alcohol, beta blockers (e.g., metoprolol, carvedilol), and other antihypertensive agents. Ketoconazole, itraconazole, and atorvastatin increase serum concentrations of aliskiren, causing an increased antihypertensive effect. Monitor the patient's blood pressure response to the cumulative effects of antihypertensive agents. Take the blood pressure readings in the supine and standing positions.

Drugs That Reduce Therapeutic Effects. Valsartan, irbesartan, and hydrochlorothiazide reduce serum levels of aliskiren, reducing its antihypertensive effects. The dosage of aliskiren may need to be increased, or the patient may be switched to other therapy.

Hyperkalemia. Renin inhibitors may cause small increases in potassium levels by reducing aldosterone secretion. Patients should not take dietary supplements of potassium or potassium-sparing diuretics (e.g., triamterene, spironolactone, amiloride) or ACE inhibitors without specific approval from a healthcare provider. If a patient has received spironolactone or eplerenone up to several months before renin inhibitor therapy, the serum potassium level should be monitored closely because the potassium-sparing effects of spironolactone and eplerenone may persist.

DRUG CLASS: ALDOSTERONE RECEPTOR ANTAGONIST

eplerenone (ĕp-LĔR-ĕ-nōn)
　Inspra (ĬN-spră)

ACTIONS

Eplerenone represents the first of a new class of antihypertensive agents known as *aldosterone receptor blocking agents.* The RAAS plays a major role in the regulation of blood pressure. When there is a reduction in blood pressure, sodium concentration, or renal blood flow, renin is secreted by the kidneys. The renin converts angiotensinogen, which is secreted by the liver, to angiotensin I. Angiotensin I is converted by angiotensin I–converting enzyme to angiotensin II. Angiotensin II produces potent vasoconstriction by acting on receptors within blood vessels. It also promotes aldosterone secretion, which causes sodium retention by stimulation of mineralocorticoid receptors in the adrenal cortex, blood vessels, and brain. These actions result in increased blood pressure secondary to the vasoconstriction and enhanced cardiac output secondary to sodium retention. Eplerenone, the aldosterone receptor blocking agent, blocks stimulation of the mineralocorticoid receptors by aldosterone, thus preventing sodium reabsorption.

USES

Eplerenone is used in treating hypertension and heart failure, either alone or in combination with other antihypertensive agents.

THERAPEUTIC OUTCOME

The primary therapeutic outcome expected from eplerenone is reduction in blood pressure.

❖ NURSING IMPLICATIONS FOR EPLERENONE

▪ Premedication Assessment

1. Obtain baseline blood pressure readings in supine and standing positions. Hold medication if systolic blood pressure is less than 100 mm Hg or the heart rate is less than 50 beats per minute, and contact the prescriber.
2. Obtain a history of bowel elimination patterns.
3. Initiate laboratory studies as requested by the healthcare provider, including renal function tests such as BUN, serum creatinine; electrolyte, triglyceride, and cholesterol levels, liver function tests (e.g., bilirubin, aspartate aminotransferase [AST], alanine aminotransferase [ALT], gamma-glutamyl transferase [GGT], alkaline phosphatase, prothrombin time, and uric acid) that will serve as a baseline for future comparison.
4. Ask whether the patient is pregnant or likely to become pregnant. If so, discuss with a healthcare provider before initiating eplerenone therapy.

▪ Availability

PO: 25- and 50-mg tablets.

▪ Dosage and Administration

PO: Initially, 50 mg once daily, with or without food. The full therapeutic effect should be apparent within 4 weeks. For patients with an inadequate blood pressure response, the dosage may be increased to 50 mg twice daily.

⚠ Medication Safety Alert

Eplerenone therapy is contraindicated in patients with the following:
- Serum potassium level higher than 5.5 mEq/L.
- Type 2 diabetes with microalbuminuria.
- Serum creatinine level higher than 2 mg/dL in men or 1.8 mg/dL in women.
- Creatinine clearance lower than 50 mL/min.
- Patients taking potassium-sparing diuretics (e.g., amiloride, spironolactone, or triamterene).
- Patients taking strong metabolic inhibitors (e.g., ketoconazole, itraconazole).
- For patients older than 65 years, or patients with mild to moderate hepatic failure, dosages higher than 50 mg daily are not recommended. For patients taking metabolism inhibitors such as cimetidine, erythromycin, saquinavir, verapamil, diltiazem, or fluconazole, the starting dosage should be reduced to 25 mg once daily.

▪ Common Adverse Effects

Gastrointestinal

Nausea, diarrhea. These adverse effects are usually mild and tend to resolve with continued therapy. Encourage the patient not to discontinue therapy without first consulting a healthcare provider.

Neurologic

Fatigue, headache. These adverse effects are usually mild and tend to resolve with continued therapy. Encourage the patient not to discontinue therapy without first consulting a healthcare provider.

Cardiovascular

Orthostatic hypotension (dizziness, weakness, faintness). Although these adverse effects are infrequent and usually mild, certain patients, particularly those who are also receiving diuretics, may suffer some degree of orthostatic hypotension, especially when therapy is initiated.

Monitor the blood pressure in both the supine and standing positions. Anticipate the development of postural hypotension and take measures to prevent an occurrence. Teach the patient to rise slowly from a supine or sitting position and to sit or lie down if feeling faint.

▪ Serious Adverse Effects

Gynecomastia, Vaginal Bleeding. A small number of men have developed gynecomastia and a small number of women have developed vaginal bleeding while receiving eplerenone therapy. Report these conditions to a healthcare provider.

Renal

Nephrotoxicity. A small number of hypertensive patients who are receiving eplerenone, particularly those with preexisting renal impairment, have developed increases in BUN and serum creatinine levels. Renal function should be monitored during the first few weeks of therapy. Report increasing BUN and creatinine levels. Dosage reduction or discontinuation of eplerenone may be required. Eplerenone therapy is not recommended in patients with creatinine clearances lower than 50 mL/min.

Hyperkalemia. Because eplerenone inhibits aldosterone, patients may develop slight increases in serum potassium. Patients most susceptible to the development of hyperkalemia (higher than 5.5 mEq/L) are those with renal impairment or diabetes mellitus. Many symptoms associated with altered fluid and electrolyte balance are subtle and interspersed with general symptoms of drug toxicity or the disease process itself.

Gather data relative to changes in the patient's mental status (e.g., alertness, orientation, confusion), muscle strength, muscle cramps, heart rate and rhythm, tremors, nausea, and general appearance (e.g., drowsy, anxious, lethargic).

Always check the electrolyte reports for early indications of electrolyte imbalance. Keep accurate records of intake and output, daily weights, and vital signs.

Metabolic

Hypertriglyceridemia, hypercholesterolemia, hyperuricemia. Increases in serum triglyceride, cholesterol, and uric acid levels have been reported during eplerenone therapy. Report rising levels to a healthcare provider.

Gastrointestinal

Hepatotoxicity. The symptoms of hepatotoxicity are anorexia, nausea, vomiting, jaundice, hepatomegaly, splenomegaly, and abnormal liver function test results (e.g., elevated bilirubin, AST, ALT, GGT, alkaline phosphatase levels, increased prothrombin time).

■ Drug Interactions

Drugs That Enhance Therapeutic and Toxic Effects. These include diuretics, phenothiazines, ketoconazole, alcohol, beta blockers (e.g., metoprolol, carvedilol), and other antihypertensive agents. Monitor the blood pressure response to the cumulative effects of antihypertensive agents. Take the patient's blood pressure in supine and standing positions. Assess the patient for hypotension, lightheadedness, dizziness, and bradycardia. Provide for patient safety; prevent falls.

Drugs That May Induce Hyperkalemia. Concurrent use of eplerenone and the following agents may induce hyperkalemia: ACE inhibitors (e.g., lisinopril, captopril, enalapril, ramipril), ARBs (e.g., losartan, candesartan, valsartan), potassium-sparing diuretics (e.g., triamterene, amiloride, spironolactone), salt substitutes (which often contain higher concentrations of potassium for flavoring), and foods marketed as "low sodium," which often have higher concentrations of potassium for flavoring.

Lithium. Eplerenone may induce lithium toxicity. Monitor for lithium toxicity manifested by nausea, anorexia, fine tremors, persistent vomiting, profuse diarrhea, hyperreflexia, lethargy, and weakness.

Grapefruit Juice. Grapefruit juice slows the metabolism of eplerenone in a minor way. If the patient develops orthostatic hypotension, a dosage reduction in eplerenone may be required.

St. John's Wort. St. John's wort stimulates the metabolism of eplerenone. A dosage increase in eplerenone may be necessary.

DRUG CLASS: CALCIUM CHANNEL BLOCKERS

ACTIONS

Calcium channel blockers are also known variously as *calcium antagonists, calcium ion antagonists, slow channel blockers,* and *calcium ion influx inhibitors.* These agents inhibit the movement of calcium ions across a cell membrane. This results in fewer dysrhythmias, a slower rate of contraction of the heart, and relaxation of smooth muscle of blood vessels, causing vasodilation and reduced blood pressure. The calcium channel blockers are classified by structure: benzothiazepines (diltiazem), diphenylalkylamine (verapamil), and dihydropyridines (amlodipine, clevidipine, felodipine, isradipine, nicardipine, nifedipine, nimodipine, and nisoldipine).

USES

Although each of these agents acts by calcium ion inhibition, there are significant differences in clinical use because they act somewhat differently on coronary blood vessels, systemic blood vessels, pacemaker cells of the heart, and conducting tissue of the heart. Their clinical effects are also dependent on the type and severity of the patient's disease. All the available calcium channel blockers are effective antihypertensive agents, but clinicians tend to use those in the dihydropyridine group more often because they have better peripheral vasodilating effects, reducing afterload. Calcium channel blockers are more effective in patients with higher pretreatment blood pressure. They increase renal sodium excretion and are usually well tolerated. Calcium channel blockers are ideal as first- or second-line medicines in patients with hypertension and coexisting angina, and are an alternative to the use of beta blockers in patients with asthma or diabetes mellitus. They are particularly effective in African Americans and older patients with hypertension, who are more likely to have low-renin hypertension. The calcium channel blockers also do not affect gout or peripheral vascular disease. Verapamil and diltiazem are also effective dysrhythmic agents (see Chapter 23).

THERAPEUTIC OUTCOME

The primary therapeutic outcome expected from calcium channel blocker therapy is reduction in blood pressure.

❖ NURSING IMPLICATIONS FOR CALCIUM CHANNEL BLOCKERS

■ Premedication Assessment

1. Obtain baseline blood pressure readings in the supine and standing positions and apical pulse.

Hold medication if systolic blood pressure is less than 100 mm Hg or the heart rate is less than 50 beats per minute, and contact the prescriber.

2. Obtain baseline weight.
3. If the patient is taking digoxin concurrently, initiate close monitoring for potential digitalis toxicity.

■ **Availability, Dosage, and Administration**
See Table 22-7.

Dosage Adjustments. See individual drug monographs for dosage parameters. Adjustments are made based on the individual patient's response to therapy.

■ **Serious Adverse Effects**
Cardiovascular, Circulatory
Hypotension and syncope. Caution the patient that hypotension and syncope may occur during the first week of therapy. These adverse effects decline once the

Table 22-7 Calcium Channel Blockers Used to Treat Hypertension

GENERIC NAME	BRAND NAME	AVAILABILITY	DOSAGE RANGE
amlodipine ⇄ *Do not confuse amlodipine with amiloride or amiodarone.*	Norvasc ⇄ *Do not confuse Norvasc with Navane, Altace, Nolvadex, Norflex, or Vasotec.*	Tablets: 2.5, 5, 10 mg	PO: Initial: 5 mg once daily; adjust over 7-14 days to a maximum of 10 mg/day
diltiazem	Cardizem ⇄ *Do not confuse Cardizem with Cardene or Clonidine.*	Tablets: 30, 60, 90, 120 mg Tablets, extended release (24 hr): 120, 180, 240, 300, 360, 420 mg Capsules, sustained release (24 hr): 120, 180, 240, 300, 360, 420 mg IV: 5 mg/mL in 5-, 10-, 25-mL vials Powder for injection: 100 mg	PO: Initial: 60-120-mg sustained release capsule twice daily; adjust as needed after 14 days Maintenance: 240-360 mg daily Maximum: 480 mg once daily,
felodipine	Plendil	Tablets, extended release (24 hr): 2.5, 5, 10 mg	PO: Initial: 5 mg daily; adjust after 14 days Maintenance: 2.5-10 mg daily Maximum:10 mg daily
isradipine	DynaCirc ⇄ *Do not confuse DynaCirc with Dynabac or Dynacin.*	Capsules: 2.5, 5 mg Tablets, extended release (24 hr): 5, 10 mg	PO: Initial: 2.5 mg twice daily Maximal response may require 2-4 wk Maintenance: 10 mg daily Maximum: 20 mg daily
nicardipine	Cardene ⇄ *Do not confuse Cardene with Cardizem, Cardura, or codeine.*	Capsules: 20, 30 mg Capsules, extended release (12 hr): 30, 45, 60 mg IV: 2.5 mg/mL in 10-mL vial; 0.1 and 0.2 mg/mL in 200-mL premixed containers	PO: Immediate release: Initial: 20 mg three times daily Maximal response may require 2 wk of therapy Adjust dosage by measuring blood pressure about 8 hr after last dose Peak effect is determined by measuring blood pressure 1-2 hr after dose administration Maintenance: 20-40 mg three times daily Maximum: 120 mg daily Extended release: Initial: 30 mg twice daily Maximum: 120 mg daily IV: 5 mg/hr by continuous infusion May titrate by 2.5 mg/hr every 15 min Maximum: 15 mg/hr

Continued

Table 22-7 Calcium Channel Blockers Used to Treat Hypertension—cont'd

GENERIC NAME	BRAND NAME	AVAILABILITY	DOSAGE RANGE
nifedipine	Procardia ⇄ Do not confuse Procardia with Provera or Peri-Colace.	Capsules: 10, 20 mg Tablets, sustained release (24 hr): 30, 60, 90 mg	PO: Initial: 30-60 mg once daily of extended-release formulation. Immediate-release (IR) formulation not indicated for hypertension management Maximum: sustained-release tablets, 120 mg daily
nisoldipine	Sular	Tablets, sustained release (24 hr): 8.5, 17, 20, 25.5, 30, 34, 40 mg	PO: Initial: 17 mg once daily; adjust over 7-14 days by 10 mg/wk Maintenance: 17-34 mg once daily
verapamil ⇄ Do not confuse verapamil with Verelan.	Calan ⇄ Do not confuse Calan with Colace. Isoptin ⇄ Do not confuse Isoptin with Isordil or Ismo.	Tablets: 40, 80, 120 mg Tablets, sustained release (24 hr): 120, 180, 240 mg Capsules, sustained release (24 hr): 100, 120, 180, 200, 240, 300, 360 mg IV: 2.5 mg/mL in 2- and 4-mL ampules and syringes	PO: Initial: 80 mg three or four times daily Sustained-release tablets and capsules: 120-240 mg once daily in the morning Maintenance: 240-480 mg daily Administer with food

dosage is stabilized. Take blood pressure readings every shift in the hospitalized patient and stress the need for the patient to monitor blood pressure after discharge. Prevent hypotensive episodes by instructing the patient to rise slowly from a supine or sitting position and perform exercises to prevent blood pooling when standing or sitting in one position for a prolonged period. If faintness occurs, instruct the patient to sit or lie down.

Edema. Assess the patient for development of edema. Perform daily weights at the same time, in similar clothing, and on the same scale. Report increases in weight to a healthcare provider for further evaluation. Edema is more common with diltiazem and the dihydropyridine calcium channel blockers.

■ **Drug Interactions**

Drugs That Enhance Therapeutic and Toxic Effects. These include diuretics, phenothiazines, alcohol, beta blockers (e.g., metoprolol, carvedilol), histamine-2 (H₂) antagonists (e.g., cimetidine, ranitidine), and other antihypertensive agents. Monitor the blood pressure response to the cumulative effects of antihypertensive agents. Take the blood pressures in supine and standing positions. Assess the patient for hypotension, lightheadedness, dizziness, and bradycardia. Provide for patient safety; prevent falls.

Grapefruit Juice. Grapefruit juice (approximately 200 mL) may elevate serum concentrations of felodipine, verapamil, nisoldipine, nifedipine, nicardipine, and possibly amlodipine, potentially causing hypotension. Grapefruit juice should not be consumed within

2 hours before or 4 hours after administration of affected calcium channel blockers.

Digoxin. Calcium channel blockers may increase serum levels of digoxin. Monitor the patient for symptoms of anorexia, nausea, vomiting, headaches, blurred or colored vision, and bradycardia. The healthcare provider may order a digoxin serum level.

DRUG CLASS: ALPHA-1 ADRENERGIC BLOCKING AGENTS

ACTIONS

Alpha-1 blockers—doxazosin, prazosin, and terazosin—act by blocking postsynaptic alpha-1 adrenergic receptors to produce arteriolar and venous vasodilation, reducing peripheral vascular resistance without reducing cardiac output or inducing a reflex tachycardia. They produce a decrease in standing blood pressure slightly greater than in supine blood pressure. These agents also have a modest positive effect on serum lipid levels, increasing HDL cholesterol and reducing LDL cholesterol, total cholesterol, and triglyceride concentrations.

Alpha-1 blockers do not increase catecholamines; therefore there is no increase in heart rate or myocardial oxygen consumption. They also have no effect on uric acid concentrations.

Because of the presence of alpha-1 receptors on the prostate gland and certain areas of the bladder, terazosin and doxazosin are also able to reduce urinary outflow resistance in men with enlarged prostate glands.

USES

Alpha-1 blockers may be used alone or in combination with other antihypertensive agents in the treatment of stage 1 or 2 hypertension, particularly in men with benign prostatic hyperplasia. They have additive effects with beta blockers and diuretics. Blood pressure response with alpha-1 blockers appears to be similar in African American and white patients. These agents can be used safely in patients with angina, gout, and hyperlipidemia. The three alpha-1 blockers have similar antihypertensive effects and adverse effects. Doxazosin and terazosin have a longer duration of action and can be administered once daily. Prazosin is often used with diuretic therapy because of its tendency to cause sodium and water retention.

Doxazosin and terazosin are also used to reduce mild to moderate urinary obstruction manifestations (e.g., hesitancy, terminal dribbling of urine, interrupted stream, impaired size and force of stream, sensation of incomplete bladder emptying) in men with benign prostatic hyperplasia (see Chapter 40).

THERAPEUTIC OUTCOMES

The primary therapeutic outcomes expected from alpha-1 blocker therapy are reduction of blood pressure and reduction of symptoms of benign prostatic hyperplasia with improvement in urine flow.

❖ NURSING IMPLICATIONS FOR ALPHA-1 ADRENERGIC BLOCKING AGENTS

▪ Premedication Assessment

1. Obtain baseline blood pressure readings in supine and standing positions and apical pulse. Hold medication if systolic blood pressure is less than 100 mm Hg or the heart rate is less than 50 beats per minute, and contact the prescriber.
2. Check if patient is pregnant or has a history of severe cerebral or coronary arteriosclerosis, gastritis, or peptic ulcer disease. (Reduction of blood pressure may diminish blood flow to these regions, which causes therapy to worsen the condition.)

▪ Availability, Dosage, and Administration
See Table 22-8.

[!] Medication Safety Alert

The initial doses of doxazosin, prazosin, and terazosin may cause hypotension with dizziness, tachycardia, and fainting; these adverse effects occur in less than 1% of patients starting therapy. Symptoms occur 15 to 90 minutes after administration of the initial dose and occur most often in patients who are already receiving propranolol, and presumably other beta blockers. These effects may be minimized by giving the first doses with food and limiting the initial dose to 1 mg. Patients should be warned that these adverse effects may occur, that they are transient, and that the patient should lie down immediately if symptoms develop.

▪ Common Adverse Effects
Neurologic
Drowsiness, headache, dizziness, weakness, lethargy. Tell the patient that these adverse effects may occur but that they tend to be self-limiting. Tell the patient not to stop taking the medication and to consult a healthcare provider if the problem becomes unacceptable.
Cardiovascular
Dizziness, tachycardia, fainting. These adverse effects occur in about 1% of patients when therapy is initiated. Symptoms develop 15 to 90 minutes after the first few doses are taken. To decrease the incidence, give the first few doses with food and limit the initial dose to 1 mg. Instruct the patient to lie down immediately if these symptoms start to occur, and provide for the patient's safety.

▪ Drug Interactions
Drugs That Enhance Therapeutic and Toxic Effects. These include diuretics, alcohol, beta blockers (e.g., metoprolol, carvedilol), and other antihypertensive agents. Monitor the blood pressure response to the cumulative effects of antihypertensive agents. Take the patient's blood pressure in supine and standing positions. Monitor for an increase in severity of adverse effects such as sedation, hypotension, and bradycardia or tachycardia.

DRUG CLASS: CENTRAL-ACTING ALPHA-2 AGONISTS

ACTIONS

Central-acting alpha-2 agonists (e.g., clonidine, guanfacine, methyldopa) act by stimulating the alpha-adrenergic receptors in the brainstem, resulting in reduced sympathetic outflow from the CNS and decreased heart rate and peripheral vascular resistance, causing a drop in both systolic and diastolic blood pressures.

USES

Alpha-2 agonists are considered adjunctive antihypertensive agents and are recommended for use only in combination with preferred or alternative antihypertensive agents. Clonidine is available as a transdermal therapeutic system (TTS) that is applied once weekly. These drugs cause more frequent adverse effects such as sedation, dizziness, dry mouth, fatigue, and sexual dysfunction. When used alone, methyldopa often causes fluid retention. They can safely be used in combination with other agents such as diuretics, vasodilators, and beta blockers.

THERAPEUTIC OUTCOME

The primary therapeutic outcome expected from the alpha-2 agonists is reduction in blood pressure.

Table 22-8 Alpha-1 Adrenergic Blocking Agents

GENERIC NAME	BRAND NAME	AVAILABILITY	DOSAGE RANGE
doxazosin ⇄ *Do not confuse doxazosin with donepezil.*	Cardura ⇄ *Do not confuse Cardura with K-Dur, Ridaura, Cardene, Cordarone, or Coumadin.*	Tablets: 1, 2, 4, 8 mg Tablets, extended release (24 hr): 4, 8 mg	Hypertension: PO: Initial: 1 mg daily AM or PM; hypotensive effects are most likely within 2-6 hr; monitor standing blood pressure Maintenance: increase to 2 mg; then, if needed, 4, 8, and 16 mg to achieve desired reduction in blood pressure Benign prostatic hyperplasia: PO: Initial: as for hypertension; increase dosage at weekly intervals to 2 mg, then 4 and 8 mg once daily Maintenance: 8 mg daily; monitor blood pressure Maximum: 16 mg daily
prazosin	Minipress	Capsules: 1, 2, 5 mg	Hypertension: PO: Initial: 1 mg two or three times daily, with first dose at bedtime to reduce syncopal episodes. Maintenance: 6-15 mg/day in two or three divided doses Maximum dosage: 40 mg/day
terazosin	Hytrin	Capsules: 1, 2, 5, 10 mg	Hypertension: PO: Initial: 1 mg at bedtime; measure blood pressure 2-3 hr after dosing and evaluate for symptoms of dizziness or tachycardia; if response is substantially diminished at 24 hr, increase dosage Maintenance: 1-5 mg daily Maximum dose: 20 mg/day Benign prostatic hyperplasia: PO: Initial: as for hypertension; gradually increase dosage in stepwise fashion to 2, 5, or 10 mg daily for acceptable urinary output Maintenance: 10 mg daily for 4-6 wk to assess urinary response Maximum dose: 20 mg/day

❖ NURSING IMPLICATIONS FOR CENTRAL-ACTING ALPHA-2 AGONISTS

▪ Premedication Assessment

1. Obtain baseline blood pressure readings in supine and standing positions and apical pulse. Hold medication if systolic blood pressure is less than 100 mm Hg or the heart rate is less than 50 beats per minute, and contact the prescriber.
2. Assess the patient's mental status; affective and cognitive behaviors should be used as a baseline for subsequent comparison. If depression is suspected, report to a healthcare provider.
3. Obtain baseline data relating to usual sleep pattern.

▪ Availability, Dosage, and Administration

See Table 22-9.

Sudden Discontinuation. Never suddenly discontinue clonidine because it could cause a rebound effect with a rapid increase in blood pressure, manifested by nervousness, agitation, restlessness, tremors, headache, nausea, and increased salivation. Rebound symptoms are most pronounced after 1 to 2 months of therapy and may begin to appear within a few hours of a missed dose. Within 8 to 24 hours, severe symptoms may develop.

When therapy is to be discontinued, a gradual reduction in dosage is necessary over 2 to 4 days, during which blood pressure must be carefully monitored.

If the clonidine transdermal patch becomes loose, the adhesive overlay should be applied directly over the patch to ensure good adhesion.

▪ Common Adverse Effects
Neurologic

Drowsiness, dizziness. Tell the patient that these symptoms may occur but that they tend to be self-limiting. Tell the patient not to discontinue the medication and to consult a healthcare provider if the adverse effects become an unacceptable problem.

⚕ Table 22-9	**Central-Acting Alpha-2 Agonists**		
GENERIC NAME	**BRAND NAME**	**AVAILABILITY**	**DOSAGE RANGE**
clonidine ⇄ *Do not confuse clonidine with colchicine, Cardizem, Klonopin, or clonazepam.*	Catapres, Catapres-TTS ⇄ *Do not confuse Catapres with Capoten or Cataflam.*	Tablets: 0.1, 0.2, 0.3 mg Transdermal patch: TTS-1 = 0.1 mg/day TTS-2 = 0.2 mg/day TTS-3 = 0.3 mg/day	PO: Initial: 0.1 mg twice daily Maintenance: 0.2-0.8 mg daily in two or three divided doses Maximum: 2.4 mg daily Transdermal: Apply to hairless area of intact skin on upper arm or torso once every 7 days; use a different site each wk Initial: Start with 0.1-mg patch; after second wk, add another 0.1-mg patch or use a larger system Maximum: Two 0.3-mg patches/wk Note: Antihypertensive effect starts 2-3 days after initiation of therapy
guanfacine	Tenex	Tablets: 1, 2 mg	Hypertension (IR only) PO: Initial: 1 mg daily at bedtime Maintenance: 1-2 mg Maximum: 3 mg daily
	Intuniv	Tablets, extended release: 1, 2, 3, 4 mg (for ADHD)	See Tenex for dosage range for hypertension Attention deficit hyperactivity disorder: PO: Initial: 1 mg daily Maintenance: 1-4 mg daily When discontinuing, taper the dose no more rapidly than 1 mg every 3-7 days
methyldopa ⇄ *Do not confuse methyldopa with levodopa or L-dopa.*	—	Tablets: 250, 500 mg IV: 50 mg/mL	PO: Initial: 250 mg two or three times daily Maintenance: 500 mg to 3 g daily in two to four doses

Gastrointestinal

Dry mouth. Tell the patient that these symptoms may occur but that they tend to be self-limiting. Tell the patient not to discontinue the medication and to consult a healthcare provider if the adverse effects become an unacceptable problem.

Genitourinary

Altered urine color. Methyldopa or its metabolites may discolor the urine, causing it to darken on exposure to air. It is to be expected and is not harmful.

Altered test reactions. Methyldopa may cause up to 20% of patients to develop a positive reaction to the direct Coombs test. Less than 0.2% of these patients will develop hemolytic anemia, however. Blood counts should be determined annually during therapy to detect hemolytic anemia.

■ Serious Adverse Effects

Psychological

Depression. Assess the patient's affect (e.g., loneliness, sadness, anxiety, anger), cognition (e.g., confusion, ambivalence, loss of interest), and other behavioral responses (e.g., agitation, irritability, altered activity level, withdrawal) before starting therapy. After starting therapy with clonidine, carefully monitor the patient for changes in usual response patterns. Assess otherwise normal emotions for an increase in duration or intensity. Note the patient's degree of socialization, response to stimulation, and changes in interactions with others. All individuals taking this drug should be monitored for development of depression, especially those with a history of depression.

Integumentary

Rash. About 10% to 15% of patients using the clonidine patch develop contact dermatitis. Patients who develop moderate or severe erythema or vesicle formation at the site of application of clonidine transdermal patches should consult a healthcare provider about the possible need to remove the patch and use alternative therapy.

■ Drug Interactions

Drugs That Enhance Therapeutic and Toxic Effects. These include digoxin, alcohol, beta blockers (e.g., metoprolol, carvedilol), verapamil, and other antihypertensive agents. Monitor the blood pressure response to the cumulative effects of antihypertensive agents. Take the patient's blood pressure in supine and standing positions. Monitor for an increase in severity of adverse effects such as sedation, hypotension, and bradycardia or tachycardia.

Drugs That Reduce Therapeutic Effects. Tricyclic antidepressants (e.g., amitriptyline, imipramine, desipramine), trazodone, and prazosin may block the antihypertensive effects of clonidine and methyldopa. Beta blockers (e.g., propranolol, atenolol, pindolol) may cause potentially life-threatening increases in blood pressure when taken with clonidine. Monitor carefully for poor blood pressure control or a gradually increasing blood pressure.

Sedative Effects. Alcohol, barbiturates, phenothiazines, benzodiazepines, tricyclic antidepressants, antihistamines, and any other drugs that cause sedation or drowsiness all potentiate the sedative effects of clonidine and methyldopa. Patients should be warned that their tolerance to alcohol and other depressants may be diminished.

Haloperidol. Methyldopa used concurrently with haloperidol may produce irritability, aggressiveness, abusive behavior, and dementia. Concurrent use is usually not recommended.

DRUG CLASS: DIRECT VASODILATORS

hydralazine (hī-DRĂL-ă-zēn)

ACTIONS

Hydralazine causes direct arteriolar smooth muscle relaxation, resulting in reduced peripheral vascular resistance. The reduction in peripheral resistance causes a reflex increase in heart rate, cardiac output, and renin release with sodium and water retention. Consequently, the hypotensive effectiveness is reduced unless the patient is also taking a sympathetic inhibitor (e.g., beta blocker) and a diuretic.

USES

Hydralazine is used to treat stage 2 hypertension and hypertension associated with renal disease and toxemia of pregnancy. It may also be used to provide symptomatic relief in patients with heart failure by reducing resistance (afterload) to left ventricular output. Because of the reflex increase in cardiac rate, hydralazine is often used in combination with a drug that inhibits tachycardia (e.g., beta blockers, clonidine, methyldopa).

A combination product (BiDil) containing hydralazine and isosorbide dinitrate has been approved by the U.S. Food and Drug Administration (FDA). This combination has been shown to reduce hospitalizations, improve quality of life, and reduce mortality in African Americans with hypertension and heart failure.

THERAPEUTIC OUTCOME

The primary therapeutic outcome of hydralazine is reduction in blood pressure.

❖ NURSING IMPLICATIONS FOR HYDRALAZINE

■ Premedication Assessment

1. Obtain baseline blood pressure readings in the supine and standing positions and apical pulse. Hold medication if systolic blood pressure is less than 100 mm Hg or the heart rate is less than 50 beats per minute, and contact the prescriber.

■ Availability

PO: 10-, 25-, 50-, and 100-mg tablets. *Intramuscular (IM), intravenous (IV):* 20 mg/mL in 1-mL vials.

■ Dosage and Administration

Adult: PO: Initially, 10 mg four times daily for the first 2 to 4 days, then 25 mg four times daily. The second week, increase the dosage to 50 mg four times daily as the patient tolerates the dosage and the blood pressure is brought under control. Maximum daily dosage is 300 mg. *IM, IV:* 10 to 20 mg IV bolus or 10 to 50 mg IM, repeated as necessary, usually every 4 to 6 hours. Monitor blood pressure often. Results usually become evident within 10 to 20 minutes.

■ Common Adverse Effects
Neurologic

Dizziness, numbness, tingling in the legs. Although these symptoms may be anticipated, they require monitoring. If severe, they should be reported so that the dosage can be adjusted appropriately.

Nausea. This symptom may be anticipated; monitoring is required. If severe, report to a healthcare provider so that the dosage can be adjusted.

Cardiovascular

Orthostatic hypotension. This may occur, particularly during initiation of therapy. Patients can usually avoid this complication by rising slowly from supine and sitting positions.

Palpitations, tachycardia. Although these symptoms may be anticipated, they require monitoring. If severe, they should be reported so that the dosage can be adjusted appropriately.

Respiratory

Nasal congestion. Nasal congestion can be treated with an antihistamine such as chlorpheniramine.

■ Serious Adverse Effects
Immunologic, Inflammatory

Fever, chills, joint and muscle pain, skin eruptions. Tell patients to report the development of these symptoms to a healthcare provider. Monitor laboratory reports for leukocyte counts and antinuclear antibody (ANA) titer.

■ Drug Interactions

Drugs That Enhance Therapeutic and Toxic Effects. These include diuretics, alcohol, beta blockers (e.g., propranolol, atenolol, pindolol), and other antihypertensive agents. Monitor the blood pressure response to the cumulative effects of antihypertensive agents. Take the patient's blood pressure in supine and standing positions. Monitor for an increase in severity of adverse effects, such as sedation, hypotension, and bradycardia or tachycardia.

nitroprusside sodium (nī-trō-PRŬS-īd)
Nitropress (NĪ-trō-prĕs)

ACTIONS

Nitroprusside is a potent vasodilator that acts directly on the smooth muscle of blood vessels. It produces both arterial and venous vasodilation, thus reducing both preload and afterload on the heart.

USES

Nitroprusside is used in patients with sudden severe hypertensive crisis and in those with refractory heart failure.

THERAPEUTIC OUTCOMES

The primary therapeutic outcomes of nitroprusside are reduction in blood pressure and improvement in symptoms associated with heart failure.

▪ Availability

IV: 25 mg/mL in 2-mL vials.

Get Ready for the NCLEX® Examination!

Key Points

- The public has made significant strides in recognizing the risk factors associated with cardiovascular disease. This awareness has led to a reduced incidence of heart attacks and strokes. Hypertension, however, is still a national health problem. Nurses can play a significant role in public education efforts, monitor for nonadherence, monitor blood pressure response to therapy, and encourage patients to make changes in lifestyle to reduce the severity of hypertension.
- Nonadherence to hypertensive therapy is a major problem, and nurses need to understand that educating the patient regarding the consequences of discontinuing therapy is not enough. Rather, the nurse must investigate the "whys" for discontinuing the therapy. Many of the reasons the patient gives may be overcome or reduced by proper interventions or a change in the type of antihypertensive agents prescribed.
- Because hypertension is a silent killer, it is important that nurses and other health professionals extend public screening programs to the community.
- Current guidelines use the systolic blood pressure as the major criterion for the diagnosis and management of hypertension in middle-aged and older Americans.
- The primary purpose for controlling hypertension is to reduce the frequency of cardiovascular disease (angina, myocardial infarction, heart failure, stroke, renal failure, retinopathy). To accomplish this goal, the ASH/ISH guidelines recommend that blood pressure must be reduced and maintained below 140/90 mm Hg in patients under the age of 80, including those with diabetes mellitus or chronic kidney disease, if possible. The goal for those patients 80 years of age or older is below 150/90 mm Hg. The target for patients with diabetes or chronic kidney disease should still be under 140/90 mm Hg.

Additional Learning Resources

SG Go to your Study Guide for additional Review Questions for the NCLEX(R) Examination, Critical Thinking Clinical Situations, and other learning activities to help you master this chapter content.

evolve Go to your Evolve website (http://evolve .elsevier.com/Clayton) for additional online resources.

Review Questions for the NCLEX® Examination

1. A patient asked the nurse about the difference between primary and secondary hypertension. Which statement by the nurse accurately answers the question?
   1. "Primary hypertension accounts for 90% of all clinical cases of high blood pressure."
   2. "It does not matter whether you have primary or secondary hypertension; your treatment plan will be the same."
   3. "Primary hypertension has no identifiable cause, and secondary hypertension is caused by some other condition. Treating the other condition may eliminate the hypertension."
   4. "Primary hypertension is curable, and secondary hypertension is only controllable."

2. The nurse was reviewing the assessments and interventions for patients with hypertension. *(Select all that apply.)*
   1. Monitoring blood pressure
   2. Listening for bowel sounds
   3. Reviewing diet history
   4. Checking laboratory values for kidney function
   5. Determining the physical activity level of the patient

3. After discussing lifestyle modifications with the patient who is hypertensive, the nurse will reinforce teaching after the patient makes the following statement:
   1. "I will weigh myself at the same time every day and report a weight gain of more than 2 pounds."
   2. "I can eat tuna and crackers for a midafternoon snack."
   3. "I will walk every day at least 20 minutes."
   4. "I think that I can keep track of my blood pressure using a journal to record it."

4. The nurse was discussing the various drug classifications used for hypertension with a new nurse during orientation and reviewed the following drug classifications in the discussion. *(Select all that apply.)*
   1. Renin inhibitors
   2. Diuretics
   3. Angiotensin II receptor blockers
   4. Anticholinergic agents
   5. Benzodiazepines

5. The nurse was explaining to a patient with newly diagnosed hypertension the initial therapy, which may include: *(Select all that apply.)*
   1. diuretics.
   2. beta blockers.
   3. aldosterone receptor antagonists.
   4. angiotensin II receptor blockers.
   5. calcium channel blockers.

6. The nurse preparing the drug irbesartan (Avapro) from the drug class angiotensin II receptor blockers knows that this drug works by:
   1. inhibiting the conversion of angiotensin I to angiotensin II.
   2. binding to and blocking angiotensin II receptor sites.
   3. preventing the release of catecholamines.
   4. blocking the stimulation of mineralocorticoid receptors.

7. The nurse is administering amlodipine (Norvasc) to a patient who asked how the drug works. The nurse's best response is:
   1. "This drug blocks the receptors that stimulate the release of renin from the kidneys."
   2. "This drug helps relax your blood vessels and slows your heart rate, which lowers your blood pressure."
   3. "This drug will help you get rid of excess water, which will lower your blood pressure."
   4. "This drug is designed to dilate your blood vessels, which in turn will lower your blood pressure."

8. The nurse is reviewing an order for the drug hydralazine that will be administered to a patient with persistent high blood pressure. The nurse recognizes this drug as a:
   1. calcium channel blocker.
   2. beta blocker.
   3. central acting alpha-2 agonist.
   4. direct vasodilator.

9. While reviewing the drug hydrochlorothiazide for a patient with hypertension, the nurse also checked this laboratory value before administration. *(Select all that apply.)*
   1. Potassium
   2. Chloride
   3. Sodium
   4. Creatinine clearance

10. After teaching the patient about the new prescription drug captopril, an ACE inhibitor, the nurse knew that further education was needed after the patient responded with this statement:
    1. "If I start to develop a cough after taking captopril, I will notify my physician."
    2. "As I understand it, I will have to get out of bed slowly to let my blood pressure stabilize."
    3. "I should take captopril with food so it will not upset my stomach."
    4. "This drug will help control my blood pressure and treat my heart failure."

Drugs Used to Treat Dysrhythmias

Objectives

1. Describe the anatomic structures and conduction system of the heart.
2. Identify the classification of drugs used to treat dysrhythmias.
3. Identify baseline nursing assessments that should be implemented during the treatment of dysrhythmias.
4. Cite common adverse effects that may be observed with the administration of antidysrhythmic drugs.
5. List the six cardinal signs of cardiovascular disease.

Key Terms

conduction system (kŭn-DŬK-shŭn SĬS-tĕm) (p. 363)
dysrhythmia (dĭs-RĬTH-mē-ă) (p. 363)
atrial flutter (Ā-trē-ŭl FLŬ-tĕr) (p. 364)
atrial fibrillation (Ā-trē-ŭl fĭb-rĭ-LĀ-shŭn) (p. 364)
paroxysmal supraventricular tachycardia (PSVT) (păr-ŏk-SĬZ-măl sū-pră-vĕn-TRĬK-yū-lăr tăk-ĕ-KĂR-dē-ă) (p. 364)

atrioventricular blocks (ă-trē-ō-vĕn-TRĬK-yū-lăr BLŎKS) (p. 364)
tinnitus (TĬ-nĭ-tŭs; tĭ-NĪ-tĭs) (p. 369)

DYSRHYTHMIAS

The function of the heart is to sustain life by rhythmically **pumping** blood to all the vital organs and the rest of the body's tissues. The **conduction system,** or electrical **system, of the** heart is the anatomic structure that controls **the sequence** of muscle contractions so that an optimal **volume** of blood is pumped from the heart with **each beat** (Figure 23-1). The conduction system is composed of nerve fibers that carry the electrical impulses to the cardiac muscle, causing it to contract.

In the normal heart, a contraction of the heart muscle begins in the pacemaker cells of the sinoatrial (SA) node. The electrical wave passes through the conduction system in the atrial muscle and causes it to contract, forcing blood from the atrial chambers into the ventricles below. The electrical current then enters the atrioventricular (AV) node, which focuses and conducts an electrical current through the bundle of His and Purkinje fibers to the ventricular muscle tissue. The muscle contracts from the apex upward, causing blood to be pumped from the right ventricle into the pulmonary artery to the lungs and from the left ventricle into the aorta to the rest of the body.

A **dysrhythmia** (sometimes called an *arrhythmia*) occurs when there is a disturbance of the normal electrical conduction, resulting in an abnormal heart muscle contraction or heart rate. All people have an occasional irregular contraction of the heart. The danger is the frequency with which the dysrhythmia occurs because the heart muscle loses its efficiency in pumping an adequate volume of blood. Thus certain types of dysrhythmias can produce additional dysrhythmias that can stop the heart from pumping even though it continues to beat for a short time (fibrillation). A person may sense an abnormal contraction (dysrhythmia) because of a flip-flop or racing of the heart. A nurse may also suspect that a patient is having dysrhythmia because of an irregular pulse. Dysrhythmias, however, must be identified with the aid of an electrocardiogram (ECG), which provides a tracing of the electrical activity of the heart.

Dysrhythmias are caused by the firing of abnormal pacemaker cells, blockage of normal electrical pathways, or a combination of both. Normally, the rate and rhythm of electrical activity and muscle contraction are regulated by the pacemaker cells of the SA node. High emotional stress, ischemia (see Chapter 24), or heart failure (see Chapter 27) may trigger normally quiet pacemaker cells in areas of the heart other than the SA or AV nodes to fire. This sends an electrical impulse out of sequence with those from the normal pacemaker cells, causing an irregular muscular contraction, sometimes sensed as a flip-flop of the heart. The second cause of a dysrhythmia is a partial obstruction of the normal conduction pathway, causing an irregular flow

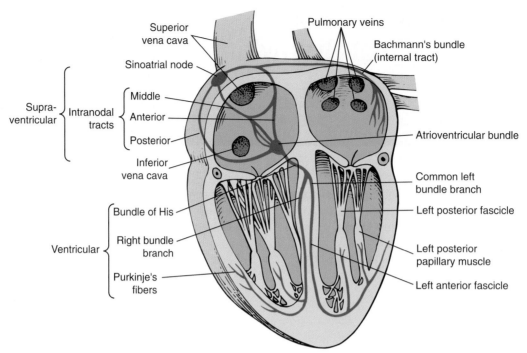

FIGURE 23-1 Schematic diagram of the heart, illustrating the conduction system. (Modified from Monahan FD, Sands JK, Neighbors M, et al: *Phipps' medical-surgical nursing: Health and illness perspectives,* ed 8, St. Louis, 2007, Mosby.)

of electrical impulses that results in an irregular pattern of muscle contractions. This is sometimes called a *reentrant dysrhythmia*. Normally, healthy heart tissue has mechanisms that protect against reentrant dysrhythmias. Various forms of heart disease cause changes in the conduction pathways that allow continuous reentrant dysrhythmias.

Dysrhythmias are most commonly classified by origin within the heart tissues. Those that develop above the bundle of His (see Figure 23-1) are called *supraventricular*. Examples of supraventricular dysrhythmias are **atrial flutter, atrial fibrillation,** premature atrial contractions (PACs), sinus tachycardia, sinus bradycardia, and **paroxysmal supraventricular tachycardia (PSVT).** Junctional dysrhythmias are those developing near or within the AV node. Dysrhythmias developing below the bundle of His are referred to as *ventricular dysrhythmias*. These include premature ventricular contractions (PVCs), ventricular tachycardia (VT), and ventricular fibrillation (VF). Dysrhythmias that result from obstruction of conduction pathways are described by location (e.g., supraventricular or ventricular, left or right bundle branches). **Atrioventricular blocks** can be subclassified by degree of block: first degree = partial block, delayed AV conduction; second degree = partial block, with occasional blocked beats; and third degree = complete block, in which the atria and ventricles function independently of each other. (It is beyond the scope of this text to describe each type of arrhythmia.) Another method of classification is based on heartbeat rate: bradyarrhythmia

(less than 60 beats/min) or tachyarrhythmia (more than 100 beats/min).

The tissues of the electrical system can be classified by conduction rate, depending on whether calcium or sodium ions create the stimulus for muscle contraction. The SA and AV nodes depend on calcium ions for electrical conduction and are referred to as *slow conduction fibers*. The atrial muscle, His-Purkinje system, and ventricular muscle depend on sodium for contraction and are sometimes referred to as *fast conduction fibers*.

TREATMENT FOR DYSRHYTHMIAS

When a dysrhythmia is suspected, a patient is often admitted to a monitored floor in an acute care setting, where wire leads are placed in appropriate locations to provide continuous electrocardiographic monitoring (telemetry). A combination of the physical examination, patient history, and electrocardiographic pattern is used to diagnose the underlying cause of the dysrhythmia. The goal of treatment is to restore normal sinus rhythm and normal cardiac function and prevent recurrence of life-threatening dysrhythmias.

DRUG THERAPY FOR DYSRHYTHMIAS

ACTIONS

Antidysrhythmic agents are complex agents with multiple mechanisms of action. They are classified according to their effects on the electrical conduction system of the heart (Table 23-1). Class I agents act as

Table 23-1	Classification of Antidysrhythmic Agents				
			EFFECT		
CLASS	**DRUGS**	**MECHANISM**	**CV**	**RP**	**AM**
Ia	quinidine (Quinidine) procainamide disopyramide (Norpace)	Na channel blockers (intermediate-acting)	↓	—	↓
Ib	lidocaine (Xylocaine) mexiletine (Mexitil)	Na channel blockers (quick-acting)	↓/↔	↓	↓
Ic	flecainide (Tambocor) propafenone (Rythmol)	Na channel blockers (slow-acting)	↓	↔	↓
II	propranolol (Inderal) esmolol (Brevibloc) metoprolol (Lopressor)	Beta blockers	↓	—	↓
III	amiodarone (Cordarone) sotalol (Betapace) ibutilide (Corvert) dofetilide (Tikosyn)	K channel blockers	/↔	—	↔
IV	verapamil (Calan) diltiazem (Cardizem)	Ca channel blockers	↓	—	↓
Miscellaneous	digoxin (Lanoxin) adenosine (Adenocard) dronedarone (Multaq)	Vagal stimulation Slows conduction	↓	↓/↔	↓

AM, automaticity; *Ca*, calcium; *CV*, conduction velocity; *Na*, sodium; *RP*, refractory period.

myocardial depressants by inhibiting sodium ion movement. The Class Ia agents prolong the duration of the electrical stimulation on cells and the refractory time between electrical impulses. Class Ib agents shorten the duration of the electrical stimulation and the time between the electrical impulses. Class Ic antidysrhythmics are the most potent myocardial depressants and slow the conduction rate through the atria and the ventricles.

Class II agents are beta-adrenergic blocking agents (beta blockers). Many dysrhythmias are caused by stimulation of the beta cells of the sympathetic nervous system of the heart. Class III agents slow the rate of electrical conduction and prolong the time interval between contractions by blocking potassium channels. Class IV agents block calcium ion flow, prolonging duration of the electrical stimulation and slowing AV node conduction.

USES

See individual drug monographs for uses of antidysrhythmic agents.

❖ NURSING IMPLICATIONS FOR ANTIDYSRHYTHMIC AGENTS

The information that nurses assess relative to the cardinal signs of cardiovascular disease can provide a basis for subsequent evaluation of the patient's response to the therapeutic modalities prescribed.

■ Assessment

Dysrhythmias are initially assessed by electrocardiographic monitoring. Various types of telemetry monitoring equipment are available. It is vitally important for the nurse not to rely completely on computerized systems, but rather to perform frequent patient assessments while viewing the telemetry system as an adjunct to astute nursing observations. A 24-hour ambulatory ECG (Holter monitor), electrophysiologic studies (EPS), exercise electrocardiography, and laboratory values are used to analyze and diagnose the patient's myocardial status.

Patients may be admitted to the coronary care unit, where specialized monitoring equipment is available for continuous surveillance of the patient. The nurses in this care unit have advanced education in cardiac physiology and the nursing care of these individuals. (See a general medical-surgical nursing text or critical care textbook for an in-depth explanation of care of the patient with a dysrhythmia.)

Medication History. Obtain details of all medications prescribed and being taken. Tactfully find out if the prescribed medications are being taken regularly and, if not, why.

History of Six Cardinal Signs of Cardiovascular Disease

- *Dyspnea (difficulty in breathing):* Record if dyspnea occurs while resting or during exertion. Is the patient affected by position, such as lying down? Does he or she awaken from sleep at night?
- *Chest pain:* Record data as to the time of onset, frequency, duration, and quality of the chest pain. Note any conditions that the patient has found that either aggravate or relieve the chest pain. Are there any associated symptoms with the pain such as sweating, ashen gray or pale skin, heart skipping a

beat, shortness of breath, nausea or vomiting, or racing of the heart? (Not all patients with a dysrhythmia have chest pain.)

- *Fatigue:* Determine whether fatigue occurs only at specific times of the day, such as evening. Ask the patient if fatigue decreases in relation to a decrease in activity level or if it is present at about the same time daily. Can he or she keep up with family and coworkers?

- *Edema:* Record the presence or absence of edema. If present, record location of edema, assessment data (e.g., degree of pitting present; ankle, midcalf, or thigh circumference), and any measures that the patient has used to eliminate edema. Chart the time of day that the edema is present (e.g., when rising in the morning, later in the evening) and the specific parts where it is present on the body. When performing daily weights, use the same scale, at the same time of day, with the patient in a similar type of clothing.

- *Syncope:* Ask the patient about conditions surrounding any episodes of syncope (faintness or dizziness). Record the degree of symptoms such as general muscle weakness, inability to stand upright, feeling of faintness, or loss of consciousness. Record what activities, if any, bring on these syncopal episodes.

- *Palpitations:* Record the patient's description of palpitations, such as "my heart skips some beats" or "it began to feel as if it were racing." Ask if these conditions are preceded by mild or strenuous exercise and how long the palpitations last.

Basic Mental Status. Identify the person's level of consciousness and clarity of thought. Both of these factors are indicators of adequate or inadequate cerebral perfusion. Subsequent regular observations for these data should be made so that apparent improvement or deterioration can be assessed. Schedule basic neurologic assessments at least once per shift.

Vital Signs. Vital signs should be taken as often as necessary to monitor the patient's status.

- *Blood pressure:* Blood pressure readings should be performed at least twice daily in stable cardiac patients and more often if indicated by the patient's symptoms or the healthcare provider's orders. Be sure to use the proper-sized blood pressure cuff and have the patient's arm at heart level.

- *Record the blood pressure in both arms:* A systolic pressure variance of 5 to 10 mm Hg is normal; readings reflecting a variance of more than 10 mm Hg should be reported for further evaluation. Always report a narrowing pulse pressure (difference between systolic and diastolic readings).

- *Pulse:* Assess bilaterally the rhythm, quality, equality, and strength of the pulses (carotid, brachial, radial, femoral, popliteal, posterior tibial, and dorsalis pedis). If any pulse is diminished or absent, record the level at which initial changes are noted. The usual words to describe the pulse are *absent,*

weak, normal, increased, or *bounding.* Report irregular rate, rhythm, and patient-reported palpitations. Check for delayed capillary refill.

- *Respirations:* Observe and chart the rate and depth of respirations. Check breath sounds at least every shift, making specific notations regarding the presence of abnormal breath sounds such as crackles or wheezes. Observe the degree of dyspnea that occurs and whether it happens with or without exertion.

- *Temperature:* Record the patient's temperature at least every shift.

- *Oxygen saturation:* Record the patient's O_2 saturation using a pulse oximeter with each vital sign measurement.

Auscultation and Percussion. Nurses with advanced skills can perform auscultation and percussion to note changes in heart size and heart and lung sounds. (See a medical-surgical nursing text for details about performing these skills.) As appropriate to nursing skills, note changes in cardiac rhythm, heart rate, changes in heart sounds, or murmurs.

Laboratory and Diagnostic Tests. Review laboratory tests and report abnormal results to the healthcare provider promptly. Such tests may include levels of serum electrolytes, especially potassium, calcium, magnesium, and sodium; arterial blood gases such as pH, Po_2, Pco_2, and HCO_3^-; coagulation studies to evaluate the blood clotting; serum enzyme levels, including aspartate aminotransferase (AST), creatine kinase (CK-MB), troponin, D-dimer, and lactic dehydrogenase (LDH); serum lipid levels (e.g., cholesterol, triglycerides); electrocardiography; chest radiography; nuclear cardiography; cardiac catheterization; EPS testing; and exercise treadmill.

Examine urinalysis reports and perform hourly monitoring of intake and output (I&O) as ordered. Report output that is less than intake or below 30 to 50 mL per hour for an adult patient. Monitor other renal function tests such as the blood urea nitrogen (BUN) and serum creatinine. Abnormalities of these tests or insufficient hourly output may indicate inadequate renal perfusion.

■ **Implementation**

- Monitor electrocardiographic tracings on a continuum (telemetry).
- Perform physical assessments of the patient in accordance with the clinical setting's policies (e.g., every 4 to 8 hours, depending on the patient's status).
- Assist the patient, as needed, to perform activities of daily living (ADLs). Make note of the degree of impairment or dyspnea seen with and without exertion.
- Administer oxygen as ordered and as necessary (PRN).
- Be aware of the policy for calling "codes," location of the emergency cart, and procedures used to check

the emergency cart supplies. Know the procedure for defibrillation and cardioversion.

- Administer prescribed medications and treatments per the Advanced Cardiac Life Support (ACLS) protocol that can best alleviate the patient's symptoms and provide the maximum level of comfort.
- Encourage physical activity as prescribed. Do not allow the patient to overexert or become fatigued.
- Institute measures to reduce anxiety. Support the patient in a calm manner, even if he or she responds in a hostile or confrontational way.

■ **Patient Education**
- Review the patient's history to identify modifiable coronary artery disease factors. Design an individualized approach to help the patient modify factors that are within his or her control.
- Cooperatively discuss and practice using coping mechanisms to handle the individual's anxiety.
- Teach the patient to take his or her own pulse and blood pressure, and emphasize signs and symptoms that should be reported.

Fostering Health Maintenance
- Throughout the course of treatment, discuss medication information and how it will benefit the patient.
- Drug therapy is one component of the treatment of dysrhythmias, and it is critical that the medications be taken as prescribed. Provide the patient and significant others with the important information contained in the specific drug monograph for the drugs prescribed. Additional health teaching and nursing interventions for drug adverse effects to expect and report will be found in each drug monograph.
- Seek cooperation and understanding of the following points so that medication compliance is increased: name of medication, dosage, route and times of administration, and common and serious adverse effects.

Patient Self-Assessment. Enlist the patient's aid in developing and maintaining a written record of monitoring parameters (e.g., pulse rate, blood pressure, degree of dyspnea and precipitating causes, chest pain, edema). See the Patient Self-Assessment Form for Cardiovascular Agents on the Evolve website. Complete the Premedication Data column for use as a baseline to track response to drug therapy. Ensure that the patient understands how to use the form and instruct the patient to bring the completed form to follow-up visits. During follow-up visits, focus on issues that will foster adherence to the therapeutic interventions prescribed.

DRUG CLASS: CLASS IA ANTIDYSRHYTHMIC AGENTS

disopyramide (dī-sō-PĬR-ă-mīd)
  Norpace (NŎR-pās)

ACTIONS
Disopyramide is a class Ia antidysrhythmic agent.

USES
Disopyramide is used to treat life-threatening premature ventricular tachycardia and ventricular tachycardia. It may be used in digitalized and nondigitalized patients. It is a useful drug alternative to quinidine or procainamide when patients develop an intolerance to, or serious adverse effects from, these agents. It should not be used in cardiogenic shock, second- or third-degree block (without a pacemaker already in place), or Q-T prolongation.

THERAPEUTIC OUTCOME
The primary therapeutic outcome expected from disopyramide therapy is conversion of dysrhythmia to normal sinus rhythm.

❖ NURSING IMPLICATIONS FOR DISOPYRAMIDE
■ **Premedication Assessment**
1. Obtain data relating to the six cardinal signs of cardiovascular disease, vital signs, and pulse oximetry levels to be used as a baseline for subsequent evaluation of response to therapy.
2. Assess usual pattern of urination and defecation.

■ **Availability**
PO: 100- and 150-mg capsules; 100- and 150-mg controlled-release (12-hr) capsules.

■ **Dosage and Administration**
PO: Dosage is individualized, but is usually 400 to 800 mg/day. Initial dosage is 100 mg every 6 to 8 hours. Making adjustments gradually, the recommended adult dosage schedule is 150 mg every 6 hours. If body weight is less than 110 lb (50 kg), the recommended dosage is 100 mg every 6 hours. Therapeutic blood level is 2 to 4 mg/L.

■ **Common Adverse Effects**
Oropharyngeal
Dry mouth, nose, throat. Suggest frequent mouth rinses or sucking on ice chips or hard candy to relieve symptoms.

■ **Serious Adverse Effects**
Cardiovascular
Myocardial toxicity. Hold the medication and report bradycardia or increasing signs of heart failure. Monitoring of the ECG for various types of dysrhythmias may be indicated as ordered by the healthcare provider.
Genitourinary
Urinary hesitancy. Tell the patient that hesitancy in starting to urinate may occur. Suggest running tap water or immersing hands in water as a means to

stimulate urination. Report decreased urinary output and bladder distention. In the hospitalized patient, record input and output. Palpate the area of the symphysis pubis to assess for distention.

Gastrointestinal

Constipation with distension and flatus. Report difficulties in defecation to a healthcare provider. Assess distention by measuring abdominal girth, as appropriate. Assess ability to expel flatus.

▪ Drug Interactions

Drugs That Enhance Therapeutic and Toxic Effects. These include procainamide, quinidine, digoxin, erythromycin, clarithromycin, fluoroquinolones (e.g., ciprofloxacin), ziprasidone, and beta blockers (e.g., propranolol, atenolol). Monitor for increases in severity of drug effects such as bradycardia and hypotension. Do not administer disopyramide within 48 hours before or 24 hours after administration of verapamil.

Drugs That Reduce Therapeutic Effects. These include phenytoin, barbiturates, primidone, and rifampin. Monitor for an increase in the frequency of the patient's dysrhythmia.

Drugs That Increase Hypotensive Effects. These include diuretics and antihypertensive agents. Instruct the patient to rise slowly from a supine position. If symptoms become more severe, report to a healthcare provider.

---

quinidine (KWĬN-ĭ-dēn)
 Do not confuse quinidine with quinacrine or quinine.

ACTIONS

Quinidine, originally obtained from cinchona bark, has been used as an antidysrhythmic agent for several decades. It is classified as a class Ia antidysrhythmic agent, working on the muscle of the heart and stabilizing the rate of conduction of impulses. It slows the heart and changes a rapid irregular pulse to a slow regular pulse.

USES

Quinidine is used most often to suppress atrial fibrillation, atrial flutter, PSVT and ventricular tachycardia, and life-threatening PVCs. Use with extreme caution in patients with digitalis intoxication or heart block.

THERAPEUTIC OUTCOME

The primary therapeutic outcome expected from quinidine therapy is conversion of a dysrhythmia to normal sinus rhythm.

❖ NURSING IMPLICATIONS FOR QUINIDINE

▪ Premedication Assessment

1. Obtain data relating to the six cardinal signs of cardiovascular disease, vital signs, and pulse oximetry

level to be used as a baseline for subsequent evaluation of response to therapy.

2. Assess and record data relating to the patient's usual pattern of bowel elimination.

▪ Availability

Quinidine sulfate: *PO:* 200- and 300-mg tablets; 300-mg sustained-release tablets.

Quinidine gluconate: *PO:* 324-mg sustained-release tablets; *IM, IV:* 80 mg/mL quinidine in 10-mL vials.

⚠ Medication Safety Alert

Do not confuse quinidine and quinine. They are both administered in dosages of 300 mg.

▪ Dosage and Administration

Adult

Quinidine sulfate: *PO:* 200 to 300 mg every 6 to 8 hours. Higher doses may be used, but the maximum single dose should not exceed 600 mg. Administer with food or milk if gastric irritation develops.

Quinidine gluconate: *IM:* not recommended.

Quinidine gluconate: *IV:* 0.25 mg/kg/min until sinus rhythm is achieved. Maximum is 10 mg/kg.

⚠ Medication Safety Alert

Intravenous administration of quinidine is extremely hazardous. Blood pressure and ECG readings should be monitored continuously because hypotension and dysrhythmia may occur. Therapeutic blood levels are 2 to 6 mg/L.

Serum levels of quinidine are determined to measure the amount in the bloodstream. Blood should be drawn before the daily dose of medication is given or at least 6 hours after administration. It is important to be consistent in the time of drawing the blood and administering the dose if more than one serum level is to be drawn from the same patient.

▪ Common Adverse Effects

Gastrointestinal

Diarrhea. Diarrhea is common during initiation of therapy. It usually subsides, but occasionally a different medication may need to be administered because of this adverse effect. Chart the frequency and consistency of the diarrhea, and monitor the patient for dehydration and electrolyte imbalance.

Neurologic

Dizziness, faintness. Dizziness or faintness may occur, particularly during initiation of therapy. These effects usually subside within a few days. Instruct the patient to rise slowly from a supine position. Monitor the patient's blood pressure.

■ **Serious Adverse Effects**

Hypersensitivity

Cinchonism. Monitor patients for signs of cinchonism and report the development of rash, chills, fever, **tinnitus** (ringing in the ears), and increasing mental confusion.

Cardiovascular

Hypotension with diuretics and antihypertensive agents. Instruct the patient to rise slowly from a supine position. If symptoms become excessive (e.g., the systolic blood pressure remains below 100 mm Hg), report to a healthcare provider.

■ **Drug Interactions**

Drugs That Enhance Therapeutic and Toxic Effects. These include cimetidine, diltiazem, phenothiazines, procainamide, digoxin, verapamil, amiodarone, ketoconazole, fluoroquinolones (e.g., ciprofloxacin), ziprasidone, and beta-adrenergic blocking agents (e.g., propranolol, atenolol). Monitor for increases in severity of drug effects such as bradycardia, tachycardia, and hypotension.

Drugs That Reduce Therapeutic Effects. These include rifampin, barbiturates, nifedipine, phenytoin, sucralfate, and disopyramide. Monitor for an increase in the frequency of dysrhythmia.

Neuromuscular Blockade, Respiratory Depression. Quinidine may prolong the effects of the surgical muscle relaxants (e.g., tubocurarine, succinylcholine) and aminoglycoside antibiotics (e.g., gentamicin, tobramycin, kanamycin). Monitor the patient's respiratory rate and depth. Observe for signs of cyanosis and additional dysrhythmias. Patients who are on respirators may require additional time to be weaned from ventilatory assistance.

Digoxin. Quinidine may increase the effects of digoxin. Monitor the patient for symptoms of anorexia, nausea, vomiting, headaches, blurred or colored vision, and bradycardia. A digoxin serum level and quinidine serum level may be ordered by a healthcare provider.

Warfarin. Quinidine may increase the anticoagulant effects of warfarin. Monitor for signs of increased bleeding: bleeding gums, increased menstrual flow, petechiae, and bruises. Monitor the laboratory report and notify the physician immediately if the prothrombin time or the international normalized ratio (INR) is abnormally high.

DRUG CLASS: CLASS IB ANTIDYSRHYTHMIC AGENTS

lidocaine (LĪ-dō-kān)
    Xylocaine (ZĪ-lō-kān)

ACTIONS

Lidocaine is a class Ib agent.

USES

Lidocaine is used in the treatment of life-threatening PVCs, VT, and ventricular fibrillation.

THERAPEUTIC OUTCOME

The primary therapeutic outcome expected from lidocaine therapy is conversion of dysrhythmia to normal sinus rhythm. Due to infrequency of use, no additional information is being presented on lidocaine.

Life Span Considerations

Lidocaine

Lidocaine for IV use to treat dysrhythmias, often used for older adults, is different from lidocaine used as a local anesthetic. For use with dysrhythmias, check the label carefully to ensure that it says "lidocaine (or Xylocaine) for cardiac dysrhythmia." Serious dysrhythmias may result if lidocaine with preservatives or lidocaine with epinephrine is administered intravenously to the patient.

DRUG CLASS: CLASS IC ANTIDYSRHYTHMIC AGENTS

flecainide acetate (flĕ-KĀN-īd Ă-sĭ-tāt)
    Tambocor (TĂM-bō-kŏr)

ACTIONS

Flecainide acetate is a class Ic antidysrhythmic agent that may be taken orally.

USES

Flecainide may be used in the prevention of paroxysmal atrial fibrillation/flutter (PAF) associated with disabling symptoms, PSVTs, and prevention of life-threatening ventricular dysrhythmias such as sustained VT. Flecainide is usually used for more serious ventricular dysrhythmias that have not responded to more traditional therapy. In addition to its therapeutic activity, a particular advantage is its twice-daily dosing schedule. Flecainide has a negative inotropic effect and may cause or worsen heart failure, particularly in patients with preexisting severe heart failure. This adverse effect may take hours to months to develop. New or worsened heart failure occurs in approximately 5% of patients. Flecainide may also aggravate an existing dysrhythmia and precipitate new ones, especially in patients with underlying heart disease.

THERAPEUTIC OUTCOME

The primary therapeutic outcome expected from flecainide therapy is conversion of dysrhythmia to normal sinus rhythm.

❖ NURSING IMPLICATIONS FOR FLECAINIDE

▪ Premedication Assessment

1. Obtain data relating to the six cardinal signs of cardiovascular disease, vital signs, and pulse oximetry levels to be used as a baseline for subsequent evaluation of response to therapy.
2. If any symptoms of heart failure are present, notify a healthcare provider before starting therapy.

▪ Availability

PO: 50-, 100-, and 150-mg tablets.

▪ Dosage and Administration

Adult:

PSVT, PAF: *PO:* Initially, 50 mg every 12 hours, increasing 50 mg twice daily every 4 days. Maximum daily dosage is 300 mg.

Sustained VT: *PO:* Initially, 100 mg every 12 hours; increase in 50-mg increments twice daily every 4 days. Most patients respond at 150 mg twice daily. Maximum daily dosage is 400 mg.

 Medication Safety Alert

Reduce dose of flecainide 50% when administered with amiodarone.

Flecainide should not be used in patients with second- or third-degree AV block in the absence of an artificial ventricular pacemaker and must be used with caution in patients with known heart failure. Monitor the ECG before and during initiation of therapy.

▪ Common Adverse Effects

The more frequent adverse effects that occur with flecainide therapy are dizziness, lightheadedness, faintness, and unsteadiness (19%); visual disturbances, such as blurred vision, difficulty in focusing, and spots before the eyes (16%); dyspnea (1%); headache (10%); nausea (9%); fatigue (8%); constipation (5%); edema (3%); and abdominal pain.

Neurologic

Dizziness, headache. These adverse effects are usually mild and tend to resolve with continued therapy. Encourage the patient not to discontinue therapy without first consulting a healthcare provider.

Gastrointestinal

Constipation, nausea. These adverse effects are usually mild and tend to resolve with continued therapy. Encourage the patient not to discontinue therapy without first consulting a healthcare provider.

▪ Serious Adverse Effects

Sensory

Visual disturbances. Provide for patient safety during temporary visual impairment. Caution the patient to avoid temporarily any tasks that require visual acuity, such as driving or operating power machinery. Instruct the patient not to rub the eyes with force when tearing. These adverse effects are usually mild and tend to resolve with continued therapy. Encourage the patient not to discontinue therapy without first consulting a healthcare provider.

Cardiovascular

Increasing dyspnea, exercise intolerance, edema. Flecainide may induce or aggravate preexisting heart failure. If these symptoms become more pronounced, the patient should be instructed to contact a healthcare provider for further evaluation.

Dysrhythmias. Flecainide may induce or aggravate preexisting dysrhythmias. The patient should be instructed to contact a healthcare provider for further evaluation if sensations of a jumping or racing heart develop.

▪ Drug Interactions

Drugs That Enhance Therapeutic and Toxic Effects. These include amiodarone, cimetidine, verapamil, protease inhibitors (e.g., ritonavir), and disopyramide. Monitor for increases of drug effects such as dysrhythmias, heart failure, and bradycardia.

Digoxin. When multiple doses of flecainide are administered to patients stabilized on a dose of digoxin, there is a 10% to 20% increase in serum digoxin concentrations. This increase may result in signs of digitalis toxicity, such as anorexia, nausea, fatigue, blurred or colored vision, bradycardia, and dysrhythmias. Monitor serum digoxin levels, electrocardiographic readings, and the clinical course of the patient closely.

Propranolol. When flecainide and propranolol are administered concurrently, there is a 20% increase in serum flecainide levels and a 30% increase in propranolol levels, with additive pharmacologic effects from each. Monitor serum levels, electrocardiographic readings, and the clinical course of the patient closely. Dosage reductions of either one or both agents may be required.

Urinary Acidifiers. These agents (e.g., ascorbic acid, ammonium chloride) may lower the urine pH, causing an increase in the urinary excretion of flecainide. Patients should be observed for redevelopment of dysrhythmias, which may require an increase in dosage of flecainide.

---

propafenone (prō-PĂ-fĕ-nōn)
  Rythmol (RĬTH-mŏl)

ACTIONS

Propafenone is classified as a class Ic antidysrhythmic agent. It also has weak beta-blocking and calcium channel blocking effects.

USES

Propafenone is used for the treatment of paroxysmal atrial fibrillation and life-threatening ventricular dysrhythmias such as VT. Because propafenone can cause additional dysrhythmias, it is used only with patients in whom the benefits outweigh the potential risks.

THERAPEUTIC OUTCOME

The primary therapeutic outcome expected from propafenone therapy is conversion of dysrhythmia to normal sinus rhythm.

❖ NURSING IMPLICATIONS FOR PROPAFENONE

▪ Premedication Assessment

1. Obtain data relating to the six cardinal signs of cardiovascular disease, vital signs, and continuous pulse oximetry and electrocardiographic monitoring to be used as a baseline for subsequent evaluation of response to therapy.
2. Record data relating to any gastrointestinal (GI) symptoms present before initiation of therapy.

▪ Availability

PO: 150-, 225-, and 300-mg tablets; 225-, 325-, and 425-mg extended-release (12-hr) capsules.

▪ Dosage and Administration

PO: Initially, 150 mg every 8 hours. At 3- or 4-day intervals, the dosage may be increased to 225 mg every 8 hours and then 300 mg every 8 hours (900 mg/day).

> **⚠ Medication Safety Alert**
>
> Because propafenone has mild beta-adrenergic blocking properties, it should not be used in patients with asthma.
>
> Administer in divided doses around the clock. If a patient misses a dose of propafenone, the next dose should not be doubled because of an increased risk of adverse reactions.

▪ Common Adverse Effects

Neurologic

Dizziness. This may occur, particularly during the initiation of therapy. Dizziness usually subsides within a few days. Instruct the patient to rise slowly from a supine position. Monitor the patient's blood pressure.

Gastrointestinal

Nausea, vomiting, constipation. Gastrointestinal complaints occur in approximately 11% of patients, but discontinuation of therapy is rarely required. Administer with food or milk to alleviate nausea. Encourage the patient not to discontinue therapy without first consulting a healthcare provider.

▪ Serious Adverse Effects

Cardiovascular

Dysrhythmias. Propafenone may induce or aggravate dysrhythmias. Patients with more serious dysrhythmias such as sustained VT are more susceptible to myocardial toxicity. The patient should be instructed to contact a healthcare provider for further evaluation if sensations of a jumping or racing heart develop.

▪ Drug Interactions

Drugs That Enhance Therapeutic and Toxic Effects. These include quinidine, cimetidine, protease inhibitors (e.g., ritonavir), ziprasidone, fluoxetine, and fluoroquinolones (e.g., ciprofloxacin). Monitor for an increase in severity of adverse effects from propafenone such as hypotension, somnolence, bradycardia, and dysrhythmias.

Drugs That Decrease Therapeutic Effects

Rifampin. Monitor patients with concurrent therapy for increased frequency of dysrhythmias.

Digoxin. Propafenone produces dose-related increases in serum digoxin levels. Measure plasma digoxin levels and reduce digoxin dosage when propafenone is started.

Propranolol, metoprolol. Propafenone appears to inhibit the metabolism of these beta blockers. A reduction in beta blocker dosage may be necessary during concurrent therapy with propafenone.

Warfarin. Propafenone increases plasma warfarin concentrations by inhibiting warfarin metabolism, thus prolonging prothrombin time. Observe for the development of petechiae, ecchymoses, nosebleeds, bleeding gums, dark tarry stools, and bright red or coffee-ground emesis. Monitor the prothrombin time (INR) and reduce the dosage of warfarin if necessary.

DRUG CLASS: CLASS II ANTIDYSRHYTHMIC AGENTS: BETA-ADRENERGIC BLOCKING AGENTS

ACTIONS

The beta-adrenergic blocking agents (e.g., esmolol, metoprolol) are used widely as antidysrhythmic agents. These agents inhibit cardiac response to sympathetic nerve stimulation by blocking the beta receptors. As a result, the heart rate, systolic blood pressure, and cardiac output are reduced.

USES

These agents are effective in the treatment of various ventricular dysrhythmias, sinus tachycardia, PSVT, PVCs, and tachycardia associated with atrial flutter or fibrillation because AV conduction is diminished.

THERAPEUTIC OUTCOME

The primary therapeutic outcome expected from beta blocker therapy is conversion to, and maintenance of, normal sinus rhythm.

❖ NURSING IMPLICATIONS FOR BETA-ADRENERGIC BLOCKING AGENTS

See Chapter 12 for further discussion of the nursing implications associated with beta-adrenergic inhibition.

DRUG CLASS: CLASS III ANTIDYSRHYTHMIC AGENTS

amiodarone hydrochloride (ăm-ē-Ō-dă-rōn hī-drō-KLŌR-īd)

⇄ *Do not confuse amiodarone with trazodone, amantadine, or amlodipine.*

Cordarone (KŌR-dă-rōn)

⇄ *Do not confuse Cordarone with Cardura or Coumadin.*

ACTIONS

Although its mechanism of action is unknown, amiodarone is a class III agent that prolongs the action potential of atrial and ventricular tissue and increases the refractory period without altering the resting membrane potential, thus delaying repolarization. In addition, amiodarone has been shown to antagonize noncompetitively both alpha- and beta-adrenergic receptors, causing systemic and coronary vasodilation. Amiodarone is chemically related to dronedarone, but their therapeutic mechanisms as antidysrhythmic agents may not be similar.

USES

Amiodarone is being used in the management of life-threatening supraventricular tachydysrhythmias, atrial fibrillation and flutter, bradycardia-tachycardia syndromes, ventricular tachycardia and fibrillation, and hypertrophic cardiomyopathy resistant to currently available therapy.

ADVERSE EFFECTS

Adverse reactions are very common with the use of amiodarone, particularly in patients receiving more than 400 mg/day. Approximately 15% to 20% of patients discontinue therapy because of adverse effects.

THERAPEUTIC OUTCOME

The primary therapeutic outcome expected from amiodarone therapy is conversion to, and maintenance of, normal sinus rhythm.

❖ NURSING IMPLICATIONS FOR AMIODARONE

▪ Premedication Assessment

1. Obtain data relating to the six cardinal signs of cardiovascular disease, vital signs, pulse oximetry, and electrocardiographic tracings to be used as a baseline for subsequent evaluation of response to therapy.
2. Initiate requested laboratory tests to be used for evaluation of pulmonary, ophthalmic, thyroid, and liver function.
3. Record data relating to the patient's usual sleep pattern and any GI symptoms present before initiation of therapy.

▪ Availability

PO: 100-, 200-, and 400-mg tablets. *IV:* 50 mg/mL in 3-, 9-, and 18-mL ampules; 1.5 mg/mL in 100-mL and 1.8 mg/mL in 200-mL dextrose IV solutions.

▪ Dosage and Administration

The difficulty of using amiodarone effectively and safely is that it poses a significant risk to patients. Patients must be hospitalized while the loading dose is given, and the response often requires 2 weeks or more. Because absorption and elimination are variable, maintenance dose selection is difficult, and it is not unusual to require a reduction in dosage or a discontinuation of treatment. The time at which a previously controlled life-threatening dysrhythmia will recur after discontinuation or dosage adjustment is unpredictable, ranging from weeks to months. Attempts to substitute other antidysrhythmic agents when amiodarone is discontinued are made difficult by the gradually but unpredictably changing amiodarone body store. A similar problem exists when amiodarone is not effective; it still poses the risk of a drug interaction with whatever subsequent treatment is tried.

PO: Loading dose: 800 to 1600 mg daily in divided doses for 1 to 3 weeks until an initial therapeutic response occurs. After the loading dose, a dosage of 600 to 800 mg daily is given for approximately 1 month. Maintenance: The lowest effective dosage should be used, generally 400 mg daily.

IV: 150 mg intravenous piggyback (IVPB) over 10 minutes, followed by an infusion of 60 mg/hr for 6 hours, then 30 mg/hr for the next 18 hours.

 Medication Safety Alert

Amiodarone is contraindicated in patients with severe sinus node dysfunction that causes sinus bradycardia, with second- and third-degree AV block, and when episodes of bradycardia have caused syncope (except in the presence of a pacemaker).

Baseline Tests. Before the start of therapy, baseline pulmonary, ophthalmic, thyroid, and liver function tests should be completed.

Gastric Irritation. If gastric irritation occurs, administer with food or milk. If symptoms persist or increase in severity, report for healthcare provider evaluation.

▪ Serious Adverse Effects

Neurologic

Fatigue, tremors, involuntary movements, sleep disturbances, numbness and tingling, dizziness, ataxia, confusion. Many of these symptoms are dose related and resolve with reduction of dosage or discontinuation of therapy. Peripheral neuropathy may be associated with long-term therapy, although the onset and presentation of symptoms are variable. Symptoms usually resolve 1 to

4 months after the discontinuation of therapy. Teach the patient to rise slowly from a supine or sitting position, and encourage the patient to sit or lie down if feeling faint. Perform a baseline assessment of the patient's degree of alertness and orientation to name, place, and time before starting therapy. Make regularly scheduled subsequent mental status evaluations and compare findings. Report development of mental status changes. Provide for patient safety during episodes of dizziness.

Respiratory

Exertional dyspnea, nonproductive cough, pleuritic chest pain. Pulmonary interstitial pneumonitis or alveolitis has been reported in 10% to 15% of patients. Particular care should be taken not to assume that such symptoms are related to cardiac failure. Tests for diffusion capacity are most likely to show an abnormality. Symptoms gradually resolve after discontinuation of therapy. Periodic chest radiographs and clinical evaluation are recommended every 3 to 6 months.

Endocrine

Thyroid disorders. Administration of amiodarone has been associated with the development of hypothyroidism (2% to 10%) and hyperthyroidism (1% to 3%). Patients with a history of thyroid disorders appear to be more susceptible to this complication. Baseline and periodic thyroid function tests should be completed in all patients.

Sensory

Yellow-brown pigmentations in the cornea, blurred vision, halos. Corneal microdeposits have been observed by slit lamp examination as early as 2 weeks after the initiation of therapy. Symptoms of blurred vision, narrowing peripheral vision, or visual halos develop in about 10% of patients. This complication is reversible after drug withdrawal. Use of methylcellulose ophthalmic solution and a minimization of the maintenance doses may limit this complication. Provide for patient safety during temporary visual impairment. Instruct the patient not to rub the eyes with force when tearing.

Gastrointestinal

Nausea, vomiting, constipation, abdominal pain, anorexia. Gastrointestinal complaints occur in about 25% of patients but rarely require discontinuation of therapy. These adverse effects commonly occur during high-dosage administration and usually respond to a dosage reduction or divided dosages.

Hepatotoxicity. Abnormal liver function test results (e.g., AST, alanine aminotransferase [ALT]) occur in 4% to 9% of patients. Liver enzyme levels in patients on relatively high maintenance doses should be monitored on a regular basis. Persistent significant elevations in the liver enzymes or hepatomegaly are indications for considering a reduction in dosage or discontinuation of therapy. Hepatitis and other liver abnormalities may develop in 1% to 3% of patients. The symptoms of hepatotoxicity are anorexia, nausea, vomiting, jaundice, hepatomegaly, splenomegaly, and abnormal liver function tests.

Cardiovascular

Dysrhythmias. Amiodarone can cause an exacerbation of the preexisting dysrhythmia, and in 2% to 4% of patients induce other new dysrhythmias as well.

Integumentary

Photosensitivity. Amiodarone has produced photosensitivity resulting in a rash in approximately 10% of patients. The severity of the rash may depend on the degree of sun exposure. Symptoms such as burning, tingling, erythema, and blistering may occur as early as 2 hours after exposure to the sun. The use of sunscreens may minimize this adverse effect. Patients should be encouraged to wear long-sleeved shirts and to avoid wearing shorts outdoors. Photosensitivity may persist for up to 4 months after discontinuation of therapy. With long-term treatment, a blue-gray discoloration of the exposed skin may occur. The risk is increased in patients of fair complexion and those with excessive sun exposure, and may be related to cumulative dose and duration of therapy. This effect gradually subsides after discontinuation of therapy. The patient should also be instructed not to use artificial tanning lamps.

▪ Drug Interactions

Cimetidine, Fluoroquinolones, Azole-Type Antifungal Agents, Protease Inhibitors, Macrolide Antibiotics. Administration with amiodarone significantly increases serum levels of amiodarone. Reduce the dose of amiodarone and monitor closely for dysrhythmias if administered concurrently.

Rifampin. Rifampin significantly reduces the serum levels of amiodarone. The dose of amiodarone may need to be increased for therapeutic effect.

Cholestyramine. Cholestyramine significantly reduces the serum levels of amiodarone. The dose of amiodarone may need to be increased for therapeutic effect.

Fentanyl. When used concurrently, fentanyl and amiodarone may cause hypotension, bradycardia, decreased cardiac output, and sinus arrest. Monitor heart rate, ECG, and pulmonary function closely.

Digoxin. Administration of amiodarone to patients receiving digoxin therapy regularly results in an increase in the serum digoxin concentration. The dose of digoxin should be reduced by 50% or discontinued. Digoxin serum levels should be closely monitored and patients observed for clinical evidence of toxicity (e.g., anorexia, nausea, fatigue, blurred or colored vision, bradycardia, dysrhythmia).

Warfarin. Potentiation of warfarin is almost always seen within 3 to 4 days in patients receiving concomitant therapy. The dose of the anticoagulant should be reduced by one third to one half, and prothrombin times (INR) should be monitored closely. Observe for the development of petechiae; ecchymoses;

nosebleeds; bleeding gums; dark, tarry stools; and bright red or coffee-ground emesis.

Quinidine. Elevation of quinidine serum levels (32% to 50%) is often observed within 2 to 3 days. The dosage of quinidine should be reduced by one third to one half or discontinued.

Procainamide. Elevation of procainamide serum levels (50%) is often observed in less than 7 days. The dosage of procainamide should be reduced by one third or discontinued.

Phenytoin. Elevation of phenytoin serum levels (200% to 300%) is observed over several weeks. The dosage of phenytoin must be gradually reduced, based on patient response. Monitor patients undergoing concurrent therapy for signs of phenytoin toxicity: nystagmus, sedation, and lethargy. Serum levels should be monitored periodically. Phenytoin may also reduce amiodarone levels. Monitor closely for loss of therapeutic effects.

Beta Blockers, Calcium Channel Blockers. Amiodarone should be used with caution in patients receiving beta-adrenergic blocking agents (e.g., propranolol, timolol, nadolol, pindolol) or calcium channel blockers (e.g., diltiazem, verapamil, nifedipine) because of the possible potentiation of bradycardia, sinus arrest, and AV block. If necessary, amiodarone can be used after insertion of a pacemaker in patients with severe bradycardia or sinus arrest.

Theophylline. Amiodarone may increase theophylline serum levels, resulting in toxicity. Effects may not be observed until after at least 1 week of concurrent therapy. Toxicity may persist for more than 1 week after amiodarone has been discontinued.

---

dofetilide (dō-FĚT-ĭ-līd)
Tikosyn (TĚK-ō-sĭn)

ACTIONS

Dofetilide is an antidysrhythmic classified as a Vaughan-Williams class III agent. It acts by blocking the cardiac potassium ion channels, delaying repolarization, thus prolonging the refractory period in the atria and ventricles. On an ECG rhythm strip, the QT interval will be prolonged. In clinically useful doses, it has no effect on sodium channels or alpha- and beta-adrenergic receptors.

USES

Dofetilide blocks reentrant dysrhythmias such as atrial fibrillation/flutter and VT and prevents their reformation. Thus it is used to convert atrial fibrillation/flutter to normal sinus rhythm and maintain sinus rhythm after conversion.

ADVERSE EFFECTS

Prolongation of the QT interval may induce ventricular dysrhythmias, particularly torsades de pointes (a ventricular dysrhythmia associated with prolongation of the QTc interval on the ECG), syncope, and sudden death. Using only the minimal dose necessary for maintenance of normal sinus rhythm is important because the frequency of dysrhythmias is directly correlated to increase in dose and further prolongation of the QT interval.

THERAPEUTIC OUTCOME

The primary therapeutic outcome expected from dofetilide therapy is conversion to, and maintenance of, normal sinus rhythm.

❖ NURSING IMPLICATIONS FOR DOFETILIDE

■ Premedication Assessment
1. Obtain baseline blood pressure readings in supine and standing positions and apical pulse.
2. Initiate laboratory studies requested by the healthcare provider (e.g., renal function tests such as BUN, serum creatinine, and electrolyte levels) to be used as a baseline for future comparison.

■ Availability
PO: 125-, 250-, and 500-mcg capsules.

■ Dosage and Administration
Before dofetilide is initiated:
• Patients must be admitted to a unit with continuous ECG monitoring available and personnel trained in the treatment of serious ventricular dysrhythmias and the initiation of dofetilide. Therapy must be continuously monitored for at least 3 days.
• Patients with atrial fibrillation must be anticoagulated before electrical or pharmacologic cardioversion to normal sinus rhythm.
• Hypokalemia must be corrected before initiation of dofetilide therapy.
• The QTc interval must be assessed. If the interval is more than 440 to 500 milliseconds, dofetilide is contraindicated.
• The creatinine clearance must be calculated.
PO: Initially, based on creatinine clearance with continuous ECG monitoring:

CALCULATED CREATININE CLEARANCE	DOFETILIDE DOSE
>60 mL/min	500 mcg twice daily
40 to 60 mL/min	250 mcg twice daily
20 to <40 mL/min	125 mcg twice daily
<20 mL/min	dofetilide contraindicated

Dosage adjustment: 2 to 3 hours after administration of the first dose, reassess the QTc interval. If the QTc interval has increased 15% or more compared with baseline, then adjust the dose as follows.

IF THE STARTING DOSE BASED ON CREATININE CLEARANCE IS	THEN THE NEW DOSE BASED ON QTC INTERVAL IS
500 mcg twice daily	250 mcg twice daily
40 to 60 mL/min	125 mcg twice daily
20 to <40 mL/min	125 mcg daily
<20 mL/min	dofetilide contraindicated

If, after the second dose, the QTc interval is more than 500 to 550 milliseconds, dofetilide should be discontinued.

Renal function and QTc interval should be recalculated every 3 months. If creatinine clearance falls, adjust the dofetilide dose according to the initial dose. If the QTc interval is more than 500 to 550 milliseconds, dofetilide should be discontinued and patients should be monitored by ECG until the QTc returns to baseline.

If a patient misses a dose, the dose should not be doubled at the next dose. The next dose should be taken at the scheduled time.

▪ Common Adverse Effects

Cardiovascular

Dysrhythmias. Various dysrhythmias (e.g., ventricular fibrillation, ventricular tachycardia, torsades de pointes, AV block, heart block) have been reported in up to 15% of patients receiving dofetilide. Continuous ECG monitoring is crucial until the patient is stable.

Chest pain. Occurs in 10% of patients.

Gastrointestinal

Nausea, abdominal pain, diarrhea. Nausea occurs in 5% of patients, abdominal pain in 3% of patients, and diarrhea in 3% of patients. These adverse effects are usually mild and tend to resolve with continued therapy. Encourage the patient not to discontinue therapy without first consulting a healthcare provider.

Neurologic

Headache. Headache occurs in 11% of patients taking dofetilide. The headaches are usually mild and tend to resolve with continued therapy. Encourage the patient not to discontinue therapy without first consulting a healthcare provider.

Other

Dizziness, insomnia, rash. Dizziness occurs in 8% of patients, insomnia in 4%, and rash in 3%.

▪ Drug Interactions

Drugs That Enhance Toxic Effects. Cimetidine, trimethoprim, and ketoconazole inhibit urinary excretion of dofetilide, potentially causing an increase in plasma concentrations and prolongation of the QTc interval.

Other medicines that prolong the QTc interval that may cause serious toxicity when used concurrently with dofetilide: dysrhythmic agents (amiodarone, disopyramide, quinidine, sotalol) chlorpromazine, cisapride, dolasetron, droperidol, moxifloxacin, ziprasidone.

 Medication Safety Alert

Dofetilide must be discontinued at least 48 hours before the initiation of other medicines that may enhance toxic effects from dofetilide.

DRUG CLASS: CLASS IV ANTIDYSRHYTHMIC AGENTS: CALCIUM CHANNEL BLOCKING AGENTS

ACTIONS

The calcium channel blockers (e.g., verapamil, diltiazem) are used widely as antidysrhythmic agents. These agents inhibit cardiac response by blocking the L-type calcium channels in the SA and AV nodal tissue. This slows AV conduction, prolongs refractoriness, and decreases automaticity.

USES

These agents are effective in the treatment of automatic and reentrant tachycardias. They are contraindicated in systolic heart failure.

THERAPEUTIC OUTCOME

The primary therapeutic outcome expected from calcium channel blocker therapy is conversion to, and maintenance of, normal sinus rhythm.

❖ NURSING IMPLICATIONS FOR CALCIUM CHANNEL BLOCKING AGENTS

See Chapter 22 for further discussion of nursing implications associated with calcium channel blocking agents.

DRUG CLASS: MISCELLANEOUS ANTIDYSRHYTHMIC AGENTS

adenosine (ă-DĔN-ō-sēn)
  Adenocard (ă-DĔN-ō-kărd)

ACTIONS

Adenosine is a naturally occurring chemical found in every cell within the body. It is not related to other antidysrhythmic agents. It has a variety of physiologic roles, including energy transfer, promotion of prostaglandin release, inhibition of platelet aggregation, antiadrenergic effects, coronary vasodilation, and suppression of heart rate.

USES

Because of its strong depressant effects on the SA and AV nodes, adenosine is recommended for the treatment of PSVT that involves conduction in the SA node, atrium, or AV node. Adenosine does not convert atrial flutter, atrial fibrillation, or ventricular tachycardia to normal sinus rhythm.

THERAPEUTIC OUTCOME

The primary therapeutic outcome expected from adenosine therapy is conversion of supraventricular tachycardias to normal sinus rhythm.

❖ NURSING IMPLICATIONS FOR ADENOSINE

▪ Premedication Assessment

1. Obtain data relating to the six cardinal signs of cardiovascular disease, vital signs, pulse oximetry, and continuous electrocardiographic monitoring to be used as a baseline for subsequent evaluation of response to therapy.

▪ Availability

IV: 3 mg/mL in 2-, 4-, 20- and 30-mL vials.

▪ Dosage and Administration

IV: 6 mg administered by rapid IV bolus injection (over 1 to 2 seconds) followed by a saline flush. A follow-up dose of 12 mg by rapid IV bolus is recommended if the initial dose is unsuccessful in restoring a normal heart rate. The 12-mg dose may be repeated once if required. Normal saline (0.9% sodium chloride) is the diluent.

▪ Common Adverse Effect

The most commonly reported adverse reactions with adenosine include flushing of the face (18%), shortness of breath (12%), chest pressure (7%), nausea (3%), and headache and lightheadedness (2%). Because the half-life of adenosine is less than 10 seconds, adverse effects are very short-lived. Treatment of any prolonged adverse effect would include oxygen and possibly other antidysrhythmic agents.

▪ Drug Interactions

Drugs That Enhance Therapeutic and Toxic Effects. Dipyridamole and carbamazepine potentiate the effects of adenosine. Smaller doses of adenosine should be used if therapy is required.

Drugs That Reduce Therapeutic Effects. Theophylline, aminophylline, and caffeine competitively antagonize adenosine; thus larger doses of adenosine are required with concurrent use.

> **digoxin** (dĭ-JŎKS-ĭn)
> **Lanoxin** (lă-NŎKS-ĭn)

ACTIONS

Digoxin slows conduction through the AV node, reducing conduction velocity and automaticity. It has a positive inotropic effect, increasing cardiac output.

USES

As an antidysrhythmic agent, digoxin may be used to treat atrial fibrillation, atrial flutter, and paroxysmal tachycardia.

THERAPEUTIC OUTCOME

The primary therapeutic outcome expected from digoxin therapy is conversion of supraventricular tachycardias to normal sinus rhythm and increased cardiac output.

❖ NURSING IMPLICATIONS FOR DIGOXIN

See Chapter 27 for further discussion of nursing implications associated with digoxin therapy.

> **dronedarone** (drō-NĔ-dĕ-rōn)
> **Multaq** (MŬL-tăk)

ACTIONS

Dronedarone is difficult to classify as an antidysrhythmic agent because it has electrophysiologic properties that fit all four Vaughan-Williams classes for antiarrhythmics. Its specific mechanisms of action for therapeutic effects are unknown. Dronedarone is somewhat structurally and pharmacologically similar to amiodarone.

USES

Dronedarone is approved for use as an antidysrhythmic agent to reduce frequency of hospitalization in patients who are in normal sinus rhythm but who have had previous episodes of atrial fibrillation or atrial flutter. In addition to a history of these dysrhythmias, risk factors that may warrant dronedarone therapy include age greater than 70 years and presence of cardiovascular conditions such as hypertension, diabetes, enlarged left atrium, and/or left ventricle with reduced left ventricular ejection volume.

Dronedarone is contraindicated in patients with heart failure, bradycardia <50 beats per minute, pregnancy (category X), breastfeeding, and liver disease (see "Drug Interactions" on p. 377). About 12% of patients must discontinue therapy because of adverse effects, most commonly GI adverse effects (3%) and prolongation of the QT interval (1.5%).

THERAPEUTIC OUTCOME

The primary therapeutic outcome expected from dronedarone therapy is maintenance of normal sinus rhythm.

❖ NURSING IMPLICATIONS FOR DRONEDARONE

▪ Premedication Assessment

1. Obtain data relating to the six cardinal signs of cardiovascular disease, vital signs, pulse oximetry, and electrocardiographic tracings to be used as a baseline for subsequent evaluation of response to therapy.
2. Initiate requested laboratory tests to be used for evaluation of pulmonary and liver function.

3. Record data relating to the patient's usual sleep pattern and any GI symptoms present before initiation of therapy.

▪ Availability

PO: 400-mg tablets.

▪ Dosage and Administration

PO: 400-mg tablet with the morning meal and another 400-mg tablet approximately 12 hours later with the evening meal.

▪ Common Adverse Effects

Gastrointestinal

Diarrhea, nausea, abdominal pain, vomiting, dyspepsia. Diarrhea occurs in 9% of patients, nausea in 5% of patients, abdominal pain in 4% of patients, vomiting in 2% of patients, and dyspepsia in 2% of patients. Gastrointestinal complaints require discontinuation of therapy in about 3% of patients.

▪ Serious Adverse Effects

Neurologic

Fatigue, loss of strength. These conditions are reported by about 7% of patients. Teach the patient to rise slowly from a supine or sitting position, and encourage the patient to sit or lie down if feeling faint. Provide for patient safety during episodes of dizziness.

Cardiovascular

Bradycardia. Dronedarone causes bradycardia in about 3% of patients. Have patient report heart rates below 50 beats per minute.

Exertional dyspnea, nonproductive cough, pleuritic chest pain. Pulmonary interstitial pneumonitis or alveolitis has been reported in 10% to 15% of patients. Particular care should be taken not to assume that such symptoms are related to cardiac failure. Tests for diffusion capacity are most likely to show abnormality. Symptoms gradually resolve after discontinuation of therapy. Periodic chest x-ray examinations and clinical evaluation are recommended every 3 to 6 months.

Integumentary

Skin eruptions. Dronedarone has produced a variety of skin rashes (generalized, macular, maculopapular, erythematous), pruritus, eczema, or dermatitis in about 5% of patients. Report findings to a healthcare provider.

▪ Drug Interactions

Drugs That Prolong the QT Interval. Drugs that prolong the QT interval are contraindicated with concurrent administration with dronedarone. Drugs that prolong the QT interval include class I antidysrhythmics (quinidine, procainamide, disopyramide, lidocaine, mexiletine, flecainide, propafenone) and class III antidysrhythmics (amiodarone, sotalol, ibutilide, dofetilide), phenothiazines, tricyclic antidepressants, and macrolide antibiotics (azithromycin, erythromycin).

Drugs That Enhance Therapeutic and Toxic Effects. Grapefruit juice, azole-type antifungal agents (ketoconazole, itraconazole, voriconazole), protease inhibitors (ritonavir), macrolide antibiotics (clarithromycin), calcium channel blockers (verapamil, diltiazem), and nefazodone enhance effects of dronedarone. Administration with dronedarone significantly increases serum levels of dronedarone. Reduce the dose of dronedarone and monitor closely for dysrhythmias if administered concurrently.

Drugs That Decrease Therapeutic Effects. Rifampin, St. John's wort, phenobarbital, carbamazepine, and phenytoin enhance metabolism of dronedarone.

Rifampin. Rifampin significantly reduces the serum levels of dronedarone. The dose of dronedarone may need to be increased for therapeutic effect.

Digoxin. Administration of dronedarone to patients receiving digoxin therapy regularly results in an increase in the serum digoxin concentration. The dose of digoxin should be reduced by 50% or discontinued. Digoxin serum levels should be closely monitored and patients observed for clinical evidence of toxicity (e.g., anorexia, nausea, fatigue, blurred or colored vision, bradycardia, dysrhythmia).

Warfarin. Potentiation of warfarin may be observed in patients receiving concomitant therapy. There are no recommendations for warfarin dosage reduction, but prothrombin times (INR) should be monitored closely. Observe for the development of petechiae; ecchymoses; nosebleeds; bleeding gums; dark, tarry stools; and bright red or coffee-ground emesis.

Get Ready for the NCLEX® Examination!

Key Points

- Dysrhythmias are complex in origin, severity, and treatment for control.
- Many of the agents used to treat dysrhythmias have serious adverse effects and must be monitored closely.
- Nurses need to check references carefully in advance of administering these drugs for the correct method of preparation, preadministration assessments needed,

rate of administration of IV drugs, and monitoring parameters essential during drug administration. If any monitoring parameter (e.g., blood pressure) is not within desired limits, hold the medication and notify the prescriber.
- Nurses can play a significant role in public education efforts, monitoring patient response to therapy, monitoring for noncompliance, and encouraging patients to participate in their own therapy.

Review Questions for the NCLEX® Examination

1. Identify the correct order that the impulse travels in the normal conduction pathway of the heart.
   1. The Purkinje fibers
   2. The AV node
   3. The bundle of His
   4. The SA node

2. The classification(s) of drugs that can be used to treat dysrhythmias include: *(Select all that apply.)*
   1. beta-adrenergic blockers.
   2. calcium channel blockers.
   3. chloride channel blockers.
   4. sodium channel blockers.
   5. potassium channel blockers.

3. The nurse reviewing the laboratory results of a 68-year-old female patient on propafenone for paroxysmal atrial fibrillation knows the following laboratory tests are monitored. *(Select all that apply.)*
   1. PSA
   2. CK-MB
   3. AST
   4. TSH
   5. LDH

4. The nurse administering a class Ia antidysrhythmic agent to a 57-year-old male patient with a history of ventricular tachycardia knows that it is important to observe for which of these adverse effects? *(Select all that apply.)*
   1. Urinary retention
   2. Bradycardia
   3. Edema
   4. Sinus rhythm
   5. Dry mouth

5. A nurse assessing a 48-year-old male patient for signs of cardiovascular disease looks for which of these symptoms? *(Select all that apply.)*
   1. Palpitations
   2. Shortness of breath
   3. Syncope
   4. Fatigue
   5. Confusion

Drugs Used to Treat Angina Pectoris

Objectives

1. Define *angina pectoris* and identify assessment data needed to evaluate an anginal attack.
2. Differentiate between *chronic stable angina* and *unstable angina* and the drug therapy used for each type.
3. Describe the actions of nitrates, beta-adrenergic blockers, calcium channel blockers, and

angiotensin-converting enzyme inhibitors on the myocardial tissue of the heart.
4. Identify risk factor management and healthy lifestyle changes that are taught to prevent disease progression and myocardial infarction or death.

Key Terms

angina pectoris (ăn-JĬ-nă PĔK-tŏr-ĭs) (p. 379)
ischemia (ĭs-KĒ-mĭa) (p. 379)
chronic stable angina (KRŎN-ĭk STĀ-bŭl) (p. 379)

unstable angina (ŭn-STĀ-bŭl) (p. 379)
variant angina (VĂR-ē-ĕnt) (p. 379)

ANGINA PECTORIS

Coronary artery disease (CAD) is the leading cause of disability, socioeconomic loss, and death in the United States, and angina pectoris is the first clinical indication of underlying CAD in many patients. **Angina pectoris** is the name given to a feeling of chest discomfort arising from the heart because of lack of oxygen getting to the heart cells. It is a symptom of coronary artery disease, and is also called *ischemic heart disease.* **Ischemia** develops when the supply of oxygen needed by the heart cells is inadequate. The lack of oxygen occurs when blood flow through the coronary arteries is reduced by atherosclerosis or spasm of the arteries. Atherosclerosis can develop as localized plaques or as a generalized narrowing of the coronary arteries. Patients are usually asymptomatic until there is at least 50% narrowing of the artery. Coronary artery disease caused by atherosclerosis is a progressive disease; however, progression can be slowed with diet control and with the use of cholesterol-lowering agents (see Chapter 21).

The presentation of angina pectoris is highly variable. The sensation of discomfort is often described variously as squeezing, tightness, choking, pressure, burning, or heaviness. This discomfort may radiate to the neck, lower jaw, shoulder, and arm. The usual anginal attack begins gradually, reaches its peak intensity over the next several minutes, and then gradually subsides after the person stops activity and rests. Attacks can last from 30 seconds to 30 minutes. Anginal

episodes are usually precipitated by factors that require an increased oxygen supply (e.g., physical activity, such as climbing a flight of stairs or lifting). Other precipitating factors include exposure to cold temperatures, emotional stress, sexual intercourse, and eating a large meal.

Angina pectoris is classified as chronic stable, unstable, or variant angina. **Chronic stable angina** is precipitated by physical exertion or stress, lasts only a few minutes, and is relieved by rest or nitroglycerin. It is usually caused by fixed atherosclerotic obstruction in the coronary arteries. **Unstable angina** is unpredictable; it changes in ease of onset, frequency, duration, and intensity. It is probably caused by a combination of atherosclerotic narrowing, vasospasm, and thrombus formation. **Variant angina** occurs while the patient is at rest; it is characterized by specific electrocardiographic changes, and it is caused by vasospasm of a coronary artery reducing blood flow. The type of angina pectoris is diagnosed by a combination of history, electrocardiographic changes during an anginal attack, and exercise tolerance testing, with or without thallium-201 scintigraphy.

TREATMENT OF ANGINA PECTORIS

The goals for the treatment of angina pectoris are to prevent myocardial infarction and death (thereby prolonging life) and to relieve anginal pain symptoms (thereby improving the quality of life). In many cases, coronary angioplasty or coronary artery bypass surgery will be considered first because these treatments have been proven to save lives over time. The choice of therapy often depends on the patient's clinical response to initial medical therapy.

Life Span Considerations

Anginal Attacks

The goal of the treatment of an anginal attack, which most often occurs in older adults, is the relief of pain rather than simply the reduction of pain. If pain is not relieved by nitroglycerin, then the patient should immediately contact the healthcare provider or be seen in the emergency department. Analgesics should not be administered in an attempt to eliminate the patient's pain.

All patients should receive extensive patient education to help them reduce their risks related to CAD. The avoidance of activities that can precipitate attacks (e.g., strenuous exercise, exposure to cold weather, drinking caffeine-containing beverages, cigarette smoking, eating heavy meals, emotional stress) should be attempted. Risk factors (e.g., diabetes mellitus, hypertension, dyslipidemia) must also be treated. A structured exercise program designed for each patient can be successful for weight reduction among overweight patients, and it can also improve cardiovascular health. Healthy muscle tissue requires less oxygen. Medications, in combination with risk reduction and exercise, are effective in preventing ischemic attacks and myocardial infarction.

DRUG THERAPY FOR ANGINA PECTORIS

ACTIONS

The underlying pathophysiology of ischemic heart disease is an imbalance between the oxygen demands of the heart and the ability of coronary arteries to deliver the needed oxygen, the spasticity of the coronary arteries, platelet aggregation, and thrombus formation. The oxygen demand of the heart is determined by the heart rate, contractility, and ventricular volume. Therefore the pharmacologic treatment of angina is aimed at decreasing oxygen demand by decreasing heart rate, myocardial contractility, and ventricular volume without inducing heart failure. Because platelet aggregation, blood flow turbulence, and blood viscosity also play certain roles—especially with unstable angina—platelet inhibitors are also prescribed to prevent anginal attacks (see Chapter 26). Because atherosclerosis causes narrowing and closure of the coronary arteries, inducing angina and myocardial infarction, the use of the 3-hydroxy-3-methylglutaryl coenzyme A (HMG-CoA) reductase inhibitors (i.e., the statins) has also become standard therapy in preventing and treating angina pectoris (see Chapter 21).

USES

Seven groups of drugs may be used to treat angina pectoris: nitrates, beta-adrenergic blockers, angiotensin-converting enzyme (ACE) inhibitors, calcium channel blockers, statins, platelet-active agents, and fatty oxidase enzyme inhibitors. Combination therapy is beneficial for many patients. Beta blockers, calcium channel blockers, statins, long-acting nitrates, and ranolazine can prevent anginal episodes. Risk factor management, healthy lifestyle changes, antiplatelet agents, and ACE inhibitors can prevent disease progression and myocardial infarction or death.

Drug therapy for patients with angina must be individualized. Most patients will be given prescriptions for medication (e.g., nitroglycerin in the form of sublingual tablets or translingual spray) to treat acute attacks and prescriptions for therapy to prevent further ischemia and myocardial infarction (and possible death). Therapy to prevent myocardial infarction consists of statins to lower low-density lipoprotein (LDL) cholesterol level and to reduce inflammation; platelet inhibitors to prevent platelet aggregation and thrombus formation; and ACE inhibitors to help dilate coronary blood vessels and to reduce the potential for thrombus formation.

The most effective agents for relieving ischemia and angina are beta blockers, calcium channel blockers, and nitrates. The drug ranolazine, which is a fatty oxidase enzyme inhibitor, modifies metabolism in the myocardial cells to reduce the oxygen demand of the contracting heart muscles, thereby reducing symptoms of angina.

Deciding which medicine to use depends on other conditions that the patient may have and the expected adverse effects of therapy. Aspirin, clopidogrel, or ticlopidine (see Chapter 26), which are platelet-active agents, may also be considered to slow platelet aggregation. Many patients will have revascularization procedures (e.g., stent placement, coronary artery bypass grafting) to restore blood flow and to reduce symptomatology. Even after revascularization, patients will still require antianginal drug therapy.

❖ NURSING IMPLICATIONS FOR ANGINAL THERAPY

■ Assessment

History of Anginal Attacks. Ask the patient specific questions to identify the onset, duration, and intensity of the pain. Ask the patient to describe the chest sensation and the pattern of occurrence (e.g., under the sternum; in the jaw, neck, and shoulder; radiation down the left arm, the right arm, or both; into the wrist, hand, and fingers). What activities precipitate an attack? Does the pain occur with or without exertion? Is the pain relieved by rest? Does the chest pain occur shortly after eating? Does the individual experience fatigue, shortness of breath, indigestion, or nausea in relation to the anginal attack? Work with the patient to plan interventions that will minimize the factors that trigger attacks. Mutually establish goals with the patient to alter risk factors that are modifiable.

Medication History

- What medications—both prescription and nonprescription—are being taken?
- Does the patient take any herbal or dietary supplements?
- What medications are being used for the treatment of the angina?
- What effect does taking nitroglycerin have on the anginal pain? How many nitroglycerin tablets are required for the patient to obtain pain relief during an attack? How many nitroglycerin tablets are being taken daily? How old is the nitroglycerin that is being used sublingually? Is it stored properly?
- Have the prescribed medications been taken regularly? If not, determine the reasons for the patient's nonadherence. Analyze nonadherence issues, and plan interventions with the patient. Plan to review drug administration, as needed.

Central Nervous System

- *Mental status:* Determine the individual's level of consciousness and clarity of thought. Check for orientation to date, time, and place, as well as level of confusion, restlessness, or irritability. Ask the patient whether he or she has noticed any changes in memory or level of awareness; these factors are indicators of cerebral perfusion.
- *Syncope:* Ask the patient to describe the conditions surrounding any episodes of syncope. Record the degree of presenting symptoms, such as general mental weakness, inability to stand upright, feeling faint, or loss of consciousness. Record what activities, if any, bring on these episodes.
- *Anxiety:* What degree of apprehension is present? Did a stressful event precipitate the attack? Plan for stress reduction education and a discussion of effective means of coping with stressful events.

Cardiovascular System

- *Palpitations:* Record the patient's description of palpitations, such as "my heart skips some beats" or "it began to feel as if it were racing." Ask if these conditions are preceded by mild or strenuous exercise and how long the palpitations last.
- *Heart rate:* Count and record the rate, rhythm, and quality of the pulse.
- *Blood pressure:* Record the blood pressure. It may be increased or decreased during an attack. Compare with previous baseline readings.
- *Respirations:* The patient may be dyspneic. Ask whether the attack occurred while the patient was at rest or during exertion.
- *Cardiovascular history:* What concurrent cardiovascular disease does the patient have (e.g., hypertension, dyslipidemia)?

- *Peripheral perfusion:* Determine the patient's peripheral perfusion by checking the pedal pulses in the lower extremities and the skin color and temperature. Note any loss of hair on the lower legs, which denotes decreased circulation.
- *Smoking:* Does the patient smoke? How much? Does the patient understand the effects of smoking on the cardiovascular system?
- Ask what, if any, activities of daily living (ADLs) have been altered to cope with the patient's symptoms.

Nutritional History

- *Diet*: Is the patient on a special diet (e.g., low-sodium diet, low-fat diet)? Is the patient being treated for high cholesterol? Does eating cause fatigue or shortness of breath?
- *Fluids*: Does the patient have any edema, especially in the ankles? Examine the dietary history to establish whether a referral to a nutritionist would benefit the individual's understanding of the diet regimen.

■ Implementation

Obtain the patient's vital signs, and include an assessment of the individual's pain rating.

- Adequate tissue perfusion is essential. Instruct the patient to take measures to avoid fatigue and cold weather, which can cause vasoconstriction, and provide for the patient's personal safety when symptoms of hypoxia are present (e.g., lightheadedness, dyspnea, chest pain).
- When pain is present, comfort measures and prescribed pain medications must be implemented to allow the individual to decrease the pain. Fatigue may increase the perception of pain; spacing activities so that fatigue does not occur is recommended. Administer oxygen as prescribed, and check the patient's oxygen saturation.
- For information about medication administration, see the individual drug monographs.

■ Patient Education

Medications

- Teach the patient about the signs and symptoms of hypotension, which may occur when nitrates are taken. Weakness, dizziness, or faintness can usually be relieved by increasing muscular activity (i.e., alternating flexing and relaxing the muscles in the legs) or by sitting or lying down. Resting for 10 to 15 minutes after taking medication may also assist the patient with the management of hypotension. Because lightheadedness or fainting is a possibility when taking nitroglycerin, safety measures to prevent injury from transient orthostatic hypotension must be stressed.
- Explain that a headache may occur with the use of nitroglycerin, but that it should subside within 20 to 30 minutes.

- Teach specific administration techniques to the patient for the type of medication prescribed (e.g., sublingual or transmucosal tablets, translingual spray, topical ointment, transdermal patches). Refer to Chapter 7, Figures 7-2, 7-3, and 7-4 for further description of percutaneous administration of nitroglycerin.

Lifestyle Modifications. Lifestyle modifications are essential for many individuals with angina. Teach the patient about appropriate behavioral changes, such as stress management (e.g., relaxation techniques, meditation, three-part breathing).

- The patient must resume ADLs within the boundaries set by the healthcare provider. Encourage activities such as regular moderate exercise, meal preparation, the resumption of usual sexual activity, and social interactions.
- Individuals who are unable to attain the degree of activity hoped for through drug therapy may become frustrated. Allow for the verbalization of feelings, and then implement actions that are appropriate to the circumstances.
- Participation in regular exercise is essential. Follow the guidelines of the American Heart Association regarding an exercise program. Increase the patient's exercise demands gradually, and monitor the effects on his or her cardiovascular system. Changes in the level of exercise may require participation in a supervised program (e.g., cardiac rehabilitation). Tell the patient to avoid overexertion. Anginal pain may occur with exercise, and taking nitroglycerin before exercise or before performing certain activities may be recommended. Instruct the patient to always stop exercising or performing any activity when chest pain is present.
- Discuss the need for smoking cessation, and make referrals to available self-help programs in the area. Smoking causes vasoconstriction; encourage a drastic reduction in smoking and preferably complete elimination of smoking. Encourage the patient to set a date to stop smoking.
- Dietary modifications aimed at decreasing the cholesterol level and a reducing program to maintain the ideal weight are usually prescribed by the physician. Depending on coexisting conditions, other dietary modifications (e.g., a low-sodium diet) may be suggested. Discourage the use of caffeine-containing products, because they may precipitate an anginal attack when they are taken in excess.
- If hypertension accompanies the angina, stress the importance of following prescribed dietary and medicinal regimens to control the disease.
- Instruct the patient not to ingest alcohol while receiving nitroglycerin therapy. Alcohol causes vasodilation, which potentially results in postural hypotension.
- Teach the patient about the proper storage of medication (especially sublingual nitroglycerin) in a dark, airtight container. Show the patient the medication's expiration date, and stress the importance of having the prescription refilled before the expiration date.
- Always report poor pain control to the healthcare provider.

Fostering Health Maintenance

- Throughout the course of treatment, discuss medication information and how it will benefit the patient.
- Drug therapy is essential to maintain the adequate oxygenation of the myocardial cells and body tissues. Although medications can control the anginal attacks, lifestyle changes to deal with the management of precipitating factors must also occur.
- Provide the patient and his or her significant others with the important information contained in the specific drug monographs for the drugs prescribed. Additional health teaching and nursing interventions for common and serious adverse effects are described in the drug monographs later in this chapter.
- Seek cooperation and understanding with regard to the following points so that medication adherence is increased: the name of the medication; its dosage, route, and times of administration; and its common and serious adverse effects.

Patient Self-Assessment. Enlist the patient's help with developing and maintaining a written record of monitoring parameters (e.g., blood pressure, pulse, degree of pain relief, exercise tolerance, adverse effects experienced). See the Patient Self-Assessment Form for Cardiovascular Agents on the Evolve website. Complete the Premedication Data column for use as a baseline to track the patient's response to drug therapy. Ensure that the patient understands how to use the form, and instruct the patient to bring the completed form to follow-up visits. During follow-up visits, focus on issues that will foster the patient's adherence with the therapeutic interventions prescribed.

DRUG CLASS: NITRATES
ACTIONS

The nitrates are the oldest effective therapy for angina pectoris. Although they have also been called *coronary vasodilators*, these agents do not increase total coronary blood flow. First, nitrates relieve angina pectoris by inducing the relaxation of the peripheral vascular smooth muscles, which results in the dilation of the arteries and veins. This reduces venous blood return (i.e., reduced preload) to the heart, which in turn leads to decreased oxygen demands on the heart. Second, nitrates increase the myocardial oxygen supply by dilating the large coronary arteries and redistributing blood flow, thereby enhancing oxygen supply to ischemic areas.

USES

Nitroglycerin is the drug of choice for the treatment of angina pectoris. It is available in different dosages so that it can be adjusted to patient needs. Sublingual tablets dissolve quite rapidly and are used primarily for acute attacks of angina. The sustained-release tablets and capsules, ointments, and transdermal patches are used prophylactically to prevent anginal attacks. All long-acting nitrates, including isosorbide dinitrate and mononitrate, appear to be equally effective when a sufficient nitrate-free interval (as discussed later in this chapter) is incorporated into the medicine regimen. The translingual spray may be used for both the prophylaxis and acute treatment of anginal attacks.

Amyl nitrite is a volatile liquid available in small glass ampules encased in a loosely woven material so that they can be crushed easily under the patient's nostrils for inhalation. The onset of action is less than 1 minute, but the duration is about 10 minutes.

Continued use of transdermal nitroglycerin patches and frequent doses of oral nitrates and sustained-release nitrates causes tolerance and the loss of the antianginal response to develop. The best way to avoid tolerance is to have periodic 8- to 12-hour nitrate-free periods. Depending on the type of angina, patients will be told when not to use nitrates (e.g., bedtime), unless they have an acute attack. When used with beta blockers or calcium antagonists, nitrates produce greater antianginal and antiischemic effects than when they are used alone. These agents also help provide prophylaxis against attacks during nitrate-free periods.

THERAPEUTIC OUTCOMES

The primary therapeutic outcomes from nitrate therapy are as follows:
1. Relief of anginal pain during an attack
2. Reduced frequency and severity of anginal attacks
3. Increased tolerance of activities

❖ NURSING IMPLICATIONS FOR NITRATES

▪ Premedication Assessment
1. Assess the level, location, duration, intensity, and pattern of the patient's pain.
2. Ask the patient when the last dose of nitrates was taken and what degree of relief was obtained.

▪ Availability, Dosage, and Administration
See Table 24-1.

Sublingual Administration
1. Instruct the patient to sit or lie down at the first sign of an oncoming anginal attack.
2. Instruct the patient to place a tablet under the tongue and allow it to dissolve; encourage the patient not to swallow the saliva immediately.

3. The American Heart Association (O'Gara, 2013) recommends that if chest pain is not relieved with one sublingual nitroglycerin tablet within 5 minutes, the patient should seek emergency medical attention (i.e., call 911). While waiting for emergency care, the patient can take one more tablet and then take a third tablet 5 minutes later if the pain is not relieved.
4. One or two tablets may be taken prophylactically a few minutes before engaging in activities that may trigger an anginal attack.
5. Chart the patient's ability to place the sublingual medication under the tongue correctly.

Medication Deterioration. Every 6 months, the nitroglycerin prescription should be refilled and the old tablets safely discarded. (Be sure that the patient knows how to read the expiration date and have the prescription refilled.)

Medication Storage. Store nitroglycerin in its original dark-colored glass container with a tight lid.

Medication Accessibility. Nonhospitalized patients should carry nitroglycerin at all times, but not in a pocket directly next to the body, because heat hastens the deterioration of the medication. When taken, the drug should produce a slight stinging or burning sensation, which usually indicates that it is still potent.

Allow the hospitalized patient to keep the nitroglycerin at the bedside or on his or her person, if ambulatory. Check the hospital policy to see if a fresh supply of medicine should be issued rather than using the agents that the patient brought from home. (Remember that the nurse is still responsible for gathering and charting relevant data regarding all medication taken by the patient when the medication is left at the bedside.)

Sustained-Release Tablet Administration. Sustained-release nitroglycerin is usually taken on an empty stomach every 8 to 12 hours. If gastritis develops, the sustained-release tablet may be taken with food.

Translingual Spray Administration. Patients should familiarize themselves with the position of the spray orifice, which can be identified by the finger rest on top of the valve. This can be particularly helpful for administration at night. The spray is highly flammable. Instruct the patient not to use the spray where it may be ignited.
1. At the time of administration, the patient should preferably be in a sitting position.
2. The canister should be held vertically, with the valve head uppermost and the spray orifice as close to the mouth as possible. Do not shake the container, because any bubbles formed may slow the release of nitroglycerin.
3. The dose should be sprayed onto or under the tongue by pressing the button firmly.
4. The patient's mouth should be closed immediately after each dose. The spray should not be swallowed or inhaled.

Table 24-1   Nitrates

GENERIC NAME	BRAND NAME	AVAILABILITY	ONSET	DURATION	DOSAGE RANGE
amyl nitrite	—	Inhalation: 0.3-mL ampules in a woven sack for crushing	0.5 min	3-5 min	Inhalation: One ampule crushed in its sack and placed under the patient's nostrils for inhalation at time of acute attack
isosorbide dinitrate ⇄ Do not confuse isosorbide dinitrate with isosorbide mononitrate.	Isordil ⇄ Do not confuse Isordil with Ismo.	Tablets, sublingual: 2.5 mg	2-3 min	1-3 hr	Sublingual: 2.5-10 mg for acute attack
		Tablets, oral: 5, 10, 20, 30, 40 mg	30-60 min	4-6 hr	PO: 2.5-40 mg two to four times daily on empty stomach
		Tablets and capsules, sustained release: 40 mg	30-60 min	6-8 hr	PO: 20-40 mg q6-8h or 80 mg q8-12h; maximum is 160 mg/day
isosorbide mononitrate ⇄ Do not confuse isosorbide mononitrate with isosorbide dinitrate.	Monoket ⇄ Do not confuse Monoket with Monopril.	Tablets, oral: 10, 20 mg	30-60 min	N/A	PO: 20 mg twice daily, 7 hr apart
	Imdur ⇄ Do not confuse Imdur with Imuran, Inderal, or K-Dur.	Tablets, sustained release (24 hr): 30, 60, 120 mg	3-4 hr	8-12 hr	PO: 30-240 mg once daily; do not crush or chew tablets
nitroglycerin ⇄ Do not confuse nitroglycerin with glycerin.	Nitrostat	Tablets, sublingual: 0.3, 0.4, 0.6 mg	1-2 min	>30 min	Sublingual: 0.3-0.6 mg for prophylactic use before activity that may induce angina pectoris or at time of acute attack
		Capsules, oral, sustained release: 2.5, 6.5, 9 mg	30-45 min	3-8 hr	PO: 2.5-9 mg two to four times daily for prophylaxis
	Nitro-Bid	Ointment: 2%	30 min	3 hr	Topical: 0.5-2 inches of ointment using special applicator q6h for two doses, then no dose for twelve hours, followed by two doses for 6 hours each.
	Nitro-Dur	Patch, transmucosal: 0.1, 0.2, 0.3, 0.4, 0.6, 0.8 mg/hr	30-60 min	Less than 24 hr	Topical: One patch applied for 12 hr; patient should wait 12 hr after removing old patch before applying new patch
	Nitrolingual	Spray, translingual metered: 0.4 mg	2 min	30-60 min	Spray: One or two sprays onto or under tongue for acute attack; repeat if needed in 3-5 min; may be used prophylactically 5-10 min before exercise
	Nitroglycerin IV ⓘ	IV: 5 mg/mL in 10-mL vials; 100, 200, 400 mcg in 5% dextrose 250 and 500 mL	1-2 min	3-5 min	IV: Initially, 5 mcg/min through an infusion pump; adjust dosage as needed

ⓘ High-alert medication.

! Medication Safety Alert

The American Heart Association (O'Gara, 2013) now recommends that if chest pain is not relieved by one sublingual nitroglycerin dose within 5 minutes, the patient should seek emergency medical attention (i.e., call 911).

Topical Ointment Administration. See Chapter 7, Figure 7-3. Nitroglycerin ointment is usually applied on arising in the morning; 6 hours later, the first dose is removed and a second dose is applied. The second dose of the ointment is removed after 6 hours, giving a nitrate-free period of 10 to 12 hours until the next morning.

1. Apply clean gloves before administering the ointment to prevent absorbing the drug through your skin.
2. Position the dose-measuring applicator paper with the printed side down.
3. Squeeze the proper amount (usually 1 to 2 inches) of ointment onto the applicator paper.
4. Place the measuring applicator on the skin, ointment-side down, and spread the ointment in a thin, uniform layer. Do not massage the ointment or rub it in. Any area without hair may be used; however, many people prefer the chest, the flank, or the upper arm. The lower extremities are not used, especially if there is reduced peripheral perfusion. (Because of the potential for skin irritation, do not shave an area to apply the medication; instead use scissors to clip hair if needed.)
5. Help the patient to develop a site rotation schedule to prevent skin irritation. Tell the patient not to apply the ointment to an area that still shows signs of irritation. Use of the applicator allows measuring of the proper dose and prevents absorption through the fingertips.
6. Cover the area where the patch is placed with a clear plastic wrap, and then tape the plastic wrap in place. (Alert the patient that the medication may discolor clothing.)
7. Perform hand hygiene before applying and after removing gloves.
8. Close the tube tightly, and store it in a cool place.
9. When terminating the use of the topical ointment, gradually reduce the dose and frequency of application over the course of 4 to 6 weeks.
10. When removing the ointment paper, apply clean gloves, wipe the area with tissue to remove the ointment, and then reapply the ointment to a different area at the appropriate time interval for rotating sites.

Transdermal Patch Administration. See Chapter 7, Figure 7-4. The transdermal patch provides a controlled release of nitroglycerin through a semipermeable membrane for 24 hours when it is applied to intact skin. The dosage released depends on the surface area of the patch. The therapeutic effect can be observed about 30 minutes after attachment, and it continues for about 30 minutes after removal. Current recommendations are to apply the patch and leave it in place for 12 to 14 hours, followed by a 10- to 12-hour patch-free (nitrate-free) interval. The patch is then reapplied for another 12 to 14 hours.

1. Apply clean gloves.
2. The patch should be applied to a clean, dry, hairless area of skin. Do not apply the patch to shaved areas, because skin irritation may alter drug absorption. If hair is likely to interfere with patch adhesion or removal, then trim the hair but do not shave it. Optimal locations for patch placement are the upper chest or side; the pelvis; and the inner, upper arm. Avoid scars, skinfolds, and wounds. Rotate the skin sites daily. (Help the patient develop a rotation chart.)
3. Perform hand hygiene before applying and after removing gloves.
4. See individual product information to determine whether the patient's patch can be worn while swimming, bathing, or showering.
5. If the patch becomes partially dislodged, discard it and replace it with a new patch.
6. Sublingual nitroglycerin may be necessary for anginal attacks, especially while the dosage is being adjusted.
7. Dispose of used patches in a place that is out of reach of children. Discarded patches still contain enough of the active ingredient to be dangerous to children.

Intravenous Nitroglycerin Administration. Intravenous nitroglycerin is used in an acute inpatient setting (e.g., intensive care unit, cardiac telemetry unit), and it requires continuous monitoring of vital signs (i.e., blood pressure, pulse, respirations, oxygen saturation levels, and central venous pressure).

An infusion pump must be used to monitor the precise delivery of the infusion. The dose is titrated to achieve the desired clinical response. Gradual weaning is needed under controlled conditions to prevent a rebound action.

This medication is never mixed with other medications and is administered only with intravenous administration sets known as "nitro tubing," which are made specifically for use with nitroglycerin. Most other plastic administration sets absorb the drug. See the manufacturer's literature for exact directions for preparation and administration of the drug.

■ Common Adverse Effects

Cardiovascular

Excessive hypotension. Excessive hypotension is an extension of the nitrate's pharmacologic activity. Other possible adverse effects include dizziness, nausea, flushing, and, rarely, syncope. Report these adverse effects so that a more appropriate dosage adjustment may be made.

Neurologic

Prolonged headache. The most common adverse effect of nitrate therapy is headache. This can range from a mild sensation of fullness in the head to an intense and severe generalized headache. Most patients develop a tolerance within a few weeks of starting therapy. Analgesics (e.g., acetaminophen) may be used, if needed. Report these adverse effects so that a more appropriate dosage adjustment may be made.

Tolerance (Increasing Dosage to Attain Relief). Tolerance to the nitrate dosages can develop rapidly, particularly if large doses are administered frequently. Tolerance can appear within a few days, and it may be well established within a few weeks. The smallest dose needed to obtain satisfactory results should be used to minimize the development of tolerance. Tolerance is broken by withdrawing the drug for a short period of time.

■ Drug Interactions

Alcohol. Alcohol accentuates the vasodilation and postural hypotension caused by the nitrates. Patients should be warned that drinking alcohol while taking nitrates may cause hypotension.

Calcium Channel Blockers and Beta-Adrenergic Blockers. Calcium channel blockers and beta-adrenergic blockers may significantly lower blood pressure. Dosage adjustments may be necessary.

Avanafil, Sildenafil, Tadalafil, and Vardenafil. The concurrent use of nitrates and these agents used for erectile dysfunction is contraindicated. These agents potentiate the vasodilatory effects of the nitrates, which results in a significant drop in blood pressure that may be fatal.

DRUG CLASS: BETA-ADRENERGIC BLOCKERS

ACTIONS

The beta-adrenergic blockers (i.e., beta blockers) (see Table 12-3) reduce myocardial oxygen demand by blocking the beta-adrenergic receptors in the heart, thereby preventing stimulation from norepinephrine and epinephrine that would normally cause an increased heart rate. Beta blockers also reduce blood pressure (see Chapter 22).

USES

The goals of beta-blocker therapy are to reduce the number of anginal attacks, reduce nitroglycerin use, and improve exercise tolerance while minimizing adverse effects. It is recommended that a patient who is admitted to the hospital with an acute myocardial infarction receive a beta blocker on arrival and be prescribed a beta blocker on discharge.

All beta blockers are effective for the treatment of angina pectoris, so product selection should be based on other conditions that the patient may have (e.g., diabetes, chronic obstructive airway disease, peripheral vascular disease) and adherence issues. The cardioselective agents (see Chapter 12) will have less effect on the beta-2 receptors of the lungs and the peripheral vasculature, thereby minimizing the adverse effects involving these body systems. Atenolol, betaxolol, and metoprolol are examples of beta blockers that can be administered once daily to minimize anginal attacks if adherence is a problem.

Dosages of beta blockers needed to control angina are extremely patient specific; therefore therapy should start at low doses and be increased, depending on the patient's needs. Optimally, exercise stress tests should be used to determine the most appropriate dosage. Combination therapy with nitrates and beta blockers appears to be more effective than nitrates or beta blockers alone. Beta blockers may also be combined with calcium channel blockers (e.g., verapamil, diltiazem) or with long-acting dihydropyridines (see the discussion of these drugs later in this chapter).

THERAPEUTIC OUTCOMES

The primary therapeutic outcomes expected from beta-blocker therapy are as follows:
1. Decreased frequency and severity of anginal attacks
2. Increased tolerance of activities
3. Reduced use of nitroglycerin for acute anginal attacks

❖ NURSING IMPLICATIONS FOR BETA-ADRENERGIC BLOCKERS

■ Premedication Assessment

1. Obtain baseline blood pressure readings with the patient in both the supine and standing positions; assess the pulse rate.
2. Check the patient's history for respiratory disorders such as bronchospasm, chronic bronchitis, emphysema, and asthma.
3. Check the patient for a history of diabetes. If diabetes is present, determine the patient's baseline serum glucose level before starting therapy.
4. See Chapter 12 for further discussion of patient education and the nursing process associated with beta-adrenergic inhibition.

DRUG CLASS: CALCIUM CHANNEL BLOCKERS

ACTIONS

These agents are known variously as *calcium antagonists, calcium ion antagonists, slow channel blockers,* and *calcium ion influx inhibitors.* Regardless of what they are called, they all share the ability to inhibit the movement of calcium ions across a cell membrane.

Calcium channel blockers (Table 24-2) may be used to treat angina pectoris by decreasing myocardial oxygen demand (i.e., decreasing workload) and increasing myocardial blood supply by dilating the coronary arteries. By inhibiting smooth muscle contraction, calcium channel blockers dilate blood vessels and decrease their resistance to blood flow. The dilation of the peripheral vessels reduces the workload of the heart. Coronary artery dilation improves coronary blood flow.

USES

Although each of these agents acts by calcium ion inhibition, there are significant differences in clinical use. Their clinical effects also depend on the type and severity of the patient's disease. The primary calcium channel blockers used to treat angina are the long-acting dihydropyridines (e.g., amlodipine, felodipine,

nifedipine), as well as diltiazem (benzothiazepine) and verapamil (diphenylalkylamine). The overall effect of calcium channel blockers will be the combined effects of vasodilator and myocardial actions with reflex-mediated adrenergic activity. Nifedipine, a potent peripheral arterial vasodilator, reduces peripheral vascular resistance; this may cause a reflex tachycardia. Verapamil and diltiazem also have myocardial depressant effects that prevent tachycardia. However, they must be used with extreme caution in patients who may be developing heart failure.

THERAPEUTIC OUTCOMES

The primary therapeutic outcomes expected from the calcium channel blockers are as follows:
1. Decreased frequency and severity of anginal attacks
2. Increased tolerance of activities

Table 24-2   Calcium Channel Blockers Used to Treat Angina Pectoris

GENERIC NAME	BRAND NAME	AVAILABILITY	DOSAGE RANGE
amlodipine ⇄ Do not confuse amlodipine with amiloride or amiodarone.	Norvasc ⇄ Do not confuse Norvasc with Navane, Altace, Nolvadex, Norflex, or Vasotec.	Tablets: 2.5, 5, 10 mg	PO: Initial: 5 mg once daily; adjust over 7-14 days to maximum of 10 mg/day
diltiazem	Cardizem ⇄ Do not confuse Cardizem with Cardene or Clonidine.	Tablets: 30, 60, 90, 120 mg	PO: Initial: 30 mg four times daily, gradually increase to 180-360 mg in three or four divided doses
	Cardizem LA, Dilacor XR, Cardizem CD,	Tablets, sustained release (24 hr), and capsules (24 hr): 120, 180, 240, 300, 360, 420 mg	PO: Initial: 120-180 mg sustained-release capsule once daily; adjust as needed after 14 days Maintenance: 240-480 mg daily
nicardipine	Cardene ⇄ Do not confuse Cardene with Cardizem, Cardura, or codeine.	Capsules: 20, 30 mg	PO: Initial: 20 mg three times daily Maximal response may require 2 wk of therapy Allow at least 3 days between dosage adjustments Maintenance: 20-40 mg three times daily
		Capsules, sustained release (12 hr): 30, 45, 60 mg	PO: Initial: 30 mg twice daily Maintenance: 30-60 mg twice daily
nifedipine	Procardia, Adalat ⇄ Do not confuse Procardia with Provera or Peri-Colace.	Capsules: 10, 20 mg	PO: Initial: 10 mg three times daily; adjust over 7-14 days to balance antianginal and hypotensive activity Maintenance: 10-20 mg three times daily
		Tablets, sustained release (24 hr): 30, 60, 90 mg	Sustained-release tablets: 30-60 mg once daily Maximum: capsules, 180 mg daily; sustained-release tablets, 120 mg daily
verapamil ⇄ Do not confuse verapamil with Verelan.	Calan, ⇄ Do not confuse Calan with Colace.	Tablets: 40, 80, 120 mg	PO: Initial, immediate release: 40-120 mg three times daily
	Calan SR Covera-HS Isoptin SR	Tablets and capsules, sustained release (24 hr): 100, 120, 180, 200, 240, 300, 360 mg	PO: Initial: 180 mg once daily at bedtime Maintenance: 120-480 mg daily Administer with food

❖ NURSING IMPLICATIONS FOR CALCIUM CHANNEL BLOCKERS

▪ Premedication Assessment

1. Obtain baseline blood pressure readings with the patient in both the supine and standing positions.
2. Check the patient for a history of heart failure; withhold the drug and consult the prescriber if heart failure is present.
3. Check the patient's laboratory values for hepatotoxicity.

▪ Availability, Dosage, and Administration

See Table 24-2. See Chapter 22 for a further discussion of patient education and the nursing process associated with calcium channel blocker therapy.

DRUG CLASS: ANGIOTENSIN-CONVERTING ENZYME INHIBITORS

ACTIONS

Angiotensin-converting enzyme inhibitors represent a major breakthrough in the treatment of cardiovascular disease. Their action is more completely described on pp. 346–349. By inhibiting the angiotensin-converting enzyme, these drugs have significant actions on the endothelial walls of coronary arteries; they promote vasodilation and minimize platelet cell aggregation, thereby preventing thrombus formation.

USES

ACE inhibitors have been proven to reduce the incidence of myocardial infarction, and they should be used as routine secondary prevention for patients with known coronary artery disease, particularly for patients with diabetes mellitus without renal failure. ACE inhibitors are recommended for the treatment of patients with an acute myocardial infarction or heart failure with left ventricular systolic dysfunction.

THERAPEUTIC OUTCOME

The primary therapeutic outcome expected from the ACE inhibitors is a reduction in the frequency of recurrent myocardial infarction.

❖ NURSING IMPLICATIONS FOR ANGIOTENSIN-CONVERTING ENZYME INHIBITORS

▪ Premedication Assessment

1. Obtain baseline blood pressure readings with the patient in both the supine and standing positions; assess the apical pulse.
2. Obtain a history of the patient's bowel elimination patterns.
3. Initiate laboratory studies as requested by the physician (e.g., electrocardiography; renal function tests such as blood urea nitrogen [BUN], serum creatinine, and electrolyte levels; and complete blood count [CBC] to serve as a baseline for future comparison).
4. Ask if the patient has a persistent cough.

▪ Availability, Dosage, and Administration

See Table 22-5 and Chapter 22 for further discussion of patient education and the nursing process associated with ACE inhibitor therapy.

 Medication Safety Alert

The initial doses of ACE inhibitors may cause hypotension with dizziness, tachycardia, and fainting; these adverse effects occur more commonly in patients who are also receiving diuretics. Symptoms occur within 3 hours after the first several doses. This effect may be minimized by discontinuing the diuretic 1 week before initiating ACE inhibitor therapy. Patients should be warned that this adverse effect may occur, that it is transient, and that they should lie down immediately if symptoms develop.

DRUG CLASS: FATTY OXIDASE ENZYME INHIBITOR

ranolazine (răn-Ō-lă-zēn)
Ranexa (răn-ĔKS-ă)

ACTIONS

Ranolazine, a fatty oxidase inhibitor, is an enzyme modulator. Its exact mechanism of action is unknown, but it shifts the metabolism in myocardial cells to reduce the oxygen required to generate energy for muscle contractions. As the demand for oxygen is reduced, the imbalance between the oxygen supply and demand diminishes, thereby reducing myocardial ischemia and angina symptoms.

USES

Ranolazine is the first new agent in more than 20 years to be used to treat chronic stable angina. It is used in combination with a dihydropyridine calcium channel blocker (e.g., amlodipine), beta blockers, and nitrates. Unlike other antianginal medicines, ranolazine does not affect the blood pressure or heart rate. Because ranolazine prolongs the QT interval (i.e., a potentially life-threatening event), it should only be used to treat angina in patients who have not achieved an antianginal response with other agents or in those who cannot tolerate the adverse effects of the other medicines. Ranolazine will not reduce the symptoms of an acute anginal episode.

THERAPEUTIC OUTCOMES

The primary therapeutic outcomes expected from ranolazine therapy are as follows:
1. Reduced frequency and severity of anginal attacks
2. Increased tolerance of activities

3. Reduced use of nitroglycerin during acute anginal attacks

❖ NURSING IMPLICATIONS FOR RANOLAZINE

■ Premedication Assessment

Initiate laboratory studies as requested by the healthcare provider (e.g., electrocardiography; renal function tests such as blood urea nitrogen [BUN], serum creatinine, and electrolyte levels; and complete blood count [CBC]) to serve as a baseline for future comparison.

■ Availability

PO: 500- and 1000-mg extended-release (12-hr) tablets.

 Medication Safety Alert

It is recommended that ranolazine **not** be taken concurrently with other medicines that are known to prolong the QT interval, such as quinidine, dofetilide, sotalol, erythromycin, and antipsychotics (e.g., thioridazine, ziprasidone). Baseline and follow-up electrocardiograms (ECGs) should be obtained to evaluate the effects of these drugs on the patient's QT interval.

■ Dosage and Administration

Dosage is 500 mg twice daily; may be increased to 1000 mg twice daily. Ranolazine may be taken with or without food. Tablets should be swallowed whole: *do not* crush, break, or chew tablets.

■ Common Adverse Effects

Neurologic

Dizziness and headache. These adverse effects are usually mild, occurring in fewer than 5% of patients. Patients should not operate an automobile or machinery or engage in activities that require mental alertness until it is known how they will react to the medicine. Patients should withhold medicine and contact their healthcare providers if they experience palpitations or fainting spells while taking ranolazine.

Gastrointestinal

Constipation, nausea. These adverse effects are usually mild, occurring in fewer than 6% of patients.

■ Drug Interactions

Drugs That Enhance Therapeutic and Toxic Effects. Azole-type antifungals (e.g., ketoconazole, fluconazole), macrolide antibiotics (e.g., erythromycin, clarithromycin), grapefruit juice, verapamil, diltiazem, and protease inhibitors (e.g., ritonavir) significantly increase the serum levels and potential toxicity of ranolazine. In general, these agents should not be used concurrently with ranolazine. If they are used concurrently, monitor patients closely for the development of dizziness, nausea, weakness, loss of muscle strength, constipation, and headache.

Ranolazine inhibits the metabolism of HMG CoA inhibitors (statins), tacrolimus, and sirolimus. Reduce the dosage of these agents per manufacturers' recommendations.

Get Ready for the NCLEX® Examination!

Key Points

- Coronary heart disease is the leading cause of disability, socioeconomic loss, and death in the United States.
- Angina pectoris is the first clinical indication of underlying CAD in many patients.
- The frequency of anginal attacks can be reduced by controlling risk factors and avoiding precipitating causes (e.g., stress).
- Medicines such as nitrates, beta blockers, ACE inhibitors, statins, platelet inhibitors, and calcium channel blockers can help to control symptoms.
- Nurses can play a significant role in public education efforts, monitoring for noncompliance, monitoring patients' responses to therapy, and encouraging patients to make changes in their lifestyles to reduce the severity of angina pectoris.

Additional Learning Resources

SG Go to your Study Guide for additional Review Questions for the NCLEX® Examination, Critical Thinking Clinical Situations, and other learning activities to help you master this chapter content.

evolve Go to your Evolve website (http://evolve.elsevier.com/Clayton) for additional online resources.

Review Questions for the NCLEX® Examination

1. The nurse is teaching a 73-year-old female patient about precipitating factors of angina and recognizes that further teaching is needed from the following statement by the patient:
   1. "I now know that it is okay for me to be intimate with my husband."
   2. "I understand that I need to rest for 1 to 2 hours after every meal."
   3. "I should avoid being outside when it gets really cold."
   4. "I will cut back on my coffee intake, but I can still have regular Coke."
2. A nurse was caring for a 65-year-old male patient who was diagnosed with chronic stable angina and knows that the difference between chronic stable angina and unstable angina is:
   1. unstable angina is easily treated with rest.
   2. chronic stable angina occurs at unpredictable times.
   3. unstable angina is treated with nitrates.
   4. chronic stable angina lasts for more than 30 minutes.

3. The nurse is preparing to administer a calcium channel blocker to a patient with angina and will assess for the following. *(Select all that apply.)*
   1. Frequent cough
   2. Laboratory values for nephrotoxicity
   3. Baseline supine and standing blood pressure
   4. Laboratory values for hepatotoxicity
   5. History of heart failure
4. After the administration of a nitrate to a patient with angina, the nurse explained to the patient the following effects may be experienced. *(Select all that apply.)*
   1. Chronic cough
   2. Earache
   3. Hypotension
   4. Prolonged palpitations
   5. Headache
5. For the patient experiencing angina and ischemia, the most effective agents for relieving these conditions are: *(Select all that apply.)*
   1. calcium channel blockers.
   2. platelet active agents.
   3. nitrates.
   4. beta blockers.
   5. HMG-CoA reductase inhibitors.

6. The nurse was discussing risk factor management with a 58-year-old male patient who was admitted with chest pain and realized that the patient needed further education after stating the following:
   1. "I know that I should quit smoking, I have been meaning to for a while, but this really hits home that I need to."
   2. "I think maybe I should learn to cook because my wife always insists on meat and potatoes and gravy; we have such heavy meals."
   3. "I walk every day with my dog for at least 20 minutes and longer in nice weather."
   4. "I figure I don't need to do anything different; I can just take my pills for this."

Drugs Used to Treat Peripheral Vascular Disease

Objectives

1. Describe the baseline assessments needed to evaluate a patient with peripheral vascular disease.
2. Identify specific measures that the patient can use to improve peripheral circulation and prevent the complications of peripheral vascular disease.
3. Identify the systemic effects to expect when peripheral vasodilating agents are administered.
4. Explain why hypotension and tachycardia occur frequently with the use of peripheral vasodilators.
5. Cite both pharmacologic and nonpharmacologic goals of the treatment for peripheral vascular disease.

Key Terms

peripheral arterial disease (PAD) (p. 391)
arteriosclerosis obliterans (ăr-tē-rē-ō-sklĕ-RŌ-sĭs ŏ-BLĬ-tĕr-ănz) (p. 391)
intermittent claudication (ĭn-tĕr-MĬT-ĕnt klaw-dĭ-KĀ-shŭn) (p. 391)

paresthesias (păr-ĕs-THĒ-zē-ăz) (p. 391)
Raynaud's disease (rā-NŌZ) (p. 391)
vasospasm (VĂ-zō-spă-zĭm) (p. 392)

PERIPHERAL VASCULAR DISEASE

The term *peripheral vascular disease* can be applied to a variety of illnesses associated with blood vessels outside the heart, but it generally refers to diseases of the blood vessels of the arms and legs (the extremities). These illnesses can be subdivided into two types based on arterial or venous origin: (1) peripheral arterial disease (PAD); and (2) venous disorders, such as acute deep vein thrombosis (see Chapter 26). The arterial disorders are subdivided into those that result from arterial narrowing and occlusion (obstructive) and those caused by arterial spasm (vasospastic).

The most common form of obstructive arterial disease is arteriosclerosis obliterans, also called *atherosclerosis obliterans*. It results from atherosclerotic plaque formation, with narrowing of the lower aorta and the major arteries that provide circulation to the legs. As with atherosclerosis of the coronary arteries, the risk factors that play an important role in the development of this disease are high levels of low-density lipoprotein cholesterol (LDL-C), hypertension, cigarette smoking, low levels of high-density lipoprotein cholesterol (HDL-C), and diabetes mellitus.

Patients tend to remain free of symptoms until there is significant narrowing (75% to 90%) in key locations of the major arteries and arterioles of the legs. The typical pain pattern described is one of aching, cramping, tightness, or weakness that occurs during exercise.

The primary pathophysiology is obstruction of blood flow through the arteries, resulting in ischemia to the tissues supplied by those arteries. A term commonly applied to this condition is intermittent claudication; it manifests as pain secondary to lack of oxygen to the muscles during exercise. During the early stages of symptoms, the patient finds relief by stopping the exercise for a few minutes. Without treatment, as the disease progresses over time, the arteries become obstructed, resulting in thrombosis and the potential for gangrene. Additional symptoms that develop are pain at rest, numbness, and paresthesias (numbness with a tingling sensation). The disease is often accompanied by increased blood viscosity. Physical findings on the lower extremities are reduced arterial pulsations on palpation; systolic bruits over the involved arteries; waxy, pale, and dry skin; a lower temperature of the skin of the extremity; edema; and numbness to sensation.

Peripheral vascular disease caused by arterial vasospasm is known as Raynaud's disease, named after the man who first described the illness in 1862. It is unfortunate that, more than 150 years later, the pathophysiology and treatment of this condition are still not well defined. Raynaud's disease is classified as either primary, in which the cause is unknown, or as secondary, in which other conditions contribute to the symptoms. Secondary causes are frequent exposure to cold weather, obstructive arterial disease, occupational trauma (e.g., pneumatic hammer users, pianists), and certain drugs (e.g., beta blockers, imipramine, nicotine, bromocriptine, vinblastine, clonidine). Heredity may also play a role. The onset of Raynaud's disease is usually during the teenage years to the 40s, and it occurs four times more frequently in women.

Raynaud's disease is thought to be caused by **vasospasm** (vasoconstriction of blood vessels) and subsequent ischemia of the arteries of the skin of the hands, fingers, and sometimes toes. The physiologic mechanisms that trigger the vasospasm are unknown. Sudden coldness applied to the extremity, such as cold water, can induce an attack. The signs and symptoms associated with Raynaud's disease are numbness, tingling, a sense of skin tightness in the affected area, and blanching of the skin because of sudden vasoconstriction followed by cyanosis. As the attack subsides, vasodilation causes a redness, or rubor, to the pale skin. The skin appears normal except during spasm. During the early years of the illness, only the fingertips of both hands are involved. However, as the disease progresses, the skin on the hands is also affected by the arteriospasm.

TREATMENT OF PERIPHERAL VASCULAR DISEASE

The goals of treatment of arteriosclerosis obliterans are reversal of the progression of the atherosclerosis, improved blood flow, pain relief, and prevention of skin ulceration and gangrene. An important concept that must be stressed to most patients is that other diseases that they may have (e.g., diabetes, hypertension, angina, dyslipidemia) are all interrelated. Control of diet, high blood pressure, smoking, weight, and diabetes will significantly help all these diseases.

Implementation of the American Heart Association's diet—an eating plan for healthy Americans—can arrest the progression of atherosclerosis. Lipid-lowering agents can be started if diet modifications do not successfully treat the hypercholesterolemia. A daily exercise program (usually walking) can significantly improve collateral blood circulation around areas of obstruction and reduce the frequency of intermittent claudication. Proper foot care (e.g., keeping feet warm and dry, wearing properly fitting shoes), especially if the patient has diabetes, is also extremely important to prevent ulcerative complications. Other nonpharmacologic treatments for improving blood flow to the extremities include avoiding cold, elevating the head of the bed by 12 to 16 inches, and arterial angioplasty and surgery.

Most vasospastic attacks of Raynaud's disease can be stopped by avoiding cold temperatures, emotional stress, tobacco, and drugs that are known to induce attacks. Keeping the hands and feet warm with gloves and socks and using foam wraparounds when handling iced beverages can reduce exposure to cold.

DRUG THERAPY FOR PERIPHERAL VASCULAR DISEASE

ACTIONS

As the causes of peripheral vascular disease have come to be better understood, clinical studies have defined which pharmacologic therapies are truly successful. It has been shown that nonpharmacologic treatment of arteriosclerosis obliterans is substantially more successful in treating the underlying pathologic condition. Pentoxifylline has had modest success; it is classified as a hemorheologic agent. It acts by enhancing red blood cell flexibility, which reduces blood viscosity, thus providing better oxygenation to muscle tissue to stop intermittent claudication. Vasodilator therapy, the mainstay of treatment until the 1980s, has little long-term benefit in most cases. A new approach to treatment became available in the form of the platelet aggregation inhibitor cilostazol. Clopidogrel and vorapaxar, newer platelet aggregation inhibitors, are also approved for the treatment of peripheral arterial disease (see Chapter 26). When drug therapy for Raynaud's disease is required, such as when the disease interferes with an individual's ability to work, agents with a vasodilating effect are used.

USES

Pentoxifylline and cilostazol are the only agents approved by the U.S. Food and Drug Administration (FDA) that are specifically indicated for the treatment of intermittent claudication caused by chronic occlusive arterial disease of the limbs. Classes of drugs that have been somewhat successful in treating Raynaud's disease are calcium channel blockers, adrenergic antagonists, angiotensin-converting enzyme (ACE) inhibitors, and direct vasodilators.

The three calcium ion antagonists studied for the treatment of Raynaud's disease are diltiazem, verapamil, and nifedipine. Of the three, nifedipine has had the greatest success in reducing the frequency of vasospastic attack in about two thirds of patients.

Adrenergic antagonists (e.g., prazosin, reserpine, methyldopa) have been used for many years for the treatment of Raynaud's disease. Unfortunately, treatment has been only moderately successful, and many adverse effects are associated with the use of these drugs.

The ACE inhibitors cause an increase in bradykinin, a potent vasodilator. Captopril has been the most extensively tested, and it has been shown to reduce the frequency and severity of attacks.

For more than 50 years, nitroglycerin, a direct vasodilator, has been applied as an ointment base to the hands of patients with Raynaud's disease. The treatment reduces the frequency and severity of attacks, but the adverse effects of dizziness, headache, and postural hypotension limit its use.

Other vasodilators (e.g., papaverine, isoxsuprine) have been used extensively over the years to treat Reynaud's disease, but these agents have not undergone testing in controlled studies. However, they are still used occasionally as adjunctive therapy to treat peripheral vascular diseases.

❖ NURSING IMPLICATIONS FOR PERIPHERAL VASCULAR DISEASE THERAPY

■ Assessment

A baseline assessment of the patient should be completed that includes the following for evaluating the history and degree of oxygenation existing in the extremities. Subsequent regular assessments should be performed for comparison and analysis of therapeutic effectiveness or lack of response to any treatments initiated.

History of Risk Factors. Determine the patient's age, gender, and race, and obtain a family history of the incidence of symptoms of peripheral vascular disease, hypertension, and cardiac disease.

Impotence. If the patient is male, has he experienced impotence?

Hypertension. Take the patient's blood pressure in sitting and supine positions daily. Ask about medications that have been prescribed. Are the medications being taken regularly? If not, why not?

Smoking. Obtain a history of the number of cigarettes or cigars that the patient smokes daily; include other sources of nicotine, such as chewing tobacco and replacement therapy. How long has the person smoked? Has the person ever tried to stop smoking? Ask if the patient understands the effect of smoking on the vascular system. How does the individual feel about modifying his or her smoking habit?

Dietary Habits

- Obtain the patient's dietary history. Ask specific questions to obtain information about foods eaten that are high in fat, cholesterol, refined carbohydrates, and sodium. Using a calorie counter, ask the person to estimate the number of calories eaten per day. How much meat, fish, and poultry is eaten daily (size and number of servings)? Estimate the percentage of total daily calories provided by fats.
- Discuss food preparation (e.g., baked, broiled, fried). How many servings of fruits and vegetables are eaten daily? What types of oils and fats are used in food preparation? See a nutrition text for further dietary history questions.
- What is the frequency and volume of alcoholic beverages consumed?

Glucose Intolerance. Ask specific questions about whether the individual currently has or has ever had an elevated serum glucose (blood sugar) level. If yes, what dietary modifications have been made? How successful have they been? What medications are being taken for the elevated serum glucose level (e.g., oral hypoglycemic agents, insulin)?

Elevated Serum Lipid Levels. Find out whether the patient is aware of having elevated lipid, triglyceride,

or cholesterol levels. If any of these levels are elevated, what measures has the patient tried for reduction, and what effect have the interventions had on the blood levels during subsequent examinations? Review any laboratory data available (e.g., LDL, very low-density lipoprotein [VLDL], liver function tests, clotting time).

Infection. Has the individual developed any slow-to-heal or nonhealing sores?

Obesity. Weigh the patient. Ask about any recent weight gains or losses and whether it was intentional or unintentional.

Psychomotor Functions

Type of lifestyle. Ask the patient to describe his or her exercise level in terms of amount (e.g., walking three blocks), intensity (e.g., how long does it take to walk three blocks?), and frequency (e.g., walking every other day). Is the patient's job physically demanding or sedentary?

Psychological stress. How much stress does the individual estimate having in his or her life? How does the individual cope with stressful situations at home and at work?

Assessment of Tissue

Oxygenation. Observe the color of each hand, finger, leg, and foot; report cyanosis or reddish-blue areas. Does the patient have dependent cyanosis (cyanosis when the legs are in the dependent position)? Examine the skin of the extremities for any signs of ulceration.

Temperature. Feel the temperature in each hand, finger, leg, and foot. Report any paleness or coldness. (NOTE: These symptoms of poor circulation will be increased if the limb is elevated above the level of the heart.)

Edema. Assess, record, and report edema and its extent, and determine whether it is relieved or unchanged when the limb is dependent.

Peripheral pulses. Record the pedal and radial pulses (Figure 25-1) at least every 4 hours if circulatory impairment is found in that limb. Compare findings among

FIGURE 25-1 Assessing for a peripheral pulse. (From Perry AG, Potter PA, Ostendorf W: *Nursing interventions and clinical skills*, ed 6, St. Louis, 2016, Mosby.)

the extremities and report diminished or absent pulses immediately. When pulses are difficult to palpate or absent, a Doppler ultrasound device may help determine peripheral blood flow.

Limb pain. Assess pain in the patient carefully. Pain during exercise that is relieved by rest may be caused by claudication. Conversely, pain when the patient is at rest may result from sudden obstruction by a thrombus or an embolus. Check the apprehension level of the patient, pedal and radial pulses, details of onset and location of pain, and vital signs, and determine whether pain is increased by dorsiflexion of the foot (positive Homan's sign). Until the status of the patient's limb pain is established, have the patient remain on bed rest and administer an analgesic if ordered. Notify the patient's healthcare provider of any pertinent findings.

■ Implementation
- Prepare the patient for diagnostic tests (e.g., ultrasonography, pulse volume recordings, segmental limb pressure, exercise testing) and possible invasive procedures, such as arteriography.
- Do not place pillows in the popliteal space or flex the knee rest on the patient's bed. Use a cradle or footboard to prevent the bed sheets from constricting the patient's circulation.
- Always check with a healthcare provider before initiating any elevation of the patient's extremities. This action is contraindicated in patients with arterial insufficiency.
- Perform baseline assessments of tissue perfusion (e.g., skin temperature, peripheral pulses) at intervals appropriate to the patient's status (at least every 4 hours).
- Implement pain management measures.

■ Patient Education
Promoting Tissue Perfusion
- Teach the patient self-care measures that promote peripheral circulation.
- Smoking causes vasoconstriction of the blood vessels. Therefore encourage a drastic reduction in—and preferably total abstinence from—smoking. Include information about smoking cessation and available support resources.
- Encourage patients to wear nothing that constricts peripheral blood flow (e.g., tight-fitting anklets, socks, garters). Tell the patient not to elevate the extremities above the level of the heart without specific orders from a healthcare provider to do so. The healthcare provider may order the patient's head of bed to be elevated at night.
- Meticulous foot and hand care is essential. Teach the patient proper self-care of the limbs, including visual inspection techniques, and explain how to take femoral, popliteal, and pedal pulses.

- Stress the need for the patient to inspect the extremities for possible skin breakdown or signs of infection. The patient should notify a healthcare provider immediately of sudden changes in color, such as mottling or a more purplish color. Cold temperatures will increase pain or decrease sensations in the extremities. Hot tubs or showers may cause additional vasodilation that adds to the drug's effects.
- Areas of discoloration in nails, cracking of the skin, and calluses or blisters on the extremities require complete follow-up. Listen to the patient's description of any changes that have been noted. Tell the patient that going barefoot can be dangerous because of the potential for injuries to the feet.
- Because of the possible decrease in sensation in the extremities, encourage the patient to test the water temperature before immersing the hands or feet. After bathing, gently pat (i.e., do not vigorously rub) the feet and hands to dry them.
- To avoid skin breakdown, the patient should alternate pairs of shoes to allow for thorough drying between wearings, change socks or hose daily, and avoid rubber-soled shoes.
- The patient should avoid standing or sitting for prolonged periods. Patients who must sit for extended periods must have a properly fitting chair. The seat should be of the correct depth so that no pressure is exerted on the popliteal space. Encourage the patient not to sit with knees or ankles crossed and to take frequent short breaks for walks. Furthermore, those who must stand for long periods should seek out tasks of the job that can be performed while sitting in a properly fitting chair or other alternatives.

Psychomotor Functions
- Maximum mobility should be maintained. Devise a daily activity plan that includes walks and usual activities of daily living (ADLs), such as shopping and housework.
- Pain management and the psychological aspects of dealing with a prolonged illness with persistent symptoms are major challenges for both the patient and the nurse (see Chapter 19).

Environment. During periods of exposure to cold temperature, the patient should wear several layers of lightweight clothing. Caution should be exercised during exposure to the cold to avoid frostbite. Because of decreased sensation in the extremities, frostbite can occur without the patient's awareness.

Nutritional Aspects
- Dietary education is strongly indicated for the treatment of peripheral vascular disease. It is particularly important to control obesity and cholesterol and triglyceride levels.
- When ulcerations are present, encourage a high-protein diet with adequate intake of vitamins to promote the healing process.

- Unless other medical conditions contraindicate, instruct the patient to drink eight 8-ounce glasses of water daily to promote adequate hydration of body tissues. Maintaining blood volume will help reduce peripheral vasoconstriction. Check with the physician regarding recommendations for fluid or caffeine restriction.

  Medication Regimen

- Certain medications for the treatment of peripheral vascular disease cause dilation of blood vessels. As a result, orthostatic hypotension may occur. Teach the patient to rise slowly from sitting or lying positions, adjust balance for stability, flex the leg muscles, and then proceed with movement.

- Teach the patient to take and record his or her own blood pressure.

- Administer prescribed medications, and consult a healthcare provider before discontinuing any medications.

  Fostering Health Maintenance

- Throughout the course of treatment, discuss medication information, and explain how the medication will benefit the patient.

- Drug therapy is not a total solution for atherosclerosis. The patient may not be committed to the lifestyle changes needed to control the modifiable aspects of the disease. Often, setting short-term goals to control the pain and finding other interventions that will allow the patient to view efforts positively will help encourage permanent adoption of the needed changes.

- Patients who are unresponsive to lifestyle modifications and drug therapy may require surgical interventions to reestablish blood flow to the affected area. Procedures such as bypass grafting, endarterectomy, or angioplasty may be appropriate. Failure to reestablish blood flow to an extremity may result in amputation.

- Provide the patient and significant others with important information contained in the specific drug monographs for the drugs prescribed. Additional health teaching and nursing interventions for common and serious adverse effects are described in each drug monograph.

- Seek cooperation and understanding of the following points so that medication compliance is increased: name of medication; dosage, route and times of administration; and common and serious adverse effects.

  Patient Self-Assessment. Enlist the patient's help with developing and maintaining a written record of monitoring parameters (e.g., color of limb, pain in limb, temperature and pulses in limb, amount of edema present). See the Patient Self-Assessment Form for Cardiovascular Agents on the Evolve website. Complete the Premedication Data column for use as a baseline to track the patient's response to drug therapy.

Ensure that the patient understands how to use the form, and instruct the patient to bring the completed form to follow-up visits. During follow-up visits, focus on issues that will foster adherence to the therapeutic interventions prescribed.

DRUG CLASS: HEMORRHEOLOGIC AGENTS

> **pentoxifylline** (pĕn-tŏks-ĭ-FĪ-lēn)
> **Trental** (TRĔN-tŏl)
> ⇄ Do not confuse Trental with Tegretol.

ACTIONS

Pentoxifylline is not an anticoagulant, but it is thought to increase erythrocyte flexibility, decrease the concentration of fibrinogen in blood, and prevent aggregation of red blood cells and platelets. These actions decrease the viscosity of blood and improve its flow properties, resulting in increased blood flow to the affected microcirculation to enhance tissue oxygenation.

USES

Pentoxifylline is the agent approved for the treatment of intermittent claudication. Pentoxifylline therapy should be considered an adjunct to—not a replacement for—smoking cessation, weight loss, exercise therapy, surgical bypass, or removal of arterial obstructions in the treatment of peripheral vascular disease.

THERAPEUTIC OUTCOME

The primary therapeutic outcome expected from pentoxifylline is improved tissue perfusion with a reduced frequency of pain, improved tolerance to exercise, and improved peripheral pulses.

❖ NURSING IMPLICATIONS FOR PENTOXIFYLLINE

■ Premedication Assessment

1. Perform baseline gastrointestinal (GI) assessments to determine whether nausea, vomiting, dyspepsia, or intolerance to caffeine products exists.
2. Assess the patient for the presence of dizziness or headache.
3. Ask specifically about any cardiac symptoms. Report these to a healthcare provider if they are present.
4. Obtain baseline data regarding the degree of pain present.
5. Inquire about a history of stroke, bleeding in the eyes, kidney problems, recent surgery, and peptic ulcer disease.

■ Availability

PO: 400-mg extended-release tablets.

■ **Dosage and Administration**

PO: 400 mg three times daily. If adverse GI or central nervous system (CNS) effects develop, the dosage should be reduced to 400 mg twice daily. If adverse effects persist, therapy should be discontinued. Symptomatic relief may start within 2 to 4 weeks, but treatment should be continued for at least 8 weeks to achieve maximal efficacy.

■ **Common Adverse Effects**

Gastrointestinal

Nausea, vomiting, dyspepsia. Dyspepsia, nausea, and vomiting occur in about 1% to 3% of patients. Belching and flatus occur in less than 1% of patients. These adverse effects are usually mild, and they tend to resolve with continued therapy. Administration with food or milk may help minimize the patient's discomfort. Encourage the patient not to discontinue therapy without first consulting a healthcare provider.

Neurologic

Dizziness, headache. Central nervous system disturbances characterized by dizziness occur in about 2% of patients, and headache and tremor occur less frequently. These adverse effects are usually mild, and they tend to resolve with continued therapy. Provide for the patient's safety during episodes of dizziness, and encourage the patient to sit or lie down if feeling faint. Encourage the patient not to discontinue therapy without first consulting the healthcare provider.

■ **Serious Adverse Effects**

Cardiovascular

Chest pain, dysrhythmias, shortness of breath. Without causing undue alarm, strongly encourage the patient to seek a physician's attention for further evaluation.

■ **Pharmacodynamics**

Intolerance to Caffeine, Theophylline, Theobromine. Pentoxifylline is a xanthine derivative. The patient should be asked specifically about any intolerance to xanthine derivatives before starting therapy.

■ **Drug Interactions**

Antihypertensive Agents. Although pentoxifylline is not an antihypertensive agent, patients receiving pentoxifylline therapy frequently display a small reduction in systemic blood pressure. Blood pressure should be monitored to observe for hypotension. The dosage of antihypertensive therapy may have to be reduced to minimize adverse effects.

Theophylline. Concurrent use of pentoxifylline and theophylline-containing drugs leads to increased theophylline levels and theophylline toxicity in some individuals. Monitor patients closely for signs of toxicity (e.g., nausea, tachycardia), and adjust the theophylline dosage as necessary.

DRUG CLASS: PLATELET AGGREGATION INHIBITOR

cilostazol (sī-lō-STĀ-zŏl)
  Pletal (PLĔ-tăl)
   Do not confuse Pletal with Plendil.

ACTIONS

Cilostazol is a selective inhibitor of cellular cyclic adenosine monophosphate (cAMP) phosphodiesterase III (PDE III). Suppression of this enzyme causes increased levels of cAMP, resulting in vasodilation and inhibition of platelet aggregation. Other mechanisms in addition to vasodilation are thought to play a role but are not fully known at this time.

USES

Cilostazol is approved for the treatment of intermittent claudication. Cilostazol therapy should be considered an adjunct to—not a replacement for—smoking cessation, weight loss, exercise therapy, surgical bypass, or removal of arterial obstructions in the treatment of peripheral vascular disease.

> ⚠️ **Medication Safety Alert**
>
> Cilostazol should not be used to treat patients with heart failure of any severity.

THERAPEUTIC OUTCOME

The primary therapeutic outcome expected from cilostazol is singular improved tissue perfusion with a reduced frequency of pain, improved tolerance to exercise, and improved peripheral pulses.

❖ NURSING IMPLICATIONS FOR CILOSTAZOL

■ **Premedication Assessment**

1. Assess the patient for the presence of dizziness or headache.
2. Obtain a baseline assessment of the degree of pain present and any symptoms of peripheral vascular disease.
3. Ask the patient specifically about any cardiac symptoms, peptic ulcer disease, or heart failure. Report these to a healthcare provider if they are present.

■ **Availability**

PO: 50- and 100-mg tablets.

■ **Dosage and Administration**

PO: 100 mg twice daily taken 30 minutes before or 2 hours after breakfast and dinner. Symptomatic relief may start within 2 to 4 weeks, but treatment should be continued for at least 12 weeks to achieve maximum efficacy.

Medication Safety Alert

Do not administer cilostazol to patients with heart failure. Phosphodiesterase inhibitors have been reported to significantly worsen heart failure.

▪ Common Adverse Effects
Gastrointestinal

Dyspepsia, diarrhea. Dyspepsia occurs in 6% of patients, and diarrhea occurs in 19% of patients. These adverse effects are usually mild, and they tend to resolve with continued therapy. Encourage the patient not to discontinue therapy without first consulting a healthcare provider.

Neurologic

Dizziness, headache. Central nervous system disturbances characterized by dizziness occur in about 10% of patients. Headache may occur in 34% of patients, and it may be severe enough to cause the discontinuation of therapy. These adverse effects are usually mild, and they tend to resolve with continued therapy.

Provide for patient safety during episodes of dizziness. Encourage the patient to sit or lie down if feeling faint. Encourage the patient not to discontinue therapy without first consulting a healthcare provider.

▪ Serious Adverse Effects
Cardiovascular

Chest pain, palpitations, dysrhythmias, shortness of breath. Without causing undue alarm, strongly encourage the patient to seek a healthcare provider's attention for further evaluation.

▪ Drug Interactions
Diltiazem, Erythromycin, Omeprazole, Fluconazole, Fluvoxamine, Fluoxetine, Sertraline, Ketoconazole, Grapefruit Juice. These substances will inhibit the metabolism of cilostazol. If cilostazol therapy is necessary for patients who are already receiving any of the preceding drugs, the starting dose of cilostazol should be half of the normal starting dose. Monitor patients closely for an increased incidence of adverse effects.

Get Ready for the NCLEX® Examination!

Key Points

- Peripheral vascular disease is a cause of significant morbidity in the United States. Major treatable causes of peripheral vascular disease are hypertension, cigarette smoking, and atherosclerosis.
- The most cost-effective and successful forms of treatment are smoking cessation, weight reduction, exercise, and dietary modification.
- Patients should be fully informed about the significance of peripheral vascular disease, the potential complications of not participating in lifestyle modification, and the use of drug therapy.

Additional Learning Resources

SG Go to your Study Guide for additional Review Questions for the NCLEX® Examination, Critical Thinking Clinical Situations, and other learning activities to help you master this chapter content.

evolve Go to your Evolve website (http://evolve.elsevier.com/Clayton) for additional online resources.

Review Questions for the NCLEX® Examination

1. The premedication assessments that the nurse performs on patients with peripheral vascular disease include: *(Select all that apply.)*
   1. checking for renal disease.
   2. obtaining a pain rating.
   3. evaluating the peripheral pulses.
   4. checking the temperature of extremities.
   5. evaluating the level of psychological stress.

2. The nurse knows that the most significant risk factors for developing peripheral vascular disease include: *(Select all that apply.)*
   1. hypertension.
   2. cigarette smoking.
   3. low LDL levels.
   4. high LDL levels.
   5. aspirin hypersensitivity.

3. The nurse was explaining to a 52-year-old male patient the meaning of his new diagnosis of "claudication." Which is the best statement?
   1. "This condition is from poor circulation resulting in a lack of oxygen to the muscles during exercise."
   2. "When patients get this, there usually is also a deep vein thrombus in the leg."
   3. "The pain you have when walking is from a vasospasm, which will cause your skin to blanch."
   4. "Generally, you do not have to treat this condition until you get pain at rest, along with numbness and tingling in your legs."

4. The nurse teaching a patient about ways to prevent vasospasms associated with Raynaud's disease includes all of these in the instructions. *(Select all that apply.)*
   1. Avoid holding cold beverages
   2. Avoid handling hot beverages
   3. Keep hands and feet warm with gloves and socks
   4. Limit the intake of caffeine products
   5. Exercise vigorously three times a day

5. The nurse was reviewing the common adverse effects of cilostazol (Pletal) with the patient who has peripheral vascular disease and included these effects in the teaching. *(Select all that apply.)*
   1. Dizziness
   2. Rhinorrhea
   3. Diarrhea
   4. Headache
   5. Dryness of the mouth

6. The nurse teaches a patient with any venous circulation disorder that the best way to prevent venous stasis and increase venous return is to:
   1. ambulate.
   2. sit with the legs elevated.
   3. frequently rotate the ankles.
   4. continuously wear compression-gradient stockings.

7. The patient who was started on pentoxifylline (Trental) asked the nurse how the drug works; the best response by the nurse is:
   1. "Trental works by increasing the flexibility of your red blood cells so clotting does not happen so easily."
   2. "Trental acts as an anticoagulant so you will not develop clots in your legs."
   3. "Trental increases the viscosity of blood, which means it makes your blood thicker."
   4. "Trental breaks down the plaque in your blood vessels so that you will not have any blood clots develop."

Drugs Used to Treat Thromboembolic Disorders

Objectives

1. Explain the primary purposes of anticoagulant therapy.
2. Describe conditions that place an individual at risk for developing blood clots and nursing interventions used to prevent these conditions.
3. Identify the actions of platelet inhibitors, anticoagulants, thrombin inhibitors, glycoprotein IIb/IIIa inhibitors, and fibrinolytic agents.
4. Describe specific monitoring procedures and laboratory data used to detect hemorrhage in the patient taking anticoagulants.
5. Describe the nursing assessments needed to monitor therapeutic response and adverse effects from anticoagulant therapy.

Key Terms

thromboembolic diseases (thrŏm-bō-ĕm-BŎL-ĭk) (p. 399)
thrombosis (thrŏm-BŌ-sĭs) (p. 399)
thrombus (THRŎM-bŭs) (p. 399)
embolus (ĔM-bō-lŭs) (p. 399)
intrinsic clotting pathway (ĭn-TRĬN-zĭk KLŎT-ĭng PǍTH-wā) (p. 399)
extrinsic clotting pathway (ĕks-TRĬN-zĭk) (p. 399)

fibrinolytic agents (fī-brĭn-ō-LĬT-ĭk Ā-gĕntz) (p. 400)
platelet inhibitors (PLĀT-lĕt ĭn-HĬB-ĭ-tĕrz) (p. 401)
anticoagulants (ăn-tī-kō-ĂG-yū-lănts) (p. 401)
thrombin inhibitors (p. 401)
glycoprotein IIb/IIIa inhibitors (glī-cō-PRŌ-tēn ĭn-HĬ-bĭ-tĕrz) (p. 401)

THROMBOEMBOLIC DISEASES

Diseases associated with abnormal clotting within blood vessels are known as **thromboembolic diseases** and are major causes of morbidity and mortality. **Thrombosis** is the process of formation of a fibrin blood clot (**thrombus**). An **embolus** is a small fragment of a thrombus that breaks off and circulates until it becomes trapped in a capillary, causing ischemia or infarction to the area distal to the obstruction (e.g., cerebral embolism, pulmonary embolism).

Major causes of thrombus formation are immobilization with venous stasis; surgery and the postoperative period; trauma to lower limbs; certain illnesses (e.g., heart failure, vasospasm, ulcerative colitis); cancers of the lung, prostate, stomach, and pancreas; pregnancy and oral contraceptives; and heredity.

Normally, blood clot formation and dissolution constitute a fine balance within the cardiovascular system. The clotting proteins normally circulate in an inactive state and must be activated to form a fibrin clot. When there is a trigger, such as increased blood viscosity from bed rest and stasis or damage to a blood vessel wall, the clotting cascade is activated. For example, if a blood vessel is injured and collagen in the vessel wall is exposed, platelets first adhere to the site of injury and release adenosine diphosphate (ADP), leading to

additional platelet aggregation that forms a "platelet plug." At the same time platelets are forming a plug, the **intrinsic clotting pathway** is triggered by the presence of collagen activating factor XII. Activated factor XIIa activates factor XI to XIa, which activates factor IX to IXa. Factor IXa, in the presence of calcium, platelet factor 3 (PF3), and factor VIII, activates factor X. Activated factor Xa, in the presence of calcium, PF3, and factor V, stimulates the conversion of prothrombin to thrombin (Figure 26-1).

Sources outside the blood vessels, such as tissue extract or thromboplastin (tissue factor), can trigger the **extrinsic clotting pathway** by activating factor VII to VIIa. Factor VIIa can also activate factor X, which results in the formation of thrombin. After stimulation from the intrinsic or extrinsic pathway, thrombin, in the presence of calcium, activates fibrinogen to soluble fibrin. With time and the presence of factor XIII, the loose fibrin mesh is converted to a tight, insoluble fibrin mesh clot. Thrombin also stimulates platelet aggregation and stimulates further activity of factors V, VIIa, VII, and Xa. As the fibrin clot is being formed, it also triggers the release of fibrinolysin, an enzyme that dissolves fibrin, preventing the clot from spreading.

Historically, thrombi have been classified into red and white blood clots. A red thrombus is actually a

Intrinsic Clotting Pathway   **Extrinsic Clotting Pathway**

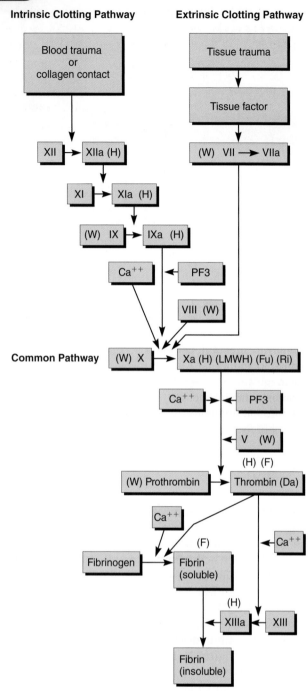

FIGURE 26-1 The clotting cascade. *Da*, site of dabigatran; *F*, site of fibrinolytic action; *Fu*, fondaparinux; *H*, site of heparin action; *LMWH*, site of low-molecular-weight heparins; *PF3*, platelet factor 3; *W*, site of warfarin action.

subsequently causing life-threatening pulmonary emboli. White thrombi develop in arteries and are composed of platelets and fibrin. This type of thrombus forms in areas of high blood flow in response to injured vessel walls. Coronary artery occlusion leading to myocardial infarction is an example of a white thrombus.

TREATMENT OF THROMBOEMBOLIC DISEASES

Diseases caused by intravascular clotting (e.g., deep vein thrombosis, myocardial infarction, dysrhythmias with clot formation, coronary vasospasm leading to thrombus formation) are major causes of death. When thrombosis is suspected, patients are admitted to the hospital where they can be closely observed for further signs and symptoms of thrombosis formation and progression, and anticoagulant or fibrinolytic therapy can be started. A combination of physical examination, patient history, Doppler ultrasound, phlebography, radiolabeled fibrinogen studies, and angiography is used to diagnose the presence and cause of a thrombus and embolism. Routine laboratory tests that are run to assess the clotting process and ensure that occult bleeding is not present are platelet count, hematocrit, prothrombin time (PT) reported as the international normalized ratio (INR), activated partial thromboplastin time (aPTT), activated clotting time (ACT), urinalysis, and stool guaiac test.

Nonpharmacologic prevention and treatment of thromboembolic disease include patient education on how to prevent venous stasis (e.g., leg exercises, leg elevation) and clinical use of sequential compression devices (SCDs). If a patient having a heart attack (myocardial infarction, acute coronary syndrome) can be transported to a cardiac intensive care facility soon after symptoms develop, revascularization treatment to reopen the coronary arteries may be performed. **Fibrinolytic agents** may be used to dissolve the arterial clot before it is permanently attached to vessel walls, causing complete obstruction. Revascularization procedures used may be a percutaneous coronary intervention (PCI) or coronary artery bypass graft (CABG). In PCI, also known as angioplasty, a catheter is inserted into the femoral artery and advanced up the aorta into the site of the coronary artery obstruction. The tip of the catheter can be equipped with different types of devices, such as a balloon to dilate the artery obstruction, or blades or lasers to reduce or remove the obstruction. A vascular stent is then often placed in the artery to keep the formerly obstructed area open. If a patient has multiple narrowed or obstructed arteries, a CABG procedure is performed, wherein a segment of the saphenous vein from the leg is harvested and attached to the coronary artery above and below the obstruction, forming a bypass for perfusion to the myocardial tissues below. The internal mammary artery can also be used in this procedure. The major

venous thrombus and is composed almost entirely of fibrin and erythrocytes (red blood cells), with a few platelets. Venous thrombi generally form in response to venous stasis after immobility or surgery. The poor circulation prevents the dilution of activated coagulation factors that normally occurs by rapidly circulating blood. The most common location of red thrombus formation is deep vein thrombosis of the lower extremities. These thrombi may extend upward into the veins of the thigh and have the potential of fragmenting, pharmacologic treatments used in the prevention and treatment of thromboembolic diseases are platelet inhibitors, anticoagulants, thrombin inhibitors, glycoprotein IIb/IIIa inhibitors, and fibrinolytic agents.

DRUG THERAPY FOR THROMBOEMBOLIC DISEASES

ACTIONS

The pharmacologic agents used to treat thromboembolic disease act either to prevent platelet aggregation or inhibit a variety of steps in the fibrin clot formation cascade (see Figure 26-1). See individual drug monographs for a more detailed discussion of mechanisms of action.

USES

Agents used in the prevention and treatment of thromboembolic disease can be divided into **platelet inhibitors, anticoagulants, thrombin inhibitors, glycoprotein IIb/IIIa inhibitors,** and fibrinolytic agents. Antiplatelet agents (e.g., aspirin, clopidogrel, prasugrel, ticagrelor) are used preventively to reduce arterial clot formation (white thrombi) by inhibiting platelet aggregation. Anticoagulants (e.g., apixaban, warfarin, fondaparinux, rivaroxaban, heparin, heparin derivatives [enoxaparin, dalteparin]) are also used prophylactically to prevent the formation of arterial and venous thrombi in predisposed patients. The heparin derivatives are also known as low-molecular-weight heparins (LMWHs). The primary purpose of anticoagulants is to prevent the formation of new clots or the extension of existing clots. They cannot dissolve an existing (white or red) clot. Dabigatran, an oral direct thrombin inhibitor, is used to prevent strokes and systemic emboli in patients with atrial fibrillation. The glycoprotein IIb/IIIa inhibitors (e.g., abciximab, eptifibatide, tirofiban) are used to prevent clot formation during PCI procedures. Fibrinolytic agents (e.g., streptokinase, alteplase) are used to dissolve arterial (fibrin-rich, white) thromboemboli once formed.

LABORATORY TESTS FOR MONITORING ANTICOAGULANT THERAPY

While receiving anticoagulant therapy, the patient will undergo regular monitoring of coagulation studies, including monitoring of the PT reported as the INR, ecarin clotting time (ECT), thrombin time (TT), aPTT, and platelet counts. These laboratory studies monitor the time it takes for the blood to clot. Results of these studies may be used as guidelines for drug dosing by the prescriber.

❖ NURSING IMPLICATIONS FOR ANTICOAGULANT THERAPY

■ Assessment

History. Ask specific questions to determine whether the patient or family members have a history of any type of vascular difficulty. Patients at greater risk for clot formation are those with a history of clot formation; those who have recently undergone abdominal, thoracic, or orthopedic surgery; and those on prolonged bed rest or anticoagulant therapy. Does the patient have any disease processes that could potentially increase the risk of bleeding (e.g., ulcer disease, concurrent chemotherapy, or radiation therapy)?

Current Symptoms

- Ask the patient to describe the symptoms. Is the patient currently taking, or has the patient recently taken, anticoagulants? Individualize further questioning to obtain data that would support or rule out thrombosis formation or progression of thrombosis.
- Collect data about reduced tissue perfusion (e.g., symptoms relating to cerebral, cardiopulmonary, or peripheral vascular disease, depending on the underlying pathophysiology). Perform a focused assessment at appropriate intervals that are consistent with the patient's status to detect further signs and symptoms of thrombosis formation or progression.
- To prevent thrombus extension or progression, SCDs (plastic sleeves placed around the legs) are used. These devices inflate and deflate to promote venous return from the legs. Sequential compression devices are removed when ambulating and discontinued when the patient resumes full activity.

Medications

- Obtain a thorough medication history of both prescribed and over-the-counter medications being taken.
- Ask specific questions relating to medicines being taken that affect clotting.
- Ask whether the patient has been complying with medication regimens and if any dosage adjustment has taken place. If anticoagulants are being taken, has the patient reported for scheduled laboratory studies? Has the patient had any reactions to the medication?

Basic Assessment

- Obtain vital signs and auscultation of breath sounds. Observe for dyspnea at rest or with exertion.
- Check mental status (e.g., orientation to date, time, and place; alertness; confusion). Use as a baseline for future comparison.
- Assess for specific signs of reduced tissue perfusion. Perform a focused assessment depending on the underlying pathologic condition (e.g., cardiopulmonary, cerebral, or peripheral vascular disease). If the presence of a thrombus is suspected in an extremity, complete a comparative assessment of the unaffected extremity.
- Collect data about any pain experienced.
- Ask specific questions about the patient's state of hydration. Review intake and output.

Diagnostic Studies. Review completed diagnostic studies and laboratory data (e.g., PT, aPTT, INR), hematocrit, platelet count, Doppler studies, exercise testing, serum triglyceride levels, arteriogram, cardiac enzyme studies.

■ **Implementation**
Techniques for Preventing Clot Formation
- Provide early, regular ambulation after surgery. Use active or passive leg exercises for patients on bed rest or restricted activity.
- Develop and follow a specific turning schedule for patients on complete bed rest to prevent tissue breakdown and blood stasis. Implement regular back care and deep breathing and coughing exercises as part of general nursing care.
- Do not flex the patient's knees or place pressure against the popliteal space with pillows.
- Do not allow the patient to stand or sit motionless for prolonged periods.
- Use properly fitted thromboembolic disease (TED) deterrent stockings only when ordered. Remove stockings and inspect the skin on every shift. Make sure that they are being worn properly and remain wrinkle-free.
- Apply SCDs as ordered and indicated. Make sure that they are applied properly.

Patient Assessment. Monitor vital signs and mental status every 4 to 8 hours or more frequently, depending on the patient's status. Observe for signs and symptoms of bleeding caused by medications (e.g., blurred vision, hematuria, ecchymosis, occult blood in the stools, change in mentation).

Nutritional Status
- The dietary regimen will depend on the patient's diagnosis and clinical status.
- Adequate hydration to promote fluidity of the blood is important. Unless coexisting diagnoses prohibit, give at least six to eight 8-ounce glasses of liquid daily.

Laboratory and Diagnostic Data. Monitoring and reporting laboratory results to the prescriber are essential during anticoagulant therapy. Coagulation tests that might be ordered include the following: whole blood clotting time (WBCT), ECT, TT, PT, aPTT, and ACT. The PT, reported as INR, is routinely used to monitor warfarin therapy, and the aPTT is most commonly used to monitor heparin therapy. The ECT and TT are used to monitor dabigatran therapy.

Medication Administration. Never administer an anticoagulant without first checking the chart for the most recent laboratory results. Be certain that the anticoagulant to be administered is ordered after the most recent results have been reported to a healthcare provider. Follow policy statements regarding checking of anticoagulant doses with other qualified professionals.

Reduce localized bleeding at the injection site by using the smallest needle possible for injections, and rotate injection sites. See individual drug monographs for specific administration techniques related to a particular medicine.

■ **Patient Education**
Nutritional Status
- While receiving anticoagulant therapy, patients should maintain their normal intake of green leafy vegetables that contain vitamin K. (Vitamin K inhibits the action of warfarin.) Patients should not start a major change in diet without discussing it with their prescriber, pharmacist, and nutritionist.
- Unless comorbidities prohibit, instruct the patient to drink six to eight 8-ounce glasses of liquid daily.

Exercise and Activity
- Discuss the level of exercise prescribed by a healthcare provider. Walking may be prescribed to promote venous blood flow. Elevation of the legs when seated may be encouraged to promote venous blood flow.
- Stress the need to prevent body injury while taking anticoagulants. Tell the patient to avoid using power equipment, use care in stepping up or down from curbs, not participate in contact sports, use only an electric razor, and brush teeth gently with a soft-bristled toothbrush.

Medication Regimen
- Instruct the patient to take the dosage of the medication exactly as prescribed. Explain the importance of returning for laboratory blood tests to determine its effectiveness and the need to adjust medicine dosages. Tell the patient to resume a regular schedule if one dose of warfarin is missed. If two or more doses are missed, the patient should consult the prescriber.
- Tell the patient to wear a medical alert bracelet.
- Explain symptoms that the patient should report, such as nosebleeds, tarry stools, coffee-ground or blood-tinged vomitus, petechiae (tiny purple or red spots occurring in various sites on the skin), ecchymoses (bruises), hematuria (blood in the urine), bleeding from the gums or any other body opening, or cuts or injuries from which the bleeding is difficult to control. Check dressings periodically for bleeding. Report excessive menstrual flow.
- In some cases, a healthcare provider may want the patient to perform guaiac testing to detect blood in the stool. If ordered, specific patient education should be done to teach the patient or support person how to perform the test.
- Tell patients that because not all bleeding is clearly visible, they should report immediately a rapid weak pulse, deep rapid respirations, moist clammy skin, and a general feeling of weakness or faintness.

Drugs Used to Treat Heart Failure

Objectives

1. Explain heart failure in terms of the body's compensatory mechanisms.
2. Identify the goals of treatment for heart failure.
3. Identify the primary actions on heart failure of digoxin, angiotensin-converting enzyme inhibitors, and beta blockers.
4. Describe digoxin toxicity and ways to prevent it.
5. Identify essential assessment data and nursing interventions needed for a patient with heart failure.

Key Terms

systolic dysfunction (sĭs-TŎL-ĭk dĭs-FŬNK-shŭn) (p. 419)
diastolic dysfunction (dī-ă-STŎL-ĭk dĭs-FŬNK-shŭn) (p. 419)
inotropic agents (ĭn-ō-TRŌ-pĭk Ā-jĕnts) (p. 421)

digitalis toxicity (dĭ-jĭ-TĂL-ĭs tŏk-SĬS-ĭ-tē) (p. 426)
positive inotropy (PŎZ-ĭ-tĭv Ī-nō-TRŌ-pē) (p. 428)
negative chronotropy (NĔG-ĕ-tĭv krō-nō-TRŌ-pē) (p. 428)
digitalization (dĭ-jĭ-tăl-ĭ-ZĀ-shŭn) (p. 428)

HEART FAILURE

The incidence of heart failure (previously known as *congestive heart failure*)—unlike that of other cardiovascular diseases—continues to increase as a result of population aging and improved survival after acute myocardial infarction. The lifetime risk of developing heart failure is 20% for Americans older than 40 years of age. It is estimated that 2% of people older than age 65 and 8% of those older than age 85 experience heart failure. Some 5.1 million Americans have this disabling condition; more than 650,000 patients develop symptoms annually, and more than 200,000 people die from heart failure each year. The 5-year mortality rate for heart failure is approximately 50%. The economic burden is staggering, with an estimated total cost of $30 billion for managing heart failure as a primary diagnosis in the United States in 2013 (Yancy, 2013). More of the Medicare budget is spent on heart failure than any other diagnosis.

Heart failure involves a cluster of signs and symptoms that arise when the left or right ventricle or both ventricles lose the ability to pump enough blood to meet the body's circulatory needs. The most common type of heart failure is **systolic dysfunction** (also known as *contracting dysfunction*). Normally, the heart pumps at a rate that supports the body's need for blood flow and oxygenation of the vital organs and muscles. Systolic heart failure results when the heart lacks sufficient force to pump all the blood (resulting in decreased cardiac output) with which it is presented to meet the body's oxygenation needs (causing decreased tissue perfusion). Early clinical symptoms are decreased exercise tolerance and poor perfusion to the peripheral tissues. As the condition progresses, the left ventricle chamber enlarges (left ventricular hypertrophy), and an increase in blood volume is required to fill the expanding ventricle to maintain cardiac output. Causes of systolic dysfunction are those that cause damage to the heart muscle itself. The most common is coronary artery disease that leads to myocardial infarction. Other causes include dysrhythmias, cardiomyopathies, and congenital heart disease. Usually, the left ventricle fails first and as the disease progresses, the right ventricle also enlarges due to increased pulmonary resistance, and it eventually fails.

Diastolic dysfunction (or *filling dysfunction*) causes heart failure because the left ventricle develops a "stiffness" and fails to relax enough between contractions to allow adequate filling before the next contraction. Symptoms of diastolic dysfunction include pulmonary congestion and peripheral edema. There are many reasons why diastolic dysfunction develops, including constrictive pericarditis, ventricular muscle hypertrophy caused by chronic hypertension, valvular heart disease that results in flow resistance, and aortic stenosis.

The general pathogenesis of heart failure is diagrammed in Figure 27-1. When the vital organs and peripheral tissues are not adequately perfused, compensatory mechanisms begin to overcome the inadequate output of the heart. The sympathetic nervous

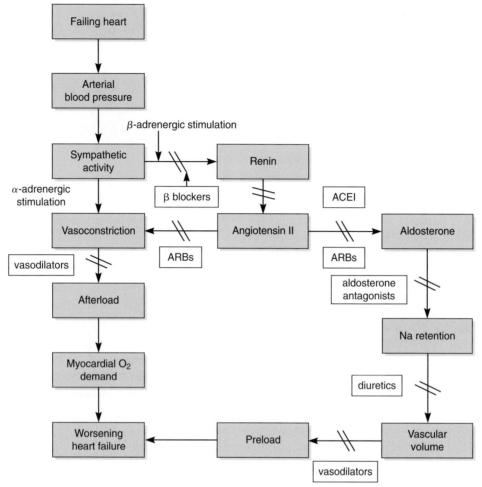

FIGURE 27-1 Pathway showing how heart failure develops and how specific classes of medicines block physiologic mechanisms to reduce the worsening of heart failure. Cardiac glycosides and phosphodiesterase inhibitors are also used to increase myocardial contractility. *ACEI*, Angiotensin-converting enzyme inhibitors; *ARBs*, angiotensin II receptor blockers; *β blockers*, beta-adrenergic blocking agents.

system releases epinephrine and norepinephrine, which produce tachycardia and increase contractility. The increased sympathetic stimulation also increases peripheral vasoconstriction, which results in an increased afterload against which the heart must pump, causing a further decrease in cardiac output (see Figure 27-1). The renin-angiotensin-aldosterone system stimulates renal distal tubule sodium and water retention in an effort to increase circulating blood volume, which increases preload to the heart. There is also an increased production of vasopressin (antidiuretic hormone) from the pituitary gland that increases water recovery from the kidneys and increases intravascular volume and preload. With decreased perfusion secondary to low cardiac output, the kidneys also increase sodium reabsorption in the proximal tubules to help expand circulating blood volume. The increased intravascular volume initially improves tissue perfusion; however, over time, excessive amounts of sodium and water are retained, causing increased pressure within the capillaries resulting in edema formation.

Early symptoms of heart failure vary depending on the underlying cause of the disease. Traditionally, the signs and symptoms of heart failure have been classified on the basis of whether failure is developing in the right ventricle or the left ventricle. However, it has been found that the symptoms overlap to such an extent because of the complexity of the syndrome that it is difficult to attribute a particular clinical indicator to a specific ventricle. It is also important to recognize that the clinical indicators vary considerably over time in response to the treatments being applied (Box 27-1).

TREATMENT OF HEART FAILURE

The overall goals for treating heart failure are to reduce the signs and symptoms associated with fluid overload, increase exercise tolerance, improve quality of life, and prolong life. If the heart failure is acute, the patient must be hospitalized for a diagnostic workup to determine the underlying cause. A combination of the American College of Cardiology Foundation and the American Heart Association (ACCF/AHA) and the New York Heart Association Functional Classification System (NYHA) is commonly used to group

FIGURE 28-1 Sites of actions of diuretics within the nephron.

Assessment

History of Related Causative Disorders and Factors. Ask the patient questions relating to any history of disorders that contribute to fluid volume excess: heart disorders (e.g., myocardial infarction, heart failure, valvular disease, dysrhythmias); liver disease (e.g., ascites, cirrhosis, cancer); renal disease (e.g., renal failure); and factors such as immobility, hypertension, pregnancy, and use of corticosteroid agents.

History of Current Symptoms. Ask the patient questions to ascertain information relating to the onset, duration, and progression of specific symptoms relating to edema, weakness, fatigue, dyspnea, productive cough, and weight gain.

Pattern of Urination. Ask the patient to describe his or her current urination pattern and to cite any changes. Details such as frequency, dysuria, incontinence, changes in the stream, hesitancy when starting to void, hematuria, nocturia, and urgency are all significant. Provide assistance with voiding for people with impaired mobility, fatigue, or other impairments.

Medication History. Obtain information from the patient about all prescribed and over-the-counter medications being taken. Tactfully ask questions about adherence to the medication regimen.

Hydration Status. Obtain the patient's baseline vital signs. Note a pulse that is bounding and full or irregular (i.e., indicating possible dysrhythmias); check the respiratory rate and quality; listen to the lung sounds to detect the presence of crackles; ask the patient about a history of recent weight gain or loss; assess for edema of the extremities; and assess for neck vein distention. Blood pressure may also be elevated.

Dehydration. Assess, report, and record significant signs of dehydration in the patient. Observe for inelastic skin turgor, sticky oral mucous membranes, a shrunken or deeply furrowed tongue, crusted lips, weight loss, deteriorating vital signs, soft or sunken eyeballs, weak pedal pulses, delayed capillary filling, excessive thirst, a high urine specific gravity (or no urine output), and possible mental confusion.

Skin turgor. Check the patient's skin turgor by gently pinching the skin together over the sternum, on the forehead, or on the forearm. Elasticity is present when the skin rapidly returns to a flat position in the well-hydrated patient. In dehydrated patients, the skin will remain in a peaked or pinched position and return very slowly to the flat, normal position. Skin turgor is not a reliable indicator in older adults because of the natural aging changes of the skin (see description under "Dehydration" above).

Oral mucous membranes. With adequate hydration, the membranes of the mouth feel smooth and glisten. With dehydration, they appear dull and are sticky. Assess skin turgor, oral mucosa, and firmness of eyeballs.

Laboratory changes. The patient's hematocrit, hemoglobin, blood urea nitrogen (BUN), creatinine, osmolality, and electrolytes will appear to fluctuate, based on the state of hydration. When the patient is overhydrated, the values appear to drop as a result of hemodilution. A dehydrated patient will show higher values because of hemoconcentration.

Overhydration. Increases in abdominal girth, weight gain, neck vein distention, and circumference of the medial malleolus indicate overhydration. Daily measurements should be obtained of the patient's abdominal girth at the umbilical level and the extremities bilaterally at a level approximately 5 cm above the medial malleolus. The development of crackles during lung auscultation is also a sign of overhydration, especially in patients with heart failure. Weigh the patient daily using the same scale, at the same time of day, with the patient wearing similar clothing.

Edema. *Edema* is a term used to describe excess fluid accumulation in the extracellular spaces, particularly in the lower limbs. Edema is considered "pitting" when an indentation remains in the tissue after pressure is exerted against a bony part, such as the shin, ankle, or sacrum. The degree is usually recorded as +1 (slight) to +4 (deep).

Pale, cool, tight, shiny skin is another sign of edema. Also listen to lung sounds to detect the presence of excess fluid (crackles) in the lungs.

Assess for the presence of edema and record the degree of pitting. Obtain a baseline measurement of abdominal girth when edema is present, and check for the presence of fluid waves in the abdomen.

Electrolyte imbalance. Because the symptoms of most electrolyte imbalances are similar, the nurse should obtain information related to changes in the patient's mental status (i.e., alertness, orientation, confusion), muscle strength, muscle cramps, tremors, nausea, and general appearance.

Susceptible people. Those who are particularly susceptible to the development of electrolyte disturbances frequently have a history of renal or cardiac disease, hormonal disorders, or massive trauma or burns, or are receiving diuretic or steroid therapy. Review the patient's available electrolyte studies.

Hypokalemia. This is indicated by a serum potassium (K^+) level of less than 3.5 mEq/L. Hypokalemia is especially likely to occur when a patient exhibits vomiting, diarrhea, or heavy diuresis. All diuretics, except the potassium-sparing type, are likely to cause hypokalemia.

Hyperkalemia. This is indicated by a serum potassium (K^+) level of more than 5.5 mEq/L. Hyperkalemia occurs most commonly when a patient is given excessive amounts of potassium supplementation, either intravenously or orally. It may also occur as an adverse effect of potassium-sparing diuretics or with renal disease.

Hyponatremia. This is indicated by a serum sodium (Na^+) level of less than 135 mEq/L. Remember the following phrase: "Where sodium goes, water goes." Because diuretics act by excreting sodium as well as water, monitor the patient for hyponatremia during and after diuresis.

Hypernatremia. This is indicated by a serum sodium (Na^+) level of more than 145 mEq/L. Hypernatremia occurs most frequently when a patient is given intravenous (IV) fluids in excess of the fluid excreted.

■ **Implementation**

Intake and Output. Intake and output (I&O) should be recorded accurately every shift and totaled every 24 hours for all patients having renal evaluations or receiving diuretics. Remember to administer diuretics in the morning whenever possible to prevent nocturia. Measure abdominal girth every shift, record degree of edema present in legs every shift, and obtain a daily weight.

Intake. Measure and record *accurately* all fluids taken (e.g., oral, parenteral, rectal, via tubes). Ice chips and foods such as gelatin that turn to a liquid state must be included. Irrigation solutions should be carefully measured so that the difference between what is instilled and what is returned can be recorded as intake.

Remember to enlist the help of the patient, family, and other visitors in this process. Ask them to keep a record of how many glasses or cups of liquids (e.g., water, juice, soda, tea, coffee) are consumed. The nurse then converts the household measurements to milliliters.

Nutrition. Patients with edema are routinely placed on a restricted sodium diet to help control edema associated with heart failure. Depending on the type of diuretic prescribed (potassium sparing or non–potassium sparing), the patient may be placed on potassium restrictions or potassium supplements.

Diet therapy for renal disease is directed at keeping a normal equilibrium of the body while decreasing the excretory load on the kidneys. See a nutrition text for modifications specific to acute and chronic renal failure.

Output. Record all output from the mouth, urethra, rectum, wounds, and tubes (e.g., surgical drains, nasogastric tubes, indwelling catheters). Liquid stools should be recorded according to consistency, color, and quantity. Urine output should include information on quantity, color, pH, odor, and specific gravity.

All other secretions should be characterized by color, consistency, volume, and changes from previous collections, if possible.

Daily output is usually 1200 to 1500 mL, or 30 to 50 mL/hr for the adult patient. Always report urine output below this hourly rate. Low hourly output may indicate dehydration, renal failure, or cardiac disease.

Keep the urinal or bedpan readily available. Tell patients and their visitors the importance of not dumping the bedpan or urinal. Instruct them to use the call light and allow the hospital personnel to empty and record all output.

Renal Diagnostics. Many laboratory tests are ordered throughout the treatment of renal dysfunction (e.g., BUN, serum creatinine, creatinine clearance, serum osmolalities, urine osmolalities). Plan schedules for appropriate timing of collections of blood and urine samples.

Serum Electrolytes. Monitor serum electrolyte reports; notify the healthcare provider of deviations from normal values.

Nutrition. Order a prescribed special diet, depending on the underlying pathologic condition. If fluid restrictions are prescribed, state the amount of fluid to be taken on each tray and the amount that may be taken orally each shift in the computer, and have this information posted at the head of the patient's bed.

▪ Patient Education
Purposes of Diuresis

- If the disease process is hypertension, stress the importance of following the prescribed methods to deal with emotions and the dietary and medicinal regimens that can control the disease (see discussion of the nursing process for hypertensive therapy in Chapter 22).
- Teach the patient and significant others the functional changes that are caused by hypertension and heart failure. Emphasize the need for lifelong treatment and adherence to drug therapy, diet, and exercise regimens to obtain maximum control of the disease process.
- Diuretics are used in the treatment of several disease processes—for example, hypertension, glaucoma, ascites, hypercalcemia, heart failure, and renal disease. Be certain that the patient understands the medication administration schedule and desired therapeutic outcome for the prescribed therapy.

Medication Considerations

- Diuretics should be taken in the morning to avoid nocturia.
- When the diuretic is prescribed on a scheduled pattern other than daily, assist the patient with developing ways to remember when to take the medication (e.g., using a calendar on which to mark dosages or using a medication holder marked with the days of the week that is loaded weekly with the medications to be taken).
- Instruct the patient to perform daily weights using the same scale, in similar clothing, and at the same time daily, usually before breakfast. Record and report significant weight changes because weight gains and losses are the best indicator of fluid loss or gain. Usually a gain of 2 pounds in 2 days should be reported.
- Potassium supplements may be prescribed concurrently with diuretics other than potassium-sparing diuretics.
- Diuretic therapy may produce postural hypotension. Teach the patient to rise slowly from a supine or sitting position, and encourage the patient to sit or lie down if feeling faint.

Nutrition

- The healthcare provider usually prescribes dietary modifications appropriate to the underlying pathologic condition, such as weight reduction or sodium restriction.
- Patients receiving potassium-sparing diuretics should be taught which foods are high in potassium content. These foods should be moderately restricted but not withheld from the diet. Salt substitutes should be avoided because they are high in potassium.
- When taking diuretics other than the potassium-sparing type, the patient is required to eat potassium-rich foods.

Fostering Health Maintenance

- Throughout the course of treatment, discuss medication information and how it will benefit the patient. Stress the importance of nonpharmacologic interventions and the long-term effects that compliance with the treatment regimen can provide.
- Provide the patient and significant others with important information contained in the specific drug monograph for the medicines prescribed. Additional health teaching and nursing interventions for the common and serious adverse effects are described in the drug monographs that follow.
- Seek cooperation and understanding of the following points so that medication compliance is increased: name of medication, dosage, route, times of administration, and common and serious adverse effects.

Patient Self-Assessment. Enlist the patient's aid in developing and maintaining a written record of monitoring parameters (see Patient Self-Assessment Form for Diuretics on the Evolve website). Complete the Pre-medication Data column for use as a baseline to track response to drug therapy. Ensure that the patient understands how to use the form, and instruct the patient to bring the completed form to follow-up visits. During follow-up visits, focus on issues that will foster adherence with the therapeutic interventions prescribed.

DRUG CLASS: CARBONIC ANHYDRASE INHIBITOR

acetazolamide (ă-sē-tă-ZOL-ă-mīd)
  Diamox (Dī-ă-mŏks)

ACTIONS

Acetazolamide is a weak diuretic that acts by inhibiting the enzyme carbonic anhydrase in the kidney, brain, and eye. As a diuretic, it promotes the excretion of sodium, potassium, water, and bicarbonate.

USES

Acetazolamide is not used frequently as a diuretic because of the availability of more effective medications.

However, it is used to reduce intraocular pressure in patients with glaucoma (Chapter 42).

DRUG CLASS: SULFONAMIDE-TYPE LOOP DIURETICS

ACTIONS

The loop diuretics are potent diuretics that act primarily by inhibiting sodium and chloride reabsorption from the ascending limb of the **loop of Henle** in the kidneys enhancing sodium, potassium, chloride, phosphate, magnesium, and bicarbonate excretion into the urine.

Furosemide also acts to increase renal blood flow and glomerular filtration rate and inhibits electrolyte absorption in the proximal and distal tubule. The maximum diuretic effect occurs 1 to 2 hours after oral administration and lasts for 4 to 6 hours. (The brand name "Lasix" is derived from "lasts six hours.") Diuresis occurs 5 to 10 minutes after IV administration, peaks within 30 minutes, and lasts approximately 2 hours.

Bumetanide also acts by increasing renal blood flow into the glomeruli and inhibiting electrolyte absorption in the proximal tubule, but does not act on the distal tubule. Its diuretic activity starts 30 to 60 minutes after oral administration, peaks within 1 to 2 hours, and lasts 4 to 6 hours. Following intravenous injection, diuresis begins within minutes and reaches maximum levels in 15 to 30 minutes.

Torsemide does not appear to affect glomerular filtration rate, renal blood flow or block reabsorption of sodium from the proximal or distal tubules. Maximum diuretic effect occurs 1 to 2 hours after oral administration and lasts 6 to 8 hours. Diuresis occurs 5 to 10 minutes after IV administration, peaks within 60 minutes, and lasts up to 6 hours.

USES

Bumetanide, furosemide, and torsemide are used to treat edema resulting from heart failure, cirrhosis of the liver, and renal disease, including nephrotic syndrome. Furosemide and torsemide may also be used for the treatment of hypertension, alone or in combination with other antihypertensive therapy. Furosemide is also used in combination with 0.9% sodium chloride infusions to enhance the excretion of calcium in patients with hypercalcemia and to treat edema and heart failure.

THERAPEUTIC OUTCOME

The primary therapeutic outcome associated with sulfonamide loop diuretic therapy is diuresis, with reduction of edema and improvement in symptoms related to excessive fluid accumulation. Reduction of blood pressure is an outcome also expected of furosemide and torsemide.

❖ NURSING IMPLICATIONS FOR SULFONAMIDE-TYPE LOOP DIURETICS

■ Premedication Assessment

1. Obtain baseline data such as vital signs, lung sounds, weight, degree of edema present, and laboratory studies (e.g., serum electrolytes, liver and renal function tests) before initiating therapy.
2. Obtain data relating to the patient's mental status (orientation, alertness, confusion), muscle strength, muscle cramps, tremors, nausea, and general appearance.
3. Patients with diabetes require baseline measurement of blood glucose levels.
4. Check for symptoms of acute gout. If present, notify the healthcare provider.
5. Note any reduction in hearing.

■ Availability

See Table 28-1.

■ Dosage and Administration

Adult: PO: Do not exceed the maximum dosages identified in Table 28-1. Administer with food or milk to reduce gastric irritation. *Do not* administer after midafternoon to prevent nocturia.

Table 28-1   Sulfonamide-Type Loop Diuretics

GENERIC NAME	BRAND NAME	DOSAGE FORMS AVAILABLE	DOSAGE RANGE
bumetanide	—	Tablets: 0.5, 1, 2 mg Injection: 0.25 mg/mL in 2-, 4-, and 10-mL vials	0.5-10 mg
furosemide ⇄ *Do not confuse furosemide with famotidine, fluoxetine, fosinopril, or minoxidil.*	Lasix ⇄ *Do not confuse Lasix with Lanoxin or Luvox.*	Tablets: 20, 40, 80 mg Oral solution: 8, 10 mg/mL IV: 10 mg/mL in 2-, 4-, and 10-mL vials	20-600 mg
torsemide ⇄ *Do not confuse torsemide with topiramate.*	Demadex ⇄ *Do not confuse Demadex with Demerol.*	Tablets: 5, 10, 20, and 100 mg Injection: 10 mg/mL in 2- and 5-mL vials	5-200 mg

Adult: IM or IV:

- Bumetanide: The IV and oral doses are equivalent. Administer IV doses over 1 to 2 minutes.
- Furosemide: The IV dose is half the oral dose. Administer slowly over 2 to 4 minutes.

■ Common Adverse Effects

Gastrointestinal

Oral irritation, dry mouth. Start regular oral hygiene measures when the therapy is initiated. Suggest the use of 1 teaspoon of hydrogen peroxide in 6 to 8 ounces of water as a mouthwash. Commercial mouthwashes contain alcohol, which may cause further drying and oral irritation. Another method to alleviate dryness is sucking on ice chips or hard candy.

Cardiovascular

Orthostatic hypotension. Although **orthostatic hypotension** (e.g., dizziness, weakness, faintness associated with a drop in blood pressure) is infrequent and generally mild, all diuretics may cause it to some degree, particularly when therapy is being initiated. Monitor the blood pressure daily in both the supine and standing positions. Anticipate the development of postural hypotension, and take measures to prevent an occurrence. Teach the patient to rise slowly from a supine or sitting position, and encourage the patient to sit or lie down if feeling faint.

■ Serious Adverse Effects

Gastrointestinal

Gastric irritation, abdominal pain. If gastric irritation occurs, administer with food or milk. If symptoms persist or increase in severity, report for physician evaluation.

Metabolic, Renal

Electrolyte imbalance, dehydration. The electrolytes most commonly altered are potassium (K^+), sodium (Na^+), and chloride (Cl^-). Hypokalemia and hyponatremia are most likely to occur. Many symptoms associated with fluid and **electrolyte imbalance** are subtle and interspersed with general symptoms of drug toxicity or the disease process itself. Gather data about changes in the patient's mental status (alertness, orientation, confusion), muscle strength, muscle cramps, tremors, nausea, and general appearance. Always check the electrolyte reports for early indications of electrolyte imbalance. Keep accurate records of I&O, daily weights, and vital signs.

Hyperuricemia. Furosemide may inhibit the excretion of uric acid, resulting in **hyperuricemia**. Patients who have had previous attacks of gouty arthritis are particularly susceptible to additional attacks as a result of hyperuricemia. Monitor the laboratory reports for early indications of hyperuricemia. Report this to the healthcare provider, who may then add a uricosuric agent or allopurinol to the patient's medication regimen.

Hyperglycemia. Diabetic or prediabetic patients must be monitored for the development of hyperglycemia, particularly during the early weeks of therapy. Assess regularly for hyperglycemia with a fingerstick blood sample and home glucometer, and report if it occurs with any frequency. Patients receiving oral hypoglycemic agents or insulin may require an adjustment in dosage.

Hypersensitivity

Hives, pruritus, rash. Report symptoms for further evaluation by the healthcare provider. Pruritus may be relieved by adding baking soda to the bath water.

 Medication Safety Alert

Patients who are allergic to sulfonamides may also be allergic to sulfonamide-type loop diuretics. Use cautiously in these patients.

■ Drug Interactions

Alcohol, Sedative Hypnotics, Narcotics. Orthostatic hypotension associated with sulfonamide-type loop diuretic therapy may be aggravated by these agents.

Digoxin. Sulfonamide-type loop diuretics may cause excessive potassium excretion, leading to hypokalemia. If the patient is also receiving digoxin, monitor closely for digitalis toxicity (anorexia, nausea, fatigue, blurred or colored vision, bradycardia, dysrhythmias).

 Clinical Goldmine

Remember, low potassium levels may cause digitalis toxicity. **Always check potassium levels for patients receiving diuretics prior to administration of digoxin.**

Aminoglycosides. The potential for ototoxicity from the aminoglycosides (e.g., gentamicin, tobramycin, amikacin) is increased. Assess the patient for gradual, often subtle, changes in hearing. Note whether the patient seems to speak more loudly, asks for statements to be repeated, or turns the television or radio progressively louder.

Cisplatin. The potential for ototoxicity from the combination of cisplatin and the sulfonamide-type loop diuretics is increased. Assess the patient for gradual, often subtle, changes in hearing. Note whether the patient seems to speak more loudly, asks for statements to be repeated, or turns the television or radio progressively louder.

Nonsteroidal Antiinflammatory Drugs. Nonsteroidal antiinflammatory drugs (NSAIDs) (e.g., indomethacin, ibuprofen, naproxen) inhibit the diuretic activity of the sulfonamide-type loop diuretics. The dose of diuretic may have to be increased or the NSAID discontinued. Maintain accurate I&O records and monitor for a decrease in diuretic activity.

Corticosteroids. Corticosteroids (e.g., prednisone) may enhance the loss of potassium. Check potassium levels and monitor more closely for hypokalemia when these two agents are used concurrently.

Metolazone. When used concurrently, there is a considerably greater diuresis than when either agent is used alone. Monitor closely for dehydration and electrolyte imbalance.

---

ethacrynic acid (ĕth-ă-KRIN-ĭk)
Edecrin (Ĕ-dĕ-krĭn)

ACTIONS

Ethacrynic acid is another diuretic that acts primarily on the ascending limb of the loop of Henle but also the proximal and distal tubules to prevent sodium and chloride reabsorption. Ethacrynic acid does not appear to affect renal blood flow or the glomerular filtration rate. Its diuretic activity begins within 30 minutes, peaks in approximately 2 hours, and lasts 6 to 8 hours.

USES

Ethacrynic acid is used to treat edema resulting from heart failure, cirrhosis of the liver, renal disease, and malignancy and for hospitalized pediatric patients with congenital heart disease. It is thought that because ethacrynic acid inhibits the reabsorption of sodium to a much greater extent than other diuretics, it may be more effective for patients with significant renal failure. It is also used in conjunction with 0.9% sodium chloride infusions to enhance excretion of calcium in patients with hypercalcemia.

THERAPEUTIC OUTCOME

The primary therapeutic outcome associated with ethacrynic acid therapy is diuresis with reduction of edema and improvement in symptoms related to excessive fluid accumulation.

❖ NURSING IMPLICATIONS FOR ETHACRYNIC ACID

■ Premedication Assessment

1. Obtain baseline data such as vital signs, lung sounds, weight, degree of edema present, and laboratory studies (e.g., serum electrolytes, liver and renal function tests) before initiating therapy.
2. Obtain data relating to the patient's mental status (orientation, alertness, confusion), muscle strength, muscle cramps, tremors, nausea, and general appearance.
3. Patients with diabetes require baseline measurement of blood glucose levels.

■ Availability

PO: 25-mg tablets; *IV:* 50 mg/vial.

■ Dosage and Administration

Adult: PO: 50 to 100 mg initially, followed by 50 to 200 mg daily. *Do not* exceed 400 mg/day. Administer with food or milk to reduce gastric irritation. *Do not* administer after midafternoon to prevent nocturia.

Adult: IV: 50 mg or 0.5 to 1 mg/kg. Add 50 mL of dextrose 5% or saline solution to 50 mg of ethacrynic acid. This solution is stable for 24 hours. Administer over several minutes through the tubing of a running infusion or by direct IV line. Occasionally, the addition of a diluent may result in a cloudy solution. These solutions should not be used. Do not mix with blood derivatives.

Pediatric: PO: 1 mg/kg PO once daily. May increase up to 3 mg/kg/day PO. Adjust dosage at intervals of 2 to 3 days. Always monitor vital signs and I&O at regular intervals when administering this agent intravenously. Report blood pressure that decreases steadily or a narrowing pulse pressure, which may indicate hypovolemia.

■ Common Adverse Effects
Cardiovascular

Orthostatic hypotension. Although this effect is infrequent and generally mild, all diuretics may cause some degree of orthostatic hypotension (dizziness, weakness, faintness associated with a drop in blood pressure), particularly when therapy is initiated or dosages are increased. Monitor the blood pressure daily in both the supine and standing positions. Anticipate the development of postural hypotension and take measures to prevent its occurrence. Teach the patient to rise slowly from a supine or sitting position, and encourage the patient to sit or lie down if feeling faint.

■ Serious Adverse Effects
Metabolic, Renal

Electrolyte imbalance, dehydration. The electrolytes most commonly altered are potassium (K^+), sodium (Na^+), and chloride (Cl^-). Hypokalemia and hyponatremia are most likely to occur. Many symptoms associated with electrolyte imbalance are subtle and interspersed with general symptoms of drug toxicity or the disease process itself. Gather data about changes in the patient's mental status (alertness, orientation, confusion), muscle strength, muscle cramps, tremors, nausea, and general appearance. Always check the electrolyte reports for early indications of electrolyte imbalance. Keep accurate records of I&O, daily weights, and vital signs.

Dizziness, deafness, tinnitus. People with impaired renal function may experience these symptoms. Assess the patient for gradual, often subtle, changes in balance and hearing. Note whether the patient seems more unsteady when standing, speaks loudly, asks for statements to be repeated, or turns the television or radio progressively louder.

Gastrointestinal

Gastrointestinal bleeding. Observe for coffee-ground vomitus or dark tarry stools, particularly in patients receiving IV therapy.

Diarrhea. Diarrhea may become severe. Report to the healthcare provider, and monitor the patient for dehydration and fluid and electrolyte imbalance.

Endocrine

Hyperglycemia. Diabetic or prediabetic patients must be monitored for the development of hyperglycemia, particularly during the early weeks of therapy. Assess regularly for hyperglycemia with a fingerstick blood sample and a glucometer, and report if it occurs with any frequency. Patients receiving oral hypoglycemic agents or insulin may require an adjustment in dosage.

■ **Drug Interactions**

Aminoglycosides. The potential for ototoxicity from the aminoglycosides (e.g., gentamicin, tobramycin, amikacin) is increased. Assess the patient for gradual, often subtle, changes in hearing. Note whether the patient seems to speak loudly, asks for statements to be repeated, or turns the television or radio progressively louder.

Nonsteroidal Antiinflammatory Drugs. Nonsteroidal antiinflammatory drugs (e.g., indomethacin, ibuprofen, naproxen) inhibit the diuretic activity of ethacrynic acid. The dose of ethacrynic acid may have to be increased or the NSAID discontinued. Maintain accurate I&O records, and monitor for a decrease in diuretic activity.

Digoxin. Ethacrynic acid may cause excess potassium excretion, leading to hypokalemia. If the patient is also receiving digoxin, monitor closely for digitalis toxicity (anorexia, nausea, fatigue, blurred or colored vision, bradycardia, dysrhythmias).

Corticosteroids. Corticosteroids (e.g., prednisone) may enhance the loss of potassium. Check potassium levels and monitor more closely for hypokalemia when these two agents are used concurrently.

DRUG CLASS: THIAZIDE DIURETICS

ACTIONS

Benzothiadiazides, more commonly called thiazides, have been an important and useful class of diuretic and antihypertensive agents since the 1960s. As diuretics, thiazides act primarily on the distal tubules of the kidney to block the reabsorption of sodium and chloride ions from the tubule. The sodium and chloride ions that are not reabsorbed are passed into the collecting ducts, taking molecules of water with them, resulting in a diuresis.

USES

Thiazides are used as diuretics in the treatment of edema associated with heart failure, renal disease, hepatic disease, pregnancy, obesity, premenstrual syndrome, and administration of adrenocortical steroids. The antihypertensive properties of thiazides result from a direct vasodilatory action on the peripheral arterioles (see Chapter 22). Thiazide diuretics tend to lose their diuretic action after about 6 weeks of therapy, but the antihypertensive properties continue. Thiazide diuretics also tend to lose their diuretic effect when creatinine clearance is less than 30 mL/minute.

THERAPEUTIC OUTCOMES

The primary therapeutic outcomes associated with thiazide therapy are diuresis with reduction of edema and improvement in symptoms related to excessive fluid accumulation, and reduction in elevated blood pressure.

❖ **NURSING IMPLICATIONS FOR THIAZIDE DIURETICS**

■ **Premedication Assessment**

1. Obtain baseline data such as vital signs, lung sounds, weight, degree of edema present, and laboratory studies (e.g., serum electrolytes, liver and renal function tests) before initiating therapy.
2. Obtain data relating to the patient's mental status (orientation, alertness, confusion), muscle strength, muscle cramps, tremors, nausea, and general appearance.
3. Patients with diabetes require baseline measurement of blood glucose levels.
4. Note any reduction in hearing.
5. Check for any symptoms of acute gout. If present, notify the physician.

■ **Availability**

Tables 28-2 and 28-3 list thiazide diuretics and diuretics chemically related to the thiazides. Most of the diuretics listed are administered in divided daily dosages for the treatment of hypertension. However, a single daily dosage may be most effective for mobilization of edema fluid.

■ **Dosage and Administration**

See Tables 28-2 and 28-3. Administer with food or milk to reduce gastric irritation. *Do not* administer after midafternoon to prevent nocturia.

■ **Common Adverse Effects**

Cardiovascular

Orthostatic hypotension. Although orthostatic hypotension (dizziness, weakness, faintness associated with a drop in blood pressure) is infrequent and generally mild, all diuretics may cause some degree of orthostatic hypotension, particularly when therapy is being initiated. Monitor the blood pressure daily in both the supine and standing positions. Anticipate the development of postural hypotension, and take measures to prevent it. Teach the patient to rise slowly from a supine or sitting position, and encourage the patient to sit or lie down if feeling faint.

■ **Serious Adverse Effects**

Gastrointestinal

Gastric irritation, nausea, vomiting, constipation. If gastric irritation occurs, administer with food or milk.

Table 28-2 Thiazide Diuretics

GENERIC NAME	BRAND NAME	DOSAGE FORMS AVAILABLE	DOSAGE RANGE
chlorothiazide	Diuril	Tablets: 250, 500 mg Oral suspension: 250 mg/5 mL Injection: 500 mg/20 mL	500 to 1000 mg once or twice daily
hydrochlorothiazide ⇄ Do not confuse hydrochlorothiazide with hydroxychloroquine.	HydroDIURIL	Tablets: 12.5, 25, 50 mg Capsules: 12.5 mg	12.5-200 mg
methyclothiazide	—	Tablets: 5 mg	2.5-10 mg

Table 28-3 Thiazide-Related Diuretics

GENERIC NAME	BRAND NAME	DOSAGE FORMS AVAILABLE	DOSAGE RANGE
chlorthalidone ⇄ Do not confuse chlorthalidone with chlorpromazine or chlorothiazide.		Tablets: 25, 50, 100 mg	50-200 mg
indapamide	—	Tablets: 1.25, 2.5 mg	2.5-5 mg
metolazone ⇄ Do not confuse metolazone with medroxyprogesterone, metaxalone, methotrexate, metoclopramide, or metoprolol.	Zaroxolyn ⇄ Do not confuse Zaroxolyn with Zyprexa.	Tablets: 2.5, 5, 10 mg	2.5-10 mg

If symptoms persist or increase in severity, report to the healthcare provider for evaluation.

Metabolic, Renal

Electrolyte imbalance, dehydration. Use of thiazides may cause or aggravate electrolyte imbalance; therefore patients should be observed regularly for signs such as dry mouth, drowsiness, confusion, muscular weakness, and nausea. The electrolytes most commonly altered are potassium (K^+), sodium (Na^+), and chloride (Cl^-). Hypokalemia is most likely to occur, and supplementary potassium is often prescribed to prevent or treat it. Many symptoms associated with altered fluid and electrolyte balance are subtle and interspersed with general symptoms of drug toxicity or the disease process itself. Gather data about changes in the patient's mental status (alertness, orientation, confusion), muscle strength, muscle cramps, tremors, nausea, and general appearance. Always check the electrolyte reports for early indications of electrolyte imbalance. Keep accurate records of I&O, daily weights, and vital signs.

Hyperuricemia. The plasma uric acid level is frequently elevated by the thiazides, which inhibit the excretion of uric acid. Patients who have had previous episodes of hyperuricemia or attacks of gouty arthritis are particularly susceptible to additional attacks when receiving thiazide therapy. Monitor the laboratory reports for early indications of hyperuricemia. Report to the healthcare provider, who may then add a uricosuric agent or allopurinol to the patient's medication regimen.

Endocrine

Hyperglycemia. The thiazides may induce hyperglycemia and aggravate cases of preexisting diabetes mellitus. Diabetic or prediabetic patients must be monitored for the development of hyperglycemia, particularly during the early weeks of therapy. Assess regularly for hyperglycemia using a fingerstick blood sample and glucometer, and report if it occurs with any frequency. Dosages of oral hypoglycemic agents and insulin may need adjustment in patients with diabetes mellitus who also require diuretic therapy.

Hypersensitivity

Hives, pruritus, rash. Report symptoms for further evaluation by the healthcare provider. Pruritus may be relieved by adding baking soda to the bath water.

▪ Drug Interactions

Digoxin. Thiazide diuretics may cause excessive excretion of potassium, resulting in hypokalemia. If the patient is also receiving digoxin, monitor closely for signs of digitalis toxicity (e.g., anorexia, nausea, fatigue, blurred or colored vision, bradycardia, dysrhythmias).

Corticosteroids. Corticosteroids (e.g., prednisone) may enhance the loss of potassium. Check potassium levels and monitor more closely for hypokalemia when these two agents are used concurrently.

Lithium. Thiazide diuretics may induce lithium toxicity. Monitor patients for lithium toxicity manifested by nausea, anorexia, fine tremors, persistent vomiting, profuse diarrhea, hyperreflexia, lethargy, and weakness.

Nonsteroidal Antiinflammatory Drugs. Nonsteroidal antiinflammatory drugs (e.g., indomethacin, ibuprofen, naproxen) inhibit the diuretic activity of this agent. The dose of thiazide may have to be increased or the NSAID discontinued. Maintain accurate I&O records, and monitor for a decrease in diuretic activity.

Oral Hypoglycemic Agents, Insulin. Because of the hyperglycemic effects of the thiazide diuretics, dosage adjustments of insulin and oral hypoglycemic agents are often required.

DRUG CLASS: POTASSIUM-SPARING DIURETICS

amiloride (ă-MIL-ōr-īd)
Midamor (MĪ-dă-mōr)

ACTIONS

Amiloride is a potassium-sparing diuretic that also has weak antihypertensive activity. Its mechanism of action is unknown, but it acts at the distal renal tubule to retain potassium and excrete sodium, resulting in a mild diuresis.

USES

Amiloride is usually used in combination with other diuretics in patients with hypertension or heart failure to help prevent hypokalemia that may result from other diuretic therapy.

THERAPEUTIC OUTCOME

The primary therapeutic outcome associated with amiloride therapy is diuresis with reduction of edema and improvement in symptoms related to excessive fluid accumulation.

❖ NURSING IMPLICATIONS FOR AMILORIDE

- **Premedication Assessment**
1. Obtain baseline data such as vital signs, lung sounds, weight, degree of edema present, and laboratory studies (e.g., serum electrolytes, liver and renal function tests) before initiating therapy.
2. Obtain data relating to the patient's mental status (orientation, alertness, confusion), muscle strength, muscle cramps, tremors, nausea, and general appearance.

- **Availability**
PO: 5-mg tablets.

- **Dosage and Administration**
Adult: *PO:* Initially, 5 mg daily. Dosages may be increased in 5-mg increments up to 20 mg daily with close monitoring of electrolytes. Administer with food or milk to reduce gastric irritation. *Do not* administer after midafternoon to prevent nocturia.

- **Common Adverse Effects**
Gastrointestinal
Anorexia, nausea, vomiting, flatulence. These adverse effects should be mild, particularly if the dose is administered with food. Persistent nausea and vomiting should be evaluated for other causes, as well as for the development of electrolyte imbalance.
Neurologic
Headache. Monitor the blood pressure at regularly scheduled intervals because amiloride is used for hypertension. Additional readings should be taken during headaches to determine if headaches are caused by the agents or by hypertension. Report persistent headaches.

- **Serious Adverse Effects**
Metabolic, Cardiovascular
Electrolyte imbalance, dehydration. The electrolytes most commonly altered are potassium (K⁺), sodium (Na⁺), and chloride (Cl⁻). Hyperkalemia is most likely to occur. Report potassium levels higher than 5 mEq/L. Many symptoms associated with altered fluid and electrolyte balance are subtle and interspersed with general symptoms of drug toxicity or the disease process itself. Gather data about changes in the patient's mental status (alertness, orientation, confusion), muscle strength, muscle cramps, tremors, nausea, and general appearance. Always check the electrolyte reports for early indications of electrolyte imbalance. Keep accurate records of I&O, daily weights, and vital signs.

- **Drug Interactions**
Lithium. Amiloride may induce lithium toxicity. Monitor patients who take lithium for lithium toxicity as manifested by nausea, anorexia, fine tremors, persistent vomiting, profuse diarrhea, hyperreflexia, lethargy, and weakness.
Potassium Supplements, Salt Substitutes. Amiloride inhibits potassium excretion. *Do not* administer with potassium supplements or use salt substitutes high in potassium because of the potentially dangerous effects of hyperkalemia.
Hyperkalemia. Angiotensin-converting enzyme (ACE) inhibitors (e.g., captopril, lisinopril, ramipril), angiotensin II receptor blockers (ARBs; e.g., losartan, candesartan) and aldosterone receptor blocking agents (e.g., eplerenone, spironolactone) inhibit aldosterone. Patients may develop hyperkalemia (K⁺ above 5.7 mEq/L). Most cases resolve without discontinuation of therapy. Patients most susceptible to the development of hyperkalemia are those with renal impairment or diabetes mellitus and those already receiving a potassium supplement. In general,

potassium-sparing diuretics (e.g., amiloride, triamterene) should not be taken concurrently with these antihypertensive agents.

Nonsteroidal Antiinflammatory Drugs. Nonsteroidal antiinflammatory drugs (e.g., indomethacin, ibuprofen, naproxen) inhibit the diuretic activity of amiloride. The dose of amiloride may have to be increased or the NSAID discontinued. Maintain accurate I&O records and monitor for a decrease in diuretic activity.

---

spironolactone (spī-rō-nō-LĂK-tōn)
Aldactone (ăl-DĂK-tōn)

ACTIONS

Spironolactone blocks the sodium-retaining and potassium-excreting and magnesium-excreting properties of aldosterone, resulting in a loss of water with the increased sodium excretion.

USES

Spironolactone is a diuretic that is particularly useful in relieving edema and ascites that do not respond to the usual diuretics. It may be given with thiazide diuretics to increase its effect and reduce the hypokalemia often induced by the thiazides. Spironolactone has also been shown to further reduce morbidity and mortality for patients with heart failure who are also being treated with an ACE inhibitor and a loop diuretic.

THERAPEUTIC OUTCOME

The primary therapeutic outcome associated with spironolactone therapy is diuresis, with reduction of edema and improvement in symptoms related to excessive fluid accumulation and heart failure.

❖ NURSING IMPLICATIONS FOR SPIRONOLACTONE

■ **Premedication Assessment**
1. Obtain baseline data such as vital signs, lung sounds, weight, degree of edema present, and laboratory studies (e.g., serum electrolytes, liver and renal function tests) before initiating therapy.
2. Obtain data relating to the patient's mental status (orientation, alertness, confusion), muscle strength, muscle cramps, tremors, nausea, and general appearance.
3. Tactfully ask about any preexisting problems with libido.

■ **Availability**
PO: 25-, 50-, and 100-mg tablets.

■ **Dosage and Administration**
Adult: PO: Initially, 100 mg daily. Maintenance dosage is usually 25 to 200 mg daily, but doses up to 400 mg may be prescribed. Administer with food or milk to reduce gastric irritation. *Do not* administer after midafternoon to prevent nocturia.
Pediatric: PO: 1.5 to 3.3 mg/kg/day in divided doses every 6 to 24 hours. Readjust the dosage every 3 to 5 days.

■ **Common and Serious Adverse Effects**
Neurologic
Mental confusion. Perform a baseline assessment of the patient's alertness; drowsiness; lethargy; and orientation to time, date, and place before starting drug therapy. Compare subsequent mental status and assess on a regular basis.

Headache. Monitor blood pressure at regularly scheduled intervals because this agent is used for hypertension. Additional readings should be taken during headaches to determine if headaches are caused by the agent or the hypertension. Report persistent headaches.

Gastrointestinal
Diarrhea. The onset of new symptoms occurring after initiating the drug therapy requires evaluation if persistent.

Metabolic
Electrolyte imbalance, dehydration. The electrolytes most commonly altered are potassium (K^+), sodium (Na^+), and chloride (Cl^-). Hyperkalemia is most likely to occur. Report potassium levels higher than 5 mEq/L. Many symptoms associated with altered fluid and electrolyte balance are subtle and interspersed with general symptoms of drug toxicity or the disease process itself. Gather data about changes in the patient's mental status (alertness, orientation, confusion), muscle strength, muscle cramps, tremors, nausea, and general appearance. Always check the electrolyte reports for early indications of electrolyte imbalance. Keep accurate records of I&O, daily weights, and vital signs.

Endocrine
Gynecomastia, reduced libido, breast tenderness. Because the chemical structure of spironolactone is similar to that of estrogen hormones, an occasional male patient will report gynecomastia, reduced libido, and diminished erection. Women may complain of breast soreness and menstrual irregularities. These effects are reversible after therapy is discontinued.

■ **Drug Interactions**
Potassium Supplements, Salt Substitutes. Spironolactone inhibits potassium excretion. *Do not* administer with potassium supplements or use salt substitutes high in potassium because of potentially dangerous effects from hyperkalemia.

Hyperkalemia. Angiotensin-converting enzyme inhibitors (e.g., captopril, lisinopril, ramipril), ARBs (e.g., losartan, candesartan), and aldosterone receptor blocking agents (e.g., eplerenone, spironolactone) inhibit aldosterone. Patients may develop hyperkalemia (K^+ above 5.7 mEq/L). Most cases resolve without discontinuation of therapy. Patients most susceptible to the development of hyperkalemia are those with renal impairment or diabetes mellitus and those already receiving a potassium supplement. In general, potassium-sparing diuretics should not be taken concurrently with these antihypertensive agents.

Nonsteroidal Antiinflammatory Drugs. Nonsteroidal antiinflammatory drugs (e.g., indomethacin, ibuprofen, naproxen) inhibit the diuretic activity of spironolactone. The dosage of spironolactone may have to be increased or the NSAID discontinued. Maintain accurate I&O records and monitor for a decrease in diuretic activity.

---

triamterene (trī-ĂM-tĕr-ēn)
Dyrenium (dī-RĒ-nē-ŭm)

ACTIONS

Triamterene is a very mild diuretic that acts by blocking the exchange of potassium for sodium in the distal tubule of the kidney, resulting in retention of potassium with excretion of sodium and water.

USES

Triamterene is an effective agent to use in conjunction with the potassium-excreting diuretics, such as the thiazides, and the loop diuretics.

THERAPEUTIC OUTCOME

The primary therapeutic outcome associated with triamterene therapy is diuresis with reduction of edema and improvement in symptoms related to excessive fluid accumulation.

❖ NURSING IMPLICATIONS FOR TRIAMTERENE

▪ Premedication Assessment

1. Obtain baseline data such as vital signs, lung sounds, weight, degree of edema present, laboratory studies (e.g., serum electrolytes, liver and renal function tests) before initiating therapy.
2. Obtain data relating to the patient's mental status (orientation, alertness, confusion), muscle strength, muscle cramps, tremors, nausea, and general appearance.

▪ Availability

PO: 50- and 100-mg capsules.

▪ Dosage and Administration

Adult: PO: 50 to 100 mg twice daily. Maximum: 300 mg daily in divided doses.

▪ Common and Serious Adverse Effects

Metabolic

Electrolyte imbalance, dehydration, leg cramps, weakness. The electrolytes most commonly altered are potassium (K^+), sodium (Na^+), and chloride (Cl^-). Hyperkalemia is most likely to occur. Report potassium levels higher than 5 mEq/L. Many symptoms associated with altered fluid and electrolyte balance are subtle and interspersed with general symptoms of drug toxicity or the disease process itself. Gather data about changes in the patient's mental status (alertness, orientation, confusion), muscle strength, muscle cramps, tremors, nausea, and general appearance (drowsy, anxious, lethargic). Always check the electrolyte reports for early indications of electrolyte imbalance. Keep accurate records of I&O, daily weights, and vital signs.

Gastrointestinal

Nausea, vomiting. These adverse effects should be mild, particularly if the dose is administered with food. Persistent nausea and vomiting should be evaluated for other causes, as well as for the development of electrolyte imbalance.

Hypersensitivity

Hives, pruritus, rash. Report symptoms for further evaluation by the prescriber. Pruritus may be relieved by adding baking soda to the bath water.

▪ Drug Interactions

Salt Substitutes, Potassium Supplements. Triamterene inhibits potassium excretion. *Do not* administer with potassium supplements or use salt substitutes high in potassium because of the potentially dangerous effects from hyperkalemia.

Hyperkalemia. Angiotensin-converting enzyme inhibitors (e.g., captopril, lisinopril, ramipril), ARBs (e.g., losartan, candesartan), and aldosterone receptor blocking agents (e.g., eplerenone, spironolactone) inhibit aldosterone. Patients may develop hyperkalemia (K^+ above 5.7 mEq/L). Most cases resolve without discontinuation of therapy. Patients most susceptible to the development of hyperkalemia are those with renal impairment or diabetes mellitus and those already receiving a potassium supplement. In general, potassium-sparing diuretics should not be taken concurrently with these antihypertensive agents.

Nonsteroidal Antiinflammatory Drugs. Nonsteroidal antiinflammatory drugs (e.g., indomethacin, ibuprofen, naproxen) inhibit the diuretic activity of triamterene. The dosage of triamterene may have to be increased or the NSAID discontinued. Maintain accurate I&O records and monitor for a decrease in diuretic activity.

DRUG CLASS: COMBINATION DIURETIC PRODUCTS

A common problem associated with thiazide diuretic therapy is hypokalemia. In an attempt to minimize this adverse effect, several products have been manufactured that contain a potassium-sparing diuretic

Table 28-4 Combination Diuretics

GENERIC NAME	BRAND NAME	DOSAGE RANGE
spironolactone 25 mg, hydrochlorothiazide 25 mg	Aldactazide-25	1-8 tablets daily
spironolactone 50 mg, hydrochlorothiazide 50 mg	Aldactazide-50	1-4 tablets daily
triamterene 37.5 mg, hydrochlorothiazide 25 mg	Dyazide	1 or 2 capsules twice daily after meals
triamterene 37.5 mg, hydrochlorothiazide 25 mg	Maxzide-25 mg	1 or 2 tablets twice daily after meals
triamterene 50 mg, hydrochlorothiazide 25 mg	—	1 or 2 capsules once or twice daily after a meal
triamterene 75 mg, hydrochlorothiazide 50 mg	Maxzide	1 tablet daily
amiloride 5 mg, hydrochlorothiazide 50 mg	Moduretic	1 or 2 tablets daily with meals

with a thiazide diuretic (Table 28-4). The goal of the combination products is to promote diuresis and antihypertensive effect through different mechanisms of action while maintaining normal serum potassium levels. Patients receiving a combination product are at risk for adverse effects resulting from any of the component drugs. Many cases of hyperkalemia and hyponatremia have been reported after the use of the combination products.

Combination products should not be used as initial therapy for edema or hypertension. Therapy with individual products should be adjusted for each patient. If the fixed combination represents the appropriate dosage for each component, the use of a combination product may be more convenient for patient compliance. Patients must be reevaluated periodically for appropriateness of therapy and to prevent electrolyte imbalance.

Get Ready for the NCLEX® Examination!

Key Points

- Diuretics are drugs that act at various locations in the nephron to increase the flow of urine.
- The purpose of diuretics is to increase the net loss of water.
- Diuretics are mainstays in the symptomatic treatment of heart failure, hypertension, and renal disease.
- Diuretics also have a variety of other medical uses, such as reducing cerebral edema, intraocular pressure, ascites, and hypercalcemia.
- The information that the nurse obtains about the patient's general clinical symptoms is important to the healthcare provider when analyzing data for diagnosis and success of therapy.

Additional Learning Resources

SG Go to your Study Guide for additional Review Questions for the NCLEX® Examination, Critical Thinking Clinical Situations, and other learning activities to help you master this chapter content.

evolve Go to your Evolve website (http://evolve .elsevier.com/Clayton) for additional online resources.

Review Questions for the NCLEX® Examination

1. The nurse is assessing a patient taking diuretics for signs of dehydration. What should the nurse assess for? *(Select all that apply.)*
   1. Elastic skin turgor
   2. Lower lab values of hematocrit and hemoglobin from baseline
   3. Dry and sticky oral mucous membranes
   4. Lab values of hematocrit and hemoglobin elevated from baseline
   5. Pitting edema around the ankles

2. The nurse reviewed the following laboratory results for a patient with a diuretic prescribed. Which of the following laboratory values support the diagnosis of hyponatremia and hypokalemia?
   1. A serum potassium level of 5.6 and a serum sodium level of 152
   2. A serum potassium level of 3.2 and a serum sodium level of 130
   3. A serum potassium level of 3.6 and a serum sodium level of 135
   4. A serum potassium level of 4.6 and a serum sodium level of 145

3. A nurse is assessing a patient receiving diuretic therapy for signs of electrolyte imbalance. Which of the following are signs or symptoms of electrolyte imbalance? *(Select all that apply.)*
   1. Peripheral edema
   2. Muscle cramps
   3. Nausea with episodes of vomiting
   4. Confusion
   5. Crackles in the lungs

4. The nurse was discussing the possible adverse effects of thiazide diuretic therapy with a patient. After the patient stated the following, the nurse recognized further education was needed:
   1. "I understand that since I am taking this hydrochlorothiazide that I can expect my kidneys to shut down."
   2. "So you are saying that if my ears start to ring continuously then I need to let my doctor know."
   3. "I will need to get my blood work done periodically to determine if this drug is making my potassium level drop."
   4. "I know that I am taking this for my high blood pressure, so I should expect that it will control it better once I get started on this."

5. The nurse reviews these laboratory tests to determine the status of renal function:
   1. Serum creatinine and BUN
   2. Blood sugar and A1$_C$
   3. Uric acid and serum calcium
   4. Serum potassium and chloride

6. The nurse was caring for a patient who asked for a pain pill (ibuprofen) for a recent arm fracture and was currently taking the diuretic furosemide. What would be an appropriate response by the nurse?
   1. "Sure, no problem; the two medications do not interact."
   2. "Since these two medications have a known interaction, I will not be allowed to give you any for pain."
   3. "If I give you the pain pill, it will affect the diuretic and you will have an increased effect from the diuretic."
   4. "The dosage of the pain medication will require an increased dosage of the diuretic."

7. The nurse knows that individuals with impaired renal function, cirrhosis of the liver, or diabetes mellitus need to be given diuretics cautiously because: *(Select all that apply.)*
   1. diabetic patients may experience hyperglycemia.
   2. patients with cirrhosis of the liver may develop orthostatic hypotension.
   3. patients with renal disease tend to develop electrolyte imbalances.
   4. diabetic patients may experience hypoglycemia.
   5. patients with renal disease will develop edema secondary to diuretics.

8. The nurse knows that when patients are treated for heart failure, the purpose of using diuretics is to:
   1. reduce cerebral edema and headaches.
   2. relieve symptoms associated with pulmonary congestion and edema.
   3. reduce ascites associated with liver congestion.
   4. relieve symptoms of renal dysfunction.

chapter

29

Drugs Used to Treat Upper Respiratory Disease

Objectives

1. Describe the function of the respiratory system and list the common upper respiratory diseases.
2. Discuss the causes of allergic rhinitis, nasal congestion and rhinitis medicamentosa.
3. Explain the major actions (effects) of sympathomimetic, antihistaminic and corticosteroid decongestants and cromolyn.
4. Explain why all decongestant products should be used cautiously by people with hypertension, hyperthyroidism,

diabetes mellitus, cardiac disease, increased intraocular pressure or prostatic disease.
5. Discuss the premedication assessments and nursing assessments needed during therapy to monitor the therapeutic response to and the common and serious adverse effects of decongestant drug therapy.

Key Terms

rhinitis (rī-NĪ-tĭs) (p. 447)
sinusitis (sī-nyū-SĪ-tĭs) (p. 448)
allergic rhinitis (ă-LĔR-jĭk rī-NĪ-tĭs) (p. 448)
antigen-antibody (ĂN-tĭ-jĕn ĂN-tĭ-bŏ-dē) (p. 448)
histamine (HĬS-tă-mēn) (p. 448)
rhinorrhea (rī-nō-RĒ-ă) (p. 448)

decongestants (dē-kŏn-JĔS-tănts) (p. 448)
rhinitis medicamentosa (rī-NĪ-tĭs mĕd-ĭ-kŏ-mĕn-TŌ-să) (p. 448)
antihistamines (ăn-tĭ-HĬS-tă-mēnz) (p. 449)
antiinflammatory agents (ăn-tĭ-ĭn-FLĂ-mă-tō-rē) (p. 450)

UPPER RESPIRATORY TRACT ANATOMY AND PHYSIOLOGY

The respiratory system is a series of airways that start with the nose and mouth and end at the alveolar sacs within the lungs. The upper respiratory tract is composed of the nose and its turbinates, the sinuses, the nasopharynx, the pharynx, the tonsils, the Eustachian tubes, and the larynx (Figure 29-1). The nose and its structures serve two functions: olfactory (i.e., smell) and respiratory. The olfactory region is located in the upper part of each nostril. It is an area of specialized tissue cells (i.e., olfactory cells) that contain microscopic hairs that react to odors in the air and then stimulate the olfactory cells. The olfactory cells in turn send signals to the brain, which processes the sensation that people perceive as a particular smell.

The respiratory function of the nose is to warm, humidify, and filter the air inhaled to prepare it for the lower respiratory airways. Both nasal passages have folds of skin called *turbinates* that significantly increase the surface area of the passages and contain massive numbers of blood vessels. The blood circulating

through the membranes lining the turbinates warms and humidifies inhaled air. The inhaled air is also filtered of particulate matter. The hairs at the entrance to the nostrils remove large particles, and the turbinates and narrowness of the nasal passages cause turbulence of the airflow passing through with each inhalation. All of the surfaces of the nose are coated with a thin layer of mucus, which is secreted by goblet cells. Because of the turbulence of the airflow, particles are thrown against the walls of the nasal passages and become trapped in the mucosal secretions. The epithelial cells lining the posterior two thirds of the nasal passages contain cilia that sweep the particulate matter back toward the nasopharynx and pharynx. Once in the pharynx, the particulate matter is expectorated or swallowed. The warming, humidification, and filtration processes continue as the air passes into the trachea, bronchi, and bronchioles.

The nasal structures are innervated by the autonomic nervous system. Cholinergic stimulation causes vasodilation of the blood vessels lining the nasal mucosa, and sympathetic (primarily alpha-adrenergic) stimulation causes vasoconstriction. The cholinergic

FIGURE 29-1 The upper respiratory tract.

fibers also innervate the secretory glands. When stimulated, they produce serous and mucous secretions within the nostrils.

The paranasal sinuses are hollow, air-filled cavities in the cranial bones on both sides and behind the nose. There are eight sinuses (four on each side). The purpose of the paranasal sinuses appears to be to act as resonating chambers for the voice and as a means of lightening the bones of the head. The sinuses are lined with the same mucous membranes and ciliated epithelia as those of the upper respiratory tract. The sinuses are connected to the nasal passages by ducts that drain into the nasal cavity from activity of the ciliated cells.

On either side of the oral pharynx is a pharyngeal tonsil, a collection of lymphoid tissue that is called the *adenoids* when enlarged. The tonsils are located in an area where mucus laden with particulate matter (e.g., virus particles, bacteria) accumulates from the ciliary action of cells in the nasopharynx above. The lymphoid tissue is rich in immunoglobulins, and is thought to play a role in the immunologic defense mechanisms of the upper airway.

Sneezing is a physiologic reflex used by the body to clear the nasal passages of foreign matter. The sneeze reflex is initiated by irritation of the nasal mucosa by foreign particulate matter. It is similar to the cough reflex, which clears the lower respiratory airways of secretions and foreign matter.

COMMON UPPER RESPIRATORY DISEASES

Rhinitis is inflammation of the nasal mucous membranes. Signs and symptoms include sneezing, nasal discharge, and nasal congestion. Rhinitis is often subclassified as acute or chronic on the basis of the duration of the signs and symptoms. The most common causes of acute rhinitis are the common cold (viral infection), bacterial infection, presence of a foreign body, and drug-induced congestion (rhinitis medicamentosa). Common causes of chronic rhinitis are allergy, nonallergic perennial rhinitis, chronic sinusitis, and a deviated septum.

The common cold is actually a viral infection of the upper respiratory tissues. When considering the amount of time lost from school and work and the number of healthcare provider office visits that this condition causes annually, it is probably the single most expensive illness in the United States. Seasons in which viral infections reach near-epidemic proportions are midwinter, spring, and early fall (i.e., a few weeks after school starts). Six different virus families, including 120 to 200 subtypes, cause coldlike symptoms; the most common are the rhinoviruses and coronaviruses. Viruses are spread from person to person by direct contact and sneezing. The earliest symptoms of a cold are a clear, watery nasal discharge and sneezing. Nasal congestion from engorgement of the nasal blood vessels and swelling of nasal turbinates quickly follows. Over the next 48 hours, the discharge becomes cloudy and much more viscous. Other symptoms include coughing, a "scratchy" or mildly sore throat (pharyngitis), and hoarseness (laryngitis). Other symptoms that occur less frequently are headache, malaise, chills, and fever. A few patients may develop a fever up to 100°F (37.8° C). Symptoms should subside within 5 to 7 days.

Complications occasionally develop as a result of the challenge to the body's immune system initiated by cold viruses. Complications can also arise from thick, tenacious mucus obstructing the sinus ducts or the Eustachian tubes to the middle ears. Bacteria are easily trapped behind these obstructions in the sinuses and ears, resulting in bacterial **sinusitis** or otitis media (infection of the middle ear). Viral infections are also a common cause of exacerbations of obstructive lung disease and of acute asthmatic attacks in susceptible individuals. If symptoms of the cold do not begin to resolve after several days or if symptoms become worse or additional symptoms appear (e.g., temperature higher than 100° F (37.8° C), earache), a healthcare provider should be consulted.

Allergic rhinitis is inflammation of the nasal mucosa as a result of an allergic reaction. Patients with allergic rhinitis have had previous exposure to one or more allergens (e.g., pollens, grasses, house dust mites) and have developed antibodies to those allergens. After this exposure, when the person inhales the allergen, an **antigen-antibody** reaction occurs, causing inflammation and swelling of the nasal passages. One of the major causes of symptoms associated with an allergy is the release of histamine during the antigen-antibody reaction.

Histamine is a compound derived from an amino acid called *histidine* that is stored in small granules in most body tissues. Its physiologic functions are not completely known, but it is released in response to allergic reactions and tissue damage caused by trauma or infection.

When histamine is released in the area of tissue damage or at the site of an antigen-antibody reaction (e.g., a pollen inhaled into the nose of a patient who is allergic to that specific pollen), it reacts with the histamine-1 (H_1) receptors in the area, and the following reactions take place: (1) the arterioles and capillaries in the region dilate, allowing increased blood flow to the area that results in redness; (2) the capillaries become more permeable, resulting in the outward passage of fluid into the extracellular spaces, causing edema (this is manifested by congestion in the mucous membranes and turbinates of the patient's nose); and (3) nasal, lacrimal, and bronchial secretions are released, resulting in a runny nose **(rhinorrhea)** and watery eyes (conjunctivitis) noted in patients with allergies. Patients with allergic rhinitis also complain of itching of the palate, ears, and eyes. Most patients

with asthma have an allergic component to the disease that triggers acute asthma attacks.

When large amounts of histamine are released (e.g., during a severe allergic reaction), there is extensive arteriolar dilation. Blood pressure drops (hypotension), the skin becomes flushed and edematous, and severe itching (urticaria) develops. Constriction (narrowing) and spasm of the bronchial tubes make respiratory effort more difficult (dyspnea), and copious amounts of pulmonary and gastric secretions are released.

Allergies may be seasonal or perennial. Seasonal allergies occur when a particular allergen is abundant—tree pollen is prevalent from late March to early June; ragweed is abundant from early August until the first hard freeze in October; and grasses pollinate from the middle of May to the middle of July. Weather conditions (e.g., rainfall, humidity, temperature) affect the amount of pollen produced during a particular year but not the actual onset or termination of the specific allergen's season. It is common for a person to be allergic to more than one allergen simultaneously, so seasonal allergies may overlap or may occur more than once per year. People who have allergies to multiple antigens (e.g., smoke, molds, animal dander, feathers, house dust mites, pollens) have varying degrees of symptoms all year round and are said to have *perennial allergies*. Allergy symptoms need to be treated, not only for symptomatic relief, but also to prevent irreversible changes within the nose, such as thickening of the mucosal epithelium, loss of cilia, loss of smell, recurrent sinusitis and otitis media, growth of connective tissue, and development of nasal or sinus polyps that aggravate rhinitis and secondary infections.

Overuse of topical **decongestants** may lead to a rebound of nasal secretions known as *rhinitis medicamentosa*. This secondary congestion is thought to be caused by excessive vasoconstriction of the blood vessels and by direct irritation of the nasal membranes by the solution. When the vasoconstrictor effects wear off, the irritation causes excessive blood flow to the passages, causing swelling and engorgement to reappear; the nose feels stuffier and more congested than it did before treatment. Over the following few weeks, a vicious cycle develops, involving more frequent use of the topical decongestant to relieve nasal passage swelling and obstruction. Rhinitis medicamentosa may develop as early as 3 to 5 days after use of long-acting topical decongestants such as oxymetazoline and xylometazoline, but it usually does not develop until after 2 to 3 weeks of regular use of short-acting topical decongestants such as phenylephrine.

TREATMENT OF UPPER RESPIRATORY DISEASES

COMMON COLD

Treatment of the common cold is limited to relieving the symptoms associated with rhinitis and, if present, pharyngitis and laryngitis; reducing the risk of complications; and preventing the spread of viral infection to others. Decongestants are the most effective agent for relieving nasal congestion and rhinorrhea.

Life Span Considerations

Decongestants

Sympathomimetic amines, more commonly called *decongestants*, and antihistamines are frequently used in combination with analgesics in cold and flu remedies. People are often not fully aware of the ingredients of over-the-counter (OTC) combination products.

Patients with diabetes mellitus, hypertension, or ischemic heart disease should use products containing decongestants only if advised to do so by a healthcare provider or pharmacist.

A paradoxical effect from antihistamines often seen in young children and older adults is central nervous system stimulation rather than sedation, which may cause insomnia, nervousness, and irritability. Antihistamines may also cause urinary retention and should be used with caution by older men who have an enlarged prostate gland.

The use of **antihistamines** (H_1-receptor antagonists) for symptomatic relief of cold symptoms has been controversial. Studies indicate that preschool-age children do not benefit from the use of antihistamines; however, older children, adolescents, and adults do receive some benefit.

Depending on whether fever, pharyngitis, or cough is present, patients may also benefit from the use of analgesics, antipyretics (see Chapter 19), expectorants, and antitussive agents (see Chapter 30). Laryngitis should be treated by resting the vocal cords as much as possible. Inhaling cool mist vapor several times daily to humidify the larynx may be beneficial, but putting medication into the inhaled vapor is of no value. Lozenges and gargles do nothing to relieve hoarseness, because they do not reach the larynx.

ALLERGIC RHINITIS

The first steps in treating allergic rhinitis are to (1) identify the allergens—through skin testing—and (2) avoid exposure, if possible. Unfortunately, it often is not possible to eliminate exposure to many allergens without severe lifestyle restrictions. Medicines must then be used to block the allergic reaction or treat the symptoms. The pharmacologic agents typically used include antihistamines, decongestants, and intranasal corticosteroid antiinflammatory agents. Saline nasal sprays can be effective in reducing nasal irritation between doses of other pharmacologic agents. If the patient is physically able, vigorous exercise for 15 to 30 minutes once or twice daily increases sympathetic output and induces vascular vasoconstriction.

Mild allergic rhinitis can be well treated by an oral second-generation antihistamine (e.g., loratadine, des-

loratadine, cetirizine, fexofenadine) or a nasal corticosteroid alone. Patients who have moderate to severe symptoms of allergic rhinitis with nasal congestion often require both an oral second-generation antihistamine and a nasal corticosteroid. Immunotherapy may be required if symptoms are only partially controlled, if high doses of intranasal or oral corticosteroids are required, or if the allergic rhinitis is complicated by asthma or sinusitis. Therapy should be started before the anticipated appearance of allergens and continue during the time of exposure.

RHINITIS MEDICAMENTOSA

The best treatment of rhinitis medicamentosa is prevention. Unfortunately, most patients are not aware of the condition until it becomes a problem. Following the directions for a daily dosage and limiting the duration of therapy to that described on the topical decongestant product are the best ways to avoid the condition.

Several strategies have been successful in treating rhinitis medicamentosa. Regardless of the approach used, the patient must understand what caused the rebound congestion and why it is important to eliminate the problem. One method is to withdraw the topical decongestant completely at once. The patient is likely to be congested and uncomfortable for the next week, but use of a saline nasal spray can help moisturize irritated nasal tissues. Nasal steroid solutions can also be used, but they still take several days to reduce inflammation and congestion. Probably the most successful approach, although the longest to complete, is to have the patient work to clear one nostril at a time. Start by reducing the strength and frequency of the decongestant used in the left nostril, while continuing with the normal dosage in the right nostril. Saline or corticosteroid nasal spray can be used every other dose in the left nostril. Eventually, the saline can be used more frequently and the decongestant can be discontinued in the left nostril. Once the patient can breathe normally through the left nostril, the same approach can be started in the right nostril. Frequent follow-up with the patient and reinforcement of progress made are important to the success of this treatment.

DRUG THERAPY FOR UPPER RESPIRATORY DISEASES

ACTIONS AND USES

Antihistamines, or H_1-receptor antagonists, are the drugs of choice for treating allergic rhinitis. Because they are administered orally and thus distributed systemically, they also reduce the symptoms of nasal itching, sneezing, rhinorrhea, lacrimation, and conjunctival itching. However, antihistamines do not reduce nasal congestion.

Decongestants are alpha-adrenergic stimulants that cause vasoconstriction of the nasal mucosa, which significantly reduces nasal congestion. When treating allergic rhinitis, decongestants are often administered in conjunction with antihistamines to reduce nasal congestion and counteract the sedation caused by many antihistamines.

Antiinflammatory agents administered intranasally are used to treat nasal symptoms resulting from mild to moderate allergic rhinitis. In general, antiinflammatory agents are not used to treat symptoms associated with a cold because the symptoms start to resolve before the antiinflammatory agents can become effective. The antiinflammatory agents used to treat allergic rhinitis are corticosteroids and cromolyn sodium.

❖ NURSING IMPLICATIONS FOR UPPER RESPIRATORY DISEASES

Nasal congestion, allergic rhinitis, and sinusitis are treated with prescription or OTC medicines. The roles of the nurse in the healthcare provider's office are to perform the initial assessment of symptoms and then focus on teaching the proper techniques for self-administering and monitoring of the medication therapy. Always review the patient's history for other diseases currently being treated (e.g., hypertension, glaucoma, asthma, prostatic hyperplasia) that may contraindicate the concurrent use of some upper respiratory medications used as OTC or prescribed treatments.

■ Assessment
Description of Symptoms
- Which symptoms are present (e.g., frequency of sneezing or coughing, hoarseness, nasal congestion, presence of nasal secretions and type [watery, viscous, color])?
- When did the symptoms start?
- Does the patient have a history of allergies? If yes, what are the known allergens? Are the symptoms associated with a particular time of year or the release of pollen from plants? Are the symptoms triggered by exposure to household environmental factors (e.g., animal dander, dust, molds, certain foods)?
- Has the individual recently been exposed to someone with a common cold or upper respiratory tract infection?
- Is the individual having pain or discomfort? What are the specific areas affected and the degree of pain?

History of Treatment
- What prescribed or OTC medicines have been used? Have any been effective?
- When allergies are suspected, has skin or blood testing been completed to determine what specific allergens are initiating the attacks?
- If pain is present, how has pain relief been obtained? Is the degree of pain relief satisfactory?

History of Concurrent Medical Problems. Ask specific questions to determine whether the patient has concurrent medical problems (e.g., glaucoma, prostatic hyperplasia, asthma, hypertension, diabetes mellitus) as described in the drug monograph preassessments.

■ Patient Education
- Make sure that the patient understands the importance of adequate rest, hydration, and personal hygiene (i.e., handwashing) to prevent the spread of infection, when present.
- Discuss the specific medications prescribed, the therapeutic effects that can be expected, and when to contact a healthcare provider if therapy does not yield the expected benefit. Explain which symptoms should be reported to the healthcare provider that would indicate a poor response to therapy (e.g., escalation of symptoms, pain, or fever with sinusitis).
- Make sure that the patient understands when to take the medicine (e.g., if treating symptoms of allergy, antihistamines should be taken 45 to 60 minutes before exposure to the allergen).
- Proper technique is important to therapy success. Explain the procedures for proper instillation of nose drops or nasal sprays associated with the prescribed treatment regimen. Document and verify that the patient can self-administer the medication as recommended.
- Teach the patient to monitor temperature, pulse, respirations, and blood pressure as appropriate to the underlying diagnosis and the medicines used to treat the diagnosed condition.

Fostering Health Maintenance
- Throughout the course of treatment, discuss medication information and how it will benefit the patient. Recognize that nonadherence may occur, especially when treatment response is not immediate.
- Seek cooperation and understanding regarding the following points so that medication adherence is increased: the name of the medication; its dosage, route, and times of administration; and its common and serious adverse effects. Numerous OTC preparations may be contraindicated when other medications or coexisting diseases are present. For example, patients taking antihypertensive medicines should not take decongestants. (See the individual drug monographs for details.)

DRUG CLASS: SYMPATHOMIMETIC DECONGESTANTS

ACTIONS

Sympathomimetic nasal decongestants (Table 29-1) stimulate the alpha-adrenergic receptors of the nasal mucous membranes, causing vasoconstriction. This constriction reduces blood flow in the engorged nasal

Table 29-1   Nasal Decongestants

GENERIC NAME	BRAND NAME	AVAILABILITY	ADULT DOSAGE RANGE
epinephrine ⇄ *Do not confuse epinephrine with ephedrine.*	Adrenalin	Solution: 0.1%	Nasal: 1-2 drops in each nostril q4-6h
naphazoline	Privine	Solution: 0.05%	Nasal: 1-2 sprays or drops in each nostril q6h (maximum)
oxymetazoline	Afrin, Duration	Solution: 0.05%	Nasal: 2-3 drops or sprays twice daily
phenylephrine ⇄ *Do not confuse phenylephrine with phenytoin or norepinephrine.*	Neo-Synephrine ⇄ *Do not confuse Neo-Synephrine with epinephrine.*	Solution: 0.125%, 0.25%, 0.5%, 1%	Nasal: 2-3 drops or sprays in each nostril q4h (maximum)
pseudoephedrine ⇄ *Do not confuse pseudoephedrine with prednisone.*	Sudafed Sudafed 12 hr Sudafed 24 hr	Tablets or capsules: 15, 30, 60, 120, 240 mg Liquid: 15, 30 mg/5 mL Drops: 7.5 mg/0.8 mL; Gel: 15 mg/5 ml	PO: 30-60 mg q4-6h; do not exceed 240 mg/24 hr
tetrahydrozoline	Tyzine	Solution: 0.05%, 0.1%	Nasal: 2-4 drops of 0.1% solution q4-6h
xylometazoline	Triaminic Nasal & Sinus Congestion	Solution: 0.05%	Nasal: 1-3 sprays in each nostril q8-10h

area, resulting in shrinkage of the engorged turbinates and mucous membranes and promoting sinus drainage, improving nasal air passage, and relieving the feelings of stuffiness and obstruction.

USES

Decongestants are the drugs of choice for relieving congestion associated with rhinitis caused by the common cold. They are also often used in conjunction with antihistamines when treating allergic rhinitis to reduce nasal congestion and to counteract the sedation caused by many antihistamines.

Decongestants can be administered orally or applied directly to the nose (topically) in the form of nasal sprays or drops to treat rhinitis. An advantage of topical administration is that it has essentially no systemic effects. Disadvantages of nasal sprays and drops are their lack of effect on conjunctival symptoms, their inconvenience, and their potential to cause rhinitis medicamentosa.

Nasal decongestants provide temporary relief of symptoms, but it is important for the patient to follow the directions on the label carefully. Initially, the stuffiness or blocked sensation will be relieved. However, misuse—including excessive use or frequency of administration—may cause a rebound swelling (i.e., rhinitis medicamentosa) of the nasal passages.

Alpha-adrenergic agents used as nasal decongestants can stimulate alpha receptors at other sites in the body as well. Therefore they should be used with caution when taken orally by patients with hyper-

tension, hyperthyroidism, diabetes mellitus, cardiac disease, increased intraocular pressure, or prostatic hyperplasia.

Many states have enacted laws regulating and tracking the amount of pseudoephedrine-containing decongestants that can be purchased by an individual. Pseudoephedrine is one of the ingredients used in the manufacturing of methamphetamine, an illicit drug with significant potential for abuse.

THERAPEUTIC OUTCOME

The primary therapeutic outcome associated with sympathomimetic decongestant therapy is reduced nasal congestion with easier breathing.

❖ NURSING IMPLICATIONS FOR SYMPATHOMIMETIC DECONGESTANTS

■ Premedication Assessment

1. Check the patient's history for evidence of hypertension, hyperthyroidism, diabetes mellitus, cardiac dysrhythmias, glaucoma, or prostatic hyperplasia. If any one of these conditions is present, consult the healthcare provider before initiating therapy.
2. Inquire about urinary pattern, particularly in male patients over the age of 55 who may be developing prostatic hyperplasia.
3. Obtain the patient's baseline vital signs.

■ Availability, Dosage and Administration

See Table 29-1; see Chapter 7 for techniques for administering nose drops and nasal spray.

■ Common Adverse Effects

Respiratory

Mild nasal irritation. Burning or stinging may be felt when sympathomimetic decongestants are administered to the nasal membranes. This may be avoided by using a weaker solution.

■ Serious Adverse Effects

Urinary Retention.

Some patients, particularly males with prostatic hyperplasia, may develop difficulty with urinary partial obstruction—starting a stream of urine—when taking oral decongestants. The obstruction is dose related and will resolve with metabolism of the drug. This adverse effect can be eliminated by using only topical decongestants rather than oral decongestants.

Cardiovascular

Hypertension. Excessive use of decongestants may result in significant hypertension. Patients already receiving antihypertensive therapy should avoid using decongestants. When sympathomimetic decongestants are used, blood pressure monitoring should be initiated; the healthcare provider should be contacted if the patient's blood pressure becomes elevated.

■ Drug Interactions

Drugs That Enhance Toxic Effects. Monoamine oxidase inhibitors (e.g., tranylcypromine, phenelzine, isocarboxazid) may enhance the toxic effects of sympathomimetic decongestants and result in significant hypertension.

Methyldopa and Reserpine. Frequent decongestant use inhibits the antihypertensive activity of methyldopa and reserpine. Concurrent therapy is not recommended.

DRUG CLASS: ANTIHISTAMINES

ACTIONS

Antihistamines, or H_1-receptor antagonists, are chemical agents that compete with the allergy-liberated histamine for H_1-receptor sites in the patient's arterioles, capillaries, and secretory glands in the mucous membranes. Antihistamines do not prevent histamine release, but they reduce the symptoms of an allergic reaction if the concentration of the antihistamine exceeds the concentration of histamine at the receptor site. Antihistamines are therefore more effective if they are taken before histamine is released or when symptoms first appear.

USES

Antihistamines are the drugs of choice for the systemic treatment of allergic rhinitis and conjunctivitis. These agents reduce rhinorrhea, lacrimation, nasal and conjunctival pruritus, and sneezing. However, antihistamines do not stop nasal congestion. The antihistamines shown in Table 29-2 have similar histamine-blocking effects when they are taken in recommended dosages, but they vary in duration of action, sedative effects, and anticholinergic effects. Occasionally, a patient may develop a tolerance to the antihistaminic effects; changing to another antihistamine is usually effective when this occurs.

Antihistamines work best if taken on a scheduled basis rather than as needed during the allergy season. These agents are much more effective if they are taken before exposure to the allergen (e.g., 45 to 60 minutes before going outdoors during pollen season).

There is no evidence that one agent is particularly better than another at treating symptoms of allergic rhinitis, although there are differences among products regarding their frequency and type of associated adverse effects. The most common adverse effect of many antihistaminic agents is sedation. Most patients acquire a tolerance to this effect with continued therapy. Reducing the dosage or changing to another antihistamine may occasionally be necessary. The most sedating antihistamines are diphenhydramine, cyproheptadine, clemastine, and doxylamine (doxylamine and diphenhydramine are the active ingredients in OTC sleep aids). The least sedating antihistamines are fexofenadine, loratadine, and desloratadine. Although some patients do not feel a sense of sedation after taking an antihistamine, their cognitive functions (e.g., attention, memory, coordination, psychomotor performance) can be significantly impaired. A disturbing observation by these patients is that they often are not aware that their cognitive abilities are impaired. This is particularly important when patients who are taking antihistamines perform potentially dangerous activities (e.g., driving).

All antihistamines display anticholinergic adverse effects, particularly when higher dosages are used. Symptoms include dry mouth, stuffy nose, blurred vision, constipation, and urinary retention. Patients with asthma, prostatic enlargement, or glaucoma should take antihistamines only with a healthcare provider's supervision. The drying effects may also make respiratory mucus more viscous and tenacious. Antihistamines should be used with caution in patients who have a productive cough. If the cough continues but becomes nonproductive, consider additional hydration and discontinue the antihistamine.

THERAPEUTIC OUTCOME

The primary therapeutic outcome associated with antihistamine therapy is reduced symptoms of allergic rhinitis (e.g., rhinorrhea, lacrimation, itching, conjunctivitis).

❖ NURSING IMPLICATIONS FOR ANTIHISTAMINES

■ Premedication Assessment

1. Review the patient's history for evidence of glaucoma, prostatic hyperplasia, or asthma. If any one

Table 29-2   Antihistamines*

GENERIC NAME	BRAND NAME	AVAILABILITY	SEDATION†	ADULT DOSAGE RANGE	MAXIMUM DAILY DOSAGE
azelastine	Astelin	Nasal spray	−	2 sprays per nostril twice daily	—
cetirizine ⇄ *Do not confuse cetirizine with cyclobenzaprine.*	Zyrtec ⇄ *Do not confuse Zyrtec with Zantac, Zestril, or Zyprexa.*	Tablets, oral solution, capsules, syrup	±	5-10 mg once daily	10 mg
chlorpheniramine maleate	Chlor-Trimeton	Tablets, capsules, syrup	+	4 mg three to six times daily	24 mg
clemastine fumarate	Tavist	Tablets, syrup	+++	1.34-2.68 mg two or three times daily	8 mg
cyproheptadine hydrochloride ⇄ *Do not confuse cyproheptadine with cyclobenzaprine.*	—	Tablets, syrup	+	4 mg three times daily	32 mg
desloratadine	Clarinex	Tablets, syrup	±	5 mg once daily	5 mg
diphenhydramine hydrochloride ⇄ *Do not confuse diphenhydramine with dicyclomine or dipyridamole.*	Benadryl, Compoz	Injection, capsules, tablets, syrup, elixir	+++	25-50 mg four to six times daily	300 mg
fexofenadine	Allegra ⇄ *Do not confuse Allegra with Adalat-CC, Asacol, or Viagra.*	Tablets, oral suspension	±	180 mg extended-release formulation daily	180 mg
ipratropium	Atrovent ⇄ *Do not confuse Atrovent with Alupent, Azmacort, Flovent, Natru-Vent, or Serevent.*	Nasal spray, inhaler	−	Spray: 2 sprays per nostril two to four times daily Inhaler: 2 inhalations four times daily	—
levocetirizine	Xyzal	Tablets, oral solution	±	2.5-5 mg once daily in the evening	5 mg
loratadine ⇄ *Do not confuse loratadine with losartan.*	Claritin	Tablets, syrup	±	10 mg daily	10 mg
olopatadine	Patanase	Nasal spray	−	2 sprays per nostril two times daily	No established dosage
promethazine hydrochloride‡ ⇄ *Do not confuse promethazine with phenazopyridine or prochlorperazine.*	Phenergan	Injection, tablets, syrup, suppository	+++	6.25-12.5 mg three or four times daily	100 mg

*Many of these antihistamines are also available in combination with decongestants.
†Sedation index: +++, high; ++, moderate; +, low; ±, low to none; −, none.
‡Promethazine is a phenothiazine with antihistaminic properties.

of these is present, consult the healthcare provider before initiating therapy.

2. Inquire about urinary pattern, particularly in male patients over the age of 55 who may be developing prostatic hyperplasia.

3. Assess the patient's work environment and consider whether drowsiness will affect safety and work performance.

4. Because antihistamines are prescribed for a variety of symptoms (e.g., hay fever, dermatologic reactions, drug hypersensitivity, rhinitis, transfusion reactions), it is necessary to individualize the patient assessments with regard to the underlying pathologic condition.

▪ Availability, Dosage, and Administration
See Table 29-2.

▪ Common Adverse Effects
Neurologic

Sedative effects. The types of antihistamines ordered can produce varying degrees of sedation. Tolerance may be produced over time, thus diminishing the effect. Operating machinery or motor vehicles may be hazardous. Warn the patient to be cautious.

Cognitive impairment. Although newer antihistamines are less sedating, patients should still be cautioned about the possibility of impaired memory, coordination, and psychomotor performance. In many states it is a crime to operate a motor vehicle while under the influence of medicines (in addition to alcohol). Operating machinery or motor vehicles may be hazardous. Caution patients to watch closely for signs of impairment (e.g., forgetfulness, poor coordination) in these situations.

Respiratory

Drying effects. Monitor the patient's cough and degree of sputum production when antihistamines are used. Because of their drying effects, antihistamines may impair expectoration. Give adequate fluids concurrently with the use of antihistamines. Maintain fluid intake at eight to ten 8-ounce glasses daily.

Anticholinergic

Blurred vision; constipation; urinary retention; dryness of mouth, throat, and nose mucosa. These symptoms are the anticholinergic effects produced by antihistamines. Patients taking these medications should be monitored for these effects.

Mucosa dryness may be alleviated by sucking hard candy or ice chips or by chewing gum. Caution the patient that blurred vision may occur, and make appropriate suggestions for the personal safety of the individual.

▪ Serious Adverse Effects
Urinary Retention. Some patients, particularly males with prostatic hyperplasia, may develop diffi-culty with urinary partial obstruction—starting a stream of urine—when taking oral antihistamines, particularly with first-generation antihistamines (e.g., diphenhydramine). The obstruction is dose related and will resolve with metabolism of the drug. This adverse effect can be eliminated by using only topical antihistamines (e.g., azelastine) or second-generation antihistamines (e.g., loratadine, desloratadine, fexofenadine) rather than first-generation antihistamines.

▪ Drug Interactions
Central Nervous System Depressants. Central nervous system depressants—including sleep aids, analgesics, tranquilizers, and alcohol—will potentiate the sedative effects of antihistamines. People who work around machinery, operate motor vehicles, or perform other duties that require constant mental alertness should be particularly cautious until they know how the medication affects them and should not take these medications while working.

DRUG CLASS: RESPIRATORY ANTIINFLAMMATORY AGENTS

Intranasal corticosteroids (ĭn-tră-NĀ-zăl cor-tĭ-cō-STĔR-oydz)

ACTIONS
The exact mechanism by which corticosteroids reduce inflammation is unknown.

USES
Patients with allergic seasonal rhinitis who do not respond to antihistamines and sympathomimetic agents may be given corticosteroids to relieve the symptoms of their allergies. Corticosteroids—whether they are applied topically or administered systemically—have been shown to be highly effective for the treatment of allergic rhinitis. Intranasal corticosteroids are successful in controlling nasal symptoms associated with mild to moderate allergic rhinitis, but systemic steroids are required for severe cases.

Topically active aerosol steroids (e.g., beclomethasone, budesonide, fluticasone, flunisolide) are highly effective, with few adverse effects. Their therapeutic effect (i.e., the reduction of sneezing, nasal itching, stuffiness, and rhinorrhea) is usually observed by the third day, although maximal effects may not be evident for 2 weeks. If symptoms do not improve within 3 weeks, therapy is discontinued. Dexamethasone intranasal aerosol has a higher incidence of systemic adverse effects and is generally not used unless therapy with the other intranasal corticosteroids is not effective. To minimize the development of adrenal suppression, these corticosteroids should be used only for short courses of therapy for acute seasonal allergies.

Table 29-3   **Intranasal Corticosteroids**

GENERIC NAME	BRAND NAME	AVAILABILITY	ADULT DOSAGE RANGE
beclomethasone dipropionate, monohydrate	Beconase AQ ⇄ *Do not confuse Beconase with Beclovent.*	Nasal spray: 42 mcg/actuation	1 or 2 sprays (42-84 mcg) in each nostril twice daily
	Qnasl	Nasal Spray: 80 mcg/actuation	1 spray in each nostril twice daily
budesonide	Rhinocort Aqua	Nasal aerosol: 120 doses/canister	1-4 sprays in each nostril once daily
ciclesonide	Omnaris	Nasal spray: 50 mcg/actuation	2 sprays in each nostril daily
	Zetonna	Nasal Spray: 37 mcg/actuation	2-3 sprays in each nostril daily
flunisolide	—	Nasal spray: 200 doses/bottle; 29 mcg/actuation	2 sprays in each nostril two or three times daily; maximum daily dosage is 8 sprays (400 mcg) in 24 hr
fluticasone	Flonase ⇄ *Do not confuse Flonase with Flovent.*	Nasal spray: 120 actuations/bottle; 50 mcg/actuation	2 (100 mcg each) sprays in each nostril once daily
mometasone	Nasonex	Nasal spray: 120 actuations/bottle; 50 mcg/actuation	2 sprays (100 mcg) in each nostril once daily
triamcinolone	Nasacort AQ ⇄ *Do not confuse Nasacort with Azmacort.*	Nasal aerosol: 100 actuations/canister; 55 mcg/actuation	2 sprays (110 mcg each) in each nostril once daily; maximum daily dosage is 4 sprays in 24 hr

THERAPEUTIC OUTCOMES

The primary therapeutic outcomes associated with intranasal corticosteroid therapy are reduced rhinorrhea, rhinitis, itching, and sneezing.

❖ NURSING IMPLICATIONS FOR INTRANASAL CORTICOSTEROID THERAPY

▪ Premedication Assessment

1. Blocked nasal passages should be treated with a topical decongestant just before beginning intranasal corticosteroids.
2. Ask the patient to blow the nose thoroughly before administering intranasal therapy.

▪ Availability, Dosage, and Administration

See Table 29-3; see Chapter 7 for techniques for administering intranasal spray.

Counseling. The therapeutic effects—unlike those of sympathomimetic decongestants—are not immediate. This should be explained to the patient in advance to ensure cooperation and the continuation of treatment with the prescribed dosage regimen. The full therapeutic benefit requires regular use, and it is usually evident within a few days, although a few patients may require up to 3 weeks for maximum benefit.

Preparation Before Administration. Patients with blocked nasal passages should be encouraged to use a decongestant just before intranasal corticosteroid administration to ensure adequate penetration. Patients should also be advised to clear their nasal passages of secretions before use.

Maintenance Therapy. After the desired clinical effect is obtained, the maintenance dosage should be reduced to the smallest amount necessary to control the symptoms.

▪ Common Adverse Effects

Respiratory

Nasal irritation. Nasal burning is usually mild and tends to resolve with continued therapy. Encourage the patient not to discontinue therapy without first consulting the healthcare provider.

▪ Drug Interactions

No significant drug interactions have been reported.

---

cromolyn sodium (KRŌ-mō-lĭn)
   NasalCrom (NĀ-zăl-krŏm)
   ⇄ *Do not confuse NasalCrom with Nasalide.*

ACTIONS

Cromolyn sodium is a mast cell stabilizer that inhibits the release of histamine and other mediators of inflammation, making it an indirect antiinflammatory agent. It must be administered before the body receives a stimulus to release histamine, such as an antigen that initiates an antigen-antibody allergic reaction.

USES

Cromolyn is recommended for use in conjunction with other medications in treating patients with severe allergic rhinitis to prevent the release of histamine, which results in symptoms of allergic rhinitis. It is also used as part of the prophylactic management of bronchospasm and asthma.

Cromolyn has no direct bronchodilatory, antihistaminic, or anticholinergic activity, and it does not relieve nasal congestion. The concomitant use of antihistamines or nasal decongestants may be necessary during initial treatment with cromolyn. A 2- to 4-week course of therapy is usually required to determine the patient's clinical response. Therapy should be continued only if there is a decrease in the severity of allergic symptoms during treatment.

THERAPEUTIC OUTCOMES

The primary therapeutic outcomes associated with cromolyn therapy are reduced rhinorrhea, itching, and sneezing and fewer incidents of bronchospasm and asthmatic exacerbations.

❖ NURSING IMPLICATIONS FOR CROMOLYN SODIUM

▪ Premedication Assessment
1. Cromolyn must be taken before exposure to the stimulus that initiates an allergic response.
2. Check to see if the concurrent use of antihistamines or nasal decongestants has been ordered by the healthcare provider, especially during the initiation of cromolyn therapy.
3. Have the patient blow his or her nose before the nasal instillation of this drug.

▪ Availability
Nasal spray: 5.2 mg/actuation in 13-mL (100 sprays) and 26-mL (200 sprays) metered-spray devices. *Inhalation with nebulizer:* 20 mg/2 mL in 2-mL plastic containers. *Oral concentrate:* 100 mg/5 mL in 5-mL ampules.

▪ Dosage and Administration
See Chapter 7 for techniques to use to administer nasal spray.

Counseling. The therapeutic effects of these drugs—unlike those of sympathomimetic amines—are not immediate. This should be explained to the patient in advance to ensure cooperation and continuation of treatment with the prescribed dosage regimen. The full therapeutic benefit requires regular use, and it is usually evident within 2 to 4 weeks. Therapy must be continued even when the patient is free of symptoms.

Nasal Spray. Adult patients with blocked nasal passages should be encouraged to use a decongestant just before intranasal cromolyn administration to ensure adequate penetration. Patients should also be advised to clear their nasal passages of secretions and then inhale through the nose during administration. One spray is placed in each nostril three or four times daily at regular intervals. The maximum dosage is six sprays in each nostril daily.

▪ Common Adverse Effects
Respiratory
Nasal irritation. The most common adverse effect is irritation manifested by sneezing, nasal itching, burning, and stuffiness. Patients usually develop a tolerance to the irritation, but this is rarely a cause for discontinuing intranasal therapy.

▪ Serious Adverse Effects
Respiratory
Bronchospasm and coughing. Notify the healthcare provider if inhalation causes bronchospasm or coughing.

▪ Drug Interactions
No significant drug interactions have been reported.

Get Ready for the NCLEX® Examination!

Key Points

- Rhinitis is defined as the inflammation of the nasal mucous membranes that causes sneezing, nasal discharge, and nasal congestion.
- The most common causes of acute rhinitis are the common cold, allergies, bacterial infection, the presence of a foreign body, and drug-induced congestion (i.e., rhinitis medicamentosa).
- The roles of the nurse when working with patients with rhinitis are to perform the initial assessment of symptoms and then to focus on teaching the proper techniques for self-administering and monitoring

medication therapy. Frequent follow-up with the patient and the reinforcement of gains made are important to the success of these treatments.

Additional Learning Resources

SG Go to your Study Guide for additional Review Questions for the NCLEX® Examination, Critical Thinking Clinical Situations, and other learning activities to help you master this chapter content.

evolve Go to your Evolve website (http://evolve.elsevier.com/Clayton) for additional online resources.

Review Questions for the NCLEX® Examination

1. A patient asked the nurse about the frequent upper respiratory illnesses that he was experiencing. The best response by the nurse would be:
   1. "Your respiratory system is designed to warm, filter, and humidify the air you breathe, as well as allow you to smell things. When you have an infection, the normal functioning can be impaired. Avoid irritants such as smoke, chemicals, or allergens that might make your nasal passages more susceptible to infections."
   2. "Sometimes when this happens your respiratory system will stop working properly and you will need to get a flu shot to get it back on track."
   3. "Studies show that once you get an infection, it never really leaves your system, so you will be having this problem regularly."
   4. "Your respiratory system can become overwhelmed with too many infections and then it doesn't work anymore."

2. After explaining allergic rhinitis to the patient, the nurse realized further teaching was needed when the patient stated the following:
   1. "I have to be careful with nasal decongestants so I don't get that rebound effect, where after I take them, once the drug wears off, my nose gets stuffy again and then I wind up taking it again."
   2. "So this antihistamine will stop my running nose and itchy eyes as well as my nasal congestion."
   3. "As I understand it, I need to keep taking my antihistamine so I don't get complications such as nasal polyps from my allergy."
   4. "So my nasal congestion is caused from reacting to the pollen in the air, which I will get every season."

3. The nurse is teaching a patient about an antihistamine that was prescribed. Which statement by the patient indicates that further teaching is needed?
   1. "I should drink 8 to 10 glasses of water every day."
   2. "If my vision starts to blur, I will need to call my doctor.'
   3. "I can suck on candy or chew gum when my mouth gets dry from this drug."
   4. "I will be able to drive without any problem because I will know when I am impaired."

4. The nurse knows that intranasal corticosteroids are used for short periods to treat seasonal allergies, and explains to the patient that the following needs to be done: (Select all that apply.)
   1. Rinse mouth prior to application
   2. Blow nose prior to application
   3. Use nose drops of topical decongestants if ordered prior to application
   4. Suck on hard candy or ice chips after application
   5. Blow nose after application

5. Before initiating antihistamine medications, the nurse knows that the patient's history should be checked for which of the following: (Select all that apply.)
   1. Hypertension
   2. Hypothyroidism
   3. Glaucoma
   4. Urinary retention
   5. Prostatic hyperplasia

6. When cromolyn sodium is prescribed for patients with severe allergic rhinitis, the nurse knows this drug will have the following effect:
   1. Bronchodilator
   2. Antihistamine
   3. Indirect antiinflammatory agent
   4. Decongestant

Objectives

1. Compare the physiologic responses of the respiratory system to emphysema, chronic bronchitis, and asthma.
2. Cite nursing assessments used to evaluate the respiratory status of a patient.
3. Distinguish the mechanisms of action of expectorants, antitussives, and mucolytic agents.
4. Describe the nursing assessments needed to monitor therapeutic response and the development of adverse effects from beta-adrenergic bronchodilator therapy.
5. Discuss the nursing assessments needed to monitor therapeutic response and the development of adverse effects from anticholinergic bronchodilator therapy.
6. List the lower respiratory conditions that use anticholinergic bronchodilators and corticosteroid inhalant therapy.

Key Terms

ventilation (vĕn-tĭ-LĀ-shŭn) (p. 458)
diffusion (dĭ-FYŪ-zhun) (p. 459)
goblet cells (GŎB-lĕt SĔLZ) (p. 459)
obstructive airway diseases (ŏb-STRŬK-tĭv ĀR-wā dĭ-ZĒ-zĕz) (p. 459)
bronchospasm (BRŎN-kō-spăz-ĕm) (p. 459)
restrictive airway diseases (rē-STRĬK-tĭv ĀR-wā) (p. 460)
chronic obstructive pulmonary disease (COPD) (KRŎN-ĭk ŏb-STRŬK-tĭv PŬL-mō-nār-ē) (p. 460)
chronic airflow limitation disease (CALD) (KRŎN-ĭk ĀR-flō lĭ-mĭ-TĀ-shŭn) (p. 460)
arterial blood gases (ABGs) (ăr-TĒR-ē-ăl BLŬD GĂS-ĕz) (p. 460)

oxygen saturation (ŎKS-ĕ-jĕn să-chŭr-Ā-shŭn) (p. 460)
spirometry (spĭ-RŎM-ĕ-trē) (p. 460)
cough (KŎF) (p. 461)
asthma (ĂZ-mă) (p. 461)
bronchitis (brŏn-KĪ-tĭs) (p. 461)
emphysema (ĕm-fĭ-SĒ-mă) (p. 463)
expectorants (ĕk-SPĔK-tōr-ănts) (p. 464)
antitussives (ăn-tĭ-TUS-ĭvz) (p. 464)
mucolytic agents (myū-kō-LĬ-tĭk) (p. 464)
bronchodilators (brŏn-kō-DĪ-lā-tŏrz) (p. 465)
antiinflammatory agents (ăn-tī-ĭn-FLĂ-mă-tō-rē) (p. 465)
immunomodulators (ĭm-myū-nō-MŎD-yū-lā-tŏrz) (p. 465)

LOWER RESPIRATORY TRACT ANATOMY AND PHYSIOLOGY

The respiratory system is a series of airways that start with the nose and mouth and end at the alveolar sacs. The nose and mouth airways connect at the pharynx. Passing out of the pharynx, the airways divide into the esophagus of the gastrointestinal (GI) tract and the larynx (voice box) and trachea of the respiratory tract. The trachea divides into the right and left mainstem bronchi, which enter the lungs. The bronchi subdivide in each lung into many smaller bronchioles, which further subdivide into many smaller airways called alveolar ducts that terminate in alveolar sacs. The alveolar sacs are surrounded by capillaries of the blood circulatory system. Human lungs contain 300 to 500 million sacs for gaseous exchange and have a surface area approximately equal to that of a tennis court. The anatomic parts of the body associated with the lower respiratory system are the larynx, trachea, bronchi, bronchioles, and alveolar sacs (Figure 30-1).

The primary function of the lower respiratory tract is the ventilatory cycle. **Ventilation** is the movement of air in and out of the lungs. Inhalation is the process of transport of air containing oxygen to the alveolar sacs, exchange of oxygen for carbon dioxide across the alveolar membranes containing blood capillaries, and exhalation of "stale air," including carbon dioxide. Ventilation of the lungs is accomplished by contraction and relaxation of the diaphragmatic and intercostal muscles (muscles between the ribs). During inspiration, the diaphragmatic and intercostal muscles contract, creating a vacuum in the lungs and pulling air in through the mouth and nose. During exhalation, relaxation of the muscles allows the chest to return to its unexpanded position, forcing air out of the lungs.

Blood flow through the pulmonary arteries to the capillaries surrounding the alveoli to the pulmonary

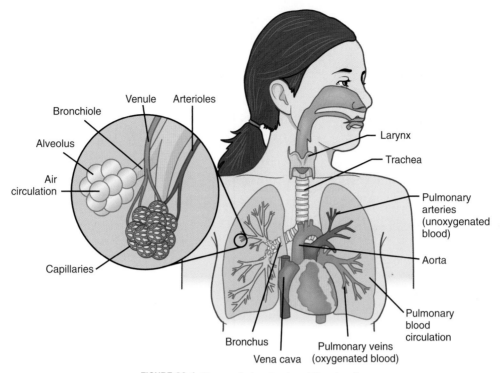

FIGURE 30-1 The respiratory tract and the alveoli.

veins is called *perfusion*. **Diffusion** is the process by which oxygen (O_2) passes across the alveolar membrane to the blood in the capillaries and carbon dioxide (CO_2) passes from the blood to the alveolar sacs for exhalation. Oxygen is transported by combining with hemoglobin in red blood cells or by dissolving in the blood plasma. Blood circulation provides distribution of oxygen to the body's cells for the sustenance of life. Ventilation and perfusion must be equal to maintain homeostasis.

The fluids of the respiratory tract originate from specialized mucous glands (**goblet cells**) and serous glands that line the respiratory tract. The goblet cells produce gelatinous mucus that forms a thin layer over the interior surfaces of the trachea, bronchi, and bronchioles. Secretion of mucus is increased by exposure to irritants, such as smoke, airborne particulate matter, and bacteria. The serous glands are controlled by the cholinergic nervous system. When stimulated, the serous glands secrete a watery fluid to the interior surface of the bronchial tree. There, the mucous secretions of the goblet cells and the watery secretions of the serous glands combine to form respiratory tract fluid.

Normally, respiratory tract fluid forms a protective layer over the trachea, bronchi, and bronchioles. Foreign bodies, such as smoke particles and bacteria, are caught in the respiratory tract fluid and are swept upward by ciliary hairs that line the bronchi and trachea to the larynx, where they are removed by the cough reflex. The expectorated (coughed up) material contains pulmonary mucous secretions, foreign particulate matter such as smoke and bacteria, and

epithelial cells sloughed from the lining of the airways. Common names given to the expectorated mass are sputum and phlegm. If too much mucus is secreted as a result of chronic irritation, cilia are destroyed by chronic inhalation of smoke, dehydration dries the mucus, or anticholinergic agents inhibit watery secretions from the serous glands, the mucus becomes viscous, forming thick plugs in the bronchiolar airways (Figure 30-2). These thick plugs are difficult to eliminate. The resultant colonization of pathogenic microorganisms in the lower respiratory tract causes inflammation and additional mucous secretions and the possible development of pneumonia from trapped bacteria.

The smooth muscle of the tracheobronchial tree is innervated by the parasympathetic and sympathetic branches of the autonomic nervous system. Stimulation of the cholinergic nerves causes bronchial constriction and increased mucus secretion. Sympathetic stimulation of adrenergic nerves causes dilation of bronchial and bronchiolar airways and inhibition of respiratory tract fluids. Both beta-1 and beta-2 adrenergic receptors are present, but the beta-2 receptors predominate.

COMMON LOWER RESPIRATORY DISEASES

Respiratory diseases are often divided into two types: obstructive and restrictive. **Obstructive airway diseases** are those that narrow air passages, create turbulence, and increase resistance to airflow. Diseases cause narrowing of the airways through smooth muscle constriction (**bronchospasm**), edema, inflammation of the

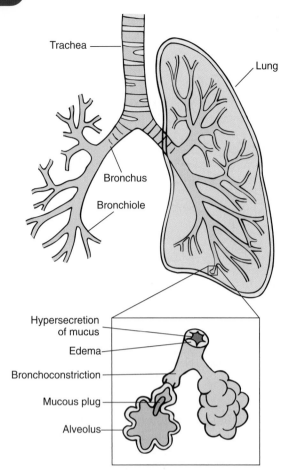

FIGURE 30-2 Factors restricting the airway. Major factors include hypersecretion of mucus, mucosal edema, and bronchoconstriction. Mucous plugs may form in the alveoli. (From Clark JB, et al: *Pharmacological basis of nursing practice*, ed 3, St. Louis, 1982, Mosby-Year Book.)

Table 30-1	Arterial Blood Gases Used to Assess Respiratory Function	
TEST	**NORMAL VALUE**	**RESULTS**
pH	7.35-7.45 (arterial)	>7.45 = Alkalosis <7.35 = Acidosis
$PaCO_2$	35-45 mm Hg	Abnormalities indicate respiratory acid-base imbalance. ↑ = Hypercapnia = respiratory acidosis ↓ = Hypocapnia = respiratory alkalosis
HCO_3	24-28 mEq/L	Abnormalities indicate metabolic acid-base imbalance. ↑ = Metabolic alkalosis ↓ = Metabolic acidosis
PaO_2	80-100 mm Hg	Measures the amount of oxygen moving through pulmonary alveoli into blood for transport to other tissues; depends on the amount of inspired oxygen. ↓ = Hypoxemia, hypoventilation ↑ = Hyperventilation
SaO_2	95%	Measures the ratio of actual oxygen content of hemoglobin compared with the hemoglobin's oxygen-carrying capacity. When decreased, either there is an impairment of oxygen binding to hemoglobin (e.g., metabolic acidosis) or inadequate amounts of oxygen are being inspired.

bronchial walls, or excess mucus secretion. Examples of obstructive lung disease are asthma and acute bronchitis. **Restrictive airway diseases** are those in which lung expansion is limited from loss of elasticity (e.g., pulmonary fibrosis) or physical deformity of the chest (e.g., kyphoscoliosis). Chronic bronchitis and emphysema are examples of both restrictive and obstructive lung diseases. Patients who have persistent airflow limitation associated with chronic inflammation in the airways and lung tissue due to noxious particles and gases are referred to as having **chronic obstructive pulmonary disease (COPD)** or **chronic airflow limitation disease (CALD)**; the terms are used interchangeably. Chronic obstructive pulmonary disease affects about 20% of U.S. adults and is the second most common cause of disability and the fourth leading cause of death.

Pulmonary function tests have been developed to assess the ventilation and diffusion capacity of the lungs to assist in diagnosis and to give an objective assessment of improvement or deterioration of the patient's clinical condition. The best indicators of overall pulmonary function (ventilation and diffusion)

are the partial pressure of **arterial blood gases (ABGs)** (e.g., PaO_2 and $PaCO_2$) and pH (Table 30-1). To determine ABGs, a sample of arterial blood must be drawn and immediately analyzed to measure the pH and partial pressures of oxygen and carbon dioxide in the blood. Another measure that is more readily available and noninvasive is the oxygen saturation of hemoglobin. **Oxygen saturation** (SaO_2) is the ratio, expressed as a percentage, of the oxygen actually bound to hemoglobin compared with the maximum amount of oxygen that could be bound to hemoglobin (see Table 30-1). Oxygen saturation is routinely used because a transcutaneous monitor (oximeter) is easily attached to the skin to measure and report oxygen saturation continuously.

Spirometry studies are routinely used to assess the capability of the patient's lungs, thorax, and respiratory muscles for moving volumes of air during inhalation and exhalation. It is recommended that spirometry

Table 30-2 Terminology Used With Spirometry

TERM	DEFINITION
Tidal volume (TV)	Volume of air inspired or expired during normal breathing
Vital capacity (VC)	Volume of air exhaled after maximal inspiration to full expiration
Residual volume (RV)	Volume of air left in lungs after maximal exhalation
Functional residual capacity (FRC)	Volume of air left in lungs after normal exhalation
Total lung capacity (TLC)	Vital capacity plus residual volume (VC + RV) = TLC
Forced expiratory volume (FEV)	Volume of air forced out of the lungs by maximal exhalation
Forced expiratory volume in 1 second (FEV_1)	Volume of air forced out in 1 sec to give the rate of flow
Forced vital capacity (FVC)	Maximal volume of air exhaled with maximal forced effort after maximal inhalation
Peak expiratory flow rate (PEFR)	Maximal rate of airflow produced during forced expiration

Box 30-1 Asthma Fact Sheet

In 2008 asthma caused:
- 10.5 million missed days of school
- 14.2 million missed days of work

In 2009 there were:
- 479,300 asthma-related hospitalizations
- 1.9 million asthma-related emergency department visits
- 8.9 million asthma-related doctor visits
- About nine people die from asthma each day. In 2009 3,388 people died from asthma.
- In the last decade, the proportion of people with asthma in the United States grew by nearly 15%

In 2010:
- 18.7 million adults had asthma, or 1 in 12 adults
- 7 million children had asthma, or 1 in 11 children

From National Center for Environmental Health, Division of Environmental Hazards and Health Effects: *Asthma's Impact on the Nation.* Data from the CDC National Asthma Control Program. Retrieved from http://www.cdc.gov/asthma/impacts_nation/asthmafactsheet.pdf.

be used to diagnose airway obstruction in symptomatic patients, but it should not be used as a screening tool for asymptomatic patients. A spirometer measures volumes of air. Terms used with spirometry are listed in Table 30-2. Patients with obstructive disease usually have a normal total lung capacity (TLC), difficulty with expiration, decreased vital capacity (VC), and increased residual capacity (RC). Patients with restrictive disease have a decrease in all measured lung volumes. The forced expiratory volume in 1 second (FEV_1) and the forced vital capacity (FVC) are the most commonly used pulmonary function tests. The FEV_1 is used to determine the reversibility of airway disease and the effectiveness of bronchodilator therapy. The peak expiratory flow rate (PEFR) meter is not as accurate but is much less costly and more readily available than other pulmonary function test equipment. This meter is routinely used by patients at home and by healthcare providers to assess the benefits of therapy for treating acute and chronic asthmatic symptoms. A patient is considered to have significant reversibility of airway obstruction if there is a 15% to 20% improvement in the FEV_1 or PEFR after bronchodilator therapy.

One of the first symptoms of a respiratory disease is the presence of a **cough**, a reflex initiated by irritation of the airway. It is a protective beneficial mechanism for clearing excess secretions from the tracheobronchial tree. The same irritants responsible for asthma or allergy may stimulate the cough receptors, or congestion of the nasal mucosa from a cold may cause a postnasal drip into the back of the throat that stimulates the cough.

A cough is productive if it helps remove accumulated secretions and phlegm from the tracheobronchial tree. A nonproductive cough results when irritants repeatedly stimulate the cough receptors but are not removed by the coughing reflex. Excessive coughing, particularly if it is dry and nonproductive, is not only uncomfortable but also tends to be self-perpetuating because the rapid air expulsion further irritates the tracheobronchial mucosa.

Asthma is a common chronic airway disease that affects more than 25 million people in the United States (Box 30-1). It is an inflammatory disease of the bronchi and bronchioles. There are intermittent periods of acute, reversible airflow obstruction (bronchoconstriction) caused by bronchiolar inflammation and hyperresponsiveness to a variety of stimuli. Examples of stimuli that trigger bronchospasm and inflammation are respiratory viral infections, inhaled allergens, cold air, dry air, emotional stress, and smoke. Symptoms of asthma include cough, wheezing, shortness of breath, tightness of the chest, and increased mucus production. The exact causes of asthma are unknown. Asthmatic patients are often subdivided into categories based on severity of disease: intermittent, mild persistent, moderate persistent, and severe persistent (Figure 30-3).

Chronic **bronchitis** is a condition in which chronic irritation causes inflammation and edema, with excessive mucus secretion leading to airflow obstruction. Chronic bronchitis refers to a chronic productive cough that is present for 3 months in each of 2 successive years and has no other identifiable cause. Common causes of chronic irritation are cigarette smoke, grain and coal dust exposure, and air pollution. A persistent productive cough present on most days is one of the earliest signs of the disease. The classic patient with chronic bronchitis has a chronic productive cough and

Clinical characteristics	Therapy (must include patient education)		Outcome

| | Quick-relief medicine | Long-term control medicine | |

Step 1
Intermittent asthma
- Intermittent brief symptoms <2 times/week
- <2 nocturnal symptoms/month
- Asymptomatic between episodes
- PEF or FEV_1
  - >80% predicted
  - <20% variability
  - FEV_1/FVC normal

- Inhaled short-acting beta-2 agonist (no more than 2 times/week)

- No daily medication
- Systemic corticosteroids for severe exacerbations separated by long periods of normal lung function

- Symptoms controlled
- PEF or FEV_1 values optimal for patient
- Reduced PEF variability
- Normal activity level
- Rarely awaken at night
- Infrequent exacerbations
- Reduced frequency of PRN inhaled beta agonist

Step 2
Mild persistent asthma
- Persistent brief symptoms
- >2 times/week but <1 time/day
- 3-4 nocturnal symptoms/month
- Exacerbations may affect activity
- PEF or FEV_1
  - ≥80% predicted
  - PEF variability 20%-30%
  - FEV_1/FVC normal

- Inhaled short-acting beta-2 agonist as needed

+ Preferred treatment:
- Low-dose inhaled corticosteroids
  OR
- Leukotriene modifier
  OR
- Inhaled cromolyn
  OR
- Sustained-release theophylline

Step 3
Moderate persistent asthma
- Daily symptoms
- Daily use of beta-2 agonist
- Exacerbations affect activity
- Exacerbations ≥2 times/week; may last days
- Nocturnal symptoms >1/week
- PEF or FEV_1
  - >60% but ≤80% predicted
  - PEF variability >30%
  - FEV_1/FVC reduced >5%

- Inhaled short-acting beta agonist (PRN, ≤3-4 times daily)

+ Preferred treatment:
- Medium-dose inhaled corticosteroids
  OR
- Low-dose inhaled corticosteroids + Long-acting beta-2 agonist
  OR
  + Leukotriene modifier or theophylline or zileuton

Note:
- Once control is sustained at any step, a step-down reduction in therapy may be cautiously attempted to achieve minimum therapy required to maintain control
- Patient must be aware of signs of worsening symptoms and how to control them

Step 4
Severe persistent asthma
- Continuous symptoms
- Limited activity level
- Frequent exacerbations
- Frequent nocturnal symptoms
- Occasional hospitalizations
- PEF or FEV_1
  - <60% predicted
  - >30% variability
  - FEV_1/FVC reduced >5%

- Inhaled short-acting beta agonist (PRN, ≤3-4 times daily)

+ Preferred treatment:
- Medium-dose inhaled corticosteroids
  AND
- Long-acting inhaled beta-2 agonist
Alternative: so high
- Medium-dose inhaled corticosteroids + tiotropium or leukotriene modifier or theophylline or zileuton

Best possible results
- Fewest symptoms
- Lowest need for PRN inhaled beta agonist
- Least limitation of activity
- Best PEF for patient
- Least PEF variability
- Fewest adverse effects from medicine

Step 5
Severe persistent asthma
- Continuous symptoms
- Limited activity level
- Frequent exacerbations
- Frequent nocturnal symptoms
- Occasional hospitalizations
- PEF or FEV_1
  - <60% predicted
  - >30% variability
  - FEV_1/FVC reduced >5%

- Inhaled short-acting beta agonist (PRN, ≤3-4 times daily)

+ Preferred treatment:
- High-dose inhaled corticosteroids + Long-acting beta-2 agonists
  AND
- Add tiotropium or
- Low-dose oral corticosteroids or
- Consider omalizumab for patients with allergies

Best possible results
- Fewest symptoms
- Lowest need for PRN inhaled beta agonist
- Least limitation of activity
- Best PEF for patient
- Least PEF variability
- Fewest adverse effects from medicine

Step 6
Severe persistent asthma
- Continuous symptoms
- Limited activity level
- Frequent exacerbations
- Frequent nocturnal symptoms
- Occasional hospitalizations
- PEF or FEV_1
  - <60% predicted
  - >30% variability
  - FEV_1/FVC reduced >5%

- Inhaled short-acting beta agonist (PRN, ≤3-4 times daily)

+ Preferred treatment:
- High-dose inhaled corticosteroids
  AND
- Long-acting inhaled beta-2 agonists
  AND
- Oral corticosteroids (2 mg/kg/day ≯60 mg/day) (reduce as symptoms allow and maintain on high-dose inhaled corticosteroids)
  AND
- Consider omalizumab for patients with allergies

Best possible results
- Fewest symptoms
- Lowest need for PRN inhaled beta agonist
- Least limitation of activity
- Best PEF for patient
- Least PEF variability
- Fewest adverse effects from medicine

FIGURE 30-3 Stepwise management of chronic asthma in adults. Therapy is stepped up to the next level of therapy if control is not achieved at the current step with proper use of medication. Step-down, or reduction of dosages, should be considered when the desired outcomes have been achieved and sustained for several weeks at the current step. Step-down therapy is desired to identify the minimum dosages of therapy required to maintain the desired outcomes. *FEV₁*, forced expiratory volume in 1 second; *PEF*, peak expiratory flow; *PRN*, as needed. (Modified from National Institutes of Health, National Heart, Lung and Blood Institute: *Expert Panel Report: guidelines for the diagnosis and management of asthma, update on selected topics-2002* (update of the NAEPP Expert Panel Report 2 [IH publication no. 97-4051A]), Washington, D.C., 1997, NIH/NHLBI; *Report 3, 2007* (updated 2012). The Global Initiative for Asthma (GINA) 2015: *Global strategy for asthma management and prevention.* Retrieved from http://www.ginasthma.org.

Table 30-4   Antitussive Agents

GENERIC NAME	BRAND NAME	AVAILABILITY	ADULT ORAL DOSAGE RANGE
benzonatate ⇄ *Do not confuse benzonatate with benazepril or benztropine.*	Tessalon Perles	Capsules: 100, 150, 200 mg	100-200 mg three times daily
codeine*	—	Tablets: 15, 30, 60 mg Solution: 30 mg/5 mL	10-20 mg q4-6h
dextromethorphan	Robitussin CoughGels ⇄ *Do not confuse Robitussin with Reglan.* Delsym	Lozenges: 5, 7.5, mg Syrup: 5, 7.5, 10, 15 mg/5 mL Liquid: 7.5, 10, 12.5, 15 mg/5 mL Suspension, extended release: 30 mg/5 mL Gel caps: 10 mg	10-20 mg q4h or 30 mg q6-8h; 60 mg q12h (sustained-release); do not exceed 120 mg per 24 hr
diphenhydramine ⇄ *Do not confuse diphenhydramine with dicyclomine or dipyridamole.*	Diphen TH Allergy Relief	Syrup, liquid: 12.5 mg/5 mL Capsules and tablets: 25, 50 mg	25 mg q4h; do not exceed 150 mg per 24 hr
hydrocodone*	—	—	5 mg q6-8h

*An ingredient in combination antitussive products.

THERAPEUTIC OUTCOME

The primary therapeutic outcome expected from acetylcysteine therapy is improved airway flow, with more comfortable breathing.

❖ NURSING IMPLICATIONS FOR ACETYLCYSTEINE THERAPY

■ Premedication Assessment
1. Record the characteristics of cough and bronchial secretions before starting therapy.
2. Obtain and record baseline vital signs, and carry out pulse oximetry.
3. Observe for and record any GI symptoms before starting therapy.
4. Perform a baseline assessment of the patient's mental status (e.g., degree of anxiety, nervousness, alertness).

■ Availability
Inhalation: 10% and 20% solutions in 4-, 10-, and 30-mL vials.

■ Dosage and Administration
Adult: Nebulization: The recommended dosage for most patients is 3 to 5 mL of the 20% solution three or four times daily. *Direct application into an intratracheal catheter or tracheostomy:* 1 to 2 mL of a 20% solution every 1 to 4 hours. After administration, the volume of bronchial secretions may increase. Some patients with inadequate cough reflex may require mechanical suctioning to maintain an open airway.

Nebulizer. This solution tends to concentrate as it is used. When three fourths of the original amount in the nebulizer is used, dilute the remaining solution with sterile water.

After therapy, wash the patient's face and hands because the drug is sticky and irritating. Thoroughly cleanse equipment used.

Storage. Store the opened solution of the drug in a refrigerator for up to 96 hours. Discard the unused portion.

Discoloration. Use medication stored only in plastic or glass containers. Contact with metals other than stainless steel can cause the solution to discolor.

■ Common Adverse Effects
Gastrointestinal

Nausea, vomiting. Acetylcysteine has a pungent odor (similar to rotten eggs) that may cause nausea and vomiting; have an emesis basin available. Do not, however, suggest it by having the basin in clear view.

■ Serious Adverse Effects
Respiratory

Bronchospasm. Acetylcysteine may occasionally cause bronchoconstriction and bronchospasm. Concurrent use of a bronchodilator may be necessary.

■ Drug Interactions
Antibiotics. Acetylcysteine inactivates most antibiotics. Do not mix together for aerosol administration. Schedule administration of inhalation antibiotics 1 hour after administration of acetylcysteine.

DRUG CLASS: BETA-ADRENERGIC BRONCHODILATING AGENTS

ACTIONS

Beta-adrenergic agonists stimulate the beta receptors in the smooth muscle of the tracheobronchial tree to relax, opening the airway passages to greater volumes of air.

USES

Beta-adrenergic bronchodilators reverse airway constriction caused by acute and chronic bronchial asthma, bronchitis, and emphysema. Agents with more selective beta-2 receptor activity (e.g., albuterol, terbutaline, formoterol, salmeterol, arformoterol, indacaterol, olodaterol, vilanterol) have more direct bronchodilating activity and fewer systemic adverse effects. (See Chapter 12 for a discussion of selective beta receptor activity.)

Unfortunately, the receptors stimulated by sympathomimetic agents causing relaxation of the smooth muscle in the tracheobronchial tree are found in other tissues as well as the pulmonary system. These receptors are also found in the muscles of the heart; blood vessels; uterus; GI, urinary, and central nervous systems. They also help regulate fat and carbohydrate metabolism. Therefore there are many adverse effects from these agents, particularly if used too frequently or in higher-than-recommended doses. Those administered by inhalation generally have fewer systemic effects because inhalation places the drug at the site of action so that smaller dosages may be used.

The short-acting beta agonists (e.g., albuterol, levalbuterol, pirbuterol, terbutaline, metaproterenol) have a rapid onset (a few minutes) and are used to treat acute bronchospasm. During acute exacerbations, these agents can be used every 3 to 4 hours. If a patient is using an increased amount of these inhaled bronchodilators on a daily basis, it is an indication of worsening asthma. Patients then must be reassessed for adherence, inhalation technique, improved environmental control, and the possible addition of corticosteroids to the therapeutic regimen.

Salmeterol, arformoterol, formoterol, indacaterol and olodaterol are long-acting inhaled bronchodilators, sometimes known as *long-acting beta-2 agonists (LABAs)*. Salmeterol and arformoterol have an onset of action in 10 to 15 minutes, with a duration of action up to 12 hours. Therefore they are administered twice daily. Salmeterol is approved for both asthma and COPD. Arformoterol is approved for use in COPD only.

Formoterol, indacaterol, and olodaterol have an onset of action in 5 to 15 minutes with a duration of action of 24 hours, and are therefore administered only 1 time daily. Formoterol is approved for use in asthma and COPD, whereas indacaterol and olodaterol are approved only for COPD. The LABAs are not used to treat acute episodes of asthma or COPD, but are used for long-term control of respiratory effort to prevent acute exacerbations of asthma and COPD.

There is concern that although LABAs decrease the frequency of asthmatic attacks, they may actually make the attacks that do occur more severe. In February 2010, the U.S. Food and Drug Administration issued an advisory on LABA use in asthma (but not COPD), stating that:

- Use of LABAs is contraindicated without the use of an asthma controller medicine such as an inhaled corticosteroid.
- Long-acting beta-2 agonists should only be used long-term in patients whose asthma cannot be adequately controlled on asthma controller medicines.
- Long-acting beta-2 agonists should be used for the shortest duration of time required to achieve control of asthma symptoms and discontinued, if possible, once asthma control is achieved. Patients should then be maintained on asthma controller medicines. Patients known to have hypertension, hyperthyroidism, diabetes mellitus, or cardiac disease with dysrhythmias may be particularly sensitive to adverse reactions and must be observed closely.

THERAPEUTIC OUTCOME

The primary therapeutic outcome associated with beta-adrenergic bronchodilator therapy is bronchodilation resulting in reduced wheezing and easier breathing.

❖ NURSING IMPLICATIONS FOR BETA-ADRENERGIC BRONCHODILATORS

▪ Premedication Assessment

1. Obtain and record baseline vital signs and pulse oximetry.
2. Assess the patient for the presence of palpitations and dysrhythmias before administration of beta-adrenergic agents. If suspected, notify the healthcare provider and ask whether therapy should be started.
3. Perform an assessment of the patient's baseline mental status (e.g., degree of anxiety, nervousness, alertness).

▪ Availability, Dosage, and Administration

See Table 30-5. Patients using inhaled bronchodilators should wait approximately 10 minutes between inhalations. This allows the medicine to dilate the bronchioles so that the second dose can be inhaled more deeply into the lungs for a more therapeutic effect. Assure that patients understand how to use the inhaler as described in the manufacturer's leaflet that accompanies the inhaler.

▪ Serious Adverse Effects

Cardiovascular

Tachycardia, palpitations. Because most symptoms are dose related, alterations should be reported to the healthcare provider. Monitor the patient's heart rate and rhythm at regular intervals throughout therapy with bronchodilators. An increase of 20 beats/min or more after treatment should be reported to the

Table 30-5 Bronchodilators

GENERIC NAME	BRAND NAME	AVAILABILITY	ADULT DOSAGE RANGE
Beta-Adrenergic Agonists			
albuterol ⇌ *Do not confuse albuterol with acebutolol.*	Proventil, Ventolin, HFA ⇌ *Do not confuse Ventolin with Benylin or Vantin.* AccuNeb	Tablets: 2, 4 mg Syrup: 2 mg/5 mL Tablets, extended release (12 hr): 4, 8 mg Aerosol: 108 mcg/actuation Solution for inhalation: 0.5-1.25 mg/3 mL	PO: 2-4 mg three or four times daily; maximum dose 32 mg daily Extended release: 8 mg q12hr; maximum dose 32 mg per 24 hr Inhale: 2 inhalations q4-6h; maximum 12 inhalations per 24 hr See manufacturer's recommendations
arformoterol	Brovana	Solution for inhalation: 15 mcg/2 mL	15 mcg twice daily
epinephrine	Micronefrin	Nebulization: 2.25% Injection: 0.1, 1 mg/mL	Nebulization: 10 drops of a 1:100 solution vial nebulizer See manufacturer's recommendations
formoterol	Foradil; Perforomist	Inhaler capsule: 12 mcg Solution for inhalation: 20 mcg/2 mL	Inhale: 1 capsule q12h using Aerolizer inhaler Nebulizer: 20 mcg q12h
indacaterol	Arcapta Neohaler	Inhalation powder: 75 mcg	Inhale: 1 capsule q24h using Neohaler inhaler at same time daily
levalbuterol	Xopenex Xopenex HFA	Solution for inhalation: 0.30, 0.63, 1.25 mg/3 mL; 1.25 mcg/0.5 mL Aerosol: 45 mcg/actuation	0.63-1.25 mg q8h Inhale: 1-2 inhalations q4-6h
metaproterenol	—	Tablets: 10, 20 mg Syrup: 10 mg/5 mL	PO: 20 mg three or four times daily
olodaterol	Striverdi Respimat	Aerosol: 2.5 mcg/actuation	Two actuations once daily at the same time of the day
pirbuterol	Maxair Autohaler	Aerosol: 200 mcg/inhalation	Inhale: 1-2 inhalations q4-6h
salmeterol	Serevent Diskus ⇌ *Do not confuse Serevent with Atrovent.* Diskus	Inhalation powder: 50 mcg/ inhalation	Inhale: 1 inhalation q12h
terbutaline ❶	Brethine	Tablets: 2.5, 5 mg Injection: 1 mg/mL	PO: 5 mg q6h Subcutaneous: 0.25 mg; repeat, if needed, in 30 min
Combination Anticholinergic and Beta-Adrenergic Bronchodilators			
umeclidinium/ vilanterol	Anoro Ellipta	Aerosol powder: meclidinium 62.5 mcg and vilanterol 25 mcg/inhalation	Inhale: 1 inhalation per 24 hr
tiotropium/ olodaterol	Spiolto Respimat	Aerosol powder: ticotropium 2.5 mcg and olodaterol 2.5 mcg/actuation	Inhale: 2 inhalations at the same time per 24 hr

❶ High-alert medication.

prescriber. Always report palpitations and suspected dysrhythmias to a healthcare provider.

Neurologic

Tremors. Tell the patient to notify the healthcare provider if tremors develop after starting any of these medications. A dosage adjustment may be necessary.

Nervousness, anxiety, restlessness, headache. Perform a baseline assessment of the patient's mental status (e.g., degree of anxiety, nervousness, alertness); compare subsequent, regular assessments with the baseline.

Dizziness. Provide for patient safety during episodes of dizziness. Report episodes of dizziness for further evaluation to a healthcare provider.

Gastrointestinal

Nausea, vomiting. Monitor all aspects of the development of these symptoms. Question the patient concerning other medications being taken and any other symptoms that have also developed. Administer the medication with food and a full glass of water or milk. Report if the symptoms are not relieved.

■ Drug Interactions

Drugs That Enhance Toxic Effects. Tricyclic antidepressants (e.g., imipramine, amitriptyline, nortriptyline, doxepin), monoamine oxidase inhibitors (e.g., tranylcypromine, pargyline), and other sympathomimetic agents (e.g., metaproterenol, isoproterenol) enhance the toxic effects of beta-adrenergic bronchodilators. Monitor for increases in severity of drug effects, such as nervousness, tachycardia, tremors, and dysrhythmias.

Drugs That Reduce Therapeutic Effects. Beta-adrenergic blocking agents (e.g., propranolol, nadolol, pindolol) reduce the therapeutic effects of beta-adrenergic bronchodilators. Higher dosages or use of another class of bronchodilator may be required.

Antihypertensive Agents. Sympathomimetic agents may reduce the therapeutic effects of antihypertensive agents. Monitor blood pressure for an indication of loss of antihypertensive control.

DRUG CLASS: ANTICHOLINERGIC BRONCHODILATING AGENTS

Anticholinergic agents have been used as bronchodilators for treating obstructive pulmonary disease for more than 200 years, but the potent anticholinergic adverse effects (e.g., throat irritation, dry mouth, reduced mucous secretions, increased secretion viscosity, mydriasis, cycloplegia, urinary retention, tachycardia) and the availability of selective sympathomimetic agents have limited their use for pulmonary disorders.

ipratropium bromide (ĭp-ră-TRŌ-pē-ŭm)
Atrovent (ĂT-rō-vĕnt), Atrovent HFA

ACTIONS

Ipratropium bromide is administered by aerosol inhalation and produces bronchodilation by competitive inhibition of cholinergic receptors on bronchial smooth muscle blocking the bronchoconstrictor action of vagal efferent impulses. The inhibition of vagal tone results in dilation of the large central airways and small airways. It has minimal effect on ciliary activity, mucus secretion, sputum volume, and viscosity.

USES

Ipratropium is used as a bronchodilator for long-term treatment of reversible bronchospasm associated with COPD. It may also be used in combination with beta-adrenergic bronchodilators in patients with asthma. Initial bronchodilation is evident within the first few minutes after inhalation, but maximal effects are seen in 1 to 2 hours. The duration of significant bronchodilation is 4 to 6 hours with usual dosages. Because its maximal effects are not seen immediately, the drug is more appropriately used for prophylaxis and mainte-nance treatment of bronchospasm associated with chronic obstructive lung disease than for acute episodes of bronchospasm associated with asthma.

Ipratropium nasal spray is used for the symptomatic relief of rhinorrhea associated with allergic and nonallergic perennial rhinitis and the common cold. It does not relieve nasal congestion, sneezing, or postnasal drip associated with these conditions.

THERAPEUTIC OUTCOMES

The primary therapeutic outcomes associated with ipratropium therapy are bronchodilation resulting in reduced wheezing and easier breathing with less effort when the inhaler is used and reduced rhinorrhea when the nasal solution is used.

❖ NURSING IMPLICATIONS FOR IPRATROPIUM

■ Premedication Assessment

1. Record baseline vital signs and pulse oximetry.
2. Check the medical record to determine whether the patient has a history of closed-angle glaucoma. If so, reconfirm the administration order with the healthcare provider before administration of ipratropium.

■ Availability

Inhalation: Aerosol canister containing approximately 200 inhalations (17 mcg/metered dose) with metered-dose inhaler mouthpiece. Nasal spray: 0.03% (21 mcg/spray; 30 mL) and 0.06% (42 mcg/spray; 15 mL) nasal spray pumps.

■ Dosage and Administration

Inhalation. The usual dose is two inhalations (34 mcg) four times daily. Patients may take additional inhalations as required, but should not exceed 12 inhalations in 24 hours. Ensure that the patient understands how to inhale the medication.

1. Clear the throat and mouth of sputum.
2. Insert the metal canister into the clear end of the mouthpiece.
3. Remove the protective cap, invert the canister, and shake thoroughly.
4. Enclose the mouthpiece with the lips. The base of the canister should be held vertically. (Keep the eyes closed because temporary blurred vision may result if the aerosol is sprayed into the eyes.)
5. Exhale deeply through the mouth or nose, then inhale slowly through the mouthpiece and at the same time firmly press once on the upended canister base; continue to inhale deeply.
6. Hold the breath for a few seconds and then remove the mouthpiece from the mouth and exhale slowly. Wait approximately 15 seconds, and repeat the second inhalation as outlined in steps 4 and 5.
7. Replace the protective cap after use.
8. Keep the mouthpiece clean. Wash with hot water. If soap is used, rinse thoroughly with plain water.

to dissolve completely. Repeat step 4 until there are no visible gelatinous particles in the solution. It is acceptable to have small bubbles or foam around the edge of the vial. Do not use if the contents of the vial do not dissolve completely within 40 minutes.

5. Invert the vial for 15 seconds to allow the solution to drain toward the stopper. Note that it is a rather viscous solution. Using a new 3-mL syringe equipped with a 1-inch, 18-gauge needle, insert the needle into the inverted vial. Position the needle tip at the very bottom of the solution in the vial when drawing the solution into the syringe. Before removing the needle from the vial, be sure to remove all the solution from the inverted vial.

6. Replace the 18-gauge needle with a 25-gauge needle for subcutaneous injection.

7. Expel air, large bubbles, and any excess solution to obtain the required 1.2-mL dose. A thin layer of small bubbles may remain at the top of the solution in the syringe. Because the solution is slightly viscous, the injection may take 5 to 10 seconds to administer.

■ Common and Serious Adverse Effects
Hypersensitivity

Injection site reactions. The most commonly reported adverse effect is injection site reaction (45%), including bruising, redness, warmth, burning, stinging, itching, hive formation, pain, indurations, mass, and inflammation. Most injection site reactions occur within 1 hour after injection, last less than 8 days, and generally decrease in frequency with subsequent dosing. Immediately report a rash or pruritus, with or without fever, and withhold additional injections until approved by the healthcare provider.

■ Drug Interactions
No drug interactions have been reported.

DRUG CLASS: MISCELLANEOUS ANTIINFLAMMATORY AGENTS

> **cromolyn sodium** (KRŌ-mō-lĭn)

ACTIONS

Cromolyn sodium is a mast cell stabilizer that inhibits the release of histamine and other mediators of inflammation, making it an indirect antiinflammatory agent. It must be administered before the body is given a stimulus to release histamine, such as an antigen that initiates an antigen-antibody allergic reaction.

USES

Cromolyn is recommended for use in conjunction with other medications for treating patients with severe bronchial asthma or allergic rhinitis to prevent the release of histamine that results in asthmatic attacks or symptoms of allergic rhinitis. It is also used for the prophylactic management of exercise-induced bronchospasm and asthma.

Cromolyn has no direct bronchodilatory, antihistaminic, or anticholinergic activity. Concomitant use of antihistamines or nasal decongestants may be necessary during initial treatment with cromolyn. A 2- to 4-week course of therapy is usually required to determine clinical response. Therapy should be continued only if there is a decrease in the severity of asthmatic symptoms.

THERAPEUTIC OUTCOME

The primary therapeutic outcome associated with cromolyn therapy is reduced frequency of episodes of allergic rhinitis, bronchospasm, and asthmatic attacks.

❖ NURSING IMPLICATIONS FOR CROMOLYN SODIUM

■ Premedication Assessment

1. This medication must be taken before exposure to the stimulus that initiates an attack of allergic rhinitis or bronchial asthma. Inhalation during an attack of bronchospasm or asthma may exacerbate symptoms.

2. Check to see whether the concurrent use of antihistamines or nasal decongestants has been ordered by the healthcare provider, especially during initiation of cromolyn therapy.

■ Availability
Inhalation: Nasal solution: 40 mg/mL in 13- and 26-mL metered device delivering 5.2 mg per actuation; solution for inhalation: 20 mg/2 mL in 60- and 120-unit dose vials and ampules.

■ Dosage and Administration
Counseling. The therapeutic effects, unlike those of beta-adrenergic decongestants, are not immediate. This should be explained to the patient in advance to ensure cooperation and continuation of treatment with the prescribed dosage regimen. Full therapeutic benefit requires regular use and is usually evident within 2 to 4 weeks. Therapy must be continued, even if the patient is symptom free.

Adult: PO: Inhalation: 20 mg via nebulizer, four times daily. Inhalation during an acute asthma attack may aggravate symptoms because the powder form of the drug can increase the irritation in the respiratory passage and result in more bronchospasm.

Intranasal: For prevention of exercise-induced bronchospasm or bronchospasm associated with cold air or environmental substances, administer two metered-dose sprays 10 to 60 minutes before exposure to the precipitating factor.

Spray one or two metered doses into each nostril. Repeat three or four times per day (every 4 to 6 hours). If needed, it may be used up to six times per day. Use every day while in contact with the allergen (e.g., pollen, molds, pets, dust). To prevent nasal allergy symptoms, use before contact with the cause of the allergy. For best results, start using up to 1 week before contact.

■ **Common Adverse Effects**

Gastrointestinal

Oral irritation, dry mouth. The most common adverse effect is irritation of the throat and trachea caused by inhaling the dry powder. This may be manifested by nasal itching and burning, nasal stuffiness, sneezing, coughing, and bronchospasm. Start regular oral

hygiene measures when the therapy is initiated. Commercial mouthwashes contain alcohol, which may cause further drying and oral irritation. Other measures to alleviate dryness include sucking on ice chips or hard candy.

■ **Serious Adverse Effects**

Respiratory

Bronchospasm, coughing. Notify the prescriber if inhalation causes bronchospasm or coughing.

■ **Drug Interactions**

No significant drug interactions have been reported.

Get Ready for the NCLEX® Examination!

Key Points

- Chronic obstructive pulmonary diseases, also known as chronic airflow limitation diseases, include chronic bronchitis and emphysema, both of which are progressive, irreversible diseases that usually cause death after a long debilitating illness.
- Asthma is an inflammatory disease that has airflow limitations; however, the episodes are intermittent and the limitations are reversible.
- Regular use of preventive medicine and removal of triggers such as allergens are key to the long-term treatment of asthma.
- Emphasize taking medications *before* exposure to a suspected trigger of an attack; treat all respiratory infections early.
- Regular use of a peak flowmeter and appropriate use of an inhaler are integral to treating asthma successfully.
- Nurses can teach patients with irreversible chronic airflow disorders techniques to manage their symptoms (e.g., adequate fluid intake to decrease secretion viscosity, breathing techniques, exercise conditioning to strengthen respiratory muscles, controlled coughing, positioning).
- Nurses can play a significant role in public education efforts, monitoring for nonadherence and encouraging patients to make changes in lifestyle to reduce the severity of CALD.
- Nurses can help the patient and/or family identify community resources available in the immediate vicinity.

Additional Learning Resources

SG Go to your Study Guide for additional Review Questions for the NCLEX® Examination, Critical Thinking Clinical Situations, and other learning activities to help you master this chapter content.

evolve Go to your Evolve website (http://evolve.elsevier.com/Clayton) for additional online resources.

Review Questions for the NCLEX® Examination

1. During a respiratory assessment of a patient, the nurse noted the patient was coughing frequently and the oxygen saturation was <90%. The following lower respiratory diseases/conditions could be the cause of these findings: *(Select all that apply.)*
   1. Pulmonary embolism
   2. Chronic obstructive pulmonary disease
   3. Asthma
   4. Pneumonia
   5. Smoking

2. During an evaluation of a patient who came into the clinic complaining of shortness of breath and increased sputum production, the nurse asks the patient for further information by the following statements: *(Select all that apply.)*
   1. "Tell me about your cough. Does it wake you at night?"
   2. "What activities would you say make you short of breath?"
   3. "When you cough up sputum, what color is it?"
   4. "Is there anyone at home to help you?"
   5. "Have you had any constipation or diarrhea recently?"

3. The nurse is preparing the antitussive agent benzonatate (Tessalon Perles) for a patient with a dry cough and knows the action of this drug will:
   1. dissolve thick sticky mucus.
   2. suppress the cough reflex response in the brain.
   3. stimulate an increase in bronchial gland secretions.
   4. reduce the release of leukotrienes.

4. The expectorant guaifenesin (Robitussin), used for relief of conditions such as the common cold and bronchitis, works by these actions: *(Select all that apply.)*
   1. Suppressing the cough reflex response in the brain
   2. Decreasing mucus viscosity
   3. Stimulating an increase in bronchial secretions
   4. Promoting ciliary action
   5. Reducing the release of leukotrienes

5. The nurse is preparing to administer the beta-adrenergic bronchodilator albuterol, but first performs the following preassessment of the patient: *(Select all that apply.)*
   1. Checks liver function test results
   2. Checks for a history of glaucoma, diabetes mellitus, or peptic ulcer disease
   3. Performs an assessment of the baseline mental status
   4. Asks about concurrent use of antihistamines or nasal decongestants
   5. Assesses for the presence of palpitations and dysrhythmias

6. The nurse was instructing the patient on the drug tiotropium bromide (Spiriva) that was being started instead of continuing ipratropium bromide (Atrovent) and included the following statements in the education: *(Select all that apply.)*
   1. "Spiriva uses the HandiHaler device for administration."
   2. "The effects of Spiriva last much longer than Atrovent so you only have to take it once a day."
   3. "This drug is used to treat acute bronchospasms."
   4. "This comes as a capsule with dry powder inside that the inhaler device will activate."
   5. "When taken correctly, this drug should result in reduced wheezing and easier breathing."

7. The nurse is preparing to administer both a bronchodilator and a steroid by inhalation and knows that this medication should be administered first:
   1. The steroid
   2. The bronchodilator
   3. It does not make a difference.
   4. Bronchodilators and steroids should not be taken together.

8. After the administration of inhaled steroid medications, the nurse instructs the patient to do the following: *(Select all that apply.)*
   1. Hold the breath for 30 seconds.
   2. Rinse the mouth and swallow.
   3. Rinse the mouth with water and spit out the water.
   4. Nothing is required.
   5. Use the bronchodilator first before the inhaled steroid when both are ordered.

Objectives

1. Explain common oral disorders and their treatments.
2. Describe therapy used for oral health.
3. Identify nursing assessments and interventions associated with treatment of mucositis.

Key Terms

cold sores (fever blisters) (KŌLD SŌRZ) (p. 484)
canker sores (KĂN-kĕr SŌRZ) (p. 485)
candidiasis (kăn-dĭ-DĪ-ă-sĭs) (p. 485)
mucositis (myū-kō-SĪ-tĭs) (p. 485)
plaque (PLĂK) (p. 485)
dental caries (DĚN-tŭl KĂR-ēz) (p. 485)

tartar (TĂR-tĕr) (p. 486)
gingivitis (jĭn-jĭ-VĪ-tĭs) (p. 486)
halitosis (hăl-ĭ-TŌ-sĭs) (p. 486)
xerostomia (zĕ-rŏs-TŌ-mē-ă) (p. 486)
dentifrices (DĚN-tĭ-frĭs-ĕz) (p. 489)
mouthwashes (MŎWTH-wăsh-ĕz) (p. 489)

ORAL ANATOMY

The mouth, or oral cavity, is the beginning of the digestive tract and contains all the essential structures needed to consume food and drink to feed the body. The mouth consists of the upper and lower lips that are outside of the oral cavity; the jaw bone; tongue; pharynx; and teeth, including the surrounding gums, the cheeks (mucus membranes inside of the mouth), the hard and soft palate (the roof of the mouth), the uvula, and the tonsils. Salivary glands are also part of the oral cavity that produce saliva to lubricate the oral cavity and to provide enzymes secreted during eating to help aid digesting of food (Figure 31-1).

MOUTH DISORDERS

Common disorders affecting the mouth are cold sores on the lip; canker sores and candidal infections of soft tissues of the tongue, cheeks, and gums; and plaque and calculus affecting the gums and teeth. Xerostomia, or lack of saliva, originates from nonoral causes. Halitosis can arise from oral or nonoral diseases. A much less common problem, but one that causes significant discomfort, is oral mucositis.

Cold sores (fever blisters) are caused by the herpes simplex type 1 virus (herpes simplex labialis) and are most commonly found at the junction of the mucous membrane and the skin of the lips or nostrils, although they can occur inside the mouth, especially affecting the gums and hard and soft palate. It is estimated that

at least half of all Americans ages 20 to 40 years have had fever blisters. Most victims were infected before 5 years of age. About half of patients will develop recurrent outbreaks of the lesions, often in the same location, separated by latent periods. The recurrence rate and extent of lesions are highly variable. Patients often predict when an outbreak may occur because of predisposing factors, such as systemic illnesses accompanied by fever, cold (hence the names fever blisters and cold sores), or flu, menstruation, extreme physical stress and fatigue, or sun and wind exposure. Chemotherapy or radiation therapy that depresses the immune system also triggers cold sores.

Patients often report that a flare-up of the sores is preceded by a prodrome of burning, itching, and/or numbness in the area where the lesion develops. The lesions first become visible as small, red papules that develop into fluid-filled vesicles (blisters) 1 to 3 mm in diameter. Smaller lesions often coalesce into larger lesions. Pain is intense, fever may be present, and increased salivation and mouth odor occur. Often, the lymph nodes in the neck are swollen because of the body's response to infection. Over the next 10 to 14 days, a crust develops over the top of many coalesced, burst vesicles; the base is erythematous. The liquid from the vesicles contains live virus that is contagious if transferred to other people by direct contact (e.g., kissing). If pus develops in the vesicles or under the crust of a cold sore, a secondary bacterial infection may be present and should be evaluated for antibiotic therapy.

Review Questions for the NCLEX® Examination

1. The nurse discussing halitosis with a patient should include these causes. *(Select all that apply.)*
   1. Smoking
   2. Canker sores
   3. Sinusitis
   4. Dimethyl sulfoxide
   5. *Candida albicans*

2. When painful oral lesions are present, the best approach to oral hygiene includes:
   1. waiting until the lesions are healed.
   2. using commercial mouthwashes for rinsing after meals and at bedtime.
   3. using normal saline, baking soda, or half-strength hydrogen peroxide rinses.
   4. giving prescribed oral or parenteral analgesic medications.

3. A patient was asking the nurse to explain canker sores. The best response(s) by the nurse includes: *(Select all that apply.)*
   1. "The causes of canker sores are not known."
   2. "Sometimes canker sores are brought on by stress and trauma to the mouth."
   3. "Canker sores are lesions that are really viral infections."
   4. "Canker sores are not contagious."
   5. "If you take aspirin, it will promote healing of the canker sores."

4. Thrush is most common in these patient demographics. *(Select all that apply.)*
   1. Infants
   2. Pregnant women
   3. Debilitated patients
   4. Teens
   5. Older adults

5. The nurse can expect that a patient who recently underwent chemotherapy will develop mucositis during this timeframe:
   1. Within 2 to 3 days
   2. Within 5 to 7 days
   3. Within 10 to 12 days
   4. Within 2 weeks

6. This drug has been approved specifically for use in preventing and treating the mucositis that develops in leukemia or lymphoma patients undergoing chemotherapy before bone marrow transplantation.
   1. Nystatin
   2. Sucralfate
   3. Viscous lidocaine
   4. Palifermin

Objectives

1. Describe the physiology of the stomach.
2. Cite common stomach disorders that require drug therapy.
3. Identify factors that prevent breakdown of the body's normal defense barriers resulting in ulcer formation.
4. Discuss the drug classifications and actions used to treat stomach disorders.
5. Identify interventions that incorporate pharmacologic and nonpharmacologic treatments for an individual with stomach disorders.

Key Terms

chief cells (CHĒF) (p. 492)
parietal cells (pă-RĪ-ĕ-tŭl) (p. 492)
hydrochloric acid (hī-drō-KLŎR-ĭk) (p. 492)
mucous cells (MŪ-kŭs SĚLZ) (p. 492)
gastroesophageal reflux disease (GERD) (găs-trō-ĕs-ŏf-ĕ-JĒ-ŭl RĒ-flŭks) (p. 492)

heartburn (HĂRT-brŭn) (p. 492)
peptic ulcer disease (PUD) (PĔP-tĭk ŬL-sŭr) (p. 493)
Helicobacter pylori (hĕl-ĭ-kō-BĂK-tŭr pī-LŎR-ē) (p. 493)

PHYSIOLOGY OF THE STOMACH

As a major part of the gastrointestinal (GI) tract, the stomach has three primary functions: (1) storing food until it can be processed in the lower GI tract; (2) mixing food with gastric secretions until it is a partially digested, semisolid mixture known as chyme; and (3) slowly emptying the stomach at a rate that allows proper digestion and absorption of nutrients and medicine from the small intestine.

Three types of secretory cells line portions of the stomach—chief, parietal, and mucus cells. The chief cells secrete pepsinogen, an inactive enzyme. Parietal cells secrete hydrochloric acid by way of a hydrogen ion pump, which activates pepsinogen to pepsin, providing the optimal pH for pepsin to start protein digestion. Stimulation of histamine-2 (H_2) receptors on the stomach's parietal cells also causes secretion of hydrochloric acid. Cholinergic nerve fibers that innervate the stomach will also increase parietal cell secretion of hydrochloric acid when stimulated by acetylcholine. Normal pH in the stomach ranges from 1 to 5, depending on the presence of food and medications. Hydrochloric acid also breaks down muscle fibers and connective tissue ingested as food and kills bacteria that enter the digestive tract through the mouth. The parietal cells also secrete intrinsic factor needed for absorption of vitamin B_{12}. The mucous cells secrete mucus, which coats the stomach wall. The 1-mm-thick coat is alkaline and protects the stomach wall from damage by hydrochloric acid and the digestive enzyme pepsin. It also contributes lubrication for food transport. Small amounts of other enzymes are also secreted in the stomach. Lipases digest fats, and gastric amylase digests carbohydrates. Other digestive enzymes are also carried into the stomach from swallowed saliva.

Prostaglandins play a major role in protecting the stomach walls from injury by stomach acids and enzymes. Prostaglandins are produced by cells lining the stomach and prevent injury by inhibiting gastric acid secretion, maintaining blood flow, and stimulating mucus and bicarbonate production.

COMMON STOMACH DISORDERS

Gastroesophageal reflux disease (GERD), more commonly referred to as *heartburn*, *acid indigestion*, or *sour stomach*, is a common stomach disorder. Approximately one third of the U.S. population experiences heartburn once each month, and 5% to 7% have heartburn daily. Common symptoms are a burning sensation, bloating, belching, and regurgitation. Other symptoms that are reported less frequently are nausea, a "lump in the throat," hiccups, and chest pain.

Gastroesophageal reflux disease is the reflux of gastric secretions, primarily pepsin and hydrochloric acid, up into the esophagus. Causes of GERD are a weakened lower esophageal sphincter, delayed gastric emptying, hiatal hernia, obesity, overeating, tight-fitting clothing, and increased acid secretion. Acid secretions are increased by smoking, alcohol, carbonated beverages, coffee, and spicy foods.

Most cases of GERD pass quickly with only mild discomfort, but frequent or prolonged bouts of acid reflux cause inflammation, tissue erosion, and ulcerations in the lower esophagus. Anyone who has recurrent or continuous symptoms of reflux, especially if the symptoms interfere with activities, should be referred to a healthcare provider. These symptoms may also accompany more serious conditions, such as ischemic heart disease, scleroderma, and gastric malignancy.

Clinical Pitfall

Nurses need to be aware that the symptoms of GERD may also accompany more serious conditions, such as ischemic heart disease, scleroderma, and gastric malignancy. It is important to do a thorough physical assessment whenever a patient presents with heartburn or acid indigestion and not simply dismiss the symptoms as GI in origin.

Peptic ulcer disease (PUD) refers to several stomach disorders that result from an imbalance between acidic stomach contents and the body's normal defense barriers, causing ulcerations in the GI tract. The most common illnesses are gastric and duodenal ulcers. It is estimated that approximately 10% of all Americans will develop an ulcer at some time in their lives. The incidence in men and women is approximately the same. Race, economic status, and psychological stress do not correlate with the frequency of ulcer disease. Often, the only symptom reported is epigastric pain, described as burning, gnawing, or aching. Patients often report that varying degrees of pain are present for a few weeks and are then gone, only to recur a few weeks later. The pain is most often noted when the stomach is empty, such as at night or between meals, and is relieved by food or antacids. Other symptoms that cause patients to seek medical attention are bloating, nausea, vomiting, and anorexia.

Ulcers appear to be caused by a combination of acid and a breakdown in the body's defense mechanisms that protect the stomach wall. Proposed mechanisms are oversecretion of hydrochloric acid by excessive numbers of parietal cells, injury to the mucosal barrier such as that resulting from prostaglandin inhibitors (nonsteroidal antiinflammatory drugs [NSAIDs], including aspirin), and infection of the mucosal wall by *Helicobacter pylori*. It had been thought that no bacterium could survive in the highly acidic environment of the stomach; however, *H. pylori* was first isolated from patients with gastritis in 1983. The bacterium seems able to live below the mucous barrier, where it is protected from stomach acid and pepsin. *H. pylori* is now thought to be associated with as many as 90% of duodenal and 70% of gastric ulcers. The exact mechanism whereby *H. pylori* contributes to ulcer formation is not known, but several hypotheses are being tested.

Several risk factors increase the likelihood of peptic ulcer disease:

1. There seems to be a genetic predisposition to PUD. Some families have a much greater history of PUD than others.
2. It is a commonly held belief that stress causes ulcers, but no well-controlled studies have supported this.
3. Cigarette smoking increases acid secretion, alters blood flow in the stomach wall, and retards prostaglandin synthesis needed for defense mechanisms.
4. Nonsteroidal antiinflammatory drugs have a twofold effect: they inhibit prostaglandins that protect the mucosa and directly irritate the stomach wall. Once ulcerations have formed, NSAIDs also slow healing.
5. It is commonly thought that certain foods (e.g., spicy foods) and alcohol contribute to ulcer formation. It is true that certain foods increase acid secretion and that alcohol irritates the stomach lining, but results from studies have not corroborated this concept.

GOALS OF TREATMENT

The goals of treatment of GERD are to relieve symptoms, decrease the frequency and duration of reflux, heal tissue injury, and prevent recurrence. The most important treatment is a change in lifestyle, which includes losing weight (if significantly over the ideal body weight), reducing or avoiding foods and beverages that increase acid production, reducing or stopping smoking, avoiding alcohol, and consuming smaller meals. Additional therapy includes remaining upright for 2 hours after meals, not eating before bedtime, and avoiding tight clothing over the abdominal area. Lozenges may be used to increase saliva production, and antacid therapy may provide relief for patients who experience infrequent heartburn. If the patient's symptoms do not improve within 2 to 3 weeks, or if the condition is severe, additional pharmacologic measures should be tried to reduce irritation. About 5% to 10% of patients with GERD require surgery.

The treatment of PUD and GERD is somewhat similar: relieve symptoms, promote healing, and prevent recurrence. Lifestyle changes that eliminate risk factors, such as cigarette smoking and foods (and alcohol) that increase acid secretion, should be initiated. Patients rarely need to be restricted to a bland diet. If NSAIDs are being taken, consideration should be given to switching to acetaminophen if feasible. For decades, ulcer treatment focused on reducing acid secretions (anticholinergic agents, H_2 antagonists, gastric acid pump inhibitors), neutralizing acid (antacids), or coating ulcer craters to hasten healing (sucralfate). Major changes in therapy have come about because of the approval of antibiotics to eradicate

H. pylori. Several large studies are under way to refine the healing and reduce ulcer recurrence rates. Various combinations of antimicrobial agents (e.g., amoxicillin, tetracycline, metronidazole, clarithromycin), bismuth, and antisecretory agents (e.g., H_2 antagonists, proton pump inhibitors [PPIs]) are used to eradicate *H. pylori.* Antibiotics are not recommended for individuals who are asymptomatic with *H. pylori* because there is concern that resistant strains of bacteria may develop.

DRUG THERAPY

ACTIONS

- Antacids neutralize gastric acid, thereby causing the gastric contents to be less acidic.
- Coating agents provide a protective covering over the ulcer crater.
- H_2 antagonists decrease the volume of hydrochloric acid produced, which increases the gastric pH and thereby results in decreased irritation to the gastric mucosa.
- Proton pump inhibitors block the formation of hydrochloric acid, reducing irritation of the gastric mucosa.
- Prokinetic agents increase the lower esophageal sphincter muscle pressure and peristalsis, hastening emptying of the stomach to reduce reflux.
- Antispasmodic agents reduce the secretion of saliva, hydrochloric acid, pepsin, bile, and other enzymatic fluids necessary for digestion and decrease GI motility and secretions.

USES

- Antacids decrease hyperacidity associated with PUD, GERD, gastritis, and hiatal hernia.
- Coating agents provide a protective barrier for the mucosal lining where hydrochloric acid may come into contact with inflamed eroded areas. They are used to treat existing ulcer craters on the gastric mucosa.
- H_2 antagonists are used to treat acute gastric and duodenal ulcers and gastroesophageal disease, as well as for maintenance to prevent ulcer recurrence.
- Proton pump inhibitors are used to treat hyperacidity conditions (e.g., GERD, Zollinger-Ellison syndrome) and peptic and gastric ulcer disease.
- Prokinetic agents are used to treat GERD.
- Antispasmodic agents decrease gastric secretions by inhibiting vagal stimulation. They are used in treating GI disorders requiring decreased gastric motility or decreased gastric secretions.

❖ NURSING IMPLICATIONS FOR AGENTS USED FOR STOMACH DISORDERS

■ Assessment

Nutritional Assessment. Obtain patient data about current height, weight, and any recent weight gain or loss. Identify the normal pattern of eating, including snacking habits. Use a food guide such as the Healthy Eating Plate (see Figure 46-3) as a guide when asking questions to identify the usual foods eaten by the individual. Ask about any nutritional or cultural restrictions associated with dietary practices. Are there any food allergies (obtain details) or foods that particularly cause gastric distress when eaten? Does the individual take any nutritional supplements? How often and how much fast food is eaten?

Esophagus, Stomach. Ask patients to describe symptoms. Question in detail what is meant by the terms *indigestion, heartburn, upset stomach, nausea,* and *belching.*

Pain, Discomfort
- Ask the patient to describe the onset, duration, location, and characteristics of pain or discomfort. Determine whether there is a relationship between the ingestion of certain types of food or drinks and the onset of pain. Ask specifically about coffee, tea, cola, chocolate, and alcohol intake.
- What has the patient done to relieve the pain or discomfort? Have there been any changes in taste (e.g., bitterness, sourness)? Record pain levels using a rating scale before and after medications are administered.

Activity, Exercise. Ask specifically what type of work or activities the individual performs that may increase intra-abdominal pressure (e.g., lifting heavy objects, bending over frequently).

History of Diseases or Disorders
- What other diagnoses have been made for diseases or disorders (e.g., ulcer, gallbladder, liver, jaundice, irritable bowel syndrome)?
- Have there been any changes in bowel elimination or stool color, consistency, or frequency?

Medication History
- What self-medications have been tried?
- What prescribed medications are being taken?
- What is the schedule of medication administration (e.g., how frequently and when are antacids taken)?

Anxiety or Stress Level. Ask the patient to describe his or her lifestyle. What does the patient think are stressors, and how often do they occur?

Smoking. What is the frequency of smoking?

■ Implementation

- Routine orders: Most healthcare providers order antacids 1 hour before meals, 2 to 3 hours after meals, and at bedtime. As-needed (PRN) medication dosages must be discussed.
- Each type of medication used to treat GERD or PUD may require somewhat different scheduling to avoid drug interactions. When developing the timeframes for administration of medications on the medication administration record (MAR), schedule the other prescribed drugs 1 hour before or 2 hours after antacids.

- Changes in diet require careful planning with the patient and the person responsible for purchasing and cooking the meals. Schedule teaching sessions appropriately. Not only may some foods need to be altered, but also the number of meals per day may need to be increased with a smaller serving at each meal.

■ **Patient Education**

Nutrition

- Implement prescribed dietary changes: eat small, more frequent meals to support optimal energy requirements and healing; avoid overdistention of the stomach; avoid any seasonings that are intolerable or that aggravate the condition; and avoid coffee, teas, colas, alcoholic beverages (including beer), carbonated beverages, peppermint, spearmint, and citric juices, which may produce discomfort in those with GERD.
- Avoid late-night snacks or meals that could result in increased gastric secretions.
- Observe for foods that aggravate the condition, and eliminate these from the diet. Drink only small amounts of fluid with the meal and drink mostly between meals. Increase protein foods and decrease fats to about 45 g/day or less; use nonfat milk.

Pain, Discomfort. Keep a written record (see Patient Self-Assessment form below) of the onset, duration, location, and precipitating factors for any pain. Sit upright at the table when eating and do not lie down for at least 2 hours after eating. When a hiatal hernia is present, elevate the head of the bed on 6- to 8-inch blocks to prevent reflux during sleep. Have the patient keep a log of the pain, including time of day, any factors that might have precipitated the pain, and degree of pain relief from medications used.

Medications

- Take prescribed medications at recommended times to promote optimal healing. See individual drug monographs for suggested scheduling.
- Avoid NSAIDs and aspirin-containing medicines that irritate the gastric mucosa. Consult the prescriber or pharmacist regarding scheduling of or discontinuation of these medications.

Lifestyle Changes

- Discuss stress and its effects on the person, and implement needed lifestyle changes.
- Encourage a significant reduction or cessation of smoking.
- Implement plans to gain sufficient rest.

Fostering Health Maintenance

- Discuss medication information and how it will benefit the course of treatment to produce an optimal response. Medications used in the treatment of hyperacidity are important measures to alleviate the irritating effects on the mucosal tissue; stress the importance of not discontinuing treatment and the need for continued medical follow-up.

- Seek cooperation and understanding of the following points so that medication adherence is increased: name of medication; dosage, route, and times of administration; and common and serious adverse effects. Stress the need to complete a full course of treatment for *H. pylori* so that the organisms are indeed killed and not only suppressed; *H. pylori* can regrow if medications are discontinued too early.

Patient Self-Assessment. Enlist the patient's aid in developing and maintaining a written record of monitoring parameters (e.g., a list of foods causing problems, degree of pain relief) (see Patient Self-Assessment form for Agents Affecting the Digestive System on the Evolve website). Complete the Premedication Data ⓔ column for use as a baseline to track response to drug therapy. Ensure that the patient understands how to use the form, and instruct the patient to bring the completed form to follow-up visits. During follow-up visits, focus on issues that will foster adherence with the therapeutic interventions prescribed.

DRUG CLASS: ANTACIDS

ACTIONS

Antacids lower the acidity of gastric secretions by buffering the hydrochloric acid (normal pH is 1 to 2) to a lower hydrogen ion concentration. Buffering hydrochloric acid to a pH of 3 to 4 is highly desired because the proteolytic action of pepsin is reduced and the gastric juice loses its corrosive effect.

USES

Antacids are commonly used for heartburn, excessive eating and drinking, and PUD. They are no longer first-line agents in the treatment of stomach disorders, but are often the first agents used by consumers to self-treat these conditions. However, nurses and patients must be aware that not all antacids are alike. They should be used judiciously, particularly by certain types of patients (e.g., those with heart failure, hypertension, renal failure). Long-term self-treatment with antacids may also mask symptoms of serious underlying diseases, such as a bleeding ulcer.

The most effective antacids available are combinations of aluminum hydroxide, magnesium oxide or hydroxide, and calcium carbonate. All act by neutralizing gastric acid. Combinations of these ingredients must be used because any compound used alone in therapeutic quantities may produce severe systemic adverse effects. Other ingredients found in antacid combination products include simethicone and bismuth. Simethicone is a defoaming agent that breaks up gas bubbles in the stomach, reducing stomach distention and heartburn. It is effective in patients who have overeaten or who have heartburn, but it is not effective in treating PUD. Bismuth compounds have little acid-neutralizing capacity and are therefore poor antacids.

The following principles should be considered when antacid therapy is planned:

- For indigestion, antacids should not be administered for more than 2 weeks. If after this time the patient is still experiencing discomfort, a healthcare provider should be contacted.
- Patients with edema, heart failure, hypertension, renal failure, pregnancy, or salt-restricted diets should use low-sodium antacids, such as Riopan or Maalox. Therapy should continue only on the recommendation of a healthcare provider.
- Antacid tablets should be used only for the patient with occasional indigestion or heartburn. Tablets *do not* contain enough antacid to be effective in treating PUD.
- A common complaint of patients consuming large quantities of calcium carbonate or aluminum hydroxide is constipation. Excess magnesium results in diarrhea. If a patient experiences these symptoms and still has stomach discomfort, a healthcare provider should be consulted.
- Effective management of acute ulcer disease requires large volumes of antacids. The selection of an antacid and the quantity to be taken depend on its neutralizing capacity. Any patient with coffee-ground emesis, bloody stools, or recurrent abdominal pain should seek medical attention immediately and not attempt to self-treat the disorder.
- Calcium carbonate and sodium bicarbonate may cause rebound hyperacidity.
- Patients with renal failure should not use large quantities of antacids containing magnesium. The magnesium ions cannot be excreted and may produce hypermagnesemia and toxicity.
- Most antacids have similar ingredients. Selection of an antacid for occasional use should be determined by quantity of each ingredient, cost, taste, and frequency of adverse effects. Patients may need to try more than one product and weigh the advantages and disadvantages of each.

THERAPEUTIC OUTCOMES

The primary therapeutic outcomes expected from antacid therapy are relief of discomfort, reduced frequency of heartburn, and healing of irritated tissues.

❖ NURSING IMPLICATIONS FOR ANTACIDS

■ Premedication Assessment
1. Check renal function test results to ensure that renal function is normal. When renal failure is present, patients should not take large quantities of antacids containing magnesium. Monitor the patient's renal function tests, including BUN (blood urea nitrogen), creatinine, and serum electrolyte levels, including magnesium and potassium. Magnesium and potassium ions cannot be excreted and may produce hypermagnesemia, hyperkalemia, and toxicity.

2. Check the pattern of bowel elimination for diarrhea or constipation.
3. Record the pattern of gastric pain being experienced; report coffee-ground emesis, bloody stools, or recurrent abdominal pain to the healthcare provider for prompt attention.
4. If the patient is pregnant or has edema, heart failure, hypertension, or salt restrictions, ensure that a low-sodium antacid has been prescribed.
5. Schedule other prescribed medications to be taken 1 hour before or 2 hours after antacids are to be administered.

Life Span Considerations
Antacids
Those older than 65 years are the most common purchasers of antacid products. Gastrointestinal disorders such as PUD, NSAID-induced ulcers, and GERD occur more often in this age group. Magnesium-containing antacids are often used as laxatives. Although the primary symptom of ulcer disease in a younger person is usually burning epigastric pain, the symptoms in an older person, if present at all, usually include complaints of vague abdominal discomfort, anorexia, and weight loss.

■ Availability, Dosage, and Administration
See Table 32-1.
- Liquid forms of antacid preparations should be used for treatment of PUD because tablets do not contain enough of the active ingredients to be effective.
- Antacid tablets may be used for occasional episodes of heartburn. They should be well chewed before swallowing for a more rapid onset of action.

■ Common Adverse Effects
Chalky Taste. A chalky taste is a common problem with antacids. Suggest a change in brands or flavors. Suggest using a liquid instead of tablets.

■ Serious Adverse Effects
Gastrointestinal
Diarrhea, constipation. Diarrhea or constipation is a common problem when antacids are used in therapeutic dosages to treat ulcers. Alternating between calcium- or aluminum-containing compounds and magnesium-containing compounds should help alleviate the problem.

■ Drug Interactions
Tetracycline Antibiotics, Fluoroquinolone Antibiotics, Phenytoin, Phenothiazines, Captopril, Ketoconazole, Corticosteroids, Digoxin, Iron Supplements. The absorption of these medicines is inhibited by antacids. These medications should be administered 1 hour before or 2 to 3 hours after antacids.
Levodopa, Valproic Acid. The absorption of levodopa is increased by magnesium-aluminum

Table 32-1   Ingredients of Commonly Used Antacids

PRODUCT	FORM	CALCIUM CARBONATE	ALUMINUM HYDROXIDE	MAGNESIUM OXIDE, HYDROXIDE OR CARBONATE	SODIUM BICARBONATE	SIMETHICONE	OTHER INGREDIENTS
Aludrox	Suspension	—	X	X	—	X	—
Baking soda	Powder	—	—	—	X	—	—
Gelusil	Tablet	—	X	X	—	X	—
Maalox Maximum Strength	Suspension	—	X	X	—	X	—
Phillip's Milk of Magnesia	Tablet, suspension	—	—	X	—	—	—
Riopan Plus	Tablet, suspension	—	—	—	—	X	magaldrate
Rolaids	Tablet	X	—	X	—	—	—
Titralac Plus	Tablet, suspension	X	—	—	—	X	—
Tums	Tablet	X	—	—	—	—	—

antacids. When antacid therapy is added, toxicity may result in the patient with Parkinson's disease whose condition is well controlled on a certain dosage of levodopa. If the patient's parkinsonism symptoms are well controlled on levodopa and antacid therapy, withdrawal of antacids may result in a recurrence of parkinsonian symptoms.

Quinidine, Amphetamines. Frequent use of sodium bicarbonate–containing antacid therapy may result in increased urinary pH. Renal excretion of quinidine and amphetamines may be inhibited, and toxicity may occur.

DRUG CLASS: HISTAMINE-2 RECEPTOR ANTAGONISTS

ACTIONS

One of the primary mechanisms of hydrochloric acid secretion has to do with histamine stimulation of histamine-2 (H_2) receptors on the stomach's parietal cells. The H_2 antagonists act by blocking the H_2 receptors, resulting in a decrease in the volume of acid secreted. The pH of the stomach contents rises as a consequence of a reduction in acid.

USES

The H_2 antagonists (cimetidine, ranitidine, nizatidine, famotidine) are used to treat GERD, duodenal ulcers, and pathologic hypersecretory conditions, such as Zollinger-Ellison syndrome, and for preventing and treating stress ulcers in critically ill patients. Unapproved uses include prevention of aspiration pneumonitis, stress ulcer prophylaxis, acute upper GI bleeding, hives, and hyperparathyroidism. All of the H_2 antago-

nists have products that are available for OTC purchase for symptomatic relief of overeating and heartburn.

Cimetidine was the first approved H_2 antagonist but differs from the other agents by its extensive liver metabolism and antiandrogenic effect that may result in gynecomastia. It also has many drug-drug interactions that are not seen with the others. Consequently, cimetidine is used less frequently than the other H_2 antagonists.

Famotidine is similar in action and use to cimetidine but has the advantages of one dose daily, fewer drug interactions, and no antiandrogenic effect. A parenteral dosage form is available.

Ranitidine is similar in action and use to cimetidine but has the advantages of twice-daily dosing, fewer drug interactions, and no antiandrogenic effect. A parenteral dosage form is also available.

Nizatidine is similar to ranitidine and famotidine but, in contrast to the other agents, is not available in a parenteral dosage form.

THERAPEUTIC OUTCOMES

The primary therapeutic outcomes expected from H_2 antagonist therapy are relief of discomfort, reduced frequency of heartburn, and healing of irritated tissues.

❖ NURSING IMPLICATIONS FOR H_2 ANTAGONISTS

■ Premedication Assessment

Perform a baseline assessment of the patient's mental status for comparison with subsequent mental status evaluations to detect central nervous system (CNS) alterations that may occur, particularly with cimetidine therapy.

Table 32-2   **Histamine-2 (H₂) Receptor Antagonists**

GENERIC NAME	BRAND NAME	AVAILABILITY	DOSAGE RANGE
cimetidine	Tagamet, Tagamet HB Apo-Cimetidine ❦	Tablets: 200, 300, 400, 800 mg Suspension: 300 mg/5 mL	*Duodenal and gastric ulcers* PO: 800-1600 mg at bedtime, 400 mg twice daily, or 300 mg four times daily *GERD* PO: 800 mg twice daily or 400 mg four times daily
famotidine ⇄ *Do not confuse famotidine with fluoxetine.*	Pepcid, Pepcid AC ⇄ *Do not confuse Pepcid with Prevacid.* ❦ Novo-Famotidine ❦	Tablets: 10, 20, 40 mg Tablets, chewable: 10, 20 mg Suspension: 40 mg/5 mL Injection: 10 mg/mL	*Duodenal and gastric ulcers* PO: 40 mg once daily at bedtime or 20 mg twice daily *GERD* PO: 20 mg twice daily
nizatidine ⇄ *Do not confuse nizatidine with tizanidine.*	Axid Apo-Nizatidine ❦	Capsules: 150, 300 mg Tablets: 75 mg Oral solution: 15 mg/mL	*Duodenal and gastric ulcers* PO: 300 mg at bedtime or 150 mg twice daily *GERD* PO: 150 mg twice daily
ranitidine ⇄ *Do not confuse ranitidine with amantadine or rimantadine.*	Zantac; Zantac 75, 150 ⇄ *Do not confuse Zantac with Xanax or Zyrtec.* PMS-Ranitidine ❦	Tablets: 75, 150, 300 mg Efferdose tablets: 25 mg Syrup: 15 mg/mL Solution: 15 mg/mL Injection: 25 mg/mL	*Duodenal and gastric ulcers* PO: 300 mg at bedtime or 150 mg twice daily *GERD* PO: 150 mg twice daily

❦ Available in Canada.

■ Availability, Dosage, and Administration

See Table 32-2.

- All may be administered with or without food.
- Because antacid therapy is often continued during early therapy of PUD, administer 1 hour before or 2 hours after the H₂-antagonist dose.

■ Common Adverse Effects

Approximately 1% to 3% of patients develop these adverse effects. They are usually mild and resolve with continued therapy. Encourage patients not to discontinue therapy without first consulting the healthcare provider.

Neurologic

Dizziness, headache, somnolence. Provide for patient safety during episodes of dizziness. If the patient develops somnolence and lethargy, encourage the use of caution when working around machinery, driving a car, or performing other duties that require mental alertness.

Gastrointestinal

Diarrhea, constipation. Maintain the patient's state of hydration, and obtain an order for stool softeners or bulk-forming laxatives if necessary. Encourage the inclusion of sufficient roughage (fresh fruits, vegetables, whole-grain products) in the diet.

■ Serious Adverse Effects

Neurologic

Confusion, disorientation, hallucinations. If high dosages (particularly of cimetidine) are used in patients with liver or renal disease or in patients older than 50 years, mental confusion, slurred speech, disorientation, and hallucinations may occur. These adverse effects dissipate over 3 or 4 days after therapy has been discontinued. Perform a baseline assessment of the patient's degree of alertness and orientation to name, place, and time before starting therapy. Make regularly scheduled subsequent mental status evaluations, and compare findings. Report alterations in mental status.

Endocrine

Gynecomastia. Mild bilateral gynecomastia and breast soreness may occur with long-term use (longer than 1 month) of cimetidine but will resolve after discontinuing therapy. Report findings of gynecomastia for further observation and possible laboratory tests.

Gastrointestinal

Hepatotoxicity. Although rare, hepatotoxicity in patients taking H₂ antagonists has been reported. The symptoms of hepatotoxicity are anorexia, nausea, vomiting, jaundice, hepatomegaly, splenomegaly, and abnormal liver function test results (elevated bilirubin, aspartate aminotransferase [AST], alanine aminotransferase [ALT], gamma-glutamyl transferase [GGT], alkaline phosphatase levels, increased prothrombin time).

■ Drug Interactions

Benzodiazepines. Cimetidine inhibits the metabolism or excretion of the following benzodiazepines: alprazolam, chlordiazepoxide, diazepam, clorazepate, flurazepam, halazepam, prazepam, and triazolam.

Patients taking cimetidine and a benzodiazepine concurrently should be observed for increased sedation; a reduction in dosage of the benzodiazepine may be required. The metabolism of oxazepam, temazepam, and lorazepam does not appear to be affected.

Theophylline Derivatives. Cimetidine inhibits the metabolism or excretion of the following xanthine derivatives: aminophylline, dyphylline, and theophylline. Patients at greater risk include those receiving larger doses of xanthine derivatives and those with liver disease. Observe for restlessness, vomiting, dizziness, and cardiac dysrhythmias. The dosage of xanthine derivative may need to be reduced.

Beta-Adrenergic Blocking Agents. Beta-adrenergic blocking agents (e.g., propranolol, labetalol, metoprolol) may accumulate as a result of inhibited metabolism. Monitor for signs of toxicity, such as hypotension and bradycardia.

Phenytoin. Cimetidine inhibits the metabolism of phenytoin. Monitor patients with concurrent therapy for signs of phenytoin toxicity: nystagmus, sedation, and lethargy. Serum levels may be ordered, and a reduced dosage of phenytoin may be required.

Lidocaine, Quinidine, Procainamide. Cimetidine may inhibit the metabolism of these agents. Monitor for signs of toxicity (e.g., bradycardia, additional dysrhythmias, hyperactivity, sedation), and reduce the dosage if necessary.

Antacids. Administer 1 hour before or 2 hours after administration of cimetidine.

Warfarin. Cimetidine may enhance the anticoagulant effects of warfarin. Observe for the development of petechiae, ecchymoses, nosebleeds, bleeding gums, dark tarry stools, and bright red or coffee-ground hematemesis. Monitor the prothrombin time (international normalized ratio [INR]), and reduce the dosage of warfarin if necessary.

Calcium Antagonists. Cimetidine may inhibit the metabolism of diltiazem, nifedipine, and verapamil. Patients should be monitored for increased effects from the calcium antagonists (e.g., bradycardia, hypotension, dysrhythmias, fatigue).

Tricyclic Antidepressants. Cimetidine may inhibit the excretion of imipramine, desipramine, and nortriptyline, usually within 3 to 5 days after the start of cimetidine therapy. If anticholinergic effects or toxicity becomes apparent, a decreased dosage of the antidepressant may be required. If cimetidine is discontinued, the patient should be monitored for a decreased response to the antidepressant.

Famotidine, Nizatidine, Ranitidine. In general, there appear to be only minor interactions with these H_2 antagonists. There are conflicting data, however. Studies indicate that patients receiving higher doses of ranitidine may be more susceptible to drug interactions with ranitidine and other drugs. When used concurrently, monitor for toxic effects of warfarin, theophylline, procainamide, and glipizide.

DRUG CLASS: GASTROINTESTINAL PROSTAGLANDIN

misoprostol (mĭs-ō-PRŎS-tŏl)
Cytotec (SĪ-tō-tĕk)

ACTIONS

Misoprostol is a synthetic prostaglandin E series drug. Prostaglandins are normally present in the GI tract to inhibit gastric acid and pepsin secretion to protect the stomach and duodenal lining against ulceration. The prostaglandin E analogues may also induce uterine contractions.

USES

Misoprostol is used to prevent and treat gastric ulcers caused by prostaglandin inhibitors (e.g., NSAIDs, including aspirin). Whereas prostaglandin inhibition is effective in reducing pain and inflammation, especially in arthritis, prostaglandin inhibition in the stomach by NSAIDs makes the patient more predisposed to peptic ulcers.

THERAPEUTIC OUTCOMES

The primary therapeutic outcomes expected from misoprostol therapy are relief of discomfort and healing of irritated tissues.

❖ **NURSING IMPLICATIONS FOR MISOPROSTOL THERAPY**

■ **Premedication Assessment**
1. Determine if the patient is pregnant. This drug is a uterine stimulant and may induce miscarriage.
2. Check the pattern of bowel elimination; misoprostol may induce diarrhea.

■ **Availability**
100- and 200-mcg tablets.

 Medication Safety Alert

Misoprostol is contraindicated during pregnancy and in women at risk of becoming pregnant. As a uterine stimulant, it may induce miscarriage.

■ **Dosage and Administration**
Adult: PO: 100- to 200-mcg tablets four times daily with food during NSAID therapy.

■ **Common Adverse Effects**
Gastrointestinal
Diarrhea. Diarrhea associated with misoprostol therapy is dose related and usually develops after approximately 2 weeks of therapy. It often resolves after about 8 days, but a few patients require discontinuation of misoprostol therapy. Diarrhea can be

minimized by taking misoprostol with meals and at bedtime and avoiding magnesium-containing antacids (e.g., Maalox liquid, Mylanta). Encourage the patient not to discontinue therapy without first consulting the healthcare provider. Encourage the patient to include sufficient roughage (fresh fruits, vegetables, whole-grain products) in the diet.

Contraindication

Pregnancy. It is crucial that therapy be discontinued if the patient is pregnant because misoprostol is a pregnancy category X drug that may cause spontaneous abortion. The patient must receive attention from the healthcare provider who prescribed the misoprostol, as well as an obstetrician. The question of alternative therapies to NSAIDs must also be considered.

▪ Drug Interactions

No significant drug interactions have been reported.

DRUG CLASS: PROTON PUMP INHIBITORS

ACTIONS

Proton pump inhibitors inhibit gastric secretion of hydrochloric acid by inhibiting the gastric acid (hydrogen ion pump) of the stomach's parietal cells. These inhibitors have no anticholinergic or H_2 receptor antagonist actions, so some hydrochloric acid continues to be secreted unless anticholinergic or histamine-2 antagonists are also administered.

USES

Proton pump inhibitors are used to treat severe esophagitis, GERD, gastric and duodenal ulcers, and hypersecretory disorders, such as Zollinger-Ellison syndrome. They may also be used in combination with antibiotics (e.g., ampicillin, amoxicillin, clarithromycin) to eradicate *H. pylori,* a common cause of PUD. Proton pump inhibitors (e.g., Nexium) are also available OTC to treat intermittent heartburn.

THERAPEUTIC OUTCOMES

The primary therapeutic outcomes expected from PPIs are relief of discomfort, reduced frequency of heartburn, and healing of irritated tissues.

❖ NURSING IMPLICATIONS FOR PROTON PUMP INHIBITOR THERAPY

▪ Premedication Assessment

Check pattern of bowel elimination; the PPIs may induce diarrhea.

▪ Availability, Dosage, and Administration

See Table 32-3. Omeprazole, lansoprazole, and esomeprazole need to be taken before a meal. Capsules and tablets should be swallowed whole; instruct the patient not to open, chew, or crush.

▪ Common Adverse Effects

The following symptoms are relatively mild and rarely result in the discontinuation of therapy. Encourage the patient not to discontinue therapy without first consulting the healthcare provider.

Gastrointestinal

Diarrhea. Maintain the patient's state of hydration. Encourage the inclusion of sufficient roughage (fresh fruits, vegetables, whole-grain products) in the diet.

Neurologic. Headache, fatigue.

Musculoskeletal. Muscle pain.

▪ Serious Adverse Effects

Skeletal

Risk of fractures. Patients who are over the age of 50 years who received high doses or used them for more than 1 year are at greater risk for fractures of the hip, wrist, and spine. Patients who continue to receive PPIs and who are at risk for osteoporosis should receive vitamin D and calcium supplementation and have their bone status monitored. Patients should not stop taking their PPI unless told to do so by their healthcare provider. Short-term, low-dose use of over-the-counter products is not likely to cause an increased risk of fractures.

Electrolytes

Hypomagnesemia. Hypomagnesemia has been reported in as little as 3 months of PPI therapy, but it more commonly occurs in patients receiving PPIs for more than 1 year. Hypomagnesemia can cause serious adverse events, including tetany, tremors, seizures, QT prolongation, and cardiac arrhythmias. Healthcare providers should consider obtaining serum magnesium levels prior to beginning long-term PPI therapy, especially in patients receiving digoxin or patients receiving diuretics or other medicines known to cause hypomagnesemia. Magnesium supplementation may resolve the hypomagnesemia, but discontinuation of the PPI may be necessary. Magnesium levels return to normal within about a week of discontinuing PPI therapy. Patients should not stop PPI therapy without first discussing it with their healthcare provider. Use of over-the-counter PPIs taken according to directions and for a limited duration has not been associated with hypomagnesemia.

Integumentary

Rash. Persistent vesicular rash from omeprazole may be cause for discontinuing therapy. Report rashes to the healthcare provider for further observation and possible laboratory tests.

▪ Drug Interactions

Diazepam, Triazolam, Flurazepam. Omeprazole and esomeprazole significantly increases the half-life of diazepam, triazolam, and flurazepam by inhibiting its metabolism. Observe patients for increased sedative effects from these medicines. Caution against

Table 32-3   Proton Pump Inhibitors

GENERIC NAME	BRAND NAME	AVAILABILITY	DOSAGE RANGE
dexlansoprazole	Dexilant	Capsules: 30, 60 mg	PO: Initial: 60 mg once daily for 4-8 wk Maintenance: 30 mg once daily
esomeprazole ⇄ *Do not confuse esomeprazole with omeprazole.*	Nexium Apo-Esomeprazole ❦	Capsules: 20, 40 mg Capsules, sustained release (24 hr): 20, 40 mg Powder for suspension: 20-, 40-mg unit dose IV: 20, 40 mg	IV, PO: Initial: 20-40 mg once daily for 4-8 wk Maintenance: 20 mg daily
lansoprazole	Prevacid ⇄ *Do not confuse Prevacid with Prinivil, Pepcid, Pravachol, Premarin, or Prilosec.* Teva-Lansoprazole ❦	Capsules, sustained release (24 hr): 15, 30 mg Tablets, dispersible: 15, 30 mg Suspension: 3 mg/mL	PO: Initial: 15-30 mg once daily 30 min before a meal for 4 wk Maintenance: 15 mg once daily Maximum: 30 mg once daily before a meal
omeprazole ⇄ *Do not confuse omeprazole with esomeprazole.*	Prilosec ⇄ *Do not confuse Prilosec with Prinivil, Prednisone, Prevacid, Prinivil, or Prozac.* Losec ❦	Capsules, sustained release: 10, 20, 40 mg Tablets, sustained release: 20 mg Suspension: 2 mg/mL in 90-, 150- and 300-mL bottles	PO: Initial: 20 mg once daily for 4 wk Maintenance: 20 mg daily *Zollinger-Ellison syndrome:* Maximum: 120 mg three times daily
pantoprazole	Protonix ⇄ *Do not confuse Protonix with Lotronex.* Pantoloc ❦	Tablets, delayed release: 20, 40 mg Powder for oral suspension: 40 mg IV: 40 mg/vial	PO: Initial: 40 mg once daily for 8 wk Maintenance: 40 mg daily IV: Initial: 40 mg once daily for up to 7-10 days; switch to oral dosages
rabeprazole	Aciphex ⇄ *Do not confuse Aciphex with Accupril, Adipex-P, Aricept, or Vioxx.* Pariet ❦	Tablets, delayed release: 20 mg Capsules, sprinkle: 5, 10 mg	PO: Initial: 20 mg daily after morning meal for up to 4 wk Maintenance: 20 mg once daily Maximum: 60 mg twice daily

❦ Available in Canada.

hazardous tasks, such as driving and operating machinery. The dosages of diazepam, triazolam, and flurazepam may have to be reduced.

Phenytoin. Omeprazole slows the metabolism of phenytoin. Observe for nystagmus, sedation, and lethargy. The dosage of phenytoin may have to be reduced.

Clopidogrel. There has been a controversy in the literature as to whether PPIs prevent conversion of clopidogrel to its active therapeutic metabolite. A consensus statement by the American Cardiology Foundation, the American Heart Association, and the American College of Gastroenterology reports that clopidogrel alone and aspirin alone and their combination are associated with an increased risk of GI bleeding; the risk of GI bleeding increases as the number of risk factors increases (such as prior GI bleeding, advanced age, concurrent use of anticoagulants); PPIs are appropriate in patients with multiple risk factors for GI bleeding who are also receiving antiplatelet therapy such as clopidogrel; a clinically significant interaction cannot be excluded in subgroups who are poor metabolizers of clopidogrel; until solid evidence exists to support staggering PPIs with clopidogrel, the dosing of PPIs should not be altered.

Warfarin. Omeprazole may reduce the rate of metabolism of warfarin. Monitor the patient closely for signs of bleeding tendencies, and monitor the prothrombin time (INR) closely. Reduction of warfarin dosage may be required.

Sucralfate. Sucralfate inhibits the absorption of PPIs. Administer the PPIs at least 30 minutes before sucralfate.

Altered Absorption. The reduction in gastric acid secretion may alter absorption of food and drugs as follows:

• *Ketoconazole, ampicillin, iron:* These medicines require an acid medium for absorption. They should be

administered at least 30 to 45 minutes before lanso-prazole therapy.
- *Insulin:* The absorption of food may be altered, and an adjustment in timing or dosage of insulin in patients with diabetes may be required.

DRUG CLASS: COATING AGENTS

> **sucralfate** (sū-KRĂL-fāt)
> **Carafate** (KĂR-ă-fāt)

ACTIONS

When swallowed, sucralfate forms a complex that adheres to the crater of an ulcer, thereby protecting it from aggravators such as acid, pepsin, and bile salts. However, sucralfate does not inhibit gastric secretions (as do the H_2 antagonists) or alter gastric pH (as do antacids).

USES

Sucralfate is used to treat duodenal ulcers, particularly in those patients who do not tolerate other forms of therapy.

THERAPEUTIC OUTCOMES

The primary therapeutic outcomes expected from sucralfate therapy are relief of discomfort and healing of irritated tissues.

❖ NURSING IMPLICATIONS FOR SUCRALFATE THERAPY

■ Premedication Assessment

Check pattern of bowel elimination; sucralfate may induce constipation.

■ Availability

PO: 1-g tablets and 1-g/10-mL suspension.

■ Dosage and Administration

Adult: PO: 1 tablet four times a day 1 hour before each meal and at bedtime, all on an empty stomach. Because antacid therapy is often continued during early therapy of ulcer disease, administer antacids at least 30 minutes before or after sucralfate.

■ Common Adverse Effects

The following adverse effects are usually mild and tend to resolve with continued therapy. Encourage the patient not to discontinue therapy without first consulting the healthcare provider.

Gastrointestinal

Constipation, dry mouth. Measures to alleviate dry mouth include sucking on ice chips or hard candy. Avoid mouthwashes that contain alcohol because they cause further drying and irritation. Maintain the patient's state of hydration, and obtain an order

for stool softeners or bulk-forming laxatives if necessary. Encourage the inclusion of sufficient roughage (e.g., fresh fruits, vegetables, whole-grain products) in the diet.

Neurologic

Dizziness. Provide patient safety during episodes of dizziness.

■ Drug Interactions

Tetracyclines. Sucralfate may interfere with the absorption of tetracycline. Administer tetracyclines 1 hour before or 2 hours after sucralfate.

Omeprazole, Lansoprazole. Sucralfate inhibits the absorption of omeprazole and lansoprazole. Administer omeprazole or lansoprazole at least 30 minutes before sucralfate.

DRUG CLASS: PROKINETIC AGENTS

> **metoclopramide** (mĕt-ō-KLŌ-pră-mīd)
> **Reglan** (RĔG-lăn)

ACTIONS

Metoclopramide is a gastric stimulant whose mechanisms of action are not fully known. It increases lower esophageal sphincter pressure, thereby reducing reflux; increases stomach contractions; relaxes the pyloric valve; and increases peristalsis in the GI tract, resulting in an increased rate of gastric emptying and intestinal transit. Metoclopramide is an antiemetic that blocks dopamine in the chemoreceptor trigger zone. It inhibits serotonin (5-HT3) when administered in higher dosages.

USES

Metoclopramide is used to relieve the symptoms of gastric reflux esophagitis and diabetic gastroparesis, as an aid in small bowel intubation, and to stimulate gastric emptying and intestinal transit of barium after radiologic examination of the upper GI tract. It is also given as an antiemetic to patients undergoing cancer chemotherapy.

THERAPEUTIC OUTCOMES

The primary therapeutic outcomes expected from metoclopramide therapy are relief of discomfort, reduced frequency of heartburn, and healing of irritated tissues.

❖ NURSING IMPLICATIONS FOR METOCLOPRAMIDE THERAPY

■ Premedication Assessment

1. Determine if other drugs being taken may induce extrapyramidal symptoms; do not administer drug concurrently.

2. Check for a history of epilepsy. If present, check with the healthcare provider before starting drug therapy.

3. Do not administer to an individual with symptoms of GI perforation, mechanical obstruction, or hemorrhage.

4. For diabetic patients, food absorption may be altered and more frequent monitoring for hypoglycemia may be required.

▪ Availability

PO: 5- and 10-mg tablets; 5-mg dispersible tablets and 5-mg/5-mL solution. *Injection:* 5 mg/mL in 2-, 10-, and 30-mL ampules.

▪ Caution

Approximately 1 in 500 patients may develop extrapyramidal symptoms manifested by restlessness, involuntary movements, facial grimacing, and possibly oculogyric crisis, torticollis, or rhythmic tongue protrusion. Children and young adults are most susceptible, as are patients receiving higher doses of metoclopramide as an antiemetic. Metoclopramide should not be used in patients with epilepsy or those receiving drugs likely to cause extrapyramidal reactions (e.g., phenothiazines) because the frequency and severity of seizures or extrapyramidal reactions may be increased. Metoclopramide must not be used in patients when increased gastric motility may be dangerous, such as with GI perforation, mechanical obstruction, or hemorrhage.

▪ Dosage and Administration

Adult

- *PO:* Diabetic gastroparesis: 10 mg four times a day 30 minutes before each meal and at bedtime. Duration of therapy depends on response and continued well-being after discontinuation of therapy.
- *IV:* Chemotherapy antiemesis: Initial two doses, 1 to 2 mg/kg, 2 mg/kg if highly emetogenic chemotherapy is being used. If vomiting is suppressed, follow with 1 mg/kg. Dilute the dose in 50 mL of parenteral solution (D5W, normal saline [0.9%], D5/0.45 saline, Ringer's solution, or lactated Ringer's solution). Infuse over at least 15 minutes, 30 minutes before beginning chemotherapy. Repeat every 2 hours for two doses, followed by one dose every 3 hours for three doses.

> **⚠ Medication Safety Alert**
>
> Rapid IV infusion of metoclopramide (Reglan) may cause sudden, intense anxiety and restlessness, followed by drowsiness. If extrapyramidal symptoms should develop, treat with diphenhydramine.

▪ Common Adverse Effects

The following adverse effects are usually mild and tend to resolve with continued therapy. Encourage the patient not to discontinue therapy without first consulting the healthcare provider.

Neurologic

Drowsiness, fatigue, lethargy, dizziness. People who work around machinery, drive a car, or perform other duties that require mental alertness should be particularly cautious. Provide patient safety during episodes of dizziness.

Gastrointestinal. Nausea.

▪ Serious Adverse Effects

Extrapyramidal Symptoms. Provide patient safety, and then report extrapyramidal symptoms to the healthcare provider immediately.

▪ Drug Interactions

Drugs That Increase Sedative Effects. Antihistamine, alcohol, analgesics, phenothiazines, and sedative-hypnotics increase the sedative effects of metoclopramide. Monitor the patient for excessive sedation, and reduce dosage if necessary.

Drugs That Decrease Therapeutic Effects. Anticholinergic agents (e.g., atropine, benztropine, antihistamines, dicyclomine) and narcotic analgesics (e.g., meperidine, morphine, oxycodone, and others) decrease the therapeutic effects of metoclopramide. Instruct the patient to avoid taking these agents while using metoclopramide.

Altered Absorption. The GI stimulatory effects of metoclopramide may alter absorption of food and drugs as follows:

- *Digoxin:* Monitor for decreased activity (e.g., return of edema, weight gain, heart failure).
- *Levodopa:* Metoclopramide may decrease the effects of levodopa. Monitor for increased parkinsonian activity (e.g., restlessness, nightmares, hallucinations, additional involuntary movements such as bobbing of head and neck, facial grimacing, active tongue movements).
- *Alcohol:* Monitor for signs of sedation and intoxication with smaller amounts of alcohol.
- *Insulin:* The absorption of food may be altered, and an adjustment in timing or dosage of insulin in patients with diabetes mellitus may be required.

DRUG CLASS: ANTISPASMODIC AGENTS

ACTIONS

Drugs used as antispasmodic agents are actually anticholinergic agents. The GI tract is heavily innervated by the cholinergic branch of the autonomic nervous system. Cholinergic fibers stimulate the GI tract, causing secretion of saliva, hydrochloric acid, pepsin, bile, and other enzymatic fluids necessary for digestion, relaxation of sphincter muscles, and peristalsis to move the contents of the stomach and bowel through the GI tract. The antispasmodic agents prevent acetylcholine from attaching to the cholinergic receptors in the GI tract. The extent of reduction of cholinergic activity depends on the amount of anticholinergic medication blocking the receptors. Inhibition of cholinergic nerve conduction results in decreased GI motility and reduced secretions.

Because cholinergic fibers innervate the entire body and these agents are not selective in their actions to the GI tract, the effects of blocking this system are seen throughout the body. To provide adequate dosages to inhibit GI motility and secretions, the following effects may also occur: reduced perspiration and oral and bronchial secretions, mydriasis (dilation of the pupils) with blurring of vision, constipation, urinary hesitancy or retention, tachycardia (possibly with palpitations), and mild transient postural hypotension. Psychiatric disturbances, such as mental confusion, delusions, nightmares, euphoria, paranoia, and hallucinations, may be indications of overdosage.

USES

Antispasmodic agents are used to treat irritable bowel syndrome, biliary spasm, mild ulcerative colitis, diverticulitis, pancreatitis, infant colic, and, in conjunction with diet and antacids, PUD. Since the advent of the H_2 antagonists and proton pump inhibitors, antispasmodic agents are used much less frequently in treating ulcers and other gastrointestinal disorders.

THERAPEUTIC OUTCOMES

The primary therapeutic outcomes expected from antispasmodic therapy are relief of discomfort, reduced frequency of heartburn, and healing of irritated tissues.

❖ NURSING IMPLICATIONS FOR ANTISPASMODIC THERAPY

■ Premedication Assessment

1. Check the patient's history to screen for the presence of closed-angle glaucoma; use of antispasmodic therapy in a patient with this condition could initiate an acute attack.
2. Perform a baseline mental status examination for future comparison of subsequent findings; these medicines may cause confusion, depression, nightmares, or hallucinations. These symptoms should be reported.
3. Obtain a baseline blood pressure and plan to monitor blood pressure for orthostatic hypotension, a common drug adverse effect.
4. Use these drugs with caution in older patients and in patients with any condition in which GI transit time is compromised because anticholinergic agents slow peristalsis.

■ Availability, Dosage, and Administration

See Table 32-4. Administer with food or milk to minimize gastric irritation.

 Medication Safety Alert

All patients should be screened for closed-angle glaucoma before initiating antispasmodic agents. Patients with open-angle glaucoma can safely use anticholinergic agents. Intraocular pressure should be monitored regularly.

■ Common Adverse Effects

Anticholinergic

Blurred vision; constipation; urinary retention; dryness of the mouth, nose, and throat. These are the anticholinergic effects produced by antispasmodic agents. Patients taking these medications should be monitored for these adverse effects. Mucosa dryness may be alleviated by sucking hard candy or ice chips or by chewing gum. If patients develop urinary hesitancy, assess for bladder distention. Report these findings to the healthcare provider for further evaluation. Give stool softeners as prescribed. Encourage adequate fluid intake and foods that provide sufficient bulk. Caution the patient that blurred vision may occur, and make appropriate suggestions for patient safety.

■ Serious Adverse Effects

Neurologic

Confusion, depression, nightmares, hallucinations. Perform a baseline assessment of the patient's degree of alertness and orientation to name, place, and time *before* initiating therapy. Make regularly scheduled subsequent mental status evaluations and compare findings. Report alterations in mental status. Provide patient safety during these episodes. Reducing the daily dosage may control these adverse effects.

Cardiovascular

Orthostatic hypotension. All antispasmodic agents may cause some degree of orthostatic hypotension, although it is infrequent and generally mild. It is manifested by dizziness and weakness, particularly when therapy is initiated. Monitor the blood pressure daily in both the supine and standing positions. Anticipate the development of postural hypotension, and take measures to prevent it. Teach the patient to rise slowly from a supine or sitting position. Encourage the patient to sit or lie down if feeling faint.

Palpitations, dysrhythmias. Report palpitations to the healthcare provider for further evaluation.

■ Drug Interactions

Amantadine, Tricyclic Antidepressants, Phenothiazines. These agents may potentiate the anticholinergic adverse effects. Confusion and hallucinations characterize excessive anticholinergic activity.

Table 32-4   Antispasmodic Agents

GENERIC NAME	BRAND NAME	AVAILABILITY	CLINICAL USES	INITIAL DOSAGE RANGE
atropine ⇄ Do not confuse atropine with Akarpine.	Atropine Sulfate	Injection: 0.25 mg/0.3 mL; 0.5 mg/0.7 mL; 0.05, 0.1, 0.4, 0.8, 1 mg/mL	Treatment of pylorospasm and spastic conditions of GI tract	PO: 0.4-0.6 mg
dicyclomine ⇄ Do not confuse dicyclomine with demeclocycline, diphenhydramine, or doxycycline.	Bentyl ⇄ Do not confuse Bentyl with Benadryl, Bumex, or Proventil. Bentylol ♣	Tablets: 20 mg Capsules: 10 mg Solution: 10 mg/5 mL Injection: 10 mg/mL	Irritable bowel syndrome Infant colic	Adults: PO: 20-40 mg three or four times daily Infants: PO: 5 mg three or four times daily
glycopyrrolate	Robinul, Cuvposa	Tablets: 1, 1.5, 2 mg Injection: 0.2 mg/mL Oral solution: 1 mg/5 mL	Peptic ulcer disease, preanesthetic	PO: 1 mg three times daily IM: 0.004 mg/kg 30-60 min before surgery
mepenzolate	Cantil	Tablets: 25 mg	Peptic ulcer disease	PO: 25-50 mg four times daily
methscopolamine	Pamine	Tablets: 2.5, 5 mg	Peptic ulcer disease	PO: 2.5 mg 30 min before meals and 2.5-5 mg at bedtime
propantheline	—	Tablets: 15 mg	Peptic ulcer disease	PO: 15 mg before meals and 30 mg at bedtime
scopolamine	Scopolamine, Transderm Scōp, Transderm-V ♣	Injection: 0.4 mg/mL Transdermal patch: 1.5 mg	GI hypermotility, pylorospasm, irritable colon syndrome	PO: 0.4-0.8 mg Preoperative: Subcutaneously or IM: 0.32-0.65 mg Patch: 1.5 mg, 72 hr duration

♣ Available in Canada.

Get Ready for the NCLEX® Examination!

Key Points

- Gastroesophageal reflux disease and PUD continue to be common illnesses that are often self-treated initially. Once medication therapy has been instituted, it is important to explain thoroughly the medications prescribed and adverse effects that should be expected or reported. Some medications taken for GERD and ulcer disease can have significant adverse effects that will need healthcare provider management.
- Solicit information about whether symptoms have decreased and whether the patient is experiencing adverse effects from therapy. Have the patient maintain a record of the pain using a standard pain rating scale. Also, have the patient record the degree of relief obtained at a specified interval after medications have been taken.
- Assess and make recommendations regarding lifestyle changes that are necessary to prevent symptom recurrence. If symptoms have not begun to diminish over 2 weeks, the nurse should encourage the person to seek medical attention.

Additional Learning Resources

SG Go to your Study Guide for additional Review Questions for the NCLEX® Examination, Critical Thinking Clinical Situations, and other learning activities to help you master this chapter content.

evolve Go to your Evolve website (http://evolve .elsevier.com/Clayton) for additional online resources.

Review Questions for the NCLEX® Examination

1. The stomach functions to digest food by secreting pepsinogen from the secretory cells known as the:
   1. parietal cells.
   2. chief cells.
   3. mucous cells.
   4. salivary cells.

2. Proton pump inhibitors and antibiotics are often used in combination to rid this common cause of PUD.
   1. *Giardia lamblia*
   2. *Clostridium difficile*
   3. *Helicobacter pylori*
   4. *Listeria monocytogenes*

3. A nurse caring for a patient with diabetes who was diagnosed with gastroparesis would expect this drug to work as a gastric stimulant.
   1. pantoprazole (Protonix)
   2. metoclopramide (Reglan)
   3. sucralfate (Carafate)
   4. misoprostol (Cytotec)

4. This statement by the patient would indicate to the nurse that further teaching is needed about how the defense mechanisms of the stomach can be compromised to cause PUD:
   1. "I should be careful about taking aspirin because it may cause damage to my stomach lining."
   2. "My doctor tells me that my stomach has an infection called *H. pylori* that caused this ulcer."
   3. "As I understand it, I have an overproduction of stomach acid that caused my ulcer."
   4. "I need to be careful about drinking too much orange juice because it is acidic and can damage my stomach lining."

5. The nurse was discussing the mechanism of action for pantoprazole with a patient diagnosed with GERD and realized further education was needed after the patient stated the following:
   1. "I understand that pantoprazole will inhibit my stomach from producing acid."
   2. "So this drug will coat the lining of my stomach so I do not get GERD symptoms."
   3. "When I take this, it will not affect how fast my food is digested."
   4. "I can expect that pantoprazole will relieve my symptoms of heartburn."

6. The nurse instructing a patient on how to reduce acid production in the stomach to prevent GERD indicated that measures to take include: *(Select all that apply.)*
   1. decrease or stop smoking.
   2. decrease the amount of coffee consumed.
   3. increase the amount of spicy foods consumed.
   4. decrease the amount of alcohol intake.
   5. increase the amount of carbonated beverages.

Drugs Used to Treat Nausea and Vomiting

http://evolve.elsevier.com/Clayton

Objectives

1. Describe the six common causes of nausea and vomiting.
2. Discuss the three types of nausea associated with chemotherapy and the nursing considerations.
3. Identify the therapeutic classes of antiemetics.
4. Discuss the scheduling of antiemetics for maximum benefit.

Key Terms

nausea (NŎ-zē-ă) (p. 507)
vomiting (VŎ-mĭt-ĭng) (p. 507)
emesis (ĔM-ĕ-sĭs) (p. 507)
retching (RĔCH-ĭng) (p. 507)
regurgitation (rē-gŭr-jĭ-TĀ-shŭn) (p. 508)
postoperative nausea and vomiting (PONV) (pōst-ŎP-ĕr-ă-tĭv) (p. 508)
hyperemesis gravidarum (hī-pĕr-ĔM-ĕ-sĭs gră-vĭ-DĂR-ŭm) (p. 509)

psychogenic vomiting (sī-kō-JĔN-ĭk) (p. 509)
chemotherapy-induced nausea and vomiting (CINV) (kē-mō-THĔR-ă-pē) (p. 509)
anticipatory nausea and vomiting (ăn-TĬS–pă-tō-rē) (p. 509)
emetogenicity (ĕ-MĔ-tō-gĕ-NĬ-sĭ-tē) (p. 509)
delayed emesis (p. 510)
radiation-induced nausea and vomiting (RINV) (p. 510)

NAUSEA AND VOMITING

Nausea is the sensation of abdominal discomfort that is intermittently accompanied by a desire to vomit. **Vomiting** is the forceful expulsion of gastric contents **(emesis)** up the esophagus and out the mouth. Nausea may occur without vomiting, and sudden vomiting may occur without prior nausea, but the two symptoms often occur together. **Retching** is the involuntary labored, spasmodic contractions of the abdominal and respiratory muscles without emesis (also known as *dry heaves*).

Nausea and vomiting accompany almost any illness, are experienced by virtually everyone at one time or another, and have a wide variety of causes (Box 33-1).

The primary anatomic areas involved in vomiting are shown in Figure 33-1. The vomiting center (VC; more recently referred to as the *central pattern generator*), located in the medulla of the brain, coordinates the vomiting reflex. Nerves from sensory receptors in the pharynx, stomach, intestines, and other tissues connect directly with the VC through the vagus and splanchnic nerves and produce vomiting when stimulated. The VC also responds to stimuli originating in other tissues, such as the cerebral cortex, vestibular apparatus of the inner ear, and blood. These stimuli travel first to the chemoreceptor trigger zone (CTZ), which then activates the VC to induce vomiting. The

CTZ is also located in the medulla. An important function of the CTZ is to sample blood and spinal fluid for potentially toxic substances and, when detected, to initiate the vomiting reflex. The CTZ cannot initiate vomiting independently, but only by stimulating the VC. Both the VC and the CTZ are much smaller than shown in Figure 33-1.

The cerebral cortex of the brain can be a source of stimulus or suppression of the VC (see Figure 33-1). Vomiting can occur as a conditioned response (e.g., see "Anticipatory Nausea and Vomiting," later in this chapter) or as a reaction to unpleasant sights and smells. Suppression of motion sickness by the person's concentration on some mental activity is an example of cortical control of the vomiting reflex. Psychological factors can play an important role (see "Psychogenic Vomiting").

When the VC is stimulated, nerve impulses are sent to the salivary, vasomotor, and respiratory centers. The vomiting reflex begins with a sudden deep inspiration that increases abdominal pressure, which is further increased by contraction of the abdominal muscles. The soft palate rises and the epiglottis closes, thus preventing aspiration of vomitus into the lungs. The pyloric sphincter contracts and the cardiac sphincter and esophagus relax, allowing stomach contents to be expelled. The flow of saliva increases to aid the expulsion. Autonomic symptoms of pallor, sweating, and

Box 33-1 Causes of Nausea and Vomiting

- Infection
- Gastrointestinal disorders (e.g., gastritis or liver, gallbladder, or pancreatic disease)
- Overeating or irritation of the stomach by certain foods or liquids
- Motion sickness
- Drug therapy (nausea and vomiting are most common adverse effects of drug therapy)
- Surgical procedures (e.g., abdominal surgery, extraocular and middle ear manipulations, testicular traction)
- Emotional disturbances and mental illness
- Pregnancy
- Pain and unpleasant sights and odors

FIGURE 33-1 Sites of action of antiemetic medicines. *1,* Cerebral cortex: anxiolytic agents; *2,* vestibular apparatus: antihistamine and anticholinergic agents; *3,* chemoreceptor trigger zone and GI tract: dopamine antagonists; *4,* serotonin receptors in GI tract and vomiting center (VC): serotonin antagonists; *5,* neurokinin receptors in VC: neurokinin-1 receptor antagonists. (Adapted from Clayton BD, Brown BK: Nausea and vomiting. In Helms RA, et al, editors: *Textbook of therapeutics: Drug and disease management,* Philadelphia, 2006, Lippincott Williams & Wilkins.)

tachycardia cause additional discomfort associated with vomiting. **Regurgitation** occurs when the gastric or esophageal contents rise to the pharynx because of greater pressure (gas bubbles, tight clothing, body position) in the stomach and should not be confused with vomiting.

COMMON CAUSES OF NAUSEA AND VOMITING

POSTOPERATIVE NAUSEA AND VOMITING

Postoperative nausea and vomiting (PONV) constitute a relatively common complication after surgery. The incidence of nausea and vomiting varies with the surgical procedure, gender, age, obesity, anesthetic procedure, and analgesia used. A previous history of motion sickness and PONV also is an indicator of the likelihood of developing this postoperative complication. Factors associated with obesity that may contribute to a higher incidence of nausea and vomiting are a larger residual gastric volume, increased esophageal reflux, and increased risk for gallbladder and gastrointestinal (GI) disease. Fat-soluble anesthetics may also accumulate in adipose tissue and continue to be released long after anesthesia is discontinued. Pain not treated with appropriate analgesia may also induce nausea and vomiting. Surgical procedures that have a higher incidence of PONV are extraocular muscle and middle ear manipulations, testicular traction, and abdominal surgery. Women have a higher incidence of PONV, possibly because of hormonal differences. Children ages 11 to 14 years have the highest incidence based on age group. Patients who have had general anesthesia have a higher incidence of PONV than those who have had regional anesthesia; spinal anesthesia is generally associated with less PONV than general anesthesia, and peripheral regional anesthesia is the least emetogenic. Analgesics (e.g., morphine, fentanyl, alfentanil) used as premedication or with regional anesthetics frequently induce nausea and vomiting. Patients under nitrous oxide anesthesia have a higher incidence of nausea and vomiting than do those under enflurane or isoflurane. Swallowed blood and gas accumulation in the stomach may also induce nausea and vomiting.

MOTION SICKNESS

Nausea and vomiting associated with motion are thought to result from stimulation of the labyrinth system of the ear, with subsequent transmission of this stimulus to the vestibular network located near the VC. When there is strong or frequent stimulation, such as from a rocking ship or airplane, the vestibular network is bombarded with an abnormally high number of impulses that radiate by cholinergic nerve impulses to the adjacent VC. Thus, drugs that inhibit the cholinergic nerve impulses from the vestibular network to the VC should be effective in treating motion sickness.

NAUSEA AND VOMITING IN PREGNANCY

The percentage of women reporting vomiting during the first 16 weeks of gestation is relatively constant at about 40%, decreasing to 20% from 17 to 20 weeks; only 9% of women report vomiting after 20 weeks of pregnancy. Vomiting is much more common among primigravidas, younger women, nonsmokers, African Americans, and obese women. Contrary to commonly held beliefs, vomiting is not more common in women who have experienced prior fetal losses or women with hypertension, proteinuria, or diabetes. There is also no association between vomiting and cohabitation; unplanned pregnancy; or gallbladder, liver, or thyroid disease.

Although traditionally described as "morning sickness," most women report that symptoms of nausea and vomiting tend to persist to varying degrees throughout the day. The cause of morning sickness is unknown, but its occurrence and severity appear to be related to the levels of free and bound estradiol and sex hormone–globulin-binding capacity.

A woman with severe persistent vomiting that interferes with nutrition, fluid, and electrolyte balance may be experiencing **hyperemesis gravidarum,** a condition in which starvation, dehydration, and acidosis are superimposed on the vomiting syndrome. Hospitalization for fluid, electrolyte and nutritional therapy may be required.

PSYCHOGENIC VOMITING

Psychogenic vomiting can be self-induced, or it can occur involuntarily in response to situations that the person considers threatening or distasteful (e.g., eating food whose origin is considered repulsive).

CHEMOTHERAPY-INDUCED NAUSEA AND VOMITING

Chemotherapy-induced nausea and vomiting (CINV) is the most unpleasant adverse effect associated with the use of cancer chemotherapy. Many patients regard it as the most stressful aspect of their disease, more so even than the prospect of dying. Because the object of cancer therapy is at least to prolong life, the effect of CINV on the quality of life must be considered.

Three types of emesis have been identified in patients receiving antineoplastic therapy: anticipatory nausea and vomiting, acute CINV, and delayed emesis.

Anticipatory nausea and vomiting is a conditioned response triggered by the sight or smell of the clinic or hospital or by the knowledge that treatment is imminent. The onset of anticipatory nausea and vomiting is usually 2 to 4 hours before treatment and is most severe at the time of chemotherapy administration. Patients who experience anticipatory nausea and vomiting are more likely to be younger and to have received about twice as many courses of chemotherapy, with

more drugs, for about three times as long as patients who do not experience this complication.

Acute CINV may be stimulated directly by chemotherapeutic agents. These agents have **emetogenicity,** which refers to having the ability to cause emesis. This type of emesis may begin 1 to 6 hours after chemotherapy has been administered and may last for up to 24 hours. The emetogenicity of antineoplastic drugs is highly variable, ranging from an incidence of almost 100% with high-dose cisplatin to less than 10% with chlorambucil. Table 33-1 summarizes

Table **33-1**	Potential of Emesis With Intravenous Antineoplastic Agents*
High (>90%)	
carmustine	epirubicin >90 mg/m^2
cisplatin	ifosfamide >10 g/m^2
cyclophosphamide >1500 mg/m^2	mechlorethamine
	procarbazine
dacarbazine	streptozotocin
doxorubicin >60 mg/m^2	
Moderate (30%-90%)	
alemtuzumab	doxorubicin <60 mg/m^2
amifostine	epirubicin <90 mg/m^2
azacitidine	idarubicin
bendamustine	ifosfamide
carboplatin	imatinib
clofarabine	irinotecan
cyclophosphamide <1500 mg/m^2	melphalan
	oxaliplatin
cytarabine >1 g/m^2	temozolomide
daunorubicin	vinorelbine
Low (10%-30%)	
bortezomib	mitoxantrone
capecitabine	paclitaxel
cetuximab	panitumamab
docetaxel	pemetrexed
etoposide	romidepsin
fludarabine	sunitinib
5-fluorouracil	thalidomide
gemcitabine	topotecan
methotrexate	trastuzumab
mitomycin	
Minimal	
bevacizumab	nelarabine
bleomycin	ofatumumab
busulfan	peginterferon
2-chlorodeoxyadenosine	rituximab
chlorambucil	sorafenib
cytarabine ≤100 mg/m^2	vinblastine
erlotinib	vincristine
fludarabine	vinorelbine
gefitinib	

Data from Roila F, Hesketh PJ, Herrstedt J, et al: Prevention of chemotherapy- and radiotherapy-induced emesis: results of the 2004 Perugia International Antiemetic Consensus Conference, *Ann Oncol* 17:20-28, 2006; Grunberg SM, Warr D, Gralla RJ, et al: Evaluation of new antiemetic agents and definition of antineoplastic agent emetogenicity—state of the art, *Support Care Cancer* 19(Suppl 1):S43-S47, 2010.
*Estimated incidence without prophylaxis.

chemotherapeutic agents in terms of emetogenicity. Emetogenicity also is influenced by dosage, duration, and frequency of administration.

Patient factors also affect acute CINV. The incidence and severity are generally higher in younger people, women, those in poor general health, and those with metabolic disorders (e.g., uremia, dehydration, infection, GI obstruction). Patients with a history of motion sickness seem to be more sensitive to the emetic effects of cytotoxic agents. The patient's outlook and attitude about cancer and therapy can significantly influence the frequency and severity of nausea and vomiting.

Delayed emesis occurs 24 to 120 hours after the administration of chemotherapy. The mechanisms are not known, but delayed emesis in patients receiving chemotherapy may be induced by metabolic byproducts of the chemotherapeutic agent or by destruction of malignant cells. The emesis experienced is usually less severe than that which occurs acutely, but it still can be significant in reducing activity, nutrition, and hydration. Patients who have incomplete control of acute emesis often experience delayed emesis. Events that often trigger delayed nausea and vomiting are brushing teeth, using mouthwash, manipulating dentures, seeing food, and quickly standing up after getting out of bed in the morning.

RADIATION-INDUCED NAUSEA AND VOMITING

Another common cause of emesis associated with the treatment of cancer is **radiation-induced nausea and vomiting (RINV)**. The use of high-energy radiation (also known as *radiotherapy*) from x-rays, gamma rays, neutrons, and other sources to kill cancer cells and shrink tumors also induces nausea and vomiting, especially when concurrent chemotherapy is used. Radiation may come from a machine outside the body (external beam radiation therapy), or it may come from radioactive material placed in the body near cancer cells (internal radiation therapy, implant radiation). The frequency of RINV depends on the treatment site, field exposure, dose of radiation delivered per fraction, and total dose delivered.

DRUG THERAPY FOR SELECTED CAUSES OF NAUSEA AND VOMITING

Control of vomiting is important for relieving the obvious distress associated with it and preventing aspiration of gastric contents into the lungs, dehydration, and electrolyte imbalance. Primary treatment of nausea and vomiting should be directed at the underlying cause. Because this is not always possible, treatment with nondrug and drug measures is appropriate. Most medicines (antiemetics) used to treat nausea and vomiting act either by suppressing the action of the VC or by inhibiting the impulses going to or coming from the center. These agents are generally more effective if administered before the onset of nausea, rather than

after it has started. The seven classes of agents used as antiemetics are dopamine antagonists, serotonin antagonists, anticholinergic agents, corticosteroids, benzodiazepines, neurokinin-1 receptor antagonists, and cannabinoids.

POSTOPERATIVE NAUSEA AND VOMITING

As noted, there is no single cause of PONV, and therefore treatment with a single pharmacologic agent for all cases is unlikely. Measures such as limiting patient movement and preventing gastric distention can reduce PONV. Adequate analgesia can also forestall this complication. Nonsteroidal antiinflammatory analgesics are not emetogenic (opioids are emetogenic) and should be given consideration if appropriate to the type of surgical procedure. Antiemetics used include dopamine antagonists, anticholinergic agents, and serotonin antagonists. The histamine-2 (H_2) antagonists (e.g., cimetidine, ranitidine) are also used to reduce gastric secretions to minimize nausea and vomiting.

Postoperative nausea and vomiting is usually managed with an as-needed (PRN) order, but patients who are considered to be at moderate to high risk should be considered for prophylactic antiemetic therapy. In addition to minimizing the risk factors listed, a multimodal treatment approach is recommended because of the variety of receptor types associated with PONV. Therapy may include hydration, supplemental oxygen, a benzodiazepine for anxiolysis, a combination of antiemetics that work by different mechanisms (e.g., droperidol, dexamethasone, serotonin antagonist), intravenous (IV) anesthesia induction agents (e.g., propofol and remifentanil), and analgesia with a nonsteroidal antiinflammatory drug (e.g., ketorolac) rather than an opioid. Nonpharmacologic techniques prior to surgery using acupuncture, transcutaneous electrical nerve stimulation, and acupressure stimulation have also been shown to reduce PONV.

The first step in treating PONV is to identify the cause. If a nasogastric (NG) tube is in place, check its patency and placement in preventing abdominal distention. Do not move an NG tube that was inserted during surgery (e.g., gastric resection); in this case, there is a danger of penetrating the suture line. Irrigation of a blocked NG tube may alleviate the nausea and vomiting. (A healthcare provider's order to irrigate the NG tube is required.) Administration of PRN antiemetics when the patient first reports nausea will often prevent vomiting.

MOTION SICKNESS

Most agents used to reduce nausea and vomiting from motion sickness are chemically related to antihistamines. The effectiveness of antihistamines in motion sickness probably results from their anticholinergic properties, not from their ability to block histamine.

NAUSEA AND VOMITING IN PREGNANCY

In most cases, morning sickness can be controlled by dietary measures alone. The woman should be advised to eat small, frequent, dry meals and to avoid fatty foods and other foods found to cause problems. Sometimes it may be difficult or impossible to work in the kitchen around food, and assistance may be required.

In about 10% to 15% of cases, dietary measures alone will be insufficient and drug therapy should be considered. Drugs that have been widely used for treating morning sickness are vitamin B_6, antihistamines (doxylamine, diphenhydramine, dimenhydrinate, meclizine), and phenothiazines such as promethazine and prochlorperazine. Ginger, an herb (see Chapter 47), is used in many cultures to treat pregnancy-induced nausea and vomiting. From a safety standpoint, vitamin B_6 and doxylamine are generally recommended first. If persistent vomiting threatens maternal nutrition, promethazine may be considered. If antidopaminergic antiemetic therapy is required, prochlorperazine is the safest time-tested medicine. Ondansetron and metoclopramide have been shown to be effective antiemetics in treating hyperemesis gravidarum and no teratogenic effects have been reported to date.

PSYCHOGENIC VOMITING

When a person has chronic or recurrent vomiting, a diagnosis of psychogenic vomiting is made after eliminating all other possible causes. The person with psychogenic vomiting usually does not lose weight and can control vomiting in certain situations (e.g., in public). Identification of the causes of psychogenic vomiting and successful resolution of the problem may not be possible. After an extensive workup eliminates other potential causes, a short course of an antiemetic drug (e.g., metoclopramide) or antianxiety drug may be prescribed, along with counseling.

ANTICIPATORY NAUSEA AND VOMITING

People with a negative attitude toward therapy, such as the belief that it will be of no benefit, are more likely to develop anticipatory nausea and vomiting. It tends to become more severe as treatments progress unless behavior therapy modifies the conditioned response. Such treatments include progressive muscle relaxation, guided imagery, hypnosis, self-hypnosis, systematic desensitization, music therapy, acupressure, and benzodiazepines (alprazolam, lorazepam). Nurses can play a significant role by maintaining a positive supportive attitude with the patient and making sure that the patient receives antiemetic therapy before each course of chemotherapy.

CHEMOTHERAPY-INDUCED NAUSEA AND VOMITING

Antiemetic therapy to minimize acute CINV is based on the emetogenic potential of the antineoplastic agents used. Combinations of antiemetics are often used, based on the assumption that antineoplastic agents produce emesis by more than one mechanism. In general, all patients being treated with chemotherapeutic agents of moderate-to-high emetogenic potential should receive prophylactic antiemetic therapy before chemotherapy is started. Combinations of ondansetron, dolasetron, granisetron or palonosetron, dexamethasone, aprepitant, and possibly lorazepam and/or an H_2 blocker (e.g., ranitidine) and/or a proton pump inhibitor (e.g., esomeprazole, pantoprazole) are often used. Antiemetic therapy should be continued for 2 to 4 days to prevent delayed vomiting. Emesis induced by moderately emetogenic agents may be treated prophylactically with a similar regimen, and therapy should be continued for 24 hours. Dexamethasone with or without a phenothiazine (prochlorperazine) or metoclopramide is recommended if the chemotherapy has low emetic potential. Lorazepam and an H_2 blocker or proton pump inhibitor (such as cited earlier) may be added to the antiemetic regimen, if necessary. Antiemetic therapy is not recommended with medications with minimum emetic risk, although prochlorperazine may be used to prevent delayed emesis. All antiemetics should be given an adequate amount of time before chemotherapy is initiated and should be continued for an appropriate time after the antineoplastic agent has been discontinued.

DELAYED EMESIS

In general, patients who have complete control of acute emesis have a much lower incidence of delayed-onset emesis. A combination of prochlorperazine, lorazepam, and diphenhydramine given orally 1 hour before meals has successfully controlled delayed emesis. Recent studies have indicated that providing optimal antiemetic therapy with the chemotherapy will significantly reduce the frequency of delayed emesis. Adding aprepitant, the neurokinin-1 (NK1) antagonist, in combination with a serotonin antagonist plus dexamethasone, significantly reduces the incidence of delayed emesis.

RADIATION-INDUCED NAUSEA AND VOMITING

Clinical guidelines recommend that patients who will be receiving radiation over a large portion of the body or those receiving single-exposure, high-dose radiation therapy to the upper abdomen should receive preventive antiemetic therapy. Granisetron and ondansetron, serotonin antagonists, with or without dexamethasone, are approved and recommended to treat RINV. Patients at low to intermediate risk for RINV should receive granisetron, ondansetron, or prochlorperazine before each dose of radiation. Rescue medicines used to treat RINV include prochlorperazine and metoclopramide. Patients who require rescue antiemetic therapy should be pretreated with a serotonin antagonist before the next dose of radiation therapy.

❖ NURSING IMPLICATIONS FOR NAUSEA AND VOMITING

Nausea and vomiting are associated with illnesses of the GI tract and other body systems and with adverse effects of medications and food intolerance. Nursing care must be individualized to the patient's diagnosis and needs at all times.

■ Assessment

History

- Obtain a history of the patient's symptoms—onset, duration, frequency, volume, and description of the vomitus (e.g., color: dark brown or black [coffee-ground emesis], greenish yellow, red-tinged; consistency, undigested food particles).
- Ask the patient's perception of precipitating factors, such as foods, odors, medications, stress, or treatment (e.g., chemotherapy, radiation therapy, surgery). Is there actual emesis, or is it primarily retching?
- Is there a history of obstruction, asthma, and/or narrow angle glaucoma?

Medications

- Ask the patient to list all current over-the-counter medications being taken (including herbal supplements) or those prescribed by a healthcare provider. Are any used to treat nausea and vomiting?
- Schedule prescribed medications on the medication profile, and requisition the medicines from the pharmacy.
- Ensure that prechemotherapy or preirradiation therapy antiemetics are marked precisely as ordered on the medication profile, along with around-the-clock or PRN orders.

Basic Assessment. Individualize the assessment procedure to the underlying cause of the symptoms if known.

- *Vital signs:* Obtain baseline vital signs, height, and weight.
- *Abdomen:* Assess bowel sounds in all four quadrants of the abdomen. Observe the size and shape of the abdomen. Note any signs of distention, ascites, or masses.
- *Hydration:* Assess and record signs of hydration, such as nonelastic skin turgor, sticky oral mucous membranes, excessive thirst, shrunken and deeply furrowed tongue, crusted lips, weight loss, deteriorating vital signs, soft or sunken eyeballs, delayed capillary filling, high urine specific gravity or no urine output, and possible mental confusion.

Laboratory Studies. Review laboratory reports for indications that include malabsorption, protein depletion, dehydration, fluid, electrolyte, blood urea nitrogen (BUN), creatinine, acid-base imbalances, and others (e.g., K^+, Cl^-, pH, PCO_2, bicarbonate, hemoglobin, hematocrit, urinalysis [specific gravity], serum albumin, total protein). The scope of laboratory data gathered will depend on the underlying cause of the nausea and vomiting and severity of the symptoms.

Nursing Considerations

- Mark the Kardex or enter data in the computer with specific parameters to be recorded: intake and output, vital signs every shift or more frequently depending on patient's status, and daily weights.
- Mark the Kardex or enter data in the computer with any requested testing of the vomitus (e.g., presence of blood, pH).
- Schedule oral hygiene measures.

■ Implementation

Nutrition

- Obtain specific orders relating to nutrition. Diet orders will depend on the underlying cause and severity of the nausea and vomiting.
- Mark the Kardex or enter data in the computer regarding nutrition status (e.g., nothing by mouth [NPO], NG suction, IV fluids, enteral or parenteral nutrition).
- As the patient's condition improves, obtain orders for a gradual progression of diet.
- Maintain hydration via oral or parenteral forms as prescribed by the prescriber.
  - *Adults:* The usual treatment includes discontinuation of solid foods and ingestion of oral rehydration solutions or clear juices. Depending on the severity of the condition or underlying cause, the patient may be NPO with an NG tube in place for decompression of the stomach to reduce the risk of vomiting. As the patient's condition improves, the diet is advanced from clear liquids to small, frequent, low-fat feedings to bland or normal diet. Generally, high-fat foods, milk products, whole grains, and raw fruits and vegetables are initially avoided.
  - *Infants:* Formula, milk products, and solid foods usually are discontinued. Fluids are offered every 30 to 60 minutes in small amounts (30 to 60 mL). The volume is gradually increased as tolerance improves. Oral rehydration solutions (e.g., Pedialyte, diluted gelatin, water, decarbonated colas, ginger ale) may be offered.
- Monitor for lactose intolerance when formula is reintroduced. Formula is generally given in a diluted form when reinitiated and gradually increased to full strength.
- Monitor hydration status using vital signs, skin turgor, daily weights, and moisture of mucous membranes, as well as intake and output.
- Perform a physical assessment every shift and a focused assessment at intervals consistent with the patient's status and underlying pathologic condition.
- Initiate hygiene measures to provide patient comfort during and after emesis. Oral hygiene should be scheduled at regular intervals, every 2 hours during

waking hours, whenever an NG tube is in place, when the patient has stomatitis, or if the condition warrants it.

- Patients with significant central nervous system (CNS) depression may have lost the gag reflex; therefore institute aspiration precautions as appropriate.
- Initiate measures to eliminate factors that contribute to nausea and vomiting (e.g., irritating foods, odors, or medications).
- Give antiemetics as prescribed or recommended. With postsurgical patients, administer when symptoms of nausea first occur. Administer before chemotherapy or radiation therapy; depending on treatment, schedule on an around-the-clock basis following chemotherapy or radiation therapy. Administer 30 to 60 minutes before undertaking an activity known to precipitate motion sickness. If a transdermal patch is to be worn during travel, it can be applied behind the ear 4 hours before departure.
- If young children experience motion sickness while riding in a car, position them so they face forward and can see the horizon; try covering the side windows with screens so they do not have to turn their heads suddenly to watch rapidly passing objects.
- Provide diversional activities.
- Monitor nutritional needs and status on a continuum.

■ **Patient Education**
Nutritional Status

- Ensure that the patient, parent, or significant other understands all aspects of the diet, fluid, and nutritional regimen during hospitalization, as well as at discharge for home management.
- Stress the importance of maintaining hydration and following the parameters that must be reported to the healthcare provider (e.g., weight loss of 2 pounds in a specified period, recurrence of nausea and vomiting).
- For patients receiving cancer treatments, the American Cancer Society has pamphlets with suggestions for supplementing dietary needs. These include, but are not limited to, giving small, frequent, low-fat meals; food temperature; and increasing protein content of meals with the use of powdered milk added to puddings, shakes made with nutritional supplements, and frozen yogurt.
- If constipation is present, help patients with cardiac disease prevent straining and the Valsalva (vasovagal) reflex by giving stool softeners or bulk-forming laxatives as needed. Ensure that bulk-forming laxatives are rehydrated with juice, water, or milk before ingestion. Maintain overall body hydration. (See Chapter 34 for more information.) For patients with degenerative neurologic disorders, a bowel program

may be necessary, usually performed every other day. Glycerin or bisacodyl suppositories or digital stimulation may be required as part of the regimen.

- Discuss ways to decrease environmental stimuli to vomit, such as removing the emesis basin from sight.
- Antiemetics cause some degree of sedation, and patients are often fatigued after receiving chemotherapy or radiation therapy; therefore caution patients not to drive or operate power equipment until these effects have subsided.

Medications. Verify the patient's and significant others' understanding of all prescribed medications to be given on a scheduled or PRN basis.

Fostering Health Maintenance

- Provide the patient and significant others with important information described in the monograph for drugs prescribed. Additional health teaching and nursing interventions, as well as common and serious adverse effects, are described in each monograph.
- Seek cooperation and understanding of the following points so that medication adherence is increased: name of medication; dosage, route, and times of administration; and adverse effects.

Patient Self-Assessment. Enlist the patient's aid in developing and maintaining a written record of monitoring parameters (e.g., weight, details of when nausea occurs and amount and appearance of vomitus, food diary of what is being eaten, which foods initiate or aggravate the symptoms) (see Appendix B: Template for Developing a Written Record for Patients to Monitor Their Own Therapy). Complete the Premedication Data column for use as a baseline to track response to drug therapy. Ensure that the patient understands how to use the form, and instruct the patient to bring the completed form to follow-up visits. During follow-up visits, focus on issues that will foster adherence with the therapeutic interventions prescribed.

DRUG CLASS: DOPAMINE ANTAGONISTS
ACTIONS

The dopamine antagonists are the phenothiazines, butyrophenones (e.g., haloperidol, droperidol), and metoclopramide. These medications inhibit dopamine receptors that are part of the pathway to the VC. Unfortunately, dopamine receptors in other parts of the brain are also blocked, potentially producing extrapyramidal symptoms of dystonia, parkinsonism, and tardive dyskinesia (see Chapters 14, 17, and 32) in some patients, especially when higher dosages are required.

USES

The phenothiazines are primarily used as antiemetics for the treatment of mild to moderate nausea and vomiting associated with anesthesia and surgery, radiation therapy, and cancer chemotherapy. Prochlorperazine and promethazine are the phenothiazines most widely used as antiemetics.

The butyrophenones also are used as antiemetics in surgery and cancer chemotherapy. These agents tend to cause less hypotension than the phenothiazines, but they produce more sedation. The most widely used butyrophenone is haloperidol. Droperidol must be administered parenterally and requires an electrocardiogram prior to and after administration because of increased risk of QT prolongation. Due to additional monitoring required, droperidol is used less frequently. Metoclopramide is an antagonist of both dopamine and serotonin receptors. In addition to acting on receptors in the brain, it acts on similar receptors in the GI tract, thus making it particularly useful for treating nausea and vomiting associated with GI cancers, gastritis, peptic ulcer, radiation sickness, gastroparesis, and migraine. High-dose metoclopramide was routinely used to treat nausea and vomiting associated with certain cancer chemotherapies until the serotonin antagonists (e.g., ondansetron) became available. In higher doses, extrapyramidal symptoms are more common with metoclopramide; therefore many cancer chemotherapy protocols now include both high-dose metoclopramide and routine doses of diphenhydramine when highly emetogenic anticancer agents are used. Metoclopramide appears to be of little value in treating motion sickness.

THERAPEUTIC OUTCOMES

The primary therapeutic outcome expected from the dopamine antagonist antiemetics is relief of nausea and vomiting.

❖ NURSING IMPLICATIONS FOR DOPAMINE ANTAGONISTS

■ **Premedication Assessment**
1. Collect data regarding emesis (type, amount, and frequency, on a continuum).
2. Assess data relative to the underlying cause of nausea and vomiting (e.g., pregnancy, postsurgical state, chemotherapy, radiation, bowel obstruction).
3. Obtain baseline data about the patient's degree of alertness before starting therapy because these medications tend to produce some degree of sedation.

■ **Availability, Dosage, Administration, and Adverse Effects**
See Table 33-2. Phenothiazines and haloperidol (see Chapter 17). Metoclopramide (see Chapter 32).

DRUG CLASS: SEROTONIN ANTAGONISTS

ACTIONS

The serotonin (5-HT$_3$) receptor antagonists have made major inroads in the treatment of emesis associated with CINV, RINV and PONV over the past few years. Serotonin receptors of the 5-HT$_3$ type are located centrally in the CTZ of the medulla and specialized cells of the GI tract and play a significant role in inducing nausea and vomiting. The serotonin antagonists block these receptors and have been shown to control nausea and vomiting associated with cisplatin and several other emetogenic chemotherapeutic agents.

USES

Studies of ondansetron and metoclopramide demonstrate that ondansetron is more effective than metoclopramide in the control of high-dose cisplatin-induced nausea and vomiting. Studies comparing the efficacy and safety of ondansetron, dolasetron, granisetron and palonosetron in the control of cisplatin-induced acute emesis and PONV conclude that there are no significant differences among the treatment groups with respect to emetic control, nausea, or adverse reactions. Granisetron and ondansetron are approved to treat nausea and vomiting associated with RINV. Palonosetron has been approved to treat acute and delayed nausea and vomiting associated with CINV and PONV. A particular advantage to this group of compounds is that there is minimal to no dopaminergic blockade, so extrapyramidal adverse effects are rare.

THERAPEUTIC OUTCOMES

The primary therapeutic outcome expected from the serotonin antagonist antiemetics is relief of nausea and vomiting.

❖ NURSING IMPLICATIONS FOR SEROTONIN ANTAGONISTS

■ **Premedication Assessment**
1. Collect data regarding emesis (type, amount, and frequency, on a continuum).
2. Assess data relative to the underlying cause of nausea and vomiting (e.g., pregnancy, postsurgical state, chemotherapy, radiation, bowel obstruction).
3. Obtain baseline data about the patient's degree of alertness before initiation of therapy because these medications tend to produce some degree of sedation.

■ **Availability, Dosage, and Administration**
See Table 33-2.

■ **Common Adverse Effects**
These adverse effects are fairly mild, especially in relation to the prevention of nausea and vomiting. Because only a few doses are administered, the frequency and duration of adverse effects are minimal.

Neurologic. Headache, sedation.

Gastrointestinal. Diarrhea, constipation.

Cardiovascular. Prolongation of the QTc interval, inducing potentially fatal dysrhythmias. This has been

Text continued on p. 521

Table 33-2 Antiemetic Agents

			ANTIEMETIC DOSAGE RANGE		
GENERIC NAME	**BRAND NAME**	**AVAILABILITY**	**ADULTS**	**CHILDREN**	**COMMENTS**
Dopamine Antagonists					
Phenothiazines					**Comments for all Phenothiazines**
chlorpromazine ⬆⬇ *Do not confuse chlorpromazine with chlordiazepoxide, chlorhexidine, chlorpropamide, or chlorthalidone.*	Teva-Chlorpromazine 🍁	Tablets: 10, 25, 50, 100, 200 mg Injection: 25 mg/mL in 1- and 2-mL ampules	PO: 10-25 mg q4-6h IM: 12.5-50 mg	PO: 0.5 mg/kg q6-8h IM: 0.5 mg/kg q6-8h (maximum IM dosage, up to 5 yr: 40 mg/day; 5-12 yr: 75 mg/day)	Phenothiazines may suppress the cough reflex. Ensure that the patient does not aspirate vomitus. Use with caution in patients, especially children, with undiagnosed vomiting. Phenothiazines can mask signs of toxicity of other drugs or mask symptoms of other diseases, such as brain tumor, Reye's syndrome, or intestinal obstruction. Use with extreme caution in patients with seizure disorders. Discontinue if rashes develop. May cause orthostatic hypotension.
prochlorperazine	Compazine, Compro, PMS-Prochlorperazine 🍁	Tablets: 5, 10 mg Rectal suppositories: 25 mg Injection: 5 mg/mL	PO: 5-10 mg q6-8h Rectal: 25 mg twice daily IM: 5-10 mg q3-4h; do not exceed 40 mg/24 hr	PO or Rectal: 20-29 lb: 2.5 mg once or twice daily (maximum of 7.5 mg daily) 30-39 lb: 2.5 mg two or three times daily (maximum of 10 mg daily) 40-85 lb: 2.5 mg three times daily or 5 mg twice daily (maximum of 15 mg daily) IM: 0.132 mg/kg three to four times per day; same oral maximum limits apply to IM dosing	
promethazine	Phenergan, Promethegan; PMS-Promethazine 🍁	Tablets: 12.5, 25, 50 mg Syrup: 6.25 mg/5 mL Suppositories: 12.5, 25, 50 mg Injection: 25, 50 mg/mL in 1-mL ampules	PO/PR: 12.5-25 mg q4-6h IM/IV: Adults: 12.5-25 mg deep IM/IV; may repeat q4-6h	PO/PR: Children >2 yr: 0.25-1 mg/kg up to 25 mg q4-6hr IM/IV: Children ≥2 years and adolescents: 0.25-1 mg/kg IM or IV (maximum: 25 mg/dose) q4-6h as needed; IVPB is preferred method of delivery	

Continued

Table 33-2 Antiemetic Agents—cont'd

GENERIC NAME	BRAND NAME	AVAILABILITY	ANTIEMETIC DOSAGE RANGE		COMMENTS
			ADULTS	CHILDREN	
Butyrophenones					
haloperidol					See earlier comments for phenothiazines.
metoclopramide					
trimethobenzamide	Tigan ⇅ Do not confuse Tigan with Tiazac.	Capsules: 300 mg Injection: 100 mg/ mL	PO: 300 mg three or four times daily IM: 200 mg three or four times daily	Trimethobenzamide is generally not recommended for use in children	Injectable form contains benzocaine. Do not use in patients allergic to benzocaine or local anesthetics. Inject in upper, outer quadrant of gluteal region. Avoid escape of solution along the route. May cause burning, stinging, pain on injection.
Serotonin Antagonists					
dolasetron	Anzemet ⇅ Do not confuse Anzemet with Aricept.	Tablets: 50, 100 mg Injection: 20 mg/ mL	PO: 100 mg within 1 hr before chemotherapy IV: 12.5 mg 15 min before cessation of anesthesia	PO: 1.8 mg/kg 60 min before chemotherapy IV: PONV: 0.35 mg/kg (max dose = 12.5 mg) 15 minutes before cessation of anesthesia	Note: PO medication is approved for chemotherapy-induced nausea and vomiting. IV medication is approved for prevention of postoperative nausea and vomiting.
granisetron	Kytril, Granisol; Apo-Granisetron ✦	Tablets: 1 mg Liquid: 1 mg/5 mL Injection: 0.1, 1 mg/mL Transdermal patch: 3.1 mg/24 hr	PO: 1 mg up to 1 hr before chemotherapy, followed by a second dose 12 hr later; or 2 mg once daily Radiation therapy: 2-mg tablet once daily or 10 mL of oral solution within 1 hr of radiation therapy IV: 10 mcg/kg infused over 5 min beginning 30 min before chemotherapy Transdermal patch: Apply one patch to the upper outer arm 24 to 48 hours before chemotherapy Patch may be worn for 7 days; do not remove for at least 24 hr after chemotherapy	IV: Children 2-16 yr: 10 mcg/kg infused over 5 minutes beginning 30 min before chemotherapy	Recommended for prevention of nausea and vomiting associated with cancer chemotherapy and radiation therapy.

Generic name	Brand names	Availability	Dosage	Uses
ondansetron	Zofran, Zofran ODT ↑↓ *Do not confuse Zofran with Reglan, Zantac, or Zosyn.* Zuplenz; Mint-Ondansetron ♦	Tablets: 4, 8, 24 mg Tablets, orally disintegrating: 4, 8 mg Injection: 2 mg/mL; 32 mg/50 mL Liquid: 4 mg/5 mL Oral film: 4, 8 mg	PO: Moderately emetogenic chemotherapy: 8 mg 30 min before chemotherapy, followed by 8 mg 8 hr later; then give 8 mg q12h for 1 to 2 days after completion of chemotherapy Highly emetogenic chemotherapy: 16 mg 30 min before chemotherapy Radiation therapy: 8 mg three times daily IV: Three 0.15-mg/kg doses: (1) 30 min before chemotherapy; (2) 4 hr later; (3) 4 more hr later *or* Single dose of 16 mg infused over 15 min, 30 min before starting chemotherapy PONV: PO: 16 mg 1 hr before induction of anesthesia IV: 4 mg just before induction anesthesia	CINV: 6 mo to 18 yr: IV: 0.15 mg/kg 30 min before chemotherapy and 0.15 mg/kg 4 and 8 hr after the first dose of ondansetron 4-11 yr: PO: 4 mg 30 min before chemotherapy and repeated 4 and 8 hr after initial dose of ondansetron, then continue q8h for 1-2 days posttreatment 12 yr: PO: 8 mg 30 min before chemotherapy and 8 hr after initial dose of ondansetron, then continue q12h for 1-2 days posttreatment PONV: IV: 1 mo to 12 yr: <40 kg: 0.1 mg/kg; >40 kg: 4 mg	Recommended for prevention of nausea and vomiting associated with cancer chemotherapy, PONV, and radiation therapy.
palonosetron	Aloxi	Injection: 0.25 mg/5 mL in 5-mL vials	IV: Chemotherapy: 0.25 mg 30 min before start of chemotherapy; *do not repeat within 2 days* PONV: 0.075 mg over 10 sec immediately before anesthesia induction	CINV: IV: 20 mcg/kg infused over 15 min beginning 30 min prior to the start of chemotherapy Not approved for PONV in children	Recommended for prevention of nausea and vomiting associated with cancer chemotherapy, prevention of delayed nausea and vomiting from chemotherapy, and PONV.

Continued

Table 33-2 Antiemetic Agents—cont'd

			ANTIEMETIC DOSAGE RANGE		
GENERIC NAME	BRAND NAME	AVAILABILITY	ADULTS	CHILDREN	COMMENTS
Anticholinergic Agents Used for Motion Sickness					
cyclizine	Marezine	Tablets: 25, 50 mg	PO: 50 mg repeated in 4-6 hr; do not exceed 200 mg daily	PO: 6-12 yr: 25 mg up to three times daily	May suppress cough reflex. Ensure that patient does not aspirate vomitus. Must be administered 30-45 min before travel.
dimenhydrinate	Dramamine; Apo-dimenhydrinate ♣	Tablets: 50 mg Injection: 50 mg/ mL	PO: 50-100 mg q4-6h; do not exceed 400 mg in 24 hr IM: 50 mg as needed	PO: 6-12 yr: 25-50 mg q6-8h; do not exceed 150 mg/24 hr 2-6 yr: up to 25 mg q6-8h; do not exceed 75 mg/24 hr	May cause sedation. Caution against operating machinery.
diphenhydramine ⇅ *Do not confuse diphenhydramine with dicyclomine or dipyridamole.*	Benadryl, Diphenhist ⇅ *Do not confuse Benadryl with benazepril or Bentyl.*	Tablets: 12.5, 25, 50 mg Orally disintegrating strips: 12.5, 25 mg Capsules: 25, 50 mg Elixir: 12.5 mg/5 mL Injection: 50 mg/ mL Liquid: 12.5, 25 mg/5 mL	PO: 25-50 mg three or four times daily IM: 10-50 mg; do not exceed 400 mg/24 hr	PO: Over 20 lb: 12.5-25 mg three or four times daily (5 mg/ kg/24 hr; do not exceed 300 mg/24 hr) IM: 5 mg/kg/24 hr, in four divided doses; do not exceed 300 mg/24 hr	
hydroxyzine ⇅ *Do not confuse hydroxyzine with hydroxyurea.*	Vistaril ⇅ *Do not confuse Vistaril with Restoril, Versed, or Zestril.* Apo-hydroxyzine ♣	Tablets: 10, 25, 50 mg Capsules: 25, 50, 100 mg Syrup: 10 mg/5 mL Liquid: 10 mg/5 mL Injection: 25, 50 mg/mL	PO: 25-100 mg three or four times daily IM: as for PO	PO: >6 yr: 10-25 mg q4-6h; under 6 yr: 10 mg q4-6h IM: as for PO	
meclizine	Antivert	Tablets: 25, 32, 50 mg	PO: 25-50 mg; may be repeated every 24 hr	Not approved for use in children under 12 yr of age	
scopolamine, transdermal	Transderm-Scop; Transderm-V ♣	Transdermal patch: 1.5 mg delivered over 72 hr	Patch: Apply to skin behind ear at least 4 hr before antiemetic effect is required; replace in 72 hr if continued therapy required. *Do not cut patches!*	Not approved for use in children	

Corticosteroids

Drug	Availability	Adult Dosage	Pediatric Dosage	Comments
dexamethasone	Tablets: 0.5, 0.75, 1, 1.5, 2, 4, 6 mg; Elixir: 0.5 mg/5 mL; Injection: 4, 10 mg/mL; Liquid: 1 mg/mL, 0.5 mg/5 mL	PO: 4-25 mg q4-6h for 1-2 days; IV: 8-20 mg before administration of chemotherapy, followed by 8 mg IV/PO on days 2 and 3	As for adults	Recommended for prevention of nausea and vomiting associated with chemotherapy.

Benzodiazepines

Drug	Availability	Adult Dosage	Pediatric Dosage	Comments
lorazepam ⇅ Do not confuse lorazepam with loperamide. — Ativan ⇅ Do not confuse Ativan with Ambien.	Tablets: 0.5, 1, 2 mg; Injection: 2, 4 mg/mL; Liquid: 2 mg/mL	PO: 1-2 mg the night before and then 45 min before chemotherapy; IV: 1.5 mg/m² (max dose 3 mg) 45 min before chemotherapy	Not recommended	Recommended for prevention and treatment of nausea and vomiting associated with chemotherapy.

Cannabinoids

Drug	Availability	Adult Dosage	Pediatric Dosage	Comments
dronabinol (THC) — Marinol	Capsules: 2.5, 5, 10 mg	PO: Initial 5 mg/m² 1-3 hr before chemotherapy, then q2-4h for a total of 4-6 doses/day; Maximum: 15 mg/m²/dose	Not recommended	Schedule III controlled substance. Common adverse effects include drowsiness, dizziness, muddled thinking, and possible impairment of coordination, sensory, and perceptual functions. Use with caution in hypertension or heart disease.
nabilone — Cesamet	Capsules: 1 mg	PO: 1-2 mg two or three times daily; Maximum: 6 mg daily in 3 doses	Not recommended	Schedule II controlled substance. Because of its potential for dysphoria, it should be used only when the patient can be supervised by a responsible individual.

Continued

Table 33-2 Antiemetic Agents—cont'd

GENERIC NAME	BRAND NAME	AVAILABILITY	ANTIEMETIC DOSAGE RANGE		COMMENTS
			ADULTS	CHILDREN	
Neurokinin-1 Receptor Inhibitor Antagonists					
aprepitant	Emend	Capsules: 40, 80, 125 mg	Chemotherapy: PO: 125 mg 1 hr before chemotherapy on day 1; 80 mg daily in the morning of days 2 and 3 PONV: PO: 40 mg within 3 hr before induction of anesthesia	Chemotherapy: Children at least 12 yr old and at least 30 kg: As for adults	In combination with other antiemetics, recommended for prevention of acute and delayed nausea and vomiting associated with initial and repeat courses of highly emetogenic cancer chemotherapy, including high-dose cisplatin. Also approved for prevention of PONV in adults.
fosaprepitant	Emend	Injection: 150 mg	Chemotherapy: IV: 150 mg administered over 15 to 20 min 30 min before chemotherapy on day 1 only	Not recommended	Same as aprepitant but not approved for PONV.
rolapitant	Varubi	Tablets: 90 mg	Chemotherapy: PO: 180 mg 1-2 hr before chemotherapy in combination with dexamethasone and a serotonin antagonist	Not recommended	Use in combination with other antiemetics for the prevention of delayed nausea and vomiting in adults receiving highly emetogenic cancer chemotherapy.

⬥ Available in Canada.
CINV, chemotherapy-induced nausea and vomiting; *IVPB,* intravenous piggyback; *PONV,* postoperative nausea and vomiting; *RINV,* radiation-induced nausea and vomiting.

reported for all drugs in the class, but is more frequently reported with ondansetron. Thus the maximum dose for ondansetron IV is 16 mg as a single dose.

■ Drug Interactions

Serotonin Antagonists (Ondansetron, Dolasetron, Granisetron, Palonosetron, Alosetron). The use of serotonin antagonists with apomorphine is contraindicated. Profound hypotension and loss of consciousness have been reported.

DRUG CLASS: ANTICHOLINERGIC AGENTS

ACTIONS

Motion sickness is thought to be caused by an excess of acetylcholine at the CTZ and the VC by cholinergic nerves receiving impulses from the vestibular network of the inner ear. Anticholinergic agents are used to counterbalance the excessive amounts of acetylcholine present.

USES

Anticholinergic agents, such as scopolamine, and antihistamines (e.g., diphenhydramine, dimenhydrinate, cyclizine, meclizine, promethazine) are used to treat motion sickness and, in the case of the antihistamines, nausea and vomiting associated with pregnancy. The choice of drug depends on both the period for which antinausea protection is required and the adverse effects. Scopolamine is the drug of choice for short periods of motion, and an antihistamine is preferred for longer periods. Of the antihistamines, promethazine is the drug of choice. Higher doses act longer, but sedation is usually a problem. Cyclizine and meclizine have fewer adverse effects than promethazine but have a shorter duration of action and are less effective for severe conditions. Diphenhydramine has a long duration, but excessive sedation is often a problem, especially after the boat, plane, or car ride is over. For very severe conditions, sympathomimetic drugs such as ephedrine are used in combination with scopolamine or an antihistamine. Anticholinergic agents are usually not effective in CINV.

THERAPEUTIC OUTCOME

The primary therapeutic outcome expected from the anticholinergic antiemetics is relief of nausea and vomiting.

❖ NURSING IMPLICATIONS FOR ANTICHOLINERGIC AGENTS

■ Premedication Assessment

1. Collect data regarding emesis (type, amount, and frequency, on a continuum).
2. Assess data relative to the underlying cause of nausea and vomiting (e.g., pregnancy, postsurgical state, chemotherapy, radiation, bowel obstruction).
3. Obtain baseline data about the patient's degree of alertness before initiation of therapy because these medications tend to produce some degree of sedation.
4. Check the patient's history to screen for presence of closed-angle glaucoma; use of an anticholinergic agent would be contraindicated.

■ Availability, Dosage, and Administration

See Table 33-2.

■ Common Adverse Effects

Neurologic

Sedative effects. Tolerance may develop over time, thus diminishing the effect. Caution patients to avoid operating power equipment or motor vehicles.

Anticholinergic Effects

Blurred vision; constipation; urinary retention; dry mucosa of the mouth, throat, and nose. These symptoms are the anticholinergic effects produced by these agents. Patients should be monitored for these adverse effects. Maintain fluid intake at eight to ten 8-ounce glasses daily. Dryness of the mucosa may be relieved by sucking hard candy or ice chips, or by chewing gum. Stool softeners, such as docusate, or the occasional use of a stimulant laxative, such as bisacodyl, may be required for constipation. Caution the patient that blurred vision may occur and make appropriate suggestions for his or her personal safety. Patients who develop urinary hesitancy should discontinue the medication and contact their healthcare provider for further evaluation.

■ Drug Interactions

Enhanced Sedation. Central nervous system depressants, including sleeping aids, analgesics, benzodiazepines, phenothiazines, and alcohol, will enhance the sedative effects of antihistamines. People who work around machinery, drive a car, or perform other duties in which they must remain mentally alert should not take these medications while working.

DRUG CLASS: CORTICOSTEROIDS

ACTIONS

Several studies have shown that dexamethasone and methylprednisolone can be effective antiemetics, either as single agents or in combination with other antiemetics. The mechanism of action is unknown. Other actions of the corticosteroids, such as mood elevation, increased appetite, and a sense of well-being, may also help in patient acceptance and control of emesis.

USES

A particular advantage of the steroids, apart from their efficacy, is their relative lack of adverse effects. Because only a few doses are administered, the usual complications associated with long-term therapy do not arise.

THERAPEUTIC OUTCOME

The primary therapeutic outcome expected from the corticosteroids as antiemetics is relief of nausea and vomiting.

❖ NURSING IMPLICATIONS FOR CORTICOSTEROIDS

■ **Premedication Assessment**
1. Collect data regarding emesis (type, amount, and frequency, on a continuum).
2. Assess data relative to the underlying cause of nausea and vomiting (e.g., pregnancy, post-surgical state, chemotherapy, radiation, bowel obstruction).
3. Obtain baseline data about the patient's degree of alertness before initiation of therapy because these medications tend to produce some degree of sedation.

■ **Availability, Dosage, and Administration**
See Table 33-2.

■ **Common and Serious Adverse Effects**
Adverse effects are infrequent because few doses are administered for nausea and vomiting. See also Chapter 37.

■ **Drug Interactions**
See Chapter 37.

DRUG CLASS: BENZODIAZEPINES

ACTIONS

Benzodiazepines act as antiemetics through a combination of effects, including sedation, reduction in anxiety, possible depression of the VC, and an amnesic effect. Of these, the amnesic effect appears to be most important in treating cancer patients, and in this respect, lorazepam and midazolam are superior to diazepam.

USES

Benzodiazepines (e.g., lorazepam, midazolam, diazepam) are effective in reducing not only the frequency of nausea and vomiting, but also the anxiety often associated with chemotherapy. Clinically, benzodiazepines are most useful in combination with other antiemetics, such as metoclopramide, dexamethasone, and serotonin antagonists.

THERAPEUTIC OUTCOME

The primary therapeutic outcome expected from benzodiazepine antiemetics is relief of nausea and vomiting.

❖ NURSING IMPLICATIONS FOR BENZODIAZEPINES

■ **Premedication Assessment**
1. Collect data regarding emesis (type, amount, and frequency, on a continuum).
2. Assess data relative to the underlying cause of the nausea and vomiting (e.g., pregnancy, postsurgical state, chemotherapy, radiation therapy, bowel obstruction).
3. Obtain baseline data about the patient's degree of alertness before initiation of therapy because these medications tend to produce some degree of sedation.

■ **Availability, Dosage, and Administration**
See Table 33-2.

■ **Common Adverse Effects, Serious Adverse Effects, and Drug Interactions**
See Chapter 15.

DRUG CLASS: CANNABINOIDS

ACTIONS

After numerous reports that smoking marijuana reduces the frequency of nausea, the antiemetic properties of the active ingredient tetrahydrocannabinol (THC) and its synthetic analogues, such as dronabinol, nabilone, and levonantradol have been studied. The cannabinoids act through several mechanisms to inhibit pathways to the VC; however, there is no dopamine antagonist activity.

USES

Cannabinoids have been shown to be more effective than placebo and equally as effective as prochlorperazine in patients receiving moderately emetogenic chemotherapy. They are less effective than metoclopramide. Because of the mind-altering effects and potential for abuse, the cannabinoids serve as antiemetics only in patients receiving chemotherapy. The cannabinoids are of more use in those younger patients who are refractory to other antiemetic regimens and in whom combination therapy may be more effective.

THERAPEUTIC OUTCOME

The primary therapeutic outcome expected from the cannabinoids is relief of nausea and vomiting.

❖ NURSING IMPLICATIONS FOR CANNABINOIDS

■ **Premedication Assessment**
1. Collect data regarding emesis (type, amount, and frequency, on a continuum).
2. Assess data relative to the underlying cause of nausea and vomiting (e.g., pregnancy, postsurgical state, chemotherapy, radiation, bowel obstruction).

3. Obtain baseline data about the patient's degree of alertness before initiation of therapy because these medications tend to produce some degree of sedation.

■ **Availability, Dosage, and Administration**

See Table 33-2.

■ **Common and Serious Adverse Effects**
Psychological

Dysphonic effects. Depressed mood, hallucinations, dreaming or fantasizing, distortion of perception, paranoid reactions, and elation are more frequent with moderate to high doses. Younger patients appear to tolerate these adverse effects better than older patients or patients who have not previously used marijuana. Patients should be specifically warned not to drive, operate machinery, or engage in any hazardous activity until it is determined that they are able to tolerate the drug and to perform such tasks safely. Patients should remain under the supervision of a responsible adult during initial use of dronabinol and after dosage adjustments.

■ **Drug Interactions**

Drugs That Increase Toxic Effects. Antihistamines, alcohol, analgesics, benzodiazepines, barbiturates, antidepressants, muscle relaxants, and sedative-hypnotics increase toxic effects. Monitor the patient for excessive sedation and reduce the dosage of the other sedative agents, if necessary.

DRUG CLASS: NEUROKININ-1 RECEPTOR ANTAGONISTS

ACTIONS

Another neurotransmitter thought to play a role in the vomiting process is substance P. Substance P is a neuropeptide found in high concentrations in the area of the CNS responsible for vomiting, and it coexists with serotonin in the enterochromaffin cells and vagal afferent nerves of the GI tract. The actions of substance P are mediated through the neurokinin-1 (NK1) receptor. NK1 antagonists block the effects of substance P in the CNS. It has no affinity for serotonin, dopamine, or corticosteroid receptors.

USES

NK1 antagonists are used for the prevention of acute and delayed CINV caused by highly emetogenic antineoplastic agents. They are used in combination with a corticosteroid and a 5-HT$_3$ receptor antagonist. They appear to have its greatest effect on reducing the frequency of delayed emesis. They do not treat CINV once it has started. Aprepitant is also used to treat pain.

THERAPEUTIC OUTCOME

The primary therapeutic outcome expected from NK1 antagonists is prevention of nausea and vomiting.

❖ **NURSING IMPLICATIONS FOR NEUROKININ-1 RECEPTOR ANTAGONISTS**

■ **Premedication Assessment**

1. Collect data regarding emesis (type, amount, and frequency, on a continuum).
2. Assess data relative to the underlying cause of nausea and vomiting (e.g., pregnancy, postsurgical state, chemotherapy, radiation therapy, bowel obstruction).
3. Assess premedication bowel pattern since diarrhea or constipation may occur posttherapy

■ **Availability**

See Table 33-2.

■ **Dosage and Administration**
Postoperative Nausea and Vomiting

See Table 33-2.

■ **Common and Serious Adverse Effects**

The most common adverse effects with NK1 antagonists are tiredness, nausea, hiccups, constipation, diarrhea, loss of appetite, headache, neutropenia, and hair loss. Because aprepitant is taken only for up to 3 days at a time, adverse effects are short-lived and rarely troublesome.

■ **Drug Interactions**

Drugs That Increase Toxic Effects With Aprepitant. Ketoconazole, itraconazole, nefazodone, clarithromycin, ritonavir, nelfinavir, cisapride, and diltiazem may inhibit the metabolism of aprepitant. Monitor the patient for signs of aprepitant toxicity.

Drugs That Reduce Therapeutic Effects of Aprepitant. Rifampin, carbamazepine, paroxetine, and phenytoin induce the metabolism of aprepitant, reducing its therapeutic effect.

Oral Contraceptives. Female patients receiving aprepitant who take oral contraceptives should be advised to use an alternative or additional method of birth control for the next month because aprepitant may enhance the metabolism of estrogens.

Dexamethasone and Methylprednisolone. Aprepitant inhibits the metabolism of these corticosteroids. Oral doses of dexamethasone and methylprednisolone should be reduced by approximately 50% when prescribed concurrently with aprepitant. Intravenous methylprednisolone dosages should be reduced by 25%.

Warfarin. Patients receiving warfarin therapy should be instructed to have an international normalized ratio (INR) checked approximately 7 to 10 days after aprepitant therapy because coadministration with aprepitant may result in increased metabolism of warfarin and a reduced INR.

Thioridazine. Concurrent use with rolapitant is contraindicated.

Key Points

- Nausea and vomiting vary from a minor inconvenience to severe debilitation.
- The six common causes of nausea and vomiting are PONV, motion sickness, nausea and vomiting in pregnancy, psychogenic vomiting, CINV, and RINV.
- Nonpharmacologic treatments, such as eliminating noxious substances, avoiding fatty or spicy foods, and restricting activity to bed and chair rest to avoid vestibular irritation, are equally important in reducing the frequency of nausea and vomiting.
- The causes of nausea and vomiting should be assessed before treatment is begun, and specific therapy should be selected for each of the causes.
- Drug therapy for treatment of nausea and vomiting include dopamine antagonists, serotonin antagonists, anticholinergic agents, corticosteroids, benzodiazepines, neurokinin-1 receptor antagonists, and cannabinoids.

Additional Learning Resources

SG Go to your Study Guide for additional Review Questions for the NCLEX® Examination, Critical Thinking Clinical Situations, and other learning activities to help you master this chapter content.

evolve Go to your Evolve website (http://evolve .elsevier.com/Clayton) for additional online resources.

Review Questions for the NCLEX® Examination

1. A 21-year-old pregnant woman comes into the clinic complaining of extreme "morning sickness." She has not been able to keep down any food or drink for 2 days. The nurse understands that these treatments are available. *(Select all that apply.)*
   1. Hospitalization with management of fluids and electrolytes by the IV route
   2. NPO until the nausea and vomiting passes
   3. Antihistamines such as diphenhydramine
   4. Ginger (herb) to treat the nausea and vomiting
   5. Scopolamine transdermal patch

2. A nurse is preparing the drug granisetron (Kytril) and explains to the patient that relief of nausea will occur as follows:
   1. "Your nausea should not be a problem if you take this drug 30 minutes before your chemotherapy."
   2. "When we administer Kytril 60 minutes before your chemotherapy, we anticipate that you will not have any nausea."
   3. "When we give you Kytril 2 hours prior to the chemotherapy, your nausea should be alleviated.
   4. "You will need to take this drug 2 hours before your chemotherapy to prevent nausea."

3. The anticholinergic agents are used to prevent this type of nausea.
   1. Anticipatory nausea and vomiting
   2. Nausea and vomiting in pregnancy
   3. Postoperative nausea and vomiting
   4. Motion sickness

4. Patients using dronabinol (THC) (Marinol) for nausea and vomiting should be taught to report these symptoms. *(Select all that apply.)*
   1. Constipation
   2. Depression
   3. Paranoia
   4. Blurred vision
   5. Hallucinations

5. The patient with chemotherapy-induced nausea and vomiting was receiving benzodiazepines because these drugs will: *(Select all that apply.)*
   1. act through several mechanisms to inhibit pathways to the vomiting center (VC).
   2. reduce anxiety associated with chemotherapy-induced nausea and vomiting.
   3. be used to counterbalance the excessive amounts of acetylcholine believed to be present.
   4. depress the VC.
   5. inhibit dopamine receptors that are part of the pathway to the VC.

6. The nurse was discussing with a patient different ways to deal with anticipatory nausea and vomiting and included in the discussion the following: *(Select all that apply.)*
   1. "We generally administer antiemetic drugs as soon as nausea develops, as this will adequately control your symptoms."
   2. "You can expect anticipatory nausea to become more severe as your chemotherapy treatments progress."
   3. "We can teach you nonpharmacologic management of your nausea that includes progressive muscle relaxation and self-hypnosis."
   4. "It is recommended that we use antiemetic therapy prior to chemotherapy so that the nausea does not occur."
   5. "The triggers for this type of nausea are often brushing teeth, seeing food, or standing up too quickly."

7. Which of these interventions help postoperative nausea and vomiting? *(Select all that apply.)*
   1. Checking patency of NG tube if one is present
   2. Limiting patient movement
   3. Ensuring adequate analgesia
   4. Advancing NG tube if one is present
   5. Administering antiemetics as ordered

Objectives

1. Explain the meaning of "normal" bowel habits and describe the underlying causes of constipation.
2. Identify the mechanism of action for the different classes of laxatives, and describe medical conditions in which laxatives should not be used.
3. Cite nine causes of diarrhea.
4. Differentiate between locally acting and systemically acting antidiarrheal agents.
5. Describe nursing assessments needed to evaluate the patient's state of hydration when suffering from either constipation or dehydration, and identify electrolytes that should be monitored whenever prolonged or severe diarrhea is present.
6. Cite conditions that generally respond favorably to antidiarrheal agents.

Key Terms

constipation (kŏn-stĭ-PĀ-shŭn) (p. 526)
laxatives (LĂKS-ĕ-tĭvz) (p. 526)
diarrhea (dī-ă-RĒ-ĕ) (p. 527)

CONSTIPATION

Constipation is defined as "a symptom-based disorder of unsatisfactory defecation and is characterized by infrequent stools or feces, difficult stool passage, or both. Difficult stool passage includes straining, a sense of difficulty passing stool, incomplete evacuation, hard/lumpy stools, prolonged time to stool defecate, or need for manual maneuvers to pass stool. Chronic constipation is defined as the presence of these symptoms for at least 3 months" (American College of Gastroenterology Chronic Constipation Task Force, 2005). Chronic constipation afflicts about 15% of North Americans and is more predominant in women, affecting two to three females for every male affected.

Constipation may result from decreased motility of the colon or from retention of feces in the lower colon or rectum. In either case, the longer the feces remain in the colon, the greater the reabsorption of water and the drier the stool becomes. The stool is then more difficult to expel from the anus. Causes of constipation include the following: improper diet, too little residue or too little fluid (e.g., lacking fruits and vegetables or high in constipating foods such as cheese and yogurt); too little fluid intake, especially considering the climate; lack of exercise and sedentary habits (e.g., "couch potato" with remote control); failure to respond to the normal defecation impulses; muscular weakness of the colon; diseases such as anemia and hypothyroidism; frequent use of constipating medications (e.g., morphine, codeine, anticholinergic agents); tumors of the bowel or pressure on the bowel from tumors; and diseases of the rectum.

Occasional constipation is not detrimental to a person's health, although it can cause a feeling of general discomfort or abdominal fullness, anorexia, and anxiety in some people. Habitual constipation leads to decreased intestinal muscle tone, increased straining at the stool as the person bears down in the attempt to pass the hardened stool, and an increased incidence of hemorrhoids. Using laxatives (medications that stimulate the bowels to evacuate stool) or enemas daily should be avoided because they decrease the muscular tone and mucus production of the rectum and may result in water and electrolyte imbalance. They also become habit forming; the weakened muscle tone adds to the inability to expel the fecal contents, which leads to the continued use of enemas or laxatives.

Many believe that even occasional failure of the bowel to move daily is abnormal and should be treated. Daily bowel movements are frequently not necessary. Many people have "normal" bowel habits even though they have only two or three bowel movements per week. As long as the patient's health is good and the stool is not hardened or impacted, this schedule is acceptable.

infectious diarrhea), and antibiotics for infection-based diarrhea.

- Initiate hygiene measures to prevent perianal skin breakdown. Cleanse the perianal area thoroughly after each stool. Apply protective ointment (e.g., zinc oxide) as prescribed; with severe diarrhea, a fecal collection apparatus may be helpful.
- Monitor vital signs, daily weights, and stool cultures and perform a focused assessment appropriate to the underlying cause of the constipation or diarrhea.

■ Patient Education
Nutritional Status

- Be certain that the individual, parent, or significant other understands all aspects of the diet and fluid orders prescribed. Ask specifically what should and should not be avoided and how much he or she should be drinking.
- Stress the inclusion of high-fiber foods and adequate fluids to maintain hydration and alleviate constipation.
- Depending on the underlying cause of the symptoms, health teaching is appropriate regarding proper food preparation, storage, and prevention of contamination.
- During travel, use bottled water when appropriate.
Activity and Exercise
- Encourage regular exercise.
Medications
- Explain the consequences of regular use of laxatives and the benefits of handling constipation with diet, exercise, and adequate fluid intake.
- When codeine or other opioids are used regularly for pain control in cancer patients, it is imperative that the patients know that stool softeners should be initiated and continued as long as constipating medications are being taken.
- If laxatives or enemas are prescribed to cleanse the intestines before diagnostic examination, be certain that the individual has written instructions for use, the time and amount to be administered, and where the laxative or enema can be purchased. Review the correct procedure for self-administering an enema with the patient, or instruct a family member.
- Emphasize the need to be in proximity to a bathroom when taking laxatives such as GoLYTELY (a polyethylene glycol electrolyte solution).
Fostering Health Maintenance
- Fecal-oral contamination may cause diarrhea. Teach proper handwashing and cleansing or disinfection of the toilet, bedpan, or commode.
- For diarrhea associated with chronic GI diseases, it is imperative to reinforce all aspects of health teaching relating to the specific disease underlying the symptomatology.
- Provide the patient and significant others with important information contained in the individual

drug monographs to identify drugs that cause constipation or diarrhea. Additional health teaching and nursing interventions for common and serious adverse effects are described in each drug monograph.

- Seek cooperation and understanding of the following points for judicious use of laxatives or antidiarrheals: name of medication; dosage, route, and times of administration; and common and serious adverse effects. For infectious diarrhea, teach the patient precautions to prevent its spread to others. For all patients with diarrhea, teach the need for adequate fluid intake and any dietary restrictions.

DRUG CLASS: LAXATIVES
ACTIONS

Laxatives are chemicals that act to promote the evacuation of the bowel. They are usually subclassified based on the mechanism of action.

Stimulant Laxatives
Stimulant laxatives (bisacodyl, sennosides A and B) act directly on the intestine, causing an irritation that promotes peristalsis and evacuation. If given orally, these agents act within 6 to 10 hours. If administered rectally, they act within 60 to 90 minutes.

Osmotic Laxatives
Osmotic laxatives (e.g., lactulose, sorbitol, polyethylene glycol, glycerin) are hypertonic compounds that draw water into the intestine from surrounding tissues. Lactulose and sorbitol have an onset of action within 24 to 48 hours. Polyethylene glycol and glycerin suppositories usually act within 1 to 2 hours.

Polyethylene glycol electrolyte solution is a relatively new approach to osmotic laxative therapy. It is a mixture of a nonabsorbable ion exchange solution and electrolytes that acts as an osmotic agent. When taken orally, it pulls electrolytes and water into the solution in the lumen of the bowel and exchanges sodium ions to replace those removed from the body. The result is a diarrhea that cleanses the bowel for colonoscopy and barium enema x-ray examination with no significant dehydration or loss of electrolytes.

Saline Laxatives
Saline laxatives (e.g., magnesium hydroxide, magnesium sulfate, magnesium citrate, sodium phosphates) are hypertonic compounds that draw water into the intestine from surrounding tissues. The accumulated water affects stool consistency and distends the bowel, causing peristalsis. These agents usually act within 1 to 3 hours and up to 6 hours for sodium phosphates. Continued use of these products significantly alters electrolyte balance and may cause dehydration.

Lubiprostone (Amitiza) induces secretion of chloride-rich intestinal fluid without altering sodium or potassium concentrations in the serum. Increasing intestinal fluid secretion increases intestinal motility with passage of feces.

Lubricant Laxatives

Lubricant laxatives (e.g., mineral oil) lubricate the intestinal wall and soften the stool, allowing a smooth passage of fecal contents. Onset of action is often 6 to 8 hours, but may be up to 48 hours because the action is highly dependent on the individual patient's normal GI transit time. Peristaltic activity does not appear to be increased. If used frequently, these oils may inhibit the absorption of fat-soluble vitamins.

Bulk-Forming Laxatives

Psyllium, calcium polycarbophil, methylcellulose, and wheat bran are approved bulk-producing laxatives. Psyllium increases stool frequency in patients with chronic constipation, but evidence is lacking for the efficacy of the other approved bulk-producing laxatives. Bulk-producing laxatives must be administered with a full glass of water. The laxative causes water to be retained within the stool. This increases bulk, which stimulates peristalsis. Onset of action is usually 12 to 24 hours, but may be as long as 72 hours, depending on the patient's GI transit time. Bulk-forming agents are usually considered the safest laxatives, even when taken routinely. Fresh fruits, vegetables, and cereals such as wheat bran are natural bulk-forming products.

Stool Softeners

Stool softeners, known as *wetting agents,* draw water into the stool, causing it to soften. Docusate calcium and docusate sodium are Food and Drug Administration (FDA)–approved, but there is little evidence that they are effective in treating chronic constipation. Psyllium is more effective in improving stool frequency than stool softeners. Stool softeners do not stimulate peristalsis and may require up to 72 hours to aid in a soft bowel movement. Action from these agents depends on the patient's state of hydration and the GI transit time.

Opioid Antagonist

Methylnaltrexone is a mu-opioid receptor antagonist that binds to opioid receptors in the GI tract, inhibiting the constipation-producing effects of opioid drugs. Because methylnaltrexone does not cross the blood-brain barrier, it does not interfere with the analgesic effects of the opioids.

USES

Stimulant, Osmotic, and Saline Laxatives

Stimulant, osmotic, and saline laxatives may be used to relieve acute constipation. Polyethylene glycol, lactulose, and lubiprostone are effective in treating chronic constipation. Lubiprostone is approved to treat chronic idiopathic constipation and irritable bowel syndrome with constipation. Smaller doses of lactulose or polyethylene glycol can be taken to regulate stool consistency and frequency. Larger doses of polyethylene glycol are routinely used as bowel preparations to remove gas and feces before radiologic examination of the kidneys, colon, intestine, or gallbladder. These products should be used only intermittently because chronic use may cause loss of normal bowel function and dependency on the agent for bowel evacuation.

Lubricant Laxatives

Lubricant laxatives are helpful for producing a soft stool without causing significant bowel spasm. Lubricants are also used prophylactically in patients who should not strain during defecation. Lubricants should not be administered to debilitated patients who are constantly in a recumbent position. The oil can be aspirated into the lungs, where it may cause lipid pneumonia. Lubricant laxatives may be used in geriatric and pregnant patients because there is little cramping accompanying their use.

Bulk-Forming Laxatives

Bulk-forming laxatives are generally considered the drug of choice for someone who is incapacitated and needs a laxative regularly. These agents may also be used in patients with irritable bowel syndrome to provide a softer consistency to the stools if a high-fiber diet is not adequate. Bulk-forming laxatives are also used to control certain types of diarrhea by absorbance of the irritating substance, thus allowing its removal from the bowel during defecation. Bulk-forming laxatives may be used in geriatric and pregnant patients because there is little cramping accompanying their use. Pediatric patients should also be treated with a change in diet to include cereals, fruits, and grains. Constipation in infants can be treated with malt soup extract, a bulk-forming laxative. It is important that bulk-forming laxatives be dispersed in a glass of water or juice before administration. If adequate volumes of water are not taken, obstruction within the GI tract may result from a bulk laxative that forms a sticky mass.

Stool Softeners

Stool softeners are routinely used for prophylactic purposes to prevent constipation or straining at stool (e.g., in patients recovering from myocardial infarction or abdominal surgery).

Opioid Antagonist

Methylnaltrexone is used for the treatment of opioid-induced constipation in patients with advanced illness who are receiving palliative care when their response to laxative therapy has not been adequate.

THERAPEUTIC OUTCOMES

The primary therapeutic outcomes expected from laxative therapy are as follows:

1. Relief from abdominal discomfort.
2. Passage of bowel contents within a few hours of administration.

❖ NURSING IMPLICATIONS FOR LAXATIVE THERAPY

▪ Premedication Assessment

1. Determine usual pattern of elimination.
2. Ask specifically about symptoms that may indicate undiagnosed abdominal pain, such as symptoms associated with intestinal obstruction or appendicitis.

> **⚠ Medication Safety Alert**
>
> Do not administer laxatives to patients with undiagnosed abdominal pain or inflammation of the GI tract, such as gastritis, appendicitis, or colitis.

▪ Availability

See Table 34-1 and individual products for dosage information.

- Lubiprostone: 8- and 24-mcg capsules.
- Methylnaltrexone: 8 mg in a 0.4-mL syringe; 12 mg in a 0.6-mL vial.

▪ Dosage and Administration

PO: Bulk-forming laxatives. Be sure to administer with adequate water to prevent esophageal, gastric, intestinal, or rectal obstruction.

Lubiprostone
- Chronic idiopathic constipation: 24 mcg taken twice daily orally with food and water.
- Irritable bowel syndrome with constipation: 8 mcg twice daily orally with food and water.

Methylnaltrexone
- Opioid-induced constipation with chronic noncancer pain: 12 mg subcutaneously once daily.
- Opioid-induced constipation with advanced illness (receiving palliative care): Treatment of opioid-induced constipation in adult patients with advanced illness (receiving palliative care) who have an inadequate response to conventional laxative regimens.

METHYLNALTREXONE	BASED ON PATIENT WEIGHT
Less than 38 kg	0.15 mg/kg
38 to 62 kg	8 mg
62 to 114 kg	12 mg
>114 kg	0.15 mg/kg

- In patients with a creatinine clearance lower than 30 mL/min, reduce the dosage by one half.
- Administer by subcutaneous injection every other day, as needed, but no more than once every 24 hours.

Table 34-1 Laxatives

GENERIC NAME	BRAND NAME	LAXATIVE TYPE
bisacodyl	Correctol	Stimulant
	Dulcolax tablets	Stimulant
docusate sodium	Colace	Stool softener
glycerin	Glycerin suppositories	Osmotic
lactulose	Constulose	Saline
lubiprostone	Amitiza	Saline
magnesium citrate	Citrate of Magnesia	Saline
magnesium hydroxide	Phillip's Milk of Magnesia	Saline
methylnaltrexone	Relistor	Opioid antagonist
mineral oil (emulsified)	Kondremul	Lubricant
polycarbophil	Fiber Con	Bulk-forming
polyethylene glycol 3350	MiraLAX	Osmotic
polyethylene glycol electrolyte solution	CoLyte GoLYTELY; MoviPrep	Osmotic Osmotic
psyllium hydrophilic mucilloid	Metamucil	Bulk-forming
sennosides A and B	Ex-Lax Peri-Colace Senokot	Stimulant Stimulant Stimulant
sodium phosphates	Fleet Phospho-Soda	Saline

▪ Common Adverse Effects

Gastrointestinal

Abdominal spasms, abdominal discomfort with flatulence, nausea. The most common adverse effect is excessive bowel stimulation that results in abdominal spasms and diarrhea. Patients who are severely constipated may develop abdominal cramps. The patient should first experience the urge to defecate, then defecate and feel a sense of relief.

▪ Serious Adverse Effects

Gastrointestinal

Abdominal tenderness, pain, bleeding, vomiting, diarrhea, increasing abdominal girth. Failure to defecate or defecation of only a small amount may indicate the presence of an impaction. These also are symptoms of an acute abdominal condition.

▪ Drug Interactions

Bisacodyl. Do not administer with milk, antacids, cimetidine, famotidine, nizatidine, or ranitidine. These products may allow the enteric coating to dissolve prematurely, resulting in nausea, vomiting, and cramping.

Psyllium. Do not administer products containing psyllium (e.g., Metamucil) at the same time as salicylates, nitrofurantoin, or digoxin, because the psyllium may inhibit absorption. Administer salicylates, nitrofurantoin, or digoxin at least 1 hour before or 2 hours after psyllium.

Mineral Oil. Daily administration of mineral oil for more than 1 to 2 weeks may cause a deficiency of the fat-soluble vitamins.

Docusate. Docusate enhances the absorption of mineral oil. Concurrent use is not recommended.

Methylnaltrexone, Lubiprostone. There are no reported drug interactions for these medications.

DRUG CLASS: ANTIDIARRHEAL AGENTS

ACTIONS

Antidiarrheal agents include a wide variety of drugs that can be divided into two broad categories—locally acting agents and systemic agents. Locally acting agents such as activated charcoal, pectin, and psyllium absorb excess water to cause a formed stool and adsorb irritants or bacteria that are causing the diarrhea. Bismuth subsalicylate acts locally to stop secretion of fluids into the GI tract that promote diarrhea; it may also have local antimicrobial effects, killing bacteria and viruses that may be inducing diarrhea.

The systemic agents act through the autonomic nervous system to reduce peristalsis and motility of the GI tract, allowing the mucosal lining to absorb nutrients, water, and electrolytes, leaving a formed stool in the colon. Representatives of the systemically acting agents are diphenoxylate, loperamide, and certain anticholinergic agents (Table 34-2).

The systemically acting agents are associated with more adverse effects (see Table 34-2) and should not be used to treat diarrhea caused by substances toxic to the GI tract, such as bacterial contaminants or other irritants. Because these agents act by reducing GI motility, the systemically acting antidiarrheals tend to allow the toxin to remain in the GI tract longer, causing further irritation.

USES

Although the ingredients of the antidiarrheal products are, in general, benign and the majority are available OTC, the decision to recommend treatment or to refer the patient to a healthcare provider is not to be taken lightly.

Antidiarrheal products are usually indicated under the following conditions:

• The diarrhea is of sudden onset, has lasted more than 2 or 3 days, and is causing significant fluid and water loss. Young children and elderly patients are more susceptible to rapid dehydration and electrolyte imbalance and therefore should start antidiarrheal therapy earlier.

• Patients with inflammatory bowel disease develop diarrhea. Rapid treatment shortens the course of the incapacitating diarrhea and allows the patient to live a more normal lifestyle. Other agents, such as adrenocorticosteroids or sulfonamides, may also be used to control the underlying bowel disease.

• Post–GI surgery patients develop diarrhea. These patients may require chronic antidiarrheal therapy to allow adequate absorption of fluids and electrolytes.

• The cause of the diarrhea has been diagnosed and the healthcare provider determines that an antidiarrheal product is appropriate for therapy. Because many cases of diarrhea are self-limiting, therapy may not be necessary.

THERAPEUTIC OUTCOME

The primary therapeutic outcome expected from antidiarrheal therapy is relief from the incapacitation and discomfort of diarrhea.

❖ NURSING IMPLICATIONS FOR ANTIDIARRHEAL AGENTS

▪ Premedication Assessment

1. Confer with patient regarding medications that may be contributing to diarrhea, including antacids containing magnesium or laxative products, antibiotics, or products containing large quantities of sorbitol.

2. Review history of onset of diarrhea and precipitating factors. Refer to healthcare provider if in doubt about administering antidiarrheal agents.

▪ Availability, Dosage and Administration

See Table 34-2. *PO:* Follow directions on the container. Be sure to give adequate water with bulk-forming agents to prevent esophageal, gastric, intestinal, or rectal obstruction.

▪ Common Adverse Effects

Gastrointestinal

Abdominal distention, nausea, constipation. Locally acting agents have essentially no adverse effects, but if used excessively, they may cause abdominal distention, nausea, and constipation.

▪ Serious Adverse Effects

Gastrointestinal

Prolonged or worsened diarrhea. This may be an indication that toxins are present in the gut and that the systemically acting antidiarrheal is causing retention of these toxins. Refer the patient for medical attention.

Table 34-2 Antidiarrheal Agents

GENERIC NAME	BRAND NAME	AVAILABILITY	ADULT DOSAGE RANGE	COMMENTS
Systemic Action				
difenoxin with atropine	Motofen	Tablets: 1 mg difenoxin with 0.025 mg atropine	PO: 2 tablets, then 1 tablet after each loose stool or every 3-4 hr as needed; do not exceed 8 tablets in 24 hr	Inhibits peristalsis Atropine added to minimize potential overdose or abuse May cause drowsiness or dizziness; use caution in performing tasks requiring alertness Do not use in children younger than 2 yr
diphenoxylate with atropine	Lomotil, Lofene	Tablets: 2.5 mg diphenoxylate with 0.025 mg atropine Liquid: 2.5 mg diphenoxylate, with 0.025 mg atropine/5 mL	PO: 5 mg three or four times daily; do not exceed 20 mg per 24 hr	Inhibits peristalsis Atropine added to minimize potential overdose or abuse May cause drowsiness or dizziness; use caution in performing tasks requiring alertness Do not use in children younger than 2 yr
loperamide	Imodium A-D	Tablets: 2 mg Capsules: 2 mg Liquid: 1 mg/5 mL; 1 mg/7.5 mL	PO: 4 mg initially, followed by 2 mg after each unformed movement; do not exceed 16 mg/day	Inhibits peristalsis Used in acute, nonspecific diarrhea and to reduce volume of discharge from ileostomy
opium (camphorated tincture) ⇄ *Do not confuse camphorated tincture of opium with deodorized tincture of opium.*	Paregoric	Liquid: 2 mg/5 mL	PO: 5-10 mL one to four times daily	Inhibits peristalsis and pain of diarrhea; 5 mL of liquid = 2 mg morphine
Local Action				
Lactobacillus acidophilus	Lactinex	Capsules, granules	PO: 2 to 4 capsules, two to four times daily, with milk Granules: 1 packet added to cereal, fruit juice, or milk three or four times daily	Bacteria used to recolonize GI tract in an attempt to treat chronic diarrhea Do not use in acute diarrhea
bismuth subsalicylate	Pepto-Bismol, Kaopectate Extra Strength	Tablets, suspension	PO: 30 mL or 2 tablets chewed every 30-60 min, up to eight doses	In the GI tract, bismuth subsalicylate dissociates; the salicylate stops secretions of fluids into the GI tract, and the bismuth has antimicrobial action against bacterial and viral enteropathogens

▪ Drug Interactions

Diphenoxylate, Difenoxin. The chemical structure of these two antidiarrheal agents is similar to meperidine. These agents should not be used in a patient receiving monoamine oxidase inhibitors (e.g., phenelzine, isocarboxazid, tranylcypromine) because of the potential for a hypertensive crisis.

Sedatives, Alcohol, Phenothiazines. Sedation caused by diphenoxylate and difenoxin is potentiated by other medications with central nervous system depressant properties.

Get Ready for the NCLEX® Examination!

Key Points

- Constipation and diarrhea are common disorders of the GI tract that most people experience occasionally throughout their lives. Most cases are self-limiting and do not require pharmacologic treatment.
- Constipation is most frequently treated by adding bulk and water to the diet and by exercising regularly. If drug treatment is required, laxatives that act by a variety of mechanisms are available: bulk formers, stimulants, osmotics, lubricants, stool softeners, and opioid antagonists.
- Acute diarrhea is usually a symptom of an underlying problem, such as a GI infection. A detailed history of recent events must be taken to assess whether to recommend treatment with antidiarrheal agents.

Additional Learning Resources

SG Go to your Study Guide for additional Review Questions for the NCLEX® Examination, Critical Thinking Clinical Situations, and other learning activities to help you master this chapter content.

evolve Go to your Evolve website (http://evolve .elsevier.com/Clayton) for additional online resources.

Review Questions for the NCLEX® Examination

1. A nurse is providing education to a patient who has complained about frequent bouts of constipation. This statement by the patient indicates further teaching is needed:
   1. "If I exercise for at least 30 minutes every day, my bowels will move more regularly."
   2. "Drinking adequate amounts of water can keep constipation from occurring."
   3. "Taking pain medications regularly will not affect my bowel habits."
   4. "Eating a diet rich in fiber should help alleviate any irregular bowel movements."

2. A nurse is preparing the drug Metamucil and explains to the patient that oral, bulk-forming laxatives will relieve constipation by this time:
   1. "You should have relief from constipation in about half an hour."
   2. "This drug takes about 1 to 3 hours to work."
   3. "Since this drug takes a while to work, do not expect results for at least 6 to 10 hours."
   4. "This drug works by absorbing water into the stool, causing a softer stool, and takes about 12 to 24 hours."

3. The patient with an ileostomy is receiving loperamide (Imodium) for treatment of diarrhea because it will: *(Select all that apply.)*
   1. soften the stool.
   2. inhibit peristalsis.
   3. absorb excess water to cause a formed stool.
   4. reduce the volume of stool discharged from the ileostomy.
   5. use an antimicrobial action.

4. The nurse was teaching a patient how the antidiarrheal agent *Lactobacillus acidophilus* (Lactinex) works. This statement by the patient indicates further teaching is needed:
   1. "When I take Lactinex, I can add it to my cereal or juice in the morning."
   2. "This drug Lactinex has a stimulating effect on my bowels."
   3. "As I understand it, I take Lactinex so that bacteria can recolonize my gut."
   4. "This drug will not have any systemic effect, so side effects are not a worry."

5. This type of laxative should not be administered to debilitated patients who are in a recumbent position most of the time.
   1. Osmotic
   2. Stimulant
   3. Lubricant
   4. Bulk forming

6. Stimulant laxatives have an onset of action of how many hours?
   1. 0.5
   2. 1 to 4
   3. 2 to 5
   4. 6 to 10

7. This antidiarrheal agent is contraindicated for use in children younger than the age of 2 years.
   1. Diphenoxylate (Lomotil)
   2. Loperamide (Imodium)
   3. Bismuth subsalicylate (Pepto-Bismol)
   4. *Lactobacillus acidophilus* (Lactinex)

8. This type of laxative may cause electrolyte imbalance and dehydration.
   1. Osmotic
   2. Stimulant
   3. Lubricant
   4. Bulk forming

Drugs Used to Treat Diabetes Mellitus

Objectives

1. Identify normal fasting blood glucose levels and differentiate between the symptoms of type 1 and type 2 diabetes mellitus.
2. Identify the major nursing considerations associated with the management of the patient with diabetes (e.g., nutritional evaluation, dietary prescription, activity and exercise, and psychological considerations).
3. Compare the signs, symptoms, and management of hypoglycemia to hyperglycemia.
4. Describe the action and use of insulin to control diabetes mellitus.
5. Discuss the action and use of oral hypoglycemic agents to control diabetes mellitus.
6. Discuss the educational needs for patients with complications from diabetes (e.g., symptoms of microvascular and macrovascular complications).

Key Terms

diabetes mellitus (dī-ă-BĒ-tēz měl-Ī-tĭs) (p. 535)
hyperglycemia (hī-pěr-glī-SĒ-mē-ă) (p. 535)
type 1 diabetes mellitus (p. 536)
type 2 diabetes mellitus (p. 536)
gestational diabetes mellitus (GDM) (jěs-TĀ-shŭn-ăl) (p. 536)
impaired glucose tolerance (IGT) (GLŬ-kōs) (p. 537)
impaired fasting glucose (IFG) (p. 537)
prediabetes (prē-dī-ă-BĒ-tēz) (p. 537)

microvascular complications (mīk-rō-VĂS-kyū-lăr) (p. 537)
macrovascular complications (măk-rō-VĂS-kyū-lăr) (p. 537)
neuropathies (nỹr-ŎP-ě-thēz) (p. 538)
paresthesia (păr-ěs-THĒ-zē-ă) (p. 538)
medical nutrition therapy (měd-ĭ-KŬL nū-TRĬSH-ěn THĚR-ě-pē) (p. 538)
hypoglycemia (hī-pō-glī-SĒ-mē-ă) (p. 538)
intensive therapy (p. 539)

DIABETES MELLITUS

Diabetes mellitus is a group of diseases characterized by **hyperglycemia** (fasting plasma glucose level >100 mg/dL) and abnormalities in fat, carbohydrate, and protein metabolism that lead to microvascular, macrovascular, and neuropathic complications. Several pathologic processes are associated with the development of diabetes, and patients often have impairment of insulin secretion, as well as defects in insulin action, resulting in hyperglycemia. It is now recognized that different pathologic mechanisms are involved that affect the development of the different types of diabetes. Diabetes is a complex, chronic illness requiring continuous medical care with multifactorial risk-reduction strategies beyond control of blood glucose (*Diabetes Care*, 38:S1, 2015).

Diabetes mellitus is occurring with increasing frequency in the United States as the population increases in weight and age. In the United States, the Centers for Disease Control and Prevention (CDC, 2014) estimates that the prevalence of diabetes in the general population is approximately 9.3% (29.1 million people, 8.1 million of whom are undiagnosed). Direct expenditures of medical care totaled $176 billion in 2012. An additional $69 billion was attributed to lost productivity at work, disability, and premature death. Diabetes is listed as the sixth leading cause of death in the United States. Most diabetes-related deaths are the result of cardiovascular disease because the risk of heart disease and stroke is two to four times greater in patients with diabetes compared with those without the disease.

Undiagnosed diabetic adults, with few or no symptoms, present a major challenge to the health profession. Because early symptoms of diabetes are minimal, many of these people do not seek medical advice. Indications of the disease are discovered only at the time of routine physical examination. Those with a predisposition to developing diabetes include people who have relatives with diabetes (they have a 2.5 times greater incidence of developing the disease), obese people (85% of all diabetic patients are overweight), and older people (four out of five diabetic patients are older than 45 years). The incidence of diabetes is higher in African Americans, Hispanics, American Indians, Native Alaskans, and women. There also appears to be a significant increase in diabetes among those younger than 20 years. The CDC has a major study underway to quantify this perception.

The National Diabetes Data Group of the National Institutes of Health and the World Health Organization Expert Committee on Diabetes (NDDG/WHO) classify diabetes by the underlying pathology causing hyperglycemia (Box 35-1).

Type 1 diabetes mellitus, formerly known as *insulin-dependent diabetes mellitus (IDDM),* is present in 5% to 10% of the diabetic population. It is caused by an autoimmune destruction of the beta cells in the pancreas. It occurs more frequently in juveniles, but patients can become symptomatic for the first time at any age. The onset of this form of diabetes usually has a rapid progression of symptoms (a few days to a few weeks) characterized by polydipsia (increased thirst), polyphagia (increased appetite), polyuria (increased urination), increased frequency of infections, loss of

weight and strength, irritability, and often ketoacidosis. Because there is no insulin secretion from the pancreas, patients require administration of exogenous insulin. Insulin dosage adjustment is easily affected by inconsistent patterns of physical activity and dietary irregularities. It is common for patients with type 1 diabetes mellitus to go into remission in the early stages of the disease, requiring little or no exogenous insulin. This condition may last for a few months and is referred to as the *honeymoon* period.

Type 2 diabetes mellitus, formerly known as *non–insulin-dependent diabetes mellitus (NIDDM),* is present in 90% to 95% of the diabetic population. In contrast to type 1 diabetes mellitus, type 2 diabetes is characterized by a decrease in beta cell activity (insulin deficiency), insulin resistance (reduced uptake of insulin by peripheral muscle cells), or an increase in glucose production by the liver. Over time, the beta cells of the pancreas fail and exogenous insulin injections may be required. Most people with type 2 diabetes mellitus also have metabolic syndrome, also known as *insulin resistance syndrome* and *syndrome X* (see Chapter 20). Type 2 diabetes onset is usually more insidious than that of type 1 diabetes. The pancreas still maintains some capability to produce and secrete insulin. Consequently, symptoms (polyphagia, polydipsia, polyuria) are minimal or absent for a prolonged period. The patient may seek medical attention several years later only after symptoms of the disease are apparent (see "Complications of Diabetes Mellitus"). Fasting hyperglycemia can be controlled by diet in some patients, but most patients require the use of supplemental insulin or oral antidiabetic agents, such as metformin or glyburide. Although the onset is usually after the fourth decade of life, type 2 diabetes can occur in younger patients who do not require insulin for control. See Table 35-1 for a comparison of the characteristics of type 1 and type 2 diabetes mellitus.

A third subclass of diabetes mellitus (see Box 35-1) includes additional types that have causes other than those that cause type 1 and type 2 diabetes mellitus. They are part of other diseases having features not generally associated with the diabetic state. Diseases that may have a diabetic component include pheochromocytoma, cystic fibrosis, acromegaly, and Cushing's syndrome. Other disorders included in this category are malnutrition, infection, drugs and chemicals that induce hyperglycemia, defects in insulin receptors, and certain genetic syndromes.

The fourth category of classification, known as *gestational diabetes mellitus (GDM),* is reserved for women who show abnormal glucose tolerance during pregnancy. Gestational diabetes is diagnosed in about 7% of all pregnancies in the United States, resulting in about 200,000 cases per year. (The range is 1% to 14%, depending on the population studied and the diagnostic criteria used.) It does not include diabetic women who become pregnant. Women with diabetes in the

---

Box 35-1	Classification of Diabetes Mellitus by Pathologic Cause

I. Type 1 diabetes (beta cell destruction, usually leading to absolute insulin deficiency)*
   • Immune mediated
   • Idiopathic
II. Type 2 diabetes (due to a progressive insulin secretory defect aggravated by insulin resistance)*
III. Other specific types
   • Genetic defects of beta cell function
   • Genetic defects in insulin action
   • Disease of the exocrine pancreas (such as cystic fibrosis)
   • Endocrinopathies
   • Drug or chemical induced (such as after organ transplantation)
   • Infections
   • Uncommon forms of immune-mediated diabetes
   • Other genetic syndromes sometimes associated with diabetes
IV. Gestational diabetes mellitus

Modified from American Diabetes Association: Classification and diagnosis of diabetes, *Diabetes Care* 38 (Suppl 1):S8, 2015.
*Patients with any form of diabetes may require insulin treatment at some stage of their disease. Such use of insulin does not, in itself, classify the patient.

Table 35-1 Features of Type 1 and Type 2 Diabetes Mellitus*

FEATURE	TYPE 1 DIABETES	TYPE 2 DIABETES
Age (yr)	<20[†]	>40[†]
Onset	Over a few days to weeks	Gradual
Insulin secretion	Falling to none	Oversecretion for years
Body image	Lean	Obese
Early symptoms	Polyuria, polydipsia, polyphagia	Often absent until complications arise
Ketones at diagnosis	Yes	No
Insulin required for treatment	Yes	No[‡]
Acute complications	Diabetic ketoacidosis	Hyperosmolar hyperglycemia
Microvascular complications at diagnosis	No	Common
Macrovascular complications at diagnosis	Uncommon	Common

*Clinical presentation is highly variable.
[†]Age of onset is most commonly younger than 20 years, but onset may occur at any age. As the rates of obesity increase, type 2 diabetes is becoming much more prevalent in children, adolescents, and young adults in all ethnic groups.
[‡]May eventually require insulin therapy over time.

Table 35-2 Criteria for Diagnosis of Diabetes Mellitus*

DIABETES MELLITUS	PREDIABETES
A1c ≥6.5% in certified laboratory using DCCT assay or	5.7%-6.4%
Symptoms of diabetes and a casual[†] plasma glucose level ≥200 mg/dL or	N/A
Fasting plasma glucose level ≥126 mg/dL[‡] or	100-125 mg/dL (IFG)
2-hour plasma glucose level ≥200 mg/dL during an OGTT	140-199 mg/dL (IGT)

Adapted from American Diabetes Association: Standards of medical care in diabetes—2015, *Diabetes Care* 38(Suppl 1):S10, 2015.
DCCT, Diabetes control and complications trial; *IFG*, impaired fasting glucose; *IGT*, impaired glucose tolerance; *OGTT*, oral glucose tolerance test.
*In the absence of unequivocal hyperglycemia, these criteria should be confirmed by repeat testing on a different day. The OGTT is not recommended for routine clinical use, but may be required in the evaluation of patients with IFG or when diabetes is still suspected despite a normal FPG, as with the postpartum evaluation of women with gestational diabetes mellitus.
[†]*Casual* is defined as any time of day without regard to time since last meal. The classic symptoms of diabetes include polyuria, polydipsia, and unexplained weight loss.
[‡]*Fasting* is defined as no caloric intake for at least 8 hours.

first trimester are classified as having type 2 diabetes. Gestational diabetes mellitus is diabetes diagnosed in the second or third trimester of pregnancy that is not clearly overt diabetes. Most gestational diabetic women have a normal glucose tolerance postpartum. Gestational diabetic patients must be reclassified 6 weeks after delivery into one of the following categories: diabetes mellitus, impaired fasting glucose, impaired glucose tolerance, or normoglycemia. Gestational diabetic patients have been put into a separate category because of the special clinical features of diabetes that develop during pregnancy and the complications associated with fetal involvement, such as neonatal macrosomia, large-for-gestational-age births, and shoulder dystocia. These women are also at a greater risk of developing diabetes 5 to 10 years after pregnancy.

There is a group of patients found to have an **impaired glucose tolerance (IGT)** or **impaired fasting glucose (IFG)**. These patients are often normally euglycemic, but develop hyperglycemia when challenged with an oral glucose tolerance test. In many of these patients, the glucose tolerance returns to normal or persists in the intermediate range for years. This intermediate stage between normal glucose homeostasis and diabetes is now known as *prediabetes.* It is now thought that patients with IGT or IFG are at a higher risk for developing type 1 or type 2 diabetes and cardiovascular disease in the future. The CDC has estimated that 79 million American adults over the age of 20 had prediabetes in 2010. Without lifestyle changes to improve their health, 15% to 30% of people with prediabetes will develop type 2 diabetes within 5 years. Categories of fasting plasma glucose (FPG) levels are the following:

- FPG less than 100 mg/dL = normal fasting glucose
- FPG at 100 mg/dL or greater but less than 126 mg/dL = IFG
- 2-hour plasma glucose level at 140 or greater but less than 199 mg/dL = IGT

See Table 35-2 for criteria for the diagnosis of types 1 and 2 diabetes mellitus.

COMPLICATIONS OF DIABETES MELLITUS

Long-standing hyperglycemia and abnormalities in fat, carbohydrate, and protein metabolism lead to microvascular, macrovascular, and neuropathic complications. **Microvascular complications** are those that arise from destruction of capillaries in the eyes, kidneys, and peripheral tissues. Diabetes has become the leading cause of end-stage renal disease and adult blindness. **Macrovascular complications** are those

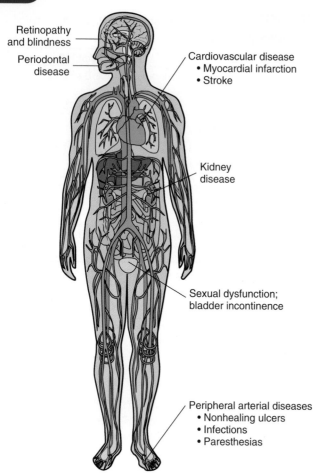

Retinopathy
and blindness

Periodontal
disease

Cardiovascular disease
• Myocardial infarction
• Stroke

Kidney
disease

Sexual dysfunction;
bladder incontinence

Peripheral arterial diseases
• Nonhealing ulcers
• Infections
• Paresthesias

FIGURE 35-1 Complications of diabetes mellitus.

associated with atherosclerosis of middle to large arteries, such as those in the heart and brain. Macrovascular complications, stroke, myocardial infarction, and peripheral vascular disease account for 75% to 80% of mortality in patients with diabetes. Complications of diabetes mellitus that often arise include the following (Figure 35-1):

• Hypertension
• Cardiovascular disease (atherosclerosis) leading to myocardial infarction and stroke
• Retinopathy leading to blindness
• Renal disease leading to end-stage renal disease and the need for dialysis
• Peripheral arterial disease leading to nonhealing ulcers, infections, and lower extremity amputations
• Neuropathies with sexual dysfunction, bladder incontinence, paresthesias, and gastroparesis
• Periodontal disease with loss of teeth

Symptoms associated with complications of diabetes may be the first indication of the disease's presence. Patients may complain of weight gain or loss. Blurred vision may indicate hyperglycemia or diabetic retinopathy. **Neuropathies** may first be observed as numb-

ness or tingling of the extremities (**paresthesia**), loss of sensation, orthostatic hypotension, impotence, vaginal yeast (candidiasis) infections, and difficulty in controlling urination (neurogenic bladder). Nonhealing ulcers of the lower extremities may indicate chronic vascular disease. Diabetic complications can be delayed or prevented with continuous normoglycemia, accomplished by monitoring blood glucose levels, drug therapy, and treatment of comorbid conditions as they arise.

TREATMENT OF DIABETES MELLITUS

Although the classification system of the NDDG/WHO was developed to facilitate clinical and epidemiologic investigation, the categorization of patients can also be helpful in determining general principles for therapy. Because a cure for diabetes mellitus is unknown at present, the minimal purpose of treatment is to prevent ketoacidosis and symptoms resulting from hyperglycemia. The long-term objective of control of the disease must involve mechanisms to stop the progression of the complications. Major determinants of success are a balanced diet, insulin or oral antidiabetic therapy, routine exercise, and good hygiene.

Patients with diabetes can lead full and satisfying lives. However, unrestricted diets and activities are not possible. Dietary treatment of diabetes using **medical nutrition therapy (MNT)** and exercise constitutes the basis for management of most patients, especially those with the type 2 form of the disease. With adequate weight reduction, exercise, and dietary control, patients may not require the use of exogenous insulin or oral antidiabetic drug therapy. People with type 1 diabetes will always require exogenous insulin injections and dietary control because the pancreas has lost the capacity to produce and secrete insulin. The aims of dietary control are the prevention of excessive postprandial hyperglycemia, the prevention of **hypoglycemia** (blood glucose level less than 60 mg/dL) in those patients being treated with antidiabetic agents or insulin, the achievement and maintenance of an ideal body weight, and a reduction of lipids and cholesterol. A return to normal weight is often accompanied by a reduction in hyperglycemia. The diet should also be adjusted to reduce elevated cholesterol and triglyceride levels in an attempt to retard the progression of atherosclerosis.

To help maintain adherence to dietary restrictions, the diet should be planned using the American Diabetes Association (ADA) MNT recommendations in relation to the patient's food preferences, economic status, occupation, and physical activity. Emphasis should be placed on what food the patient may have and what exchanges are acceptable. Food should be measured for balanced portions, and the patient should be cautioned not to omit meals or between-meal and bedtime snacks.

Patient education and reinforcement are extremely important to successful therapy. The intelligence and motivation of the diabetic patient and his or her awareness of potential complications contribute significantly to the ultimate outcome of the disease and the quality of life that the patient may lead.

All diabetic patients must receive adequate instruction on personal hygiene, especially regarding care of the feet, skin, and teeth. Infection is a common precipitating cause of ketosis and acidosis and must be treated promptly.

Patients with diabetes must also be aggressively treated for comorbid diseases (smoking cessation [including e-cigarettes], treatment of dyslipidemia, blood pressure control, antiplatelet therapy, influenza and pneumococcal vaccinations) to help prevent microvascular and macrovascular complications. The ADA and the American Association of Clinical Endocrinologists (ACCE) have developed programs of intensive diabetes self-management that applies to type 1 and type 2 diabetes mellitus. These programs include the concepts of care, the responsibilities of the patient and the healthcare provider, and the appropriate intervals for laboratory testing and follow-up. Patient education, understanding, and direct participation by the patient in his or her treatment are key components of long-term success in disease management. **Intensive therapy** describes a comprehensive program of diabetes care that includes patient-centered communication, a team approach to care, self-monitoring of blood glucose four or more times daily, MNT, exercise, and, for those patients with type 1 diabetes, three or more insulin injections daily or use of an insulin pump for continuous insulin infusion. See Table 35-3 for the treatment goals recommended by the ADA and the ACCE.

DRUG THERAPY FOR DIABETES MELLITUS

"Hyperglycemia defines diabetes, and glycemic control is fundamental to diabetes management" (*Diabetes Care*, 38: s35, 2015). The primary treatment goal of type 1 and type 2 diabetes is normalization of blood glucose levels. Insulin is required to control type 1 diabetes and other types of diabetes in patients whose blood glucose cannot be controlled by an MNT diet, exercise, weight reduction, or other antidiabetic agents. Patients normally controlled with other antidiabetic agents require insulin during situations of increased physiologic and psychological stress, such as pregnancy, surgery, and infections. The dosage of insulin is usually adjusted according to the blood glucose levels. The patient should test the blood glucose level before each meal and at bedtime while the insulin and food intake are being regulated.

The ADA now recommends that patients with prediabetes be treated to prevent or delay the onset of type 2 diabetes. Patients should be referred to an effective ongoing support program targeting weight loss of 7% of body weight and increasing physical activity to at least 150 minutes per week of moderate activity such as walking. The Medical Care in Diabetes–2015 also recommends that people should be encouraged

Table 35-3 Treatment Goals for Diabetes and Comorbid Diseases*

DISEASE	MONITORING PARAMETER	ADA THERAPEUTIC GOALS	AACE THERAPEUTIC GOALS
Diabetes	A1$_C$	<7%[†]	≤6.5%
	Preprandial plasma glucose	80-130 mg/dL	<110 mg/dL
	Postprandial plasma glucose	<180 mg/dL	<140 mg/dL
Hypertension	Blood pressure	<140/90 mm Hg	<130/80 mm Hg
Dyslipidemia	LDL cholesterol	<100 mg/dL	<70 mg/dL highest risk
			<100 mg/dL high risk
	Non-HDL cholesterol		<100 mg/dL highest risk
			<130 mg/dL high risk
	HDL cholesterol	>40 mg/dL in males	
		>50 mg/dL in females	
	Total cholesterol/		<3.5 in high risk
	HDL cholesterol		<3.0 in highest risk
	Triglycerides	<150 mg/dL	<150 mg/dL
Weight	Weight loss	BMI <25 kg/m² (see p. 319)	BMI <25 kg/m² (see p. 319)
		Asian Americans: BMI <23 kg/m²	Reduce weight at least 5%-10%; avoid weight gain

BMI, body mass index; *HDL*, high-density lipoprotein; *LDL*, low-density lipoprotein.
*Recommended by the American Diabetes Association (Standards of Medical Care in Diabetes, Diabetes Care, 38: [Suppl 1]:S4, 2015) and the American Association of Clinical Endocrinologists (AACE Comprehensive Diabetes Management Algorithm 2013, *Endocrine Practice* 19:327, 2013).
[†]The goal hemoglobin A1$_C$ level for patients in general is less than 7%, but the ideal goal for individual patients is as close to normal (<6%) as possible without significant hypoglycemia.

to limit the amount of time they spend being sedentary by breaking up extended amounts of time (>90 min) spent sitting. Metformin therapy should be considered for treatment of prediabetes, especially in those patients whose body mass index (BMI) is greater than 35 kg/m^2, are older than 60 years, and women with prior GDM. Patients should be monitored at least annually for the development of diabetes mellitus.

Other antidiabetic agents are used in the therapy of type 2 diabetes. They are recommended only for those patients whose diabetes cannot be controlled by MNT diet and exercise alone and who are not prone to develop ketosis, acidosis, or infections. Patients most likely to benefit from treatment are those who have developed diabetes after age 40 and who require less than 40 units of insulin daily.

A combination of antidiabetic agents working by different mechanisms is often required to control hyperglycemia successfully (Figure 35-2):

- *Biguanide:* The only biguanide available in the United States is metformin. Unless contraindicated, it is the initial drug of choice for treatment of type 2 diabetes. Metformin decreases hepatic glucose production by inhibiting glycogenolysis and gluconeogenesis, reducing absorption of glucose from the small intestine, and increasing insulin sensitivity, which improves glucose uptake in peripheral muscle and adipose cells. The net result is a significant decrease in fasting and postprandial blood glucose and A1$_C$ concentrations.
- *Secretogogues:* The sulfonylureas (e.g., glyburide, glipizide, glimepiride) and the meglitinides (repaglinide, nateglinide) stimulate the pancreas to secrete more insulin. The sulfonylureas also diminish hepatic glucose production and metabolism of insulin by the liver. The net effect is a normalization of insulin and glucose levels.
- *Thiazolidinediones (TZDs):* The TZDs (e.g., pioglitazone, rosiglitazone) increase tissue sensitivity to insulin, causing greater glucose uptake in muscle, adipose, and liver tissue. They also diminish glucose production by the liver.
- *Alpha-glucosidase inhibitors:* Acarbose and miglitol inhibit enzymes in the small intestine that metabolize complex carbohydrates. This slows the absorption of carbohydrates, reducing postprandial hyperglycemia.

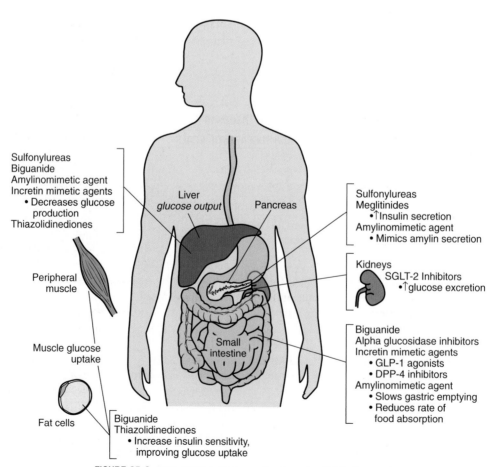

FIGURE 35-2 Sites and mechanisms of action of antidiabetic agents.

| Table 35-4 | Summary of Physiologic Effects of Antidiabetic Agents |

DRUG	INSULIN SECRETION	DECREASE IN FASTING BLOOD GLUCOSE LEVEL	EFFECT ON HEMOGLOBIN A1$_C$ LEVEL	WEIGHT GAIN
Insulin	Decrease	Significant	Significant	Yes
Sulfonylureas	Increase	40-60 mg/dL	1%-2%	Yes
Meglitinides	Increase	30 mg/dL	1.1%	Yes
Biguanide (metformin)	No change	53 mg/dL	1.4%	No; mild
Thiazolidinediones	No change	25-55 mg/dL	0.1%-0.7%	Yes
Alpha-glucosidase inhibitors	No change	20-30 mg/dL	0.5%-1%	No
Glucagon-like peptide-1 agonists	Increase	—	1.0%-1.5%	No
Dipeptidyl peptidase-4 inhibitors	Increase	—	0.5%-0.8%	No
Sodium-glucose cotransporter 2 inhibitors	Decrease	—	0.7%-1%	No

Data from the American Association of Clinical Endocrinologists: Medical guidelines for the management of diabetes mellitus. The ACCE system of intensive diabetes self-management, 2002 update, *Endocr Pract* 8(Suppl 1):52, 2002; Department of Health and Human Services and Department of Agriculture: Dietary guidelines for Americans, 2005. Retrieved from www.health.gov/dietaryguidelines.

- *Sodium-glucose cotransporter 2 inhibitors (SGLT2 inhibitors):* These agents block the reabsorption of glucose by the kidneys, causing the sugar to be excreted in the urine, lowering blood glucose. The SGLT2 inhibitors are canagliflozin, dapagliflozin, and empagliflozin.
- *Incretin-based therapy:* It is thought that patients with type 2 diabetes have a suppressed incretin hormone system. The incretin hormones act in the gastrointestinal tract to control blood glucose levels by enhancing insulin secretion, suppressing glucagon secretion from the liver, suppressing glucose output from the liver, delaying gastric emptying (thus slowing carbohydrate and lipid absorption), reducing postprandial hyperglycemia, reducing appetite, and maintaining beta cell function. There are currently two classes of agents that increase incretin activity: (1) incretin mimetics (the glucagonlike peptide-1 [GLP-1] agonists albiglutide, dulaglutide, exenatide, and liraglutide) and (2) dipeptidyl peptidase-4 (DPP-4) inhibitors (alogliptin, sitagliptin, saxagliptin, and linagliptin).

Initial antidiabetic therapy for type 2 diabetes is highly dependent on the patient's success with lifestyle modification and diet control. A consensus statement endorsed by the ADA recommends metformin in combination with MNT and exercise as initial treatment of type 2 diabetes mellitus. If the goal A1$_C$ level below 7% has not been achieved with this monotherapy within 3 to 6 months, add basal insulin (most effective) and/or a sulfonylurea (least expensive), a TZD, or an incretin-based DPP-4 inhibitor, or GLP-1 agonist. If the A1$_C$ level is still higher than 7%, insulin doses should be intensified, and another member of a drug class not already being used in the initial therapy should be added. An alpha-glucosidase inhibitor may be added if postprandial hyperglycemia is a problem. See Table 35-4 for a comparison of antidiabetic agents and their effects on lowering blood glucose levels and A1$_C$ concentrations.

❖ NURSING IMPLICATIONS FOR PATIENTS WITH DIABETES MELLITUS

A major challenge in nursing is to teach the recently diagnosed diabetic patient all the necessary information to manage self-care and the disease process and to prevent complications. The patient must be taught the entire therapeutic regimen—diet, activity level, blood or urine testing, medication, self-injection techniques, prevention of complications, illness management, and effective management of hypoglycemia or hyperglycemia. Patient education may begin in the hospital and continue for several weeks in the outpatient setting. Dietitians, nurses, diabetic nurse educators, and pharmacists are all actively involved in educating the patient and family. A referral to the ADA serves as an excellent resource in the community for the patient and family. Many diabetic patients have difficulty understanding the critical balance that must be maintained among the dietary prescription, prescribed medication and maintenance of general health. All are important to the control and effective management of the disease process.

■ Assessment and Implementation
Description of Current Symptoms
- Ask the reasons for seeking the current appointment or admission.
Patient's Understanding of Diabetes Mellitus
- Assess the individual's current knowledge of the treatment of diabetes mellitus. Gather additional data about the person's current educational needs

with regard to self-management of the disease process. Answer questions that the patient has, including rationale for actions being recommended.

- Will other family members or significant others be providing part of the care or participating in the health education portion of the individual's care?
- Patients who are readmitted must be assessed for the understanding of the treatment regimen and for adherence with the prescribed diet, medications, and exercise.
- For pregnant women, risk assessment for GDM should be performed at the first prenatal visit. High-risk women who have an initial negative testing for diabetes should be retested between 24 and 28 weeks of gestation.

Psychosocial Assessment

- *Mental status:* Ask specific information to evaluate the patient's current level of consciousness, alertness, comprehension, and appropriateness of responses. Evaluate the person's judgment capabilities and ability to solve problems about the management of the diabetes.
- *Adaptation to disease:* Ask specifically about the person's adjustment to the diagnosis of diabetes mellitus; in a recently diagnosed individual, identify prior coping mechanisms used successfully to deal with life events.
- *Feelings:* Assess for fears and the person's perspective of the impact of the disease on his or her life. Encourage expression of the patient's feelings and concerns; address the patient's concerns first. Involve support personnel, as appropriate, in the delivery of care or planning for home management of the diabetes.
- *Support system:* Obtain information regarding who can provide support for the patient. Does the individual live alone? What effect does the disease have on other members of the family structure (e.g., children who are diabetic, people with renal or visual complications)? Does the patient participate in a support group for patients with diabetes?

Nutrition

- Is the patient on a prescribed MNT diet? The recently diagnosed diabetic patient requires a thorough nutritional assessment. Information collected by the nurse or dietitian should include identification of the patient's average daily diet, the ability and willingness to prepare foods, food budget, and level of daily activity and exercise.
- Ask about diet prescription—total daily calories and distribution pattern of carbohydrates, fats, and proteins.
- Have there been any problems encountered in purchasing or preparing the foods? Has it been difficult to comply with the diet? If so, what are the problems encountered?
- How much alcohol is consumed and how often?

- Has the individual experienced any weight loss or gain recently?
- If the patient is a child, obtain data relating to the individual's growth and development patterns.

Activity and Exercise

- Does the individual experience weakness or fatigue with daily activities? Does the patient get regular exercise? What type, intensity, and duration is the exercise? Has there been any significant variation in the degree of exercise recently?
- Has the patient made any adjustments in the insulin, oral antidiabetic agents, or diet to offset an increase or decrease in exercise?
- Has there been a change in occupation that has affected the level of exercise?

Medications

- What medications have been prescribed, and what is the degree of adherence with the regimen? Monitor for common and serious adverse effects, and document associated monitoring parameters on the records (e.g., blood glucose, ketone testing). If the patient is taking insulin, ask specifically about the type and dose being taken and the times of administration. Assess the ability and accuracy to self-administer injections. If a family member gives the insulin, assess his or her ability and accuracy in giving injections.
- What over-the-counter medications (including herbal medicines) does the patient take, and how often? Does the patient consume alcohol? If so, how much and how often?

Monitoring

- Ask the patient to bring a record of self-monitoring of insulin or antidiabetic agents taken, as well as any blood glucose testing or A1$_C$ testing that was done. Has the patient done any testing for ketones? If so, what were the results? Other tests to be performed periodically include the fasting lipid profile, which includes measurement of lipid levels (high-density lipoprotein [HDL], low-density lipoprotein [LDL] cholesterol, triglycerides), serum creatinine, and microalbuminuria. When hypertension is present, perform a urinalysis and check for albuminuria. If protein is negative, microalbumin testing should be performed to determine the presence of protein in the urine. Annual monitoring of LDL, triglyceride, and A1$_C$ levels is recommended.

■ **Physical Assessment**

Generally, data are collected about all body systems to serve as a baseline for subsequent evaluations throughout the course of treatment. Periodic focused assessments are completed to detect signs and symptoms of complications commonly associated with diabetes mellitus.

- *Hypoglycemia:* Have there been any episodes of hypoglycemia? If so, obtain details of the occurrences (e.g., has the patient eaten the prescribed diet, taken the prescribed medications, or altered the exercise level?). If a hypoglycemic reaction occurs, notify the team leader or primary nurse, who will then contact the healthcare provider. The underlying cause of the hypoglycemia must be identified to prevent further occurrences. If in doubt about whether a hypoglycemic reaction is taking place, treat as though a hypoglycemic reaction is occurring to prevent neurologic damage from prolonged reduction in glucose to the nerve cells (e.g., brain cells). Record all prescription and over-the-counter medications being taken to assess whether any drug interactions may be causing the hypoglycemia.

- *Hyperglycemia:* With any hyperglycemic reaction, notify the team leader or primary nurse, who will then contact the prescriber. The goals of treatment include maintaining normal fluid and electrolyte balance and restoring a normal serum glucose level.
- *Illnesses, stress:* Have there been any recent illnesses, infections, or stressful events? If so, what treatments have been initiated? Ask specifically about any sores on the skin and feet, periodontal disease, and occurrence of urinary tract or vaginal (candidiasis) infections.
- *Vascular changes:* Obtain baseline vital signs. Does the person have any symptoms of, or is the patient being treated for, cerebrovascular, peripheral vascular, or cardiovascular disease (including hypertension), or diabetic retinopathy or nephropathy? Obtain a current history of the patient's blood pressure and details of any medications being taken to treat hypertension.
- *Neuropathy:* Ask about specific symptoms of paresthesias (numbness or tingling sensations), foot injuries and ulcerations, diarrhea, postural hypotension, impotence, or neurogenic bladder.
- *Smoking:* Obtain a history of smoking and tobacco use from all patients with diabetes mellitus.

■ Patient Education

The ADA has developed areas of diabetic education. Not all aspects of the care outlined in these recommendations are presented in the sample teaching plan for diabetics (see Chapter 5, Box 5-2). The recommendations must be adapted to the individual's needs. It may not be possible to teach the entire program during the hospitalization period. Teach the individual specifics regarding the type of diabetes that has been diagnosed.

- Type 1 diabetes mellitus results from damage to the beta cells of the pancreas, where insulin is normally produced. Insulin is needed to transport the glucose required by the body cells from the bloodstream to the individual cells to be used as an energy source. Without beta cells, no insulin is produced and the glucose accumulates in the blood (hyperglycemia).
- Type 1 diabetes mellitus requires the administration of insulin injections to replace the insulin that the body is no longer able to make. The patient must follow a prescribed diet and exercise program, perform glucose testing, and, when hyperglycemia is present, test for ketones in the urine.
- Type 2 diabetes mellitus is an illness characterized by abnormal beta cell function, resistance to insulin action, and increased hepatic glucose production. Type 2 diabetes mellitus requires a prescribed diet and exercise program, weight loss to a near-ideal body level, glucose testing, and an oral antidiabetic agent or antihyperglycemic agent if the diabetes cannot be managed with diet and exercise alone. During times of illness, or if the oral treatment stops being effective, insulin may be required. Special needs may be required for patients who are pregnant or nursing.

Psychological Adjustment

- When first diagnosed, the patient may experience varying degrees of grief, anger, denial, or acceptance. Let the patient express these concerns, and address those items that are considered to be of greatest importance first.
- Encourage the idea that the patient can control most aspects of diabetes by careful management of diet, medications, and activities. Having a sense of control is important to everyone. Stress that learning to manage the disease process is the best long-term approach.
- Discuss the individual's lifestyle, travel, work, school schedules, and activities, and individualize the care needs.
- Discuss the need for continued regular monitoring of the diabetes to minimize the effect that the disease may have on the patient and family.

Smoking. Healthcare providers should emphasize the need for smoking (including e-cigarettes) cessation as a priority of care for all patients with diabetes.

Nutrition

- Diet is used alone or in combination with insulin or oral antidiabetic agents to control diabetes mellitus. The patient with diabetes, whether type 1 or 2, must follow a prescribed diet to achieve optimal control of the disease.
- The dietary prescription is based on the nutritional and energy requirements necessary to maintain an appropriate weight, lifestyle, and normal growth and development. Diabetic patients are encouraged to maintain a reasonable body weight based on height, gender, and frame size.
- Medical nutrition therapy is now being recommended for patients with diabetes. Standardized calorie-level meal patterns based on exchange lists have traditionally been used to plan meals for hospitalized patients. Other meal planning systems include menus based on *Dietary Guidelines for Americans* (USDHHS, 2015), regular hospital menus, individualized meal plans, or menus using carbohydrate counting. A new system, called the

consistent-carbohydrate diabetes meal plan, is being developed that uses meal plans without a specific calorie level; instead, it incorporates a consistent carbohydrate content for each meal and snack. The meal plan also includes appropriate fat and protein modifications and emphasizes consistent timing of meals and snacks. A typical day's meals and snacks provide 1500 to 2000 calories with 45% to 65% of the calories from carbohydrate, 10% to 35% from protein, and 20% to 35% from fat. If a patient's nutritional needs are more or less than provided by these meal plans, individualized adjustments may be required. Patients who often require adjustments include children, adolescents, metabolically stressed patients, pregnant women, and older adult patients.

- Weight loss is recommended for all adults who are overweight (BMI = 25 to 29.9 kg/m^2) or obese (BMI ≥30 kg/m^2) or who have or are at risk for developing type 2 diabetes. The primary approach for achieving weight loss is therapeutic lifestyle change, which includes a reduction in energy (food) intake and/or an increase in physical activity. A moderate decrease in caloric balance (500 to 1000 kcal/day) will result in slow but progressive weight loss (1 to 2 lb/wk). For most patients, weight loss diets should supply at least 1000 to 1200 kcal/day for women and 1200 to 1600 kcal/day for men.

- Additional goals for MNT include maintaining a blood glucose level in the normal range to reduce the risk of complications of diabetes, a normal lipid profile to reduce the risk for microvascular disease, and normal blood pressure levels to reduce the risk for vascular disease.

- The ADA no longer endorses any single meal plan or specified percentages of macronutrients as it has in the past. The Institute of Medicine and the ADA recommend, in general, that the diet be composed of 45% to 65% carbohydrates, 15% to 20% protein (0.8 to 1 g protein/kg of body weight), and no more than 30% fat. Monounsaturated and polyunsaturated fats should be the primary fat sources; saturated fats should be limited to no more than 10% of the diet and cholesterol intake to 300 mg or less daily. *Trans*-fatty acids should be avoided when possible. Including high-fiber foods (e.g., legumes, oats, barley) assists in lowering both blood glucose and blood cholesterol levels. Reduced sodium, alcohol, and caffeine consumption is also advisable (see also Chapter 46). The ADA has several cookbooks and pamphlets on nutrition available for the diabetic person.

- Patients with diabetes, as well as all individuals, need to be encouraged to consume an adequate intake of vitamins and minerals from natural food sources.

- Inclusion of sucrose is now permitted in limited amounts in the diabetic diet; however, the amount eaten must be calculated as part of the carbohydrate intake for the day. Meal plans such as "no concentrated sweets," "no added sugar," "low sugar," and "liberal diabetic diets" are no longer appropriate. These diets do not reflect the diabetes nutrition recommendations and unnecessarily restrict sucrose. Such meal plans may perpetuate the false notion that simply restricting sucrose-sweetened foods will improve blood glucose control.

- The U.S. Food and Drug Administration (FDA) has approved the use of four artificial sweeteners as sugar substitutes: saccharin, aspartame (NutraSweet), sucralose (Splenda), and acesulfame potassium.

- Patients with diabetes should adhere to the same guidelines for ingestion of alcohol as for all Americans—no more than two drinks daily for men and one drink daily for women. People with good control of their diabetes may ingest alcohol in moderation. However, drinking can result in hypoglycemia or hyperglycemia in diabetics. The effects of alcohol are influenced by the amount ingested, if ingested on an empty stomach, or if used chronically or excessively. Many alcoholic beverages are high in sugar and should be used with caution; light beer or dry wines are alternatives. One drink is defined as 12 ounces of beer, 5 ounces of wine, or 1.5 ounces of distilled spirits, each of which contains 15 grams of alcohol. Because alcohol affects the blood sugar, it may be prudent to test the blood glucose level before and after drinking to identify how the alcohol reacts in a particular patient. Abstinence is recommended for pregnant patients, those with known medical problems aggravated by its use, and those with a history of alcohol abuse.

- Dietary considerations for children and adolescents with type 1 or 2 diabetes are similar to the needs for all other children. They need to maintain a steady intake of a balanced diet aimed at maintaining normal growth and development. It is important to obtain height and weight values and to compare these to the normal growth curve found on charts to ascertain whether the dietary intake is adequate, deficient, or excessive. The individual's meal planning must be done in such a way as to accommodate irregular meal times and schedules and the varying activity levels of the child or adolescent.

- All women have similar nutritional needs during pregnancy and lactation whether they have diabetes or not. A woman with gestational diabetes is given education on food choices that are appropriate for normal weight gain, normoglycemia, and absence of ketones. Some with gestational diabetes may require a modest restriction in carbohydrates.

- In older adults, a change in body weight of more than 10 pounds or 10% of the body weight in less than 6 months is considered sufficient reason to investigate for nutrition-related causes. In general, older people with diabetes in long-term care settings tend to be underweight rather than overweight. Administering a daily vitamin supplement to older adults, especially those with decreased energy intake, may be advisable. Specialized diets do not appear to be beneficial to the older adult in a long-term care setting, where food choices are decidedly limited. It is preferable to make medication adjustments to control blood glucose rather than implement food restrictions in the long-term care setting. Physical activity should be encouraged.

Activity and Exercise

- Maintenance of a normal lifestyle is to be encouraged. This includes exercise and activities enjoyed by the individual. The normal daily energy level is used in determining the dietary and medication requirements for the patient. The ADA recommends that initial therapy be modest, based on the patient's willingness and ability, gradually increasing the duration and frequency to 30 to 45 minutes of moderate aerobic activity 3 to 5 days per week (150 minutes per week), when possible. Greater activity levels of at least 1 hour daily of moderate (walking) or 30 minutes daily of vigorous (jogging) activity may be needed to achieve successful long-term weight loss.

- As with all individuals who are about to undertake exercise, a proper period of warm-up and cool-down consisting of 5 to 10 minutes of aerobic activity at a low intensity should be done. It is very important to maintain proper foot care in a diabetic patient who is to start exercising. Use silica gel or air midsoles, as well as polyester or cotton blend socks to prevent blisters, and keep the feet as dry as possible. Visible inspection of the feet surfaces before and after exercise is an important component of an exercise regimen and is especially important for diabetic patients who already have peripheral neuropathy. Persons with loss of protective sensation should not use step exercises, jogging, prolonged walking, or treadmills as an exercise regimen. Rather, they should substitute swimming, bicycling, rowing, chair exercises, arm exercises, or other non–weight-bearing exercises.

- Just as it is important for the patient to maintain a certain diet, it is equally important to maintain a certain activity level. Patients who suddenly increase or decrease their activity level are susceptible to developing episodes of hyperglycemia or hypoglycemia. Both dietary and medication prescriptions may require adjustment if patients do not plan to resume the previous exercise level. Patients should consult with the prescriber before initiating an exercise program.

- Additional self-monitoring of the blood glucose level may be advisable before, during, and approximately 30 minutes after exercise to provide the prescriber with data to analyze regarding the effects of exercise on the individual's blood glucose level. The ADA recommends that the diabetic not exercise if his or her glucose level is above 250 mg/dL. Conversely, exercising with hypoglycemia is not advisable. A snack high in carbohydrates (10 to 20 g) should be taken before exercising if the blood sugar is less than 100 mg/dL.

- Exercise helps the cells use glucose; therefore exercise lowers the glucose level.

- Drink sufficient fluids without caffeine when exercising to prevent dehydration.

- Stop exercising if feeling weak, sick, dizzy, or if experiencing any type of pain.

Medication

- Insulin or oral antidiabetic agent therapy may be required to control diabetes mellitus. No changes in therapy should be made without medical supervision.

- A variety of combinations of insulin or insulin and oral antidiabetic agents may be used to provide control of the blood glucose level. The goal of therapy is to consistently maintain the blood glucose level within normal range. Administration schedules have evolved over the years to accomplish this goal. The schedules commonly used are as follows:
  1. Divided doses of intermediate-acting insulin (two thirds in the morning, one third in the evening before dinner)
  2. A combination of rapid- or short-acting and intermediate-acting insulin in the morning, followed by rapid- or short-acting insulin at dinner and intermediate-acting insulin before bedtime
  3. Rapid- or short-acting insulin before each meal and intermediate-acting or long-acting insulin at bedtime
  4. Rapid-acting or short-acting and long-acting insulin before breakfast, rapid-acting or short-acting insulin before lunch, and rapid-acting or short-acting and long-acting insulin again before dinner
  5. Continuous infusion of rapid- or short-acting insulin using a small, portable insulin infusion pump

- The regimen chosen depends on each person's response to medications, schedule of daily activities, and compliance with blood glucose monitoring, insulin injections, and diet.

- Medication preparation, dosage, frequency, storage, and refilling should be discussed and taught in detail. See Figure 10-3 for administration of subcutaneous injections and Figure 9-26 for mixing of insulins. Also, discuss proper disposal of used syringes and needles in the home setting.

- Be certain that the patient understands how to refill prescriptions for insulin or oral antidiabetic agents. When purchasing insulin, ask the patient to double-check the type, concentration (usually U-100), and expiration date. Insulin types should not be changed without the approval of the prescribing healthcare provider. The insulin should be stored in the refrigerator (not the freezer) before use. Once it is opened and being used, it can be stored at room temperature for up to 1 month. The patient or nurse should date the bottle when first opened and used. The patient should always have a spare bottle of each type of insulin prescribed available for use.

- When a patient is experiencing an acute illness, injury, or surgery, hyperglycemia may result. When ill, the patient should continue with the regular diet plan and increase noncaloric fluids such as broth, water, and other decaffeinated drinks. The patient should continue to take the oral agents and/or insulin as prescribed and monitor the blood glucose level at least every 4 hours. If the glucose level is higher than 240 mg/dL, urine should be tested for ketones (see "Urine Testing for Ketones" on p. 547). If the patient is unable to eat the normal caloric intake, he or she should continue to take the same dose of oral agents and/or insulin prescribed, but supplement food intake with carbohydrate-containing fluids such as soups, regular juices, and decaffeinated soft drinks. The healthcare provider should be notified immediately if the patient is unable to "keep anything down." Patients should understand that medication for diabetes, including insulin, should not be withheld during times of illness because counterregulatory mechanisms in the body often increase the blood glucose level dramatically. Food intake is also necessary because the body requires extra energy to deal with the stress of illness. Extra insulin may also be necessary to meet the demand of illness.

- If pregnancy is suspected, consult an obstetrician as soon as possible about continuing and adjusting medication therapy during pregnancy.

- Patients with diabetes should receive an annual influenza vaccination and at least one lifetime pneumococcal vaccination before the age of 65. The vaccination should be repeated at least 5 years later and after the patient turns 65 years of age.

Hypoglycemia. Hypoglycemia, or low blood sugar, can occur from too much insulin, a sulfonylurea, insufficient food intake to cover the insulin given, imbalances caused by vomiting and diarrhea, and excessive exercise without additional carbohydrate intake.

Symptoms. Recognize and assess early symptoms of hypoglycemia; these include nervousness, tremors, headache, apprehension, sweating, cold and clammy skin, and hunger. If uncorrected, hypoglycemia progresses to blurring of vision, lack of coordination, incoherence, coma, and death. Children younger than 6 to 7 years may not have the cognitive abilities to recognize and initiate self-treatment of hypoglycemia.

Treatment. If the patient is conscious and able to swallow, give 2 to 4 ounces of fruit juice, 1 cup of skim milk, or 4 ounces of a nondiet soft drink, or give a piece of candy such as a gumdrop. An alternative is to carry a glucose-containing product (e.g., Glutose gel, Dex4 Glucose tablets) and take as recommended when hypoglycemic. Repeat in 10 to 15 minutes if relief of symptoms is not evident. Do not use hard candy if there is a danger of aspiration. If the patient is unconscious, having a seizure, or unable to swallow, administer glucagon or 20 to 50 mL of glucose 50% IV. (People taking insulin should have a family member, significant other, or coworker who is able to administer glucagon.) Obtain a blood glucose level at the time of hypoglycemia, if possible.

Hyperglycemia. Hyperglycemia (elevated blood sugar) occurs when the glucose available in the body cannot be transported into the cells for use because of a lack of insulin necessary for the transport mechanism. Hyperglycemia can be caused by nonadherence, overeating, acute illness, or acute infection.

Symptoms. Symptoms of hyperglycemia are headache, nausea and vomiting, abdominal pain, dizziness, rapid pulse, rapid shallow respirations, and a fruity odor to the breath from acetone. If untreated, hyperglycemia may also cause coma and death. Glucose levels higher than 240 mg/dL and ketones present in the urine are early indications of diabetic ketoacidosis.

Treatment. Treatment of hyperglycemia often requires hospitalization with close monitoring of hydration status; administration of IV fluids and insulin; and blood glucose, urine ketone, and potassium levels. Hyperglycemia usually occurs because of another cause; therefore the problem, often an infection, must also be identified and treated.

Prevention. The risk of hyperglycemia can be minimized by taking the prescribed dose of insulin or oral antidiabetic agent; adhering to the prescribed diet and exercise; reporting fevers, infection, or prolonged vomiting or diarrhea to the healthcare provider; and maintaining an accurate written record for the healthcare provider to analyze to determine the individual patient's needs. Self-monitoring of blood glucose results and evaluation of urine ketones can provide the prescriber with valuable information to manage the treatment of the individual effectively.

Self-Monitoring of Blood Glucose

- Home blood glucose monitoring (self-monitoring) is an accepted practice for managing diabetes mellitus. It is used to evaluate the degree of control of the blood glucose. It can also be used to evaluate when additional insulin must be taken or to determine the effect of exercise on insulin needs.

- Educate the individual using the equipment for self-monitoring that will be used at home. Teach the person all details of the operation, including calibration, care, handling, and cleansing of the glucose monitor.

- The best time to check blood glucose levels is just before meals, 1 to 2 hours after meals, before bed, and between 2 and 3 AM. The prescriber will give specific instructions regarding how often and when glucose testing should be done. When the person is ill, it is important to increase the frequency of glucose monitoring.

- A small sample of capillary blood is obtained, generally using an automatic finger-sticking lancet. The blood sample is applied to a reagent strip, which is then placed into an electronic device that reads the amount of color change and converts this into a numeric value representing the blood glucose level. There also are meters and sensors that do not use reagent strips for delivering the glucose results. "Talking" glucometers are on the market for those who are visually impaired. Written records of the blood glucose results should be maintained and taken to all follow-up visits with the healthcare provider for analysis.

Urine Testing for Ketones

- Teach the patient to perform urine testing for ketones at least four times daily during times of stress, infection, or when signs or symptoms of hyperglycemia are suspected or present. (Ketone testing should be done when the blood glucose level is consistently higher than 300 mg/dL, during pregnancy, or when symptoms of ketoacidosis, such as nausea, vomiting, or abdominal pain, are present.) The healthcare provider may suggest additional times when ketones should be monitored, depending on the type of regimen prescribed for controlling blood glucose. An accurate written record of the results should be maintained. Guidelines for reporting abnormal results to the prescriber should be discussed at the time of discharge. First morning urine tests from pregnant women and up to 30% of first morning specimens in individuals who are fasting may have positive readings. Several drugs also may interfere with the results of ketone urine testing, giving false-positive values. Blood ketone testing methods that quantify beta-hydroxybutyric acid are available for home testing and are preferred over urine ketone testing for monitoring and diagnosing ketoacidosis.
- Suggest that ketone testing be initiated when an illness occurs and the serum glucose is elevated above the individual's usual range. Explain when to call the healthcare provider. Suggest increasing fluid intake whenever ketones are positive.

Other Laboratory Glucose Testing

- The A1$_C$ test measures the percentage of hemoglobin that has been irreversibly glycosylated because of high blood sugar levels. This provides a reflection of the average blood sugar level attained over the past 2 to 3 months. This test is used in conjunction with home self-glucose monitoring to assess overall glycemic control.
- The fructosamine test measures the amount of glucose bonded to a protein, fructosamine. This reflects the average blood level attained over the past 1 to 3 weeks.

Complications Associated With Diabetes Mellitus

Cardiovascular disease. Men and women with diabetes are at an increased risk of dying from complications of cardiovascular disease. Aspirin therapy is a primary prevention strategy for both diabetic men and women with type 1 or type 2 diabetes who have a 10-year cardiovascular risk >10%. This includes most men aged >50 years or women >60 years who have at least one additional major risk factor (family history of cardiovascular disease, hypertension, smoking, dyslipidemia or albuminuria). Enteric-coated aspirin in doses of 75 to 162 mg daily is taken by individuals who do *not* have an aspirin sensitivity. Aspirin therapy is no longer recommended for those who do not meet the criteria.

Peripheral vascular disease. The person with diabetes mellitus is more likely to suffer from peripheral vascular disease than the general population. Reduced blood supply to the extremities may result in intermittent claudication, numbness and tingling, and a greater likelihood of foot infection. The following are symptoms the patient should look for in caring for the extremities:

- *Color:* Observe the color of each hand, finger, leg, and foot; report cyanosis or reddish-blue discolorations. Inspect the skin of the extremities for any signs of ulceration.
- *Temperature:* Feel the temperature in each hand, finger, leg, and foot. Report paleness and coldness. Note that these symptoms will be increased if the limbs are elevated above the level of the heart.
- *Edema:* Report edema, its extent, and whether relieved or unchanged when in a dependent position.
- *Limb pain:* Pain with exercise that is relieved by rest may be from claudication and should be reported to the healthcare provider.
- *Care:* Prevent ulcers, injury, and infection in the lower extremities with meticulous regular care. Use lotion to prevent dryness. Inspect the feet daily for any signs of skin breakdown or loss of sensation; report to the healthcare provider and do not attempt to self-treat. The presence of redness, warmth, or calluses may signal an impending breakdown. Always cut toenails straight across and seek foot care from a podiatrist if problems are noted.

Visual alterations. Visual changes are common in the patient with diabetes mellitus. These patients frequently suffer from blurred vision associated with an elevated blood sugar. Any diabetic person with intermittently blurred vision should contact the healthcare provider for a check of the blood sugar level. Once the hyperglycemia is controlled, the blurred vision usually resolves.

Blindness. In advanced stages of diabetes mellitus, the patient may suffer from changes (microangiopathies) in the small blood vessels of the eyes. Retinal hemorrhages, degeneration of retinal vascular tissue, cataracts, and eventual blindness may occur. The patient with diabetes should have regular eye examinations to allow early treatment of any apparent alterations.

Renal disease. People with diabetes mellitus are more susceptible to urinary tract infections; therefore symptoms such as burning on urination or low back pain should be evaluated promptly. Patients are also more susceptible to renal disease. Routine periodic monitoring of protein in the urine determines the presence of renal disease. In patients with type 1 or 2 diabetes who have microalbuminuria, even a small reduction in protein intake has been shown to improve the glomerular filtration rate and reduce urinary albumin excretion rates.

Infection. Any type of infection can cause a significant loss of control of diabetes mellitus. Patients should check themselves carefully for any signs of redness, tenderness, swelling, or drainage that may occur when there is any break in the skin. Patients should be taught to report immediately early signs of infection, such as fever or sore throat. During an infection, the dosage of insulin may require an adjustment to compensate for a change in metabolic rate, diet, and exercise. Contact the healthcare provider for specific directions.

Neuropathies. Explain to appropriate individuals the complication of degeneration of nerves when it exists. Ask the patient to describe sensations (e.g., numbness, tingling) in the extremities. Inspect the feet for blisters, ulcerations, ingrown toenails, or sores. Occasionally, the patient will not be aware of these lesions because of the degeneration of nerves in the area. When numbness and lack of sensation are present, always test the water temperature before immersing a limb. Because of impaired sensation, it is easy to burn the skin, and the patient may be unaware of the burn until later.

Impotence. Impotence may occur from a number of causes and should be discussed on an individual basis with the healthcare provider.

Hypertension. All patients with diabetes should have a blood pressure measurement, including orthostatic measurements, completed on every routine office visit. The ADA (2015) has developed a new set of guidelines for treatment of hypertension to work in conjunction with the American Heart Association goals for hypertension. The goal blood pressure with antihypertensive therapy in patients with diabetes is a range of 130 to 140/80 to 90 mm Hg.

Fostering Health Maintenance
- Throughout the course of treatment, discuss medication, diet, exercise, and the need to achieve and maintain good glucose control to prevent the complications associated with diabetes mellitus. The patient must achieve a high degree of understanding of diabetes mellitus and its management. The patient and family members must be included in the entire educational program.

- With shorter hospitalizations, it may be necessary to incorporate follow-up care by a health professional from a visiting nurses association or a home health agency in the discharge planning.
- Seek cooperation and understanding of the following points so that medication compliance is increased: name of medication, dosage, route and time of administration, common and serious adverse effects.

At Discharge. Develop a list of specific equipment and supplies that the patient will need when discharged. Keep in mind the cost of these supplies. Consider the following:
1. *Syringes:* Disposable syringes are convenient and presterilized but are more expensive. Be sure to tell the patient that disposable syringes are designed to be used once and then discarded. However, recent literature refers to the repeated use of the same syringe by an individual patient as long as the needle remains sharp and is kept clean and covered. *Check with the individual prescriber before instituting this practice.* Diabetics are susceptible to infection, and healing may be a problem. The newer, smaller 30- and 31-gauge needles can become bent with even one use, forming a hook at the end of the needle. If the needle is reused, the hook may result in a laceration to the tissue and lead to adverse effects. Syringes being reused should be stored at room temperature. The potential benefits of storing a syringe and needle for reuse in the refrigerator or of wiping the needle with alcohol are unknown. Cleansing the needle with alcohol may disrupt the silicone coating on the needle, resulting in increased pain at the injection site. Syringes are available in 0.3-, 0.5-, 1-, and 2-mL capacities. In some cases, the insulin pen may also be prescribed for use by appropriate individuals. Several medical devices have been developed to reduce the incidence of needlesticks and other sharp injuries. When performing patient education on the self-administration of insulin, it is important to use the type of syringe and needle device that will be used at home to ensure that the patient knows how to manipulate the device correctly. Insulin can also be administered using a jet injector for those with a phobia of needles or unable to use a syringe. They are not a routine option for use in all patients with diabetes.
2. *Insulin pumps:* An insulin pump uses regular insulin or the rapid-acting insulin analogues such as lispro, aspart, or glulisine. The use of mixtures of insulins in insulin pumps is not recommended because this approach has not been evaluated.
3. *Needles:* Disposable needles are more convenient but also more expensive. Patients usually use a 27-, 28-, 29-, 30-, or 31-gauge ½- or ⅝-inch needle, but needles should be adjusted to the individual. An obese patient may require a 1- to 1½-inch-long needle to inject the insulin properly. Several lengths

of needles are available, and blood glucose should be monitored when changing from one needle length to another. Always dispose of insulin syringes, needles, and lancets in sharps containers. (See Chapter 9 for further discussion of syringes, needles, and safety during use.)

4. *Specialized equipment:* Magni-Guides are available for the visually impaired patient. This holds the vial of insulin, acts as a guide in withdrawing insulin, and has a magnifying glass to make reading the syringe scale easier. Insulin pens are available for blind or neurologically impaired patients. A talking glucose-measuring device is also available for the visually impaired individual to perform self-monitoring of capillary blood glucose levels. Persons with diabetes desiring more information on insulin delivery aids can contact the ADA.

5. *Self-monitoring equipment for blood glucose:* Be certain that the individual has or understands where to purchase the supplies used with the specific brand of self-monitoring glucose machine to be used at home. Because a number of models of self-monitoring equipment are available, it is important that the individual be trained on the specific equipment that will be used at home.

Patient Self-Assessment. Enlist the patient's aid in developing and maintaining a written record of monitoring parameters (e.g., blood glucose, insulin dosage, pertinent stress factors, exercise level, illnesses, or major changes in diet or other routine). (See the Patient Self-Assessment Form for Antidiabetic Agents on the Ⓔ Evolve website.) Complete the Premedication Data column for use as a baseline to track response to drug therapy. Ensure that the patient understands how to use the form, and instruct the patient to bring the completed form to follow-up visits. During follow-up visits, focus on issues that will foster adherence with the therapeutic interventions prescribed.

Life Span Considerations
Children With Diabetes Mellitus

For children who have diabetes, it is essential that the appropriate faculty of the school, whether a day care, preschool, or regular school environment, be familiar with the child's health needs. Figure 35-3 is a diabetic healthcare plan for use in school and day care.

Life Span Considerations
Insulin

Almost all patients receiving insulin will experience a hypoglycemic reaction at some point. Symptoms of hypoglycemic reaction vary from patient to patient. Be aware that confusion and lethargy are signs of hypoglycemia but may sometimes be overlooked in older adult patients because slowness and confusion can be interpreted as signs of aging.

DRUG CLASS: INSULINS
ACTIONS

Insulin is a hormone produced in the beta cells of the pancreas, which is a key regulator of metabolism. Insulin is required for the entry of glucose into skeletal and heart muscle and fat. It also plays a significant role in protein and lipid metabolism. It is not required for glucose transport into the brain, kidney, gastrointestinal, or liver tissue.

The pancreas secretes insulin at a steady rate of 0.5 to 1 unit/hr. It is released in greater quantities when the blood glucose level rises above 100 mg/dL such as after a meal. The average rate of insulin secretion in an adult is 30 to 50 units daily.

Insulin deficiency reduces the rate of transport of glucose into cells, producing hyperglycemia. Other metabolic reactions also are inhibited by the lack of insulin and intracellular glucose, resulting in the conversion of protein to glucose (gluconeogenesis), hyperlipidemia, ketosis, and acidosis).

Insulins from the pancreases of different animals have similar activity and were used in human beings for many years. Biosynthetic human insulin is now used by most patients, especially people newly diagnosed with diabetes. It has fewer allergic reactions associated with it than animal-origin insulins.

USES

Three factors—onset, peak, and duration—are important in the use of insulin therapy. *Onset* is the time required for the medication to have an initial effect or action, *peak* is when the insulin will have the maximum effect, and *duration* is how long the agent remains active in the body. When monitoring insulin therapy, it is important to understand these terms and to associate them with the type of insulin being administered to ascertain when a patient is most susceptible to hyperglycemia or hypoglycemia.

Four types of insulin, based on onset, peak, and duration are in use today: rapid-acting, short-acting, intermediate-acting, and long-acting insulins (Table 35-5). The most rapid-acting insulins are the insulin analogues, newer synthetic forms called lispro, aspart, and glulisine. They are clear solutions that may be injected separately or mixed in the same syringe with an intermediate-acting insulin. Aspart and lispro are as potent as human regular insulin, but have a more rapid onset and shorter duration of activity. Glulisine has a similar onset of action to lispro and aspart, but has a shorter duration of action. Their rapid onset of action is related to a more rapid absorption rate from subcutaneous tissue than is the case with regular insulin. Aspart appears to have a slightly more rapid onset than lispro. Aspart, lispro, and glulisine are usually administered within 10 to 15 minutes of a meal. The rationale for the development and use of these newer insulins is that when a meal is ingested, the

Diabetes Care Plan for _____(name of student)_____ School _____ Effective Dates: _____

To be completed by parents/health care team and reviewed with necessary school staff. Copies should be kept in student's classrooms and school records.

Date of Birth: _____ **Grade:** _____ **Homeroom Teacher:** _____

Contact information:
Parent/guardian #1: _____ Address: _____
  Telephone - Home: _____ Work: _____ Cell Phone: _____
Parent/guardian #2: _____ Address: _____
  Telephone - Home: _____ Work: _____ Cell Phone: _____
Student's Doctor/Health Care Provider: _____ Telephone: _____
  Nurse Educator: _____ Telephone: _____
Other emergency contact: _____ Relationship: _____
  Telephone - Home: _____ Work: _____ Cell Phone: _____
Notify parent/guardian in the following situations: _____

Blood Glucose Monitoring
Target range for blood glucose: _____ mg/dL to _____ mg/dL   Type of blood glucose meter student uses: _____
Usual times to test blood glucose: _____
Times to do extra tests (check all that apply):
  _____ Before exercise   _____ When student exhibits symptoms of hyperglycemia
  _____ After exercise   _____ When student exhibits symptoms of hypoglycemia
  _____ Other (explain): _____
Can student perform own blood glucose tests?   Yes   No   Exceptions: _____
School personnel trained to monitor blood glucose level and dates of training: _____

Insulin
Times, types, and dosages of insulin injections to be given during school:
Time   Type(s)   Dosage
_____   _____   _____
_____   _____   _____
_____   _____   _____
School personnel trained to assist with insulin injection and dates of training: _____

Can student give own injections?   Yes   No
Can student determine correct amount of insulin?   Yes   No
Can student draw correct dose of insulin?   Yes   No

For Students with Insulin Pumps:
Type of pump: _____
Insulin/carbohydrate ratio: _____
Correction factor: _____

Is student competent regarding pump?   Yes   No
Can student effectively troubleshoot problems   Yes   No
(e.g., ketosis, pump malfunction)?
Comments: _____
_____
_____

Meals and Snacks Eaten at School (The carbohydrate content of the food is important in maintaining a stable blood glucose level.)
        Time   Food content/amount
Breakfast _____   _____
AM snack   _____   _____
Lunch   _____   _____
PM snack   _____   _____
Dinner   _____   _____
Snack before exercise?
  Yes   No   _____
Snack after exercise?
  Yes   No

Other times to give snacks (content/amount): _____
_____
A source of glucose such as _____
should be readily available at all times.
Preferred snack foods: _____
Foods to avoid, if any: _____
Instructions for when food is provided to the class, (e.g., as part of a class party or food sampling): _____

Hypoglycemia (Low Blood Sugar)
Usual symptoms of hypoglycemia: _____
_____
Treatment of hypoglycemia: _____
_____
School personnel trained to administer glucagon and dates of training: _____
_____
Glucagon should be given if the student is unconscious, having a seizure (convulsion), or unable to swallow. If required, glucagon should be administered promptly and then 911 (or other emergency assistance) and parents should be called.

Hyperglycemia (High Blood Sugar)
Usual symptoms of hyperglycemia: _____
_____
Treatment of hyperglycemia: _____
_____
Circumstances when urine or blood ketones should be tested: _____
_____
Treatment for ketones: _____
_____

Exercise and Sports
A snack such as _____ should be readily available at the site of exercise or sports.
Restrictions on activity, if any: _____
Student should not exercise if blood glucose is below _____ mg/dL.

Supplies and Personnel
Location of supplies: Blood glucose monitoring equipment: _____ Insulin administration supplies: _____
            Glucagon emergency kit: _____ Ketone testing supplies: _____
            Snack foods: _____
Personnel trained in the symptoms and treatment of low and high blood sugar and dates of training: _____
_____

Signatures
Reviewed by: _[student's health provider/date]_   Acknowledged/received by: _[guardian/date]_   Acknowledged/received by: _[school representative/date]_

FIGURE 35-3 Diabetes health care plan. (From American Diabetes Association: Care of children with diabetes in the school and day care setting, *Diabetes Care* 26(Suppl 1):s131-s135, 2003.)

Table 35-5 Commercially Available Forms of Insulin

TYPE OF INSULIN	MANUFACTURER	STRENGTH (Units/mL)	SOURCE	ONSET (hr)	PEAK (hr)	DURATION* (hr)	HYPERGLYCEMIA†	HYPOGLYCEMIA†
Rapid-Acting Insulin								
Insulin Analogue Injection								
NovoLog (aspart)	Novo Nordisk	100	Semisynthetic	0.2-0.33	1-3	3-5	After lunch (3)	Within 1-3 hr
Humalog (lispro)	Lilly	100	Semisynthetic	0.2-0.33	0.5-2.5	3-6.5	After lunch (3)	Within 1-3 hr
Apidra (glulisine)	Sanofi-Aventis	100	Semisynthetic	0.2-0.33	0.5-1.5	4-5	After lunch (3)	Within 1-3 hr
Short-Acting Insulin								
Insulin Injection								
Humulin R (human)	Lilly	100, 500	Semisynthetic	0.5-1	2.5-5	5-10	Early AM (1)	Before lunch (3)
Novolin R (human)	Novo Nordisk	100	Semisynthetic	0.5-1	2.5-5	8	Early AM	Before lunch
Intermediate-Acting Insulin								
Isophane Insulin Suspension (NPH)								
Humulin N (human)	Lilly	100	Semisynthetic	1-2	4-12	16-28	Before lunch (2)	3 PM to supper (3)
Novolin N (human)	Novo Nordisk	100	Semisynthetic	1-2	4-12	24	Before lunch	3 PM to supper
Isophane Insulin Suspension (NPH) and Insulin Injection (Regular)								
Humulin 50/50 (human) (50% NPH/50% regular)	Lilly	100	Semisynthetic	0.5-1	4-8	24	Before lunch	3 PM to supper
Humulin 70/30 (human) (70% NPH/30% regular)	Lilly	100	Semisynthetic	0.5-1	4-12	24	Before lunch	3 PM to supper
Novolin 70/30 (human) (70% NPH/30% regular)	Novo Nordisk	100	Semisynthetic	0.5-1	2-12	24	Before lunch	3 PM to supper
Insulin Analogue Protamine Suspension and Insulin Analogue Injection								
Humalog Mix 75/25 (75% lispro protamine/25% lispro)	Lilly	100	Semisynthetic	0.25-0.5	0.5-1.5	18-24	—	3 PM to supper
NovoLog Mix 70/30 (70% aspart protamine/30% aspart)	Novo Nordisk	100	Semisynthetic	0.2-0.33	2.4	18-24	—	3 PM to supper
Long-Acting Insulin								
Lantus (glargine)	Sanofi-Aventis	100	Semisynthetic	1.1	—‡	24	Mid-AM to mid-PM (1)	—‡
Toujeo (glargine)	Sanofi-Aventis	300	Semisynthetic	1.1	—‡	24	Mid-AM to mid-PM	—‡
Levemir (detemir)	Novo Nordisk	100	Semisynthetic	1	—‡	Up to 24	Mid-AM to mid-PM (1)	—‡

NPH, neutral protamine Hagedorn.
*The times listed are averages based on a newly diagnosed diabetic patient. Factors modifying these times include patient variation, site and route of administration, and dosage.
†Most often occurs when insulin is administered (1) at bedtime the previous night, (2) before breakfast the previous day, (3) before breakfast the same day.
‡No pronounced peak activity.

blood glucose rises for about 2 to 3 hours. After injection, regular insulin takes 30 minutes to start acting, peaks at 2½ to 5 hours, and may have a duration of 5 to 10 hours. Lispro and aspart start to act within 10 minutes of injection, peak within 1 to 2 hours, and are gone by 3 to 5 hours. Glulisine has a similar onset of action, but peaks in 30 to 90 minutes with a duration of action up to 2½ hours. Consequently, the newer rapid-acting, shorter-duration insulins are used to control hyperglycemia associated with meals without having longer-lasting effects with the potential for hypoglycemia. These insulins may also be used without any other insulin in patients with type 2 diabetes who only have hyperglycemia associated with ingestion of meals (postprandial hyperglycemia). Aspart and glulisine may also be injected intravenously.

Regular insulin has long been used for its short onset of activity and relatively short duration of action. But, as noted in Table 35-5, regular insulin is slower in its onset and longer in duration than the rapid-acting insulins. Regular insulin is approved to be injected by both IV and subcutaneous routes of administration. Human regular insulin is usually administered 30 to 60 minutes before meals.

Neutral protamine Hagedorn (NPH) insulin is an intermediate-acting insulin containing specific amounts of regular insulin and protamine. The protamine binds to the insulin. When administered subcutaneously, the insulin is slowly released from the protamine and becomes active, giving it the intermediate-acting classification.

Lispro and aspart insulin may also be mixed with protamine to prolong their duration of action. Two products are available: 75% lispro protamine suspension and 25% lispro solution (Humalog Mix 75/25) and 70% aspart protamine suspension and 30% aspart solution (NovoLog Mix 70/30). The combined effect is a rapid-acting onset with an intermediate duration of action of 12 to 24 hours.

Insulin glargine and insulin detemir are biosynthetic long-acting insulins. They are absorbed from the subcutaneous tissue in a uniform manner without large fluctuations in insulin levels, reducing the possibility of hypoglycemic reactions. Most commonly injected in the evening, these products provide a 24-hour basal source of insulin for the body. Rapid-acting insulin is then injected just before meals to control hyperglycemia secondary to the meal, or intermediate-acting NPH can be injected in the morning and late afternoon to treat hyperglycemia from meals. Neither insulin glargine nor detemir should be mixed with other insulins.

Insulin degludec is an ultra–long-acting insulin with a duration of action of approximately 40 hours. It is also a more stable insulin that can remain at room temperature for 8 weeks. It will be marketed in 2016 as a single product (Tesiba) and a 70/30 combination mix with the rapid-acting analog insulin aspart (Ryzodeg).

STORAGE OF INSULIN

Insulin should not be allowed to freeze and should not be heated above a temperature of 98° F. A general rule of thumb is that the bottle of insulin should be stored in the refrigerator (not the freezer) until opened. Because patients find it uncomfortable to inject cold insulin, the bottle (and insulin cartridges for insulin pens) may then be kept at room temperature (68° to 75° F) until gone. For all insulins other than regular, lispro, aspart, or glulisine, the vial should be gently rolled in the palms of the hands (not shaken) to warm and resuspend the insulin. Once an insulin vial is opened, it should be discarded within 30 days. Even though the insulin has not deteriorated, there is concern that the contents are no longer sterile and the vial may become a reservoir for infection, especially with patients who reuse needles.

At sustained temperatures above room temperature, insulins lose potency rapidly. Do not leave in a hot car throughout the day.

Excess agitation should be avoided to prevent loss of potency, clumping, or precipitation. When insulins are prefilled in syringes, the syringes should be stored in a refrigerator for up to 30 days in a vertical position with the needle facing upward. Prior to use, the syringe should be taken out of the refrigerator, allowed to warm to room temperature, and then gently rolled between the hands to remix the insulin before administration.

THERAPEUTIC OUTCOMES

The primary therapeutic outcomes expected from insulin therapy are as follows:
1. A decrease in both fasting blood glucose levels and $A1_C$ concentrations in the range defined as acceptable for the individual patient
2. Fewer long-term complications associated with poorly controlled diabetes mellitus

❖ NURSING IMPLICATIONS FOR INSULIN

■ Premedication Assessment
1. Confirm that a blood glucose level was recently measured and was acceptable for the individual patient.
2. Confirm that the patient has had a level of activity reasonable for that patient and that the anticipated level of activity planned for the next several hours is balanced with the insulin dose.
3. Confirm that the prescribed diet is being consumed as planned and that no changes in diet are anticipated in relation to insulin dosage over the next several hours (e.g., with patients on nothing by mouth [NPO] status, consider holding medication).

■ Availability, Dosage and Administration
See Table 35-5, Figure 9-26, and Chapter 10 for information regarding availability and administration.

Table 35-6 Compatibility of Insulin Combinations

COMBINATION	RATIO	MIX BEFORE ADMINISTRATION
regular + NPH	Any combination	2 to 3 mo
aspart + NPH	Any combination	Immediately
lispro + NPH	Any combination	Immediately
glulisine + NPH	Any combination	Immediately
glargine	Do not mix with other insulin	
detemir	Do not mix with other insulin	

Maintenance therapy for newly diagnosed diabetic patients should incorporate the following information:

- Effective control of diabetes mellitus requires a balanced food intake, exercise, blood glucose levels measured several times daily, and insulin dosage adjustments based on the blood glucose levels.
- Several methods have been developed to initiate insulin therapy. The method chosen depends on such issues as fluctuation of the patient's blood glucose; ability of the patient to measure, mix, and administer the insulin; and adherence to planned exercise and diet.
- Before starting a standardized regimen, the diet and physical exercise level must be stabilized. A standard approach is to calculate the initial total daily dose of insulin based on 0.5 to 0.8 unit/kg of whole body (not lean body) weight. NPH (human) insulin is often used to initiate therapy. This total daily dosage is then split into two doses so that two thirds are administered in the morning before breakfast and one third is administered 30 minutes before the evening meal. The insulin dosage is then adjusted over the next several weeks based on blood glucose measurements taken (usually) four times daily and on A1$_C$ levels. Diet and exercise may also require adjustment.

Mixing Insulins. Many patients with diabetes mix rapid-acting insulin with intermediate-acting or long-acting insulin to manage the hyperglycemia that follows a meal or snack. See Table 35-6 and Chapter 9 for the technique to follow when mixing insulins. When regular insulin, insulin lispro, or insulin aspart is combined with another insulin in the same syringe, the rapid-acting insulin should be drawn into the syringe first to avoid contaminating the rapid-acting insulin vial with the longer-acting insulin, which may happen if the longer-acting insulin was drawn into the syringe first and then the needle was inserted into the rapid-acting insulin to draw it into the syringe.

■ Common and Serious Adverse Effects

Metabolic

Hyperglycemia. Diabetic or prediabetic patients must be monitored for the development of hyperglycemia, particularly during the early weeks of therapy. Assess regularly for abnormal blood glucose levels and, in certain patients as requested by the healthcare provider, for glycosuria and ketones. If symptoms occur frequently, the healthcare provider should be notified and the patient's written records of the results of self-testing should be supplied to the healthcare provider for analysis. Patients receiving insulin may require an adjustment in dosage.

Hypoglycemia. Insulin overdose or decreased carbohydrate intake may result in hypoglycemia. If untreated, irreversible brain damage may occur. Hypoglycemia occurs most frequently when the administered insulin reaches its peak action (see Table 35-5). Hypoglycemia must be treated immediately. The following conditions may predispose a patient with diabetes to a hypoglycemic (insulin) reaction: improper measurement of insulin dosage, excessive exercise, insufficient food intake, concurrent ingestion of hypoglycemic drugs, and discontinuation of drugs (see "Drug Interactions") that cause hyperglycemia. Monitor the patient for the following signs of hypoglycemia: headache, nausea, weakness, hunger, lethargy, decreased coordination, general apprehension, sweating, or blurred or double vision.

Hypersensitivity, Immune System

Allergic reactions. Allergic reactions, manifested by itching, redness, and swelling at the site of injection, are common in patients receiving insulin therapy. These reactions may be caused by modifying proteins in NPH insulin, the insulin itself, the alcohol used to cleanse the injection site, the patient's injection technique, or the intermittent use of insulin.

Spontaneous desensitization frequently occurs within a few weeks. Local irritation may be reduced by changing to insulins derived from biosynthetic sources (e.g., "human" insulin), by using unscented alcohol swabs and disposable syringes and needles, and by checking the patient's injection technique. Acute rashes covering the whole body and anaphylactic symptoms are rare, but if they occur, they must be treated with antihistamines, epinephrine, and steroids.

Lipodystrophies. Rotation of injection sites is important to avoid atrophy or hypertrophy of subcutaneous fat tissue. This dermatologic condition may occur at the site of frequent insulin injections. The hypertrophic areas tend to be used more frequently by diabetic patients because the fat pad becomes anesthetized. In addition to the adverse cosmetic effects, the absorption rate of insulin from these sites becomes significantly prolonged and erratic. Loss of diabetic control may result, particularly in patients with unstable type 1 diabetes.

■ Drug Interactions

Hyperglycemia. The following medications may produce hyperglycemia, especially in prediabetic and diabetic patients (insulin dosages may require adjustment): albuterol, asparaginase, calcitonin, clozapine, olanzapine, corticosteroids, cyclophosphamide, diazoxide, diltiazem, diuretics (e.g., thiazides, furosemide, bumetanide), dobutamine, epinephrine, glucagon, isoniazid, lithium, morphine, niacin, nicotine, oral contraceptives, pentamidine, phenothiazines, phenytoin, protease inhibitors, terbutaline, somatropin, and thyroid hormones.

Diabetic or prediabetic patients must be monitored for the development of hyperglycemia, particularly during the early weeks of therapy. Assess the patient regularly for elevated blood glucose level or glycosuria and report if it occurs with any frequency.

Hypoglycemia. The following drugs may cause hypoglycemia, thereby decreasing insulin requirements, in diabetic patients: anabolic steroids, angiotensin-converting enzyme (ACE) inhibitors, alcohol, nonselective beta-adrenergic blocking agents, calcium, clonidine, disopyramide, fluoxetine, ethanol, fenfluramine, fibrates, lithium, insulin, monoamine oxidase inhibitors (MAOIs), pentamidine, pentoxifylline, pyridoxine, salicylates, sulfonamides, and sulfonylureas. Monitor for the following signs of hypoglycemia: headache, nausea, weakness, hunger, lethargy, decreased coordination, general apprehension, sweating, or blurred or double vision. Notify the healthcare provider if any of these symptoms appear.

Beta-Adrenergic Blocking Agents. Beta blockers (e.g., propranolol, nadolol, metoprolol) may mask many of the symptoms of hypoglycemia. Notify the healthcare provider if you suspect that any of these symptoms appear intermittently.

DRUG CLASS: BIGUANIDE ORAL ANTIDIABETIC AGENT

metformin (mĕt-FŎR-mĭn)
Glucophage (GLŪ-kō-fāj)
⇄ *Do not confuse metformin with metronidazole.*

ACTIONS

Metformin represents a class of oral antihyperglycemic agents known as the biguanides. It decreases hepatic glucose production by inhibiting glycogenolysis and gluconeogenesis, reduces absorption of glucose from the small intestine, and increases insulin sensitivity, improving glucose uptake in peripheral muscle and adipose cells. Metformin may also stimulate glucose metabolism by anaerobic glycolysis. The net result is a significant decrease in fasting and postprandial blood glucose and A1c concentrations. Insulin must be present for metformin to be active and therefore is not effective in type 1 diabetes.

USES

Metformin is used as an adjunct to the diet to lower blood glucose levels in patients with type 2 diabetes mellitus whose hyperglycemia cannot be controlled by diet and exercise alone. It has the particular advantage that it will not cause hypoglycemia, as can occur with insulin and the sulfonylureas. It may also be used in combination with other oral antidiabetic agents to lower blood glucose because the agents act by different mechanisms.

Metformin has two other beneficial effects: it does not cause weight gain, and actually may cause weight loss, contrary to the actions of the sulfonylureas, meglitinides, and insulin; and it also has a favorable effect on triglycerides. It produces a modest decrease in concentrations of serum triglycerides and total and LDL cholesterol, with modest increases in concentrations of HDL cholesterol. See the cautionary note in "Dosage and Administration" regarding renal function, heart failure, and liver impairment.

THERAPEUTIC OUTCOMES

The primary therapeutic outcomes expected from biguanide oral antidiabetic agent therapy are as follows:
1. A decrease in fasting blood glucose and A1c concentrations in the range defined as "acceptable" for the individual patient
2. Fewer long-term complications associated with poorly controlled type 2 diabetes mellitus

❖ NURSING IMPLICATIONS FOR METFORMIN

▪ Premedication Assessment
1. Confirm that blood glucose and A1c levels were recently measured and were acceptable for the individual patient.
2. Confirm that the prescribed diet is being consumed as planned and that no changes in diet are anticipated in relation to oral hypoglycemic agent dosage over the next several hours (e.g., in patients on NPO status, consider holding medication).

▪ Availability
PO: Tablets: 500, 850, 1000 mg; tablets, extended release (24 hr): 500, 750, 1000 mg; oral solution 500 mg/5 mL.

▪ Dosage and Administration
Adult: PO: Initially, 500 mg twice daily with the morning and evening meals. Dosage is increased by adding 500 mg to the daily dosage each week, up to 2500 mg daily. In general, most patients require at least 1500 mg daily for therapeutic effect. At dosages of 2000 mg and more, metformin should be administered three times daily (e.g., 1000 mg with breakfast, 500 mg with lunch, and 1000 mg with dinner, or 850 mg each with breakfast, lunch, and dinner). If a patient's blood glucose level is not controlled with the maximum dosage, a sulfonylurea or a TZD oral hypoglycemic agent may be added to the regimen.

Medication Safety Alert

Lactic acidosis is a rare but potentially life-threatening complication that can occur during treatment with metformin. It is recommended that metformin therapy *not* be initiated in the following patients:

- Men with a serum creatinine level of 1.5 mg/dL and women with a serum creatinine level of 1.4 mg/dL
- Patients with tissue hypoperfusion, such as in heart failure, shock, or septicemia, and patients at risk for developing metabolic acidosis
- Patients with clinical or laboratory evidence (hyperbilirubinemia, elevated aspartate aminotransferase [AST], alanine aminotransferase [ALT] level) of liver disease
- Patients scheduled to receive IV radiopaque dyes. Radiopaque dyes often induce temporary renal insufficiency, so metformin should be discontinued 24 to 48 hours before procedures in which radiopaque dye will be administered (e.g., kidney studies). Metformin should not be reinitiated for 2 to 3 days, until normal renal function has been proven.

■ Common Adverse Effects
Gastrointestinal

Nausea, vomiting, anorexia, abdominal cramps, flatulence. These adverse effects are most common and are the reason for slow dose titration. They are usually mild and tend to resolve with continued therapy. Taking the medication with meals will help reduce these adverse effects. Encourage the patient not to discontinue therapy without first consulting the healthcare provider.

■ Serious Adverse Effects
Metabolic

Malaise, myalgias, respiratory distress, hypotension. A rare adverse effect of metformin is lactic acidosis. A gradual onset of these symptoms may be an early indication of the development of lactic acidosis. Patients with reduced renal function, poor circulation, and/or excessive alcohol intake are most susceptible to developing lactic acidosis.

■ Drug Interactions
Drugs That May Enhance Toxic Effects. Amiloride, cimetidine, digoxin, furosemide, morphine, procainamide, quinidine, quinine, ranitidine, triamterene, trimethoprim, and vancomycin are excreted by the same route through the kidneys that metformin depends on for excretion. There is a possibility that these drugs block the excretion of metformin, potentially causing lactic acidosis. Monitor for signs of lactic acidosis (refer to earlier discussion).

Ethanol. Patients should be cautioned against excessive alcohol intake, acute or chronic, when taking metformin, because alcohol potentiates the effects of metformin on lactate metabolism.

Hyperglycemia. The following drugs, when used concurrently with metformin, may decrease its therapeutic effects: corticosteroids, phenothiazines, diuretics, oral contraceptives, thyroid replacement hormones, phenytoin, diazoxide, and lithium carbonate. Diabetic and prediabetic patients must be monitored for the development of hyperglycemia, particularly during the early weeks of therapy. Assess regularly for elevated blood glucose level or glycosuria and report if it occurs with any frequency.

Nifedipine. Nifedipine appears to increase the absorption of metformin. Reducing the dosage of metformin may minimize adverse effects.

DRUG CLASS: SULFONYLUREA ORAL HYPOGLYCEMIC AGENTS

ACTIONS

The sulfonylureas lower blood glucose levels by stimulating the release of insulin from the beta cells of the pancreas. The sulfonylureas also diminish glucose production and metabolism of insulin by the liver.

USES

The sulfonylureas are effective in type 2 diabetes patients in whom the pancreas still has the capacity to secrete insulin, but they are of no value in the patient with type 1 diabetes who has no beta cell function. Sulfonylureas may be effective in the treatment of type 2 diabetes mellitus that cannot be controlled by diet and exercise if the patient is not susceptible to developing ketosis, acidosis, or infections. Patients most likely to benefit from oral hypoglycemic treatment are those who develop signs of diabetes after age 40 years and who require less than 40 units of insulin per day (indicating that some insulin is still being secreted by the beta cells). Sulfonylureas may induce hypoglycemia due to overproduction of insulin.

THERAPEUTIC OUTCOMES

The primary therapeutic outcomes expected from sulfonylurea oral hypoglycemic therapy are as follows:
1. A decrease in fasting blood glucose and $A1_C$ concentrations in the range defined as acceptable for the individual patient
2. Fewer long-term complications associated with poorly controlled diabetes mellitus

❖ NURSING IMPLICATIONS FOR SULFONYLUREA ORAL HYPOGLYCEMIC AGENTS

■ Premedication Assessment
1. Confirm that blood glucose and $A1_C$ levels were recently measured and were hyperglycemic for the individual patient.
2. Confirm that the patient has had a level of activity "reasonable" for that patient and that the anticipated level of activity planned for the next several

Table 35-7   Sulfonylurea Oral Hypoglycemic Agents

GENERIC NAME	BRAND NAME	AVAILABILITY	INITIAL DOSAGE	DOSAGE RANGE	DURATION* (hr)
First Generation					
chlorpropamide ⇄ *Do not confuse chlorpropamide with chlorpromazine.*	—	Tablets: 100, 250 mg	100 mg daily	100-750 mg daily	24-72
tolazamide	—	Tablets: 250, 500 mg	100 mg daily	0.1-1 g daily	12-16
tolbutamide	—	Tablets: 500 mg	1 g twice daily	0.25-3 g daily	6-12
Second Generation					
glimepiride	Amaryl ⇄ *Do not confuse Amaryl with Altace, Avandia, Reminyl, or Symmetrel.*	Tablets: 1, 2, 4 mg	1-2 mg daily	1-8 mg daily	24
glipizide	Glucotrol	Tablets: 5, 10 mg	2.5-5 mg daily	15-40 mg daily	10-24
glipizide XL	Glucotrol XL	Extended release (24 hr): 2.5, 5, 10 mg	5-10 mg	20 mg	24
glyburide	DiaBeta ⇄ *Do not confuse DiaBeta with Zebeta.*	Tablets: 1.25, 2.5, 5 mg	1.5-3 mg daily	0.75-12 mg daily	24
	Glynase	Tablets, micronized: 1.5, 3, 6 mg	2.5-5 mg daily	1.25-20 mg daily	24

*The times listed are averages based on a newly diagnosed diabetic patient. Factors modifying these times include patient variation and dosage.

hours is balanced with the oral hypoglycemic agent dosage.

3. Confirm that the prescribed diet is being consumed as planned and that no changes in diet are anticipated in relation to the oral hypoglycemic agent dosage over the next several hours (e.g., in patients on NPO status, consider holding medication).

■ **Availability, Dosage, and Administration**

See Table 35-7. Individual dosage adjustment is essential for the successful use of oral hypoglycemic agents. A patient should receive a 1-month trial on maximum dosage of the sulfonylurea being used before the medication can be considered a primary failure. If a patient represents a secondary failure (a patient initially controlled on oral agents), changing to an alternative sulfonylurea is occasionally successful in controlling blood sugar levels.

⊞ Medication Safety Alert

In general, sulfonylureas should not be administered to patients who are allergic to sulfonamides. These patients may also be allergic to sulfonylureas.

■ **Common Adverse Effects**
Gastrointestinal
Nausea, vomiting, anorexia, abdominal cramps. These adverse effects are usually mild and tend to resolve

with continued therapy. Encourage the patient not to discontinue therapy without first consulting the healthcare provider.

■ **Serious Adverse Effects**
Metabolic
Hypoglycemia. Patients receiving oral hypoglycemic therapy are as susceptible to hypoglycemia as diabetic patients on insulin therapy. Consequently, blood glucose levels must be monitored closely, especially in the early stages of therapy. Monitor for the following signs of hypoglycemia: headache, nausea, weakness, hunger, lethargy, decreased coordination, general apprehension, sweating, or blurred or double vision. Hypoglycemia must be treated immediately. Mild symptoms may be controlled by the oral administration of a glucose source (e.g., a lump of sugar, orange juice, carbonated cola beverage [not diet], candy [not chocolate]) or ingestion of a commercially prepared product such as Glutose. Severe symptoms may be relieved by the administration of IV glucose, and parenteral glucagon may be prescribed in some cases. If in doubt about whether the patient is hypoglycemic or hyperglycemic, always treat the individual for hypoglycemia to prevent the possible neurologic complications that can occur from untreated hypoglycemia. Notify the healthcare provider immediately if any of these symptoms appear. The dosage of oral hypoglycemic agents may also have to be reduced.

Gastrointestinal

Hepatotoxicity. The symptoms of hepatotoxicity are anorexia, nausea, vomiting, jaundice, hepatomegaly, splenomegaly, and abnormal liver function (e.g., elevated bilirubin, AST, ALT, gamma-glutamyl transferase [GGT], alkaline phosphatase levels, increased prothrombin time).

Hematologic

Blood dyscrasias. Routine laboratory studies (e.g., red blood cell [RBC] and white blood cell [WBC] counts, differential counts) should be scheduled. Stress the need for the patient to return for this laboratory work.

Immune System. Monitor for the development of a sore throat, fever, purpura, jaundice, or excessive and progressively increasing weakness.

Dermatologic reactions. Report a rash or pruritus immediately. Withhold additional doses pending approval by the healthcare provider.

■ **Drug Interactions**

Hypoglycemia. The following drugs may enhance the hypoglycemic effects of the sulfonylureas: azole antifungal agents (e.g., fluconazole), fluoroquinolone antibiotics, ethanol, androgens (e.g., methandrostenolone), chloramphenicol, warfarin, beta-adrenergic blocking agents, salicylates, sulfonamides (e.g., sulfamethoxazole), and MAOIs.

Monitor the patient for the following signs of hypoglycemia: headache, nausea, weakness, hunger, lethargy, decreased coordination, general apprehension, sweating, or blurred or double vision. Notify the healthcare provider if any of these symptoms appear.

Hyperglycemia. The following drugs, when used concurrently with the sulfonylureas, may decrease the therapeutic effects of the sulfonylureas: corticosteroids, fluoroquinolone antibiotics, thiazide diuretics, phenothiazines, oral contraceptives, thyroid replacement hormones, phenytoin, diazoxide, and lithium carbonate.

Diabetic or prediabetic patients must be monitored for the development of hyperglycemia, particularly during the early weeks of therapy. Assess regularly for elevated blood glucose level or glycosuria, and notify the healthcare provider if either occurs with any frequency.

Patients receiving insulin may require an adjustment in dosage.

Beta-Adrenergic Blocking Agents. Beta blockers (e.g., propranolol, nadolol, metoprolol, carvedilol) may induce hypoglycemia, but may also mask many of the symptoms of hypoglycemia. Notify the healthcare provider if any of these symptoms appear intermittently.

Alcohol. Ingestion of alcoholic beverages during sulfonylurea therapy may infrequently result in an Antabuse-like reaction, manifested by facial flushing, pounding headache, feeling of breathlessness, and nausea.

In patients who develop an Antabuse-like reaction to alcohol, the use of alcohol and preparations containing alcohol (e.g., over-the-counter cough medications, mouthwashes) should be avoided during therapy and for up to 5 days after discontinuation of sulfonylurea therapy.

DRUG CLASS: MEGLITINIDE ORAL HYPOGLYCEMIC AGENTS

meglitinides (mĕ-GLĬ-tĭ-nīdz)

ACTIONS

The meglitinides are nonsulfonylurea oral hypoglycemic agents. They lower blood glucose levels by stimulating the release of insulin from the beta cells of the pancreas.

USES

The meglitinides are effective in patients with type 2 diabetes mellitus in whom the pancreas still has the capacity to secrete insulin, but they are of no value in patients with type 1 diabetes mellitus who have no beta cell function. The meglitinides may be effective in the treatment of type 2 diabetes mellitus that cannot be controlled by diet and exercise if the patient is not susceptible to developing ketosis, acidosis, or infections. Patients most likely to benefit from oral hypoglycemic treatment are those who develop signs of diabetes after age 40 and who require less than 40 units of insulin daily (indicating that some insulin is still being secreted by the beta cells). The meglitinides may be used alone or in combination with metformin to control hyperglycemia. The meglitinides have the advantage of having a short duration of action, thus reducing the potential for hypoglycemic reactions. On the other hand, having to take doses up to four times daily may reduce compliance. The meglitinides may be of particular use for patients normally well controlled on diet but who may have periods of transient loss of control, such as during an infection.

THERAPEUTIC OUTCOMES

The primary therapeutic outcomes expected from meglitinide oral hypoglycemic therapy are as follows:
1. A decrease in fasting blood glucose and the A1$_C$ concentrations in the range defined as "acceptable" for the individual patient
2. Fewer long-term complications associated with poorly controlled diabetes mellitus

❖ **NURSING IMPLICATIONS FOR MEGLITINIDE THERAPY**

■ **Premedication Assessment**
1. Confirm that blood glucose and A1$_C$ levels were recently measured and were hyperglycemic for the individual patient.

Table 35-8   Meglitinide Oral Hypoglycemic Agents

GENERIC NAME	BRAND NAME	AVAILABILITY	DAILY DOSAGE RANGE	MAXIMUM DAILY DOSAGE
nateglinide	Starlix	Tablets: 60, 120 mg	Initially, 60 to 120 mg before each meal	360 mg
repaglinide	Prandin ⇄ Do not confuse Prandin with Avandia.	Tablets: 0.5, 1, 2 mg	Initially, 0.5 mg before each meal	16 mg

2. Confirm that the patient has had a level of activity "reasonable" for that patient and that the anticipated level of activity planned for the next several hours is balanced with the oral hypoglycemic agent dosage.

3. Confirm that the prescribed diet is being consumed as planned and that no changes in diet are anticipated in relation to the oral hypoglycemic agent dosage over the next several hours (e.g., in patients on NPO status, consider holding medication).

■ **Availability, Dosage, and Administration**
• See Table 35-8. Doses may be administered within 1 to 30 minutes of the meal.
• Individual dosage adjustment is essential for the successful use of the meglitinides. Dosages may be adjusted weekly, based on fasting blood glucose.
• Doses may be taken preprandially two, three, or four times daily in response to changes in the patient's meal pattern.

! Medication Safety Alert

Patients should skip a scheduled dose if they skip a meal so that the risk of hypoglycemia is reduced.

■ **Common and Serious Adverse Effects**
Metabolic
Hypoglycemia. Patients receiving oral hypoglycemic therapy are as susceptible to hypoglycemia as diabetic patients on insulin therapy. Consequently, blood glucose levels must be monitored closely, especially in the early stages of therapy. Monitor for the following signs of hypoglycemia: headache, nausea, weakness, hunger, lethargy, decreased coordination, general apprehension, sweating, or blurred or double vision. Hypoglycemia must be treated immediately. Mild symptoms may be controlled by the oral administration of a glucose source (e.g., a lump of sugar, orange juice, carbonated cola beverage [not diet], candy [not chocolate]) or ingestion of a commercially prepared product such as Glutose. Severe symptoms may be relieved by administering IV glucose, and parenteral glucagon may be prescribed in some cases. If in doubt about whether the patient is hypoglycemic or hyperglycemic, always treat the individual for hypoglycemia to prevent the possible neurologic complications

that can occur from untreated hypoglycemia. Notify the healthcare provider immediately if any of these symptoms appear. The dosage of oral hypoglycemic agents also may have to be reduced.

■ **Drug Interactions**
Hypoglycemia. The following drugs may enhance the hypoglycemic effects of repaglinide and nateglinide: ethanol, erythromycin, clarithromycin, nonsteroidal antiinflammatory drugs (NSAIDs), sulfonylureas, gemfibrozil, itraconazole, ketoconazole, androgens (e.g., methandrostenolone), chloramphenicol, warfarin, salicylates, sulfonamides (e.g., sulfisoxazole), probenecid, and MAOIs.

Monitor for the following signs of hypoglycemia: headache, nausea, weakness, hunger, lethargy, decreased coordination, general apprehension, sweating, or blurred or double vision. Notify the healthcare provider if any of these symptoms appear.

Hyperglycemia. The following drugs, when used concurrently with the meglitinides, may decrease the therapeutic effects of the meglitinides: corticosteroids, phenothiazines, diuretics, estrogens, oral contraceptives, thyroid replacement hormones, niacin, sympathomimetics, calcium channel blockers, phenytoin, diazoxide, and lithium carbonate.

Beta-Adrenergic Blocking Agents. Beta blockers (e.g., propranolol, nadolol, metoprolol, carvedilol) may induce hypoglycemia, but may also mask many of the symptoms of hypoglycemia. Notify the prescriber if you suspect that any of these symptoms appear intermittently.

Carbamazepine, Barbiturates, Rifampin. These agents may increase repaglinide metabolism. Monitor blood glucose levels closely when any of these agents are started or discontinued.

Erythromycin, Clarithromycin, Ketoconazole, Miconazole. These agents may inhibit repaglinide metabolism. Monitor closely for hypoglycemia if any of these agents are started in a patient receiving repaglinide.

DRUG CLASS: THIAZOLIDINEDIONE ORAL ANTIDIABETIC AGENTS

thiazolidinediones (thī-ă-zŏl-ĭ-dēn-DĪ-ōnz)

ACTIONS

The thiazolidinediones (TZDs) lower blood glucose levels by increasing the sensitivity of muscle and fat tissue to insulin, allowing more glucose to enter the cells in the presence of insulin for metabolism. Thiazolidinediones also may inhibit hepatic gluconeogenesis and decrease hepatic glucose output. Unlike sulfonylureas or meglitinides, TZDs do not stimulate the release of insulin from the beta cells of the pancreas, but insulin must be present for these agents to work.

USES

Thiazolidinediones are effective in patients with type 2 diabetes mellitus in whom the pancreas still has the capacity to secrete insulin, but are of no value in the person with type 1 diabetes who has no beta cell function. Thiazolidinediones may be effective in the treatment of type 2 diabetes mellitus that cannot be controlled by diet and exercise if the patient is not susceptible to developing ketosis, acidosis, or infections. They are not indicated as initial therapy for patients with type 2 diabetes mellitus. Rosiglitazone and pioglitazone may be used as monotherapy (with diet and exercise) or in combination with insulin, sulfonylureas, or metformin to control blood glucose levels. Therapy often takes 4 to 6 weeks for notable effect and several months for full therapeutic effect.

THERAPEUTIC OUTCOMES

The primary therapeutic outcomes expected from TZD oral antidiabetic therapy are as follows:
1. A decrease in fasting blood glucose and A1$_C$ concentrations in the range defined as "acceptable" for the individual patient
2. Fewer long-term complications associated with poorly controlled diabetes mellitus

❖ NURSING IMPLICATIONS FOR THIAZOLIDINEDIONE THERAPY

▪ Premedication Assessment
1. Confirm that blood glucose and A1$_C$ levels were recently measured and were hyperglycemic for the individual patient.

2. Perform scheduled baseline laboratory tests. Liver function, including bilirubin, AST, ALT, GGT, and alkaline phosphatase tests, should be determined before initiation of therapy, once a month for the first year, and quarterly after the first year. A baseline test should also be completed for body weight; hemoglobin and hematocrit; WBC count; and total cholesterol, HDL cholesterol, LDL cholesterol, and triglyceride levels.
3. Confirm that the prescribed diet is being consumed as planned and that no changes in diet are anticipated in relation to the oral hypoglycemic agent dosage over the next several hours (e.g., in patients on NPO status, consider holding medication).
4. Premenopausal, anovulatory women should be informed that TZDs might induce the resumption of ovulation. These women may be at risk for pregnancy if adequate contraception is not used (see "Drug Interactions: Oral Contraceptives").

▪ Availability, Dosage, and Administration
See Table 35-9. Individual dosage adjustment is essential for the successful use of hypoglycemic agents. A patient should be given a multiweek trial (12 weeks for rosiglitazone and pioglitazone therapy) before adjusting the dosage or adding other hypoglycemic agents. In general, TZDs should not be used in patients with heart failure.

▪ Common Adverse Effects
Gastrointestinal
Nausea, vomiting, anorexia, abdominal cramps. These adverse effects are usually mild and tend to resolve with continued therapy. Encourage the patient not to discontinue therapy without first consulting the healthcare provider.

▪ Serious Adverse Effects
Metabolic
Hypoglycemia. Patients receiving TZDs are not susceptible to hypoglycemia unless they are also receiving other hypoglycemic therapy, such as insulin or sulfonylureas. If patients are receiving multiple hypoglycemic therapies, blood glucose levels must be monitored closely, especially in the early stages of therapy. Monitor for the following signs of hypoglycemia:

Table 35-9 Thiazolidinedione Oral Hypoglycemic Agents

GENERIC NAME	BRAND NAME	AVAILABILITY	DAILY DOSAGE RANGE	MAXIMUM DAILY DOSAGE
pioglitazone	Actos ⇌ Do not confuse Actos with Actonel.	Tablets: 15, 30, 45 mg	PO: Initially, 15-30 mg once daily	45 mg
rosiglitazone	Avandia ⇌ Do not confuse Avandia with Amaryl, Atacand, or Avelox.	Tablets: 2, 4, 8 mg	PO: Initially, 2 mg twice daily or 4 mg once daily	8 mg

headache, nausea, weakness, hunger, lethargy, decreased coordination, general apprehension, sweating, or blurred or double vision. Hypoglycemia must be treated immediately. Mild symptoms may be controlled by the oral administration of a glucose source (e.g., a lump of sugar, orange juice, carbonated cola beverage [not diet], candy [not chocolate]) or ingestion of a commercially prepared product such as Glutose. Severe symptoms may be relieved by IV administration of glucose, and parenteral glucagon may be prescribed in some cases. If in doubt about whether the patient is hypoglycemic or hyperglycemic, always treat the individual for hypoglycemia to prevent the possible neurologic complications that can occur from untreated hypoglycemia. Notify the healthcare provider immediately if any of the previously mentioned symptoms appear. The dosage of oral hypoglycemic agents also may have to be reduced.

Weight gain. Weight gain of a few pounds is a common adverse effect of TZD therapy. It also may be a sign of fluid accumulation and increased plasma volume. Monitor patients for signs of edema and heart failure and report to the healthcare provider if present.

Gastrointestinal

Hepatotoxicity. The symptoms of hepatotoxicity are anorexia, nausea, vomiting, jaundice, hepatomegaly, splenomegaly, and abnormal liver function (elevated bilirubin, AST, ALT, GGT, alkaline phosphatase levels, increased prothrombin time).

■ **Drug Interactions**

Hypoglycemia. The following drugs may enhance the hypoglycemic effects of TZDs: sulfonylureas, ethanol, androgens (e.g., methandrostenolone), chloramphenicol, warfarin, salicylates, sulfonamides (e.g., sulfisoxazole), and MAOIs.

Monitor for the following signs of hypoglycemia: headache, nausea, weakness, hunger, lethargy, decreased coordination, general apprehension, sweating, or blurred or double vision. Notify the healthcare provider if any of these symptoms appear.

Hyperglycemia. The following drugs, when used concurrently with TZDs, may decrease the therapeutic effects of TZDs: corticosteroids, phenothiazines, diuretics, oral contraceptives, thyroid replacement hormones, phenytoin, diazoxide, and lithium carbonate.

Diabetic or prediabetic patients need to be monitored for the development of hyperglycemia, particularly during the early weeks of therapy.

Assess regularly for elevated blood glucose level or glycosuria and report if it occurs with any frequency. Patients receiving insulin may require an adjustment in dosage.

Beta-Adrenergic Blocking Agents. Beta blockers (e.g., propranolol, nadolol, metoprolol, carvedilol) may induce hypoglycemia, but may also mask many of the symptoms of hypoglycemia. Notify the healthcare provider if you suspect that any of these symptoms appear intermittently.

Oral Contraceptives. Pioglitazone may enhance the metabolism of ethinyl estradiol and norethindrone, which may cause a resumption of ovulation in patients taking oral contraceptives. Counseling regarding alternative methods of birth control (e.g., contraceptive foam, condoms) should be planned. This interaction has not been reported with rosiglitazone.

Drugs That Inhibit Metabolism. Erythromycin, ketoconazole, itraconazole, calcium channel blockers, cisapride, corticosteroids, cyclosporine, triazolam, hydroxymethylglutaryl (HMG)-coenzyme A (CoA) reductase inhibitors (statins) may inhibit the metabolism of pioglitazone. If a TZD hypoglycemic agent is indicated for a patient already receiving one of these agents, rosiglitazone should be considered over pioglitazone because these agents do not inhibit its metabolism.

DRUG CLASS: ALPHA-GLUCOSIDASE INHIBITOR AGENTS

> **acarbose** (Ă-kăr-bōs)
> **Precose** (PRĒ-kōs)

ACTIONS

Acarbose is classified as an antihyperglycemic agent. It is an enzyme inhibitor that inhibits pancreatic alpha-amylase and gastrointestinal alpha-glucoside hydrolase enzymes used in the digestion of sugars. In patients with diabetes, this enzyme inhibition results in delayed glucose absorption and a lowering of postprandial hyperglycemia.

USES

Acarbose is used as an adjunct to the diet to lower blood glucose levels in patients with type 2 diabetes mellitus whose hyperglycemia cannot be controlled by diet and exercise alone. It has the particular advantage that it will not cause hypoglycemia, as can occur with insulin and the sulfonylureas. It also may be used in combination with the sulfonylureas or metformin to lower the blood glucose level because the agents act by different mechanisms.

THERAPEUTIC OUTCOMES

The primary therapeutic outcomes expected from acarbose therapy are as follows:

1. A decrease in postprandial blood glucose and $A1_C$ concentrations in the range defined as "acceptable" for the individual patient
2. Fewer long-term complications associated with poorly controlled type 2 diabetes mellitus

❖ **NURSING IMPLICATIONS FOR ACARBOSE**

■ **Premedication Assessment**

1. If the patient is also receiving an oral hypoglycemic agent or insulin therapy, ensure that the dosages of

these medications are well adjusted before starting acarbose therapy.

2. Review the patient's history to ensure that there is no gastrointestinal malabsorption syndrome or obstruction present.
3. Review the patient's medical history to ensure that no liver abnormalities are present.

▪ Availability
25-, 50-, and 100-mg tablets.

▪ Dosage and Administration
Adult: PO: Initially, 25 mg three times daily at the start of each main meal. The dosage is adjusted at 4- to 8-week intervals based on 1-hour postprandial blood glucose concentrations and on the severity of adverse effects. The maintenance dosage is 50 to 100 mg three times daily.

The maximum recommended dosage for patients weighing less than 60 kg (132 lb) is 50 mg three times daily. The maximum dosage for patients weighing more than 60 kg is 100 mg three times daily.

▪ Common Adverse Effects
Gastrointestinal

Abdominal cramps, diarrhea, flatulence. These adverse effects are caused by the metabolism of carbohydrates in the large intestine that were blocked from metabolism in the small intestine by acarbose. These adverse effects are usually mild and tend to resolve with continued therapy. Encourage the patient not to discontinue therapy without first consulting the healthcare provider.

▪ Serious Adverse Effects
Metabolic

Hypoglycemia. Although acarbose does not cause hypoglycemia by itself, it can enhance the hypoglycemia caused by a sulfonylurea or insulin. Consequently, blood glucose levels must be monitored closely, especially in the early stages of therapy.

Monitor for the following signs of hypoglycemia: headache, nausea, weakness, hunger, lethargy, decreased coordination, general apprehension, sweating, or blurred or double vision. Hypoglycemia must be treated immediately. Treatment should be initiated with oral dextrose (Glutose) because its metabolism is not blocked by acarbose. Do not use sucrose (table sugar) because its metabolism is blocked by acarbose. Severe symptoms may be relieved by IV administration of glucose, and parenteral glucagon may be prescribed in some cases. If in doubt about whether the patient is hypoglycemic or hyperglycemic, always treat the individual for hypoglycemia to prevent the possible neurologic complications that can occur from untreated hypoglycemia. Notify the healthcare provider immediately if any of these symptoms appear. The dosage of oral hypoglycemic agents may also have to be reduced.

Gastrointestinal

Hepatotoxicity. Acarbose has been reported to cause elevations of serum aminotransferase levels (AST and ALT). In rare cases, it causes hyperbilirubinemia. It is recommended that serum aminotransferase concentrations be checked every 3 months during the first year of treatment and periodically thereafter.

▪ Drug Interactions
Hyperglycemia. The following drugs, when used concurrently with acarbose, may decrease the therapeutic effects of acarbose: corticosteroids, phenothiazines, diuretics, oral contraceptives, thyroid replacement hormones, phenytoin, diazoxide, and lithium carbonate.

Digestive Enzymes, Intestinal Adsorbents. Digestive enzymes (e.g., amylase, pancreatin) and intestinal adsorbents (e.g., charcoal) may reduce the effect of acarbose. Concurrent therapy is not recommended.

Digoxin. Acarbose may inhibit the absorption of digoxin. Monitor serum digoxin levels and therapeutic effects to assess whether the dosage of digoxin needs to be adjusted. Monitor closely when the dosage of acarbose is increased or discontinued.

---

miglitol (MĬG-lĭ-tŏl)
  Glyset (GLĪ-sĕt)

ACTIONS
Miglitol is an enzyme inhibitor that inhibits pancreatic alpha-amylase and gastrointestinal alpha-glucoside hydrolase enzymes used in the digestion of sugars. In patients with diabetes, this enzyme inhibition results in delayed glucose absorption and a lowering of postprandial hyperglycemia.

USES
Miglitol is used as an adjunct to diet and exercise to lower blood glucose levels in patients with type 2 diabetes mellitus whose hyperglycemia cannot be controlled by diet and exercise alone. It has the particular advantage that it will not cause hypoglycemia, as can occur with insulin and the sulfonylureas. It also may be used in combination with the sulfonylureas to lower the blood glucose level because the agents act by different mechanisms.

THERAPEUTIC OUTCOMES
The primary therapeutic outcomes expected from miglitol therapy are as follows:
1. A decrease in postprandial blood glucose and A1$_C$ concentrations in the range defined as "acceptable" for the individual patient
2. Fewer long-term complications associated with poorly controlled type 2 diabetes mellitus

❖ NURSING IMPLICATIONS FOR MIGLITOL

▪ Premedication Assessment

1. If the patient is also receiving a sulfonylurea hypoglycemic agent or insulin therapy, ensure that the dosages of these medications are well adjusted before starting miglitol therapy.
2. Review the patient's history to ensure that there is no gastrointestinal malabsorption syndrome or obstruction present.
3. Review the patient's medical history to ensure that no liver abnormalities are present.

▪ Availability

25-, 50-, and 100-mg tablets.

▪ Dosage and Administration

Adult: PO: Initially, 25 mg three times daily at the start (first bite) of each main meal. Some patients may start with 25 mg daily to avoid gastrointestinal adverse effects. The dosage is adjusted at 4- to 8-week intervals based on 1-hour postprandial plasma glucose levels and A1$_C$ concentrations and on the severity of adverse effects. The maintenance dosage is 50 to 100 mg three times daily. The maximum recommended dosage is 100 mg three times daily.

▪ Common Adverse Effects

Gastrointestinal

Abdominal cramps, diarrhea, flatulence. These adverse effects are caused by the metabolism of carbohydrates in the large intestine that were blocked from metabolism in the small intestine by miglitol. These adverse effects are usually mild, especially with low initial dosages, and tend to resolve with continued therapy. Encourage the patient not to discontinue therapy without first consulting the healthcare provider.

▪ Serious Adverse Effects

Metabolic

Hypoglycemia. Although miglitol does not cause hypoglycemia by itself, it can enhance the hypoglycemia caused by a sulfonylurea or insulin. Consequently, blood glucose levels must be monitored closely, especially in the early stages of therapy.

Monitor for the following signs of hypoglycemia: headache, nausea, weakness, hunger, lethargy, decreased coordination, general apprehension, sweating, or blurred or double vision. Hypoglycemia must be treated immediately. Treatment should be initiated with oral dextrose (Glutose), because its metabolism is not blocked by miglitol. Do not use sucrose (table sugar), because its metabolism is blocked by miglitol. Severe symptoms may be relieved by IV administration of glucose, and parenteral glucagon may be prescribed in some cases. If in doubt about whether the patient is hypoglycemic or hyperglycemic, always treat the individual for hypoglycemia to prevent the

possible neurologic complications that can occur from untreated hypoglycemia. Notify the prescriber immediately if any of these symptoms appear. The dosage of oral hypoglycemic agents may also have to be reduced.

▪ Drug Interactions

Hyperglycemia. The following medications, when administered concurrently with miglitol, may decrease the therapeutic effects of miglitol: corticosteroids, phenothiazines, diuretics, oral contraceptives, thyroid replacement hormones, phenytoin, diazoxide, and lithium carbonate.

Propranolol, Ranitidine. Miglitol may interfere with the absorption of these agents. Concurrent therapy is not recommended.

Digestive Enzymes, Intestinal Adsorbents. Digestive enzymes (e.g., amylase, pancreatin) and intestinal adsorbents (e.g., charcoal) may reduce the effect of miglitol. Concurrent therapy is not recommended.

DRUG CLASS: AMYLINOMIMETIC AGENT

pramlintide (PRĂM-lĭn-tīd)
    Symlin Pen (SĬM-lĭn)

ACTIONS

Pramlintide is a synthetic analogue of amylin. Amylin is a protein secreted from pancreatic beta cells with insulin in response to food intake. Patients with a deficiency of insulin also have a deficiency of amylin. Amylin and pramlintide reduce postprandial glucose levels by the following actions:

- Suppressing glucagon secretion from the liver, thereby suppressing glucose output from the liver
- Delaying gastric emptying, thus slowing carbohydrate and lipid absorption and reducing postprandial hyperglycemia
- Suppressing the appetite, with subsequent potential weight reduction

USES

Pramlintide is used as additional therapy to reduce elevated postprandial hyperglycemia in patients with type 1 or 2 diabetes mellitus who are taking mealtime insulin, or metformin, a sulfonylurea, or a combination of metformin and a sulfonylurea but who have not achieved adequate glycemic control.

Pramlintide should **not** be used in patients with any of the following:

- Poor compliance with a current insulin therapy
- Poor compliance with self-monitoring of blood glucose level
- A1$_C$ level higher than 9%
- Recurrent episodes of severe hypoglycemia requiring assistance occurring during the previous 6 months

- Unawareness of oncoming hypoglycemic episodes
- Need for medications to stimulate gastric motility

THERAPEUTIC OUTCOMES

The primary therapeutic outcomes expected from pramlintide therapy are as follows:
1. A decrease in postprandial blood glucose and A1$_C$ concentrations in the range defined as "acceptable" for the individual patient
2. Fewer long-term complications associated with poorly controlled type 1 or 2 diabetes mellitus

❖ NURSING IMPLICATIONS FOR PRAMLINTIDE

▪ Premedication Assessment
1. Ensure that the dosages of concurrent oral antidiabetic therapy are well adjusted before starting pramlintide therapy.
2. Assess the patient's ability to self-administer injections.
3. Discuss with patients their compliance with current insulin therapy and ability to do self-monitoring of blood glucose levels.
4. Make sure that the patient and family understand the signs and symptoms of hypoglycemia and its causes.
5. Identify whether the patient is pregnant or breastfeeding.
6. Monitor the patient's weight prior to beginning therapy and on a regular basis thereafter.
7. Review the manufacturer's patient information brochure on the proper use of the Symlin pen (syringe) with the patient.

▪ Availability
Prefilled pens: 1500 mcg/1.5 mL and 2700 mcg/2.7 mL.

▪ Dosage and Administration
Adult

Subcutaneous: Pramlintide is administered subcutaneously into the abdomen or thigh. Do not use the upper arm because of variable absorption.
- Administer pramlintide and insulin as separate injections at separate sites at least 2 inches apart. Rotate sites.
- If a dose of pramlintide is missed, do not administer an additional injection. Wait until the next major meal.

NOTE: Pramlintide dosage differs depending on whether the patient has type 1 or type 2 diabetes.

Type 1 diabetes: *Subcutaneous:* Initially, 15 mcg immediately before major (≥250-kcal or ≥30-g carbohydrate) meals.
- Reduce preprandial, rapid-acting, or short-acting insulin doses, including fixed-mix insulins (e.g., 75/25), by 50%.

- Monitor blood glucose levels frequently, including before and after meals and at bedtime.
- Increase pramlintide dosage by 15 mcg when no significant nausea has occurred for at least 3 days. Maximum dose is 60 mcg before major meals.
- Adjust insulin doses to optimize blood glucose control once the target dose of pramlintide has been achieved and nausea (if experienced) has subsided.

Type 2 diabetes: *Subcutaneous:* Initially, 60 mcg immediately before major (≥250-kcal or ≥30-g carbohydrate) meals.
- Reduce preprandial, rapid-acting, or short-acting insulin doses, including fixed-mix insulins (e.g., 75/25), by 50%.
- Monitor blood glucose levels frequently, including before and after meals and at bedtime.
- Increase pramlintide dosage to 120 mcg when no significant nausea has occurred for 3 to 7 days. Maximum dose is 120 mcg before major meals.
- Adjust insulin doses to optimize blood glucose control once the target dose of pramlintide has been achieved and nausea (if experienced) has subsided.

> **!** **Medication Safety Alert**
>
> Patients should be cautioned to *not* take their dose of pramlintide if any of the following is a factor:
> - Their blood glucose level is low.
> - They plan to skip a meal.
> - They plan to eat a meal with fewer than 250 calories or 30 g of carbohydrates.
> - They are sick and cannot eat a usual meal.
> - They are having surgery or a medical test in which they must fast before the test.
> - They are pregnant or breastfeeding and have not talked to their healthcare provider.

Storage. Unopened syringes of pramlintide should be stored refrigerated at 36° to 46° F (2.2° to 7.8° C). Do not freeze or use if it has been frozen. Opened (in use) syringes may be kept refrigerated or at room temperature for up to 30 days. Opened syringes, whether or not refrigerated, should be discarded after 30 days.

▪ Common Adverse Effects
Gastrointestinal

Nausea, vomiting, indigestion. Nausea is the most common adverse effect with pramlintide. Mild nausea is more likely during the first weeks after starting therapy and usually does not last long. Starting with a low dose and building up slowly is important. These adverse effects are usually mild to moderate and tend to resolve with continued therapy. Encourage the patient not to discontinue therapy without first consulting the healthcare provider.

■ **Serious Adverse Effects**

Metabolic

Hypoglycemia. Although pramlintide does not cause hypoglycemia by itself, it can enhance the hypoglycemia that may be caused by a sulfonylurea or insulin. Consequently, blood glucose levels must be monitored closely, especially in the early stages of therapy.

Monitor for the following signs of hypoglycemia: headache, nausea, weakness, hunger, lethargy, decreased coordination, general apprehension, sweating, or blurred or double vision. Hypoglycemia must be treated immediately. Mild symptoms may be controlled by the oral administration of a glucose source (e.g., a lump of sugar, orange juice, carbonated cola beverage [not diet], candy [not chocolate]) or ingestion of a commercially prepared product such as Glutose. Severe symptoms may be relieved by IV administration of glucose, and parenteral glucagon may be prescribed in some cases. If in doubt about whether the patient is hypoglycemic or hyperglycemic, always treat the individual for hypoglycemia to prevent the possible neurologic complications that can occur from untreated hypoglycemia. Notify the healthcare provider immediately if any of these symptoms appear. The dosage of oral antidiabetic agents may also have to be reduced.

■ **Drug Interactions**

Hypoglycemia. The following drugs may enhance the hypoglycemic effects of pramlintide and insulin: sulfonylureas, meglitinides, ACE inhibitors (e.g., captopril, ramipril, lisinopril), disopyramide, fibrates (e.g., gemfibrozil), fluoxetine, MAOIs (e.g., tranylcypromine, isocarboxazid), pentoxifylline, propoxyphene, salicylates, and sulfonamide antibiotics. Monitor for the following signs of hypoglycemia: headache, nausea, weakness, hunger, lethargy, decreased coordination, general apprehension, sweating, and blurred or double vision. Notify the healthcare provider if any of these symptoms appear.

Hyperglycemia. The following medications, when used concurrently with pramlintide, may decrease its therapeutic effects: corticosteroids, phenothiazines, diuretics, oral contraceptives, thyroid replacement hormones, phenytoin, diazoxide, and lithium carbonate.

DRUG CLASS: SODIUM-GLUCOSE COTRANSPORTER 2 INHIBITORS

ACTIONS

In normal physiology, sodium-glucose cotransporter 2 (SGLT2) proteins located in the epithelial cells of the proximal tubules of the nephron (kidneys) reabsorb about 80% to 90% of the glucose filtered across the glomerulus, transporting it back into the circulating blood. In type 2 diabetes, SGLT2 is oversecreted, reabsorbing even more glucose back into the blood that may aggravate hyperglycemia. Sodium-glucose cotransporter 2 inhibitors block the secretion of the SGLT2 protein, dropping glucose reabsorption from 90% to less than 10%, causing the glucose to be excreted in the urine.

USES

Sodium-glucose cotransporter 2 inhibitors are a new class of antidiabetic agents used to treat hyperglycemia in type 2 diabetes by reducing renal glucose reabsorption in the proximal convoluted tubule, enhancing increased urinary glucose excretion. They are used as adjuncts to diet and exercise to improve blood glucose control in adults with type 2 diabetes. They may be used as monotherapy or in combination with metformin, sulfonylureas, TZDs, dipeptidyl peptidase-4 inhibitors, and insulin. With continuous use, the $A1_C$ is lowered about 0.7%, similar to other adjunctive antidiabetic agents. Patients who have type 1 diabetes or who are susceptible to ketoacidosis are not candidates for SGLT2 inhibitor therapy.

THERAPEUTIC OUTCOMES

The primary therapeutic outcomes expected from SGLT2 inhibitor therapy are as follows:
1. A decrease in postprandial blood glucose and $A1_C$ concentrations in the range defined as "acceptable" for the individual patient
2. Fewer long-term complications associated with poorly controlled type 2 diabetes mellitus

❖ **NURSING IMPLICATIONS FOR SGLT2 INHIBITORS**

■ **Premedication Assessment**
1. Ensure that the dosages of concurrent antidiabetic therapy are well adjusted before starting SGLT2 inhibitor therapy.
2. Confirm that blood glucose and $A1_C$ levels were recently measured and were hyperglycemic for the individual patient.
3. Review the estimated glomerular filtration rate (eGFR) as a renal function test to assure that the SGLT2 inhibitor being prescribed is acceptable based on the patient's glomerular filtration rate. Monitor the eGFR periodically during therapy, as SGLT2 inhibitors may reduce renal function.
4. Ensure that the patient's serum calcium level is normal before starting therapy. Patients predisposed to hyperkalemia (including those with renal impairment or taking potassium-sparing diuretics, ACE inhibitors, and ARBs) are more likely to develop hyperkalemia; monitor serum potassium level after initiation in those who are predisposed.
5. Discuss with patients their compliance with current antidiabetic therapy and ability to do self-monitoring of blood glucose levels.
6. Ensure that the patient and family understand the signs and symptoms of hypoglycemia and its causes and treatment.

Table 35-10 Sodium Glucose Cotransporter 2 Inhibitors				
GENERIC NAME	BRAND NAME	AVAILABILITY	DAILY DOSAGE RANGE	MAXIMUM DAILY DOSAGE
canagliflozin	Invokana	PO: Tablets: 100, 300 mg	PO: 100 mg once daily	300 mg; adjust dose in renal impairment; do not use in patients with a GFR of <30 mL/min/1.73 m^2
dapagliflozin	Farxiga	PO: Tablets: 5, 10 mg	PO: 5 mg once daily	10 mg; do not use in patients with GFR <60 mL/min/1.73 m^2
empagliflozin	Jardiance	PO: Tablets: 10, 25 mg	PO: mg once daily	25 mg; do not use in patients with GFR <45 mL/min/1.73 m^2

7. Discuss with both male and female patients their histories of urinary tract and genital fungal infections. Assure that the patients know the signs and symptoms of these infections and the need to report to their healthcare provider.
8. Identify whether the patient is pregnant or breastfeeding.
9. Monitor the patient's weight prior to beginning therapy and on a regular basis thereafter. This class of medicine is not associated with weight gain as are some of the other antidiabetic medicines. Weight losses of 4 to 7 pounds were reported in clinical trials.

▪ Availability, Dosage, and Administration
See Table 35-10.

▪ Common and Serious Adverse Effects
Cardiovascular
Hypotension. Sodium-glucose cotransporter 2 inhibitors may induce vascular dehydration due to excretion of water along with hypertonic concentrations of glucose in the urine. Patients may develop hypotension with low systolic blood pressure, particularly in elderly patients and those concurrently taking antihypertensive medications and diuretics for other conditions. Maintain adequate hydration, especially when initiating therapy.

Increases in low-density lipoprotein cholesterol. It was noted in clinical trials that LDL-C raised 5% to 7% in patients participating in the trials. The clinical significance of this mild elevation is unknown. The healthcare provider will decide whether or not to treat the LDL-C.

Metabolic
Hypoglycemia. Hypoglycemia is quite rare in patients using the SGLT2 inhibitors as monotherapy, but is more common in concurrent therapy with insulin and those agents that secrete insulin (secretogogues) (e.g., insulin, sulfonylureas, meglitinides). When using lower doses of insulin, the secretogogues or the SGLT2 inhibitors may be necessary to reduce the incidence of hypoglycemia.

Glycosuria. Based on the mechanism of action of SGLT2 inhibitors, patients will commonly spill glucose in the urine. Patients who test urine to monitor their diabetes should stop doing so because the results will be meaningless for monitoring.

Genitourinary
Genitourinary tract infections. All patients prescribed an SGLT2 inhibitor are at slightly greater risk of developing bacterial and fungal infections of the genitourinary tract due to glucosuria. Those patients with chronic or recurrent genitourinary infections are more likely to develop infections. Report symptoms to the healthcare provider for appropriate treatment.

Increased urination. Excretion of additional urine glucose may result in polyuria and nocturia. Incidence was low, less than 1% above those patients treated with placebo in clinical trials.

▪ Drug Interactions
Antihypertensive Agents (ACE Inhibitors, Beta Blockers, Alpha Blockers, Calcium Channel Blockers, Diuretics). Patients taking antihypertensive agents may be more susceptible to orthostatic hypotension and hypotensive episodes induced by hypovolemic dehydration caused by SGLT2 inhibitors.

INCRETIN-BASED ANTIDIABETIC THERAPY

In normal physiology there are two proteins known as incretin peptides: glucagon-like peptide-1 (GLP-1) and glucose-dependent insulinotropic polypeptide (GIP). (The term *glucose-dependent* means that they are secreted only when glucose levels start to rise.) These hormones are released from L cells in the distal ileum and colon in response to ingestion of carbohydrates and fats. The incretins help control blood glucose levels by the following mechanisms:
• Enhancing insulin secretion
• Suppressing glucagon secretion from the liver, thereby suppressing glucose output from the liver
• Delaying gastric emptying, thus slowing carbohydrate and lipid absorption and reducing postprandial hyperglycemia
• Reducing appetite
• Maintaining beta cell function
These actions result in the reduction in basal glucose concentrations and in elevations of postprandial glucose concentrations. There is also a reduced appetite, with subsequent weight reduction.

One of the pathophysiologies associated with type 2 diabetes mellitus is low incretin levels. A new approach to the treatment of this form of diabetes is to enhance the activity of incretin hormones. There are currently two classes of agents that support the incretins: the incretin mimetic agents albiglutide, dulaglutide, exenatide and liraglutide, which are GLP-1 agonists that improve GLP-1 levels, and dipeptidyl peptidase-4 inhibitors alogliptin, linagliptin, saxagliptin, and sitagliptin.

DRUG CLASS: INCRETIN MIMETIC AGENTS (GLUCAGON-LIKE PEPTIDE-1 AGONISTS)

ACTIONS

Glucagon-like peptide-1 (GLP-1) agonists mimic the actions of this incretin for self-regulating glycemic control, resulting in an increase in serum insulin and a reduction in glucose concentrations.

USES

Glucagon-like peptide-1 agonists are used as additional therapy to reduce elevated fasting and postprandial hyperglycemia in patients with type 2 diabetes mellitus who are taking metformin, a sulfonylurea, or a combination of metformin and a sulfonylurea, but who have not achieved adequate glycemic control. Particular benefits of GLP-1 agonists are that they enhance insulin secretion only in the presence of hyperglycemia, and insulin secretion decreases as the blood glucose level approaches normal levels.

Albiglutide and dulaglutide are administered once weekly, whereas liraglutide is administered once daily, and exenatide must be administered twice daily. Albiglutide must be reconstituted prior to administration, whereas dulaglutide is ready for injection.

Liraglutide causes thyroid C-cell tumors in rats and mice. It is not known whether it causes tumors in humans, but it is contraindicated in patients with a family history of thyroid cancers. As a precaution against the growth of tumors, liraglutide is not recommended as a first-line agent in the treatment of diabetes.

THERAPEUTIC OUTCOMES

The primary therapeutic outcomes expected from GLP-1 agonist therapy are as follows:
1. A decrease in fasting and postprandial blood glucose levels and $A1_C$ concentrations in the range defined as "acceptable" for the individual patient
2. Fewer long-term complications associated with poorly controlled type 2 diabetes mellitus

❖ NURSING IMPLICATIONS FOR GLP-1 AGONISTS

■ Premedication Assessment
1. Ensure that the dosages of concurrent oral antidiabetic therapy are well adjusted before starting GLP-1 therapy.
2. Assess the patient's or family member's ability to self-administer injections.

■ Availability, Dosage, and Administration
See Table 35-11. Administer GLP-1 agonists as a subcutaneous injection in the thigh, abdomen, or upper arm. Exenatide is a twice-daily administration, whereas liraglutide is a once-daily administration independent

🔖 Table 35-11 Glucagon-like Peptide-1 Agonists

GENERIC NAME	BRAND NAME	AVAILABILITY	DOSAGE RANGE	MAXIMUM DOSAGE
albiglutide	Tanzeum	Prefilled pen for one-time use: 30 mg and 50 mg	Subcutaneous: 30 or 50 mg one time weekly	50 mg; 1 injection weekly
dulaglutide	Trulicity	Prefilled pen for one-time use: 0.75 and 1.5 mg	Subcutaneous: 0.75 mg or 1.5 mg one time weekly	5 mg; 1 injection weekly
exenatide	Byetta	Prefilled pen cartridges: 1.2 mL of solution to deliver 5 mcg per injection; 2.4 mL of solution to deliver 10 mcg per injection (each prefilled pen will deliver 60 doses to provide a 30-day supply of the twice-daily medication)	Subcutaneous: 5 mcg twice daily within 60 minutes of morning and evening meals; 6 or more hours apart	10 mcg twice daily
	Bydureon	Subcutaneous suspension: 2 mg/vial		
liraglutide	Victoza	Prefilled pen cartridge: 18 mg per 3 mL	Subcutaneous: 0.6 mg once daily at any time for 1 wk May increase dose to 1.2 mg once daily May increase to 1.8 mg for glycemic control.	Use with caution in patients with renal or hepatic impairment No dosage adjustment is required for these conditions.

of meals. Do *not* administer exenatide after a meal. Based on clinical response, the dose of the agonist may be increased.

The GLP-1 agonists are used in conjunction with metformin and/or a sulfonylurea. Dosage adjustment of the metformin is not necessary, but a dosage reduction of the sulfonylurea might be necessary to reduce the risk of hypoglycemia.

Glucagon-like peptide-1 pens should be stored refrigerated at 36° to 46° F (2.2° to 7.8° C). Do not freeze or use if it has been frozen. Warm to room temperature before use. After first use, the pens may be stored at room temperature (59° to 86° F [15° to 30° C]). The pens should be discarded 30 days after first use, even if some of the drug remains in the pen.

■ Common Adverse Effects

Gastrointestinal

Nausea, vomiting, diarrhea, constipation. These adverse effects are usually mild to moderate and tend to resolve with continued therapy. Encourage the patient not to discontinue therapy without first consulting the healthcare provider.

Neurologic

Headache. These adverse effects are usually mild to moderate and tend to resolve with continued therapy. Encourage the patient not to discontinue therapy without first consulting the healthcare provider.

Immune System, Respiratory

Upper respiratory infection. In clinical trials with GLP-1 agonists there was a higher rate of upper respiratory infection in the GLP-1 agonist–treated group than in the placebo-treated group. Notify the prescriber if symptoms of nasal congestion and sore throat develop during GLP-1 therapy.

■ Serious Adverse Effects

Metabolic

Hypoglycemia. Although GLP-1 agonists do not cause hypoglycemia by themselves, they can enhance the hypoglycemia that may be caused by a sulfonylurea or other secretagogues. Consequently, blood glucose levels must be monitored closely, especially in the early stages of therapy. Monitor for the following signs of hypoglycemia: headache, nausea, weakness, hunger, lethargy, decreased coordination, general apprehension, sweating, or blurred or double vision. Hypoglycemia must be treated immediately. Mild symptoms may be controlled by the oral administration of a glucose source (e.g., a lump of sugar, orange juice, carbonated cola beverage [not diet], candy [not chocolate]) or ingestion of a commercially prepared product such as Glutose. Severe symptoms may be relieved by IV administration of glucose, and parenteral glucagon may be prescribed in some cases. If in doubt about whether the patient is hypoglycemic or hyperglycemic, always treat the individual for hypoglycemia to prevent the possible neurologic complications that can occur from untreated hypoglycemia. Notify the healthcare provider immediately if any of these symptoms appear. The dosage of oral antidiabetic agents may also have to be reduced.

Pancreatitis. Glucagon-like peptide-1 agonists may rarely cause pancreatitis, particularly when treatment is started and following increases in dosage. Observe for signs and symptoms of pancreatitis, including persistent, severe abdominal pain that may radiate around to the back and may be accompanied with vomiting. If symptoms develop, hold the dose of medication and contact the healthcare provider.

■ Drug Interactions

Hypoglycemia. The following drugs may enhance the hypoglycemic effects of the sulfonylureas and GLP-1 agonists: ethanol, androgens (e.g., methandrostenolone), chloramphenicol, warfarin, beta-adrenergic blocking agents (e.g., propranolol, metoprolol, carvedilol), salicylates, sulfonamides (e.g., sulfisoxazole), and MAOIs.

Monitor for the following signs of hypoglycemia: headache, nausea, weakness, hunger, lethargy, decreased coordination, general apprehension, sweating, and blurred or double vision.

Notify the healthcare provider if any of these symptoms appear.

Hyperglycemia. The following medications, when used concurrently with GLP-1 agonists, may decrease the therapeutic effects of GLP-1 agonists: corticosteroids, phenothiazines, diuretics, oral contraceptives, thyroid replacement hormones, phenytoin, diazoxide, and lithium carbonate.

DRUG CLASS: DIPEPTIDYL PEPTIDASE-4 INHIBITORS

ACTIONS

The incretin hormones GIP and GLP-1 are quickly metabolized by dipeptidyl peptidase-4 (DPP-4), which results in hyperglycemia. Dipeptidyl peptidase-4 inhibitors prolong the life of active GLP-1 and GIP, prolonging the beneficial effects of the incretin hormones in reducing hyperglycemia.

USES

Dipeptidyl peptidase-4 inhibitors may be used as monotherapy or as additional therapy as an adjunct to diet and exercise to reduce elevated fasting and postprandial hyperglycemia in patients with type 2 diabetes mellitus who are taking metformin, a sulfonylurea, or a combination of metformin and a sulfonylurea, but who have not achieved adequate glycemic control. Particular benefits of DPP-4 inhibitors are that they enhance insulin secretion only in the presence of hyperglycemia, and insulin secretion decreases as blood glucose approaches normal levels.

THERAPEUTIC OUTCOMES

The primary therapeutic outcomes expected from DPP-4 inhibitor therapy are as follows:

1. A decrease in fasting and postprandial blood glucose levels and $A1_C$ concentrations in the range defined as "acceptable" for the individual patient
2. Fewer long-term complications associated with poorly controlled type 2 diabetes mellitus

❖ NURSING IMPLICATIONS FOR DPP-4 INHIBITORS

▪ Premedication Assessment

Ensure that the dosages of concurrent oral antidiabetic therapy are well adjusted before starting DPP-4 inhibitor therapy.

▪ Availability, Dosage and Administration

See Table 35-12.

Adult: Administer with or without food. Adjust DPP-4 inhibitor dosage for patients with renal impairment.

> **⚠ Medication Safety Alert**
>
> Dipeptidyl peptidase-4 inhibitors do not cause hypoglycemia by themselves, but their concurrent use with an agent known to cause hypoglycemia (e.g., sulfonylureas) should be closely monitored. Use with caution when given with other agents that may also cause hypoglycemia. A lower dose of the sulfonylurea may be required.

▪ Common Adverse Effects

Gastrointestinal

Nausea, abdominal pain, diarrhea. These adverse effects are usually mild to moderate and tend to resolve with continued therapy. Encourage the patient not to discontinue therapy without first consulting the healthcare provider.

Neurologic

Headache. These adverse effects are usually mild to moderate and tend to resolve with continued therapy. Encourage the patient not to discontinue therapy without first consulting the healthcare provider.

Immunologic and Respiratory

Upper respiratory infection, nasopharyngitis. In clinical trials with DPP-4 inhibitors, there was a higher rate of upper respiratory infection and nasopharyngitis in the DPP-4 inhibitor–treated group than in the placebo-treated group. Notify the prescriber if symptoms of nasal congestion and sore throat develop during DPP-4 inhibitor therapy.

▪ Serious Adverse Effects

Metabolic

Hypoglycemia. Patients may develop hypoglycemia when DPP-4 inhibitors are used in combination with other agents that may induce hypoglycemia (e.g., sulfonylureas). Consequently, blood glucose levels must be monitored closely, especially in the early stages of therapy.

Monitor for the following signs of hypoglycemia: headache, nausea, weakness, hunger, lethargy, decreased coordination, general apprehension, sweating, or blurred or double vision.

Hypoglycemia must be treated immediately. Mild symptoms may be controlled by the oral administration of a glucose source (e.g., a lump of sugar, orange juice, carbonated cola beverage [not diet], candy [not chocolate]) or ingestion of a commercially prepared product such as Glutose. Severe symptoms may be relieved by IV administration of glucose, and parenteral glucagon may be prescribed in some cases. If in doubt about whether the patient is hypoglycemic or hyperglycemic, always treat the individual for hypoglycemia to prevent the possible neurologic complications that can occur from untreated hypoglycemia.

Notify the healthcare provider immediately if any of these symptoms appear. The dosage of oral antidiabetic agents may also have to be reduced.

Pancreatitis. Dipeptidyl peptidase-4 inhibitors infrequently cause pancreatitis, particularly when treatment is started and following increases in dosage. Observe for signs and symptoms of pancreatitis, including persistent, severe abdominal pain that may radiate around to the back and may be accompanied with vomiting. If symptoms develop, hold the dose of medication and contact the healthcare provider.

Immunologic

Hypersensitivity. With use of DPP-4 inhibitors there have been infrequent reports of hypersensitivity reactions manifested by skin rashes, angioedema, and

 Table 35-12 Dipeptidyl Peptidase-4 Inhibitors

GENERIC NAME	BRAND NAME	AVAILABILITY	DAILY DOSAGE RANGE	MAXIMUM DAILY DOSAGE
alogliptin	Nesina	PO: Tablets: 6.25, 12.5 and 25 mg	PO: 25 mg daily	25 mg; adjust dose in renal impairment
linagliptin	Tradjenta	PO: Tablets: 5 mg	PO: 5 mg once daily	5 mg
saxagliptin	Onglyza	PO: Tablets: 2.5, 5 mg	PO: 2.5-5 mg once daily	5 mg; adjust dose in renal impairment
sitagliptin	Januvia	PO: Tablets: 25, 50, 100 mg	PO: 100 mg once daily	100 mg; adjust dose in renal impairment

anaphylaxis. If symptoms develop, hold the dose of medication and contact the healthcare provider.

■ Drug Interactions

Digoxin. Patients taking sitagliptin and digoxin concurrently may experience a 20% increase in digoxin serum levels. In most patients, this is not a particular problem, but monitor for bradycardia. Hold the digoxin dose and contact the prescriber if the heart rate is below 60 beats/min.

Hypoglycemia. The following drugs may enhance the hypoglycemic effects of DPP-4 inhibitors: ethanol, androgens (e.g., methandrostenolone), chloramphenicol, warfarin, beta-adrenergic blocking agents (e.g., propranolol, metoprolol, carvedilol), salicylates, sulfonamides (e.g., sulfisoxazole), and MAOIs.

The following drugs may inhibit the metabolism of saxagliptin, enhancing hypoglycemic effects: ketoconazole, itraconazole, telithromycin, clarithromycin, nefazodone, atazanavir, indinavir, nelfinavir, ritonavir, and saquinavir.

Monitor for the following signs of hypoglycemia: headache, nausea, weakness, hunger, lethargy, decreased coordination, general apprehension, sweating, or blurred or double vision. Notify the healthcare provider if any of these symptoms appear.

Hyperglycemia. The following drugs, when used concurrently with DPP-4 inhibitors, may decrease the therapeutic effects of sitagliptin: corticosteroids, phenothiazines, diuretics, oral contraceptives, thyroid replacement hormones, phenytoin, diazoxide, and lithium carbonate.

The following drugs may enhance the metabolism of linagliptin, reducing the therapeutic effects: rifampin, phenobarbital, phenytoin, and carbamazepine. Change therapy to another DPP-4 inhibitor.

DRUG CLASS: ANTIHYPOGLYCEMIC AGENTS

glucagon (GLŬ-kă-gŏn)

ACTIONS

Glucagon is a hormone secreted by the alpha cells of the pancreas that breaks down stored glycogen to glucose, resulting in elevated blood glucose levels. Glucagon also aids in converting amino acids to glucose (gluconeogenesis). Glucagon is dependent on the presence of glycogen for its action. It has essentially no action in cases of starvation, adrenal insufficiency, or chronic hypoglycemia.

USES

Glucagon is used to treat hypoglycemic reactions in patients with diabetes mellitus.

THERAPEUTIC OUTCOME

The primary therapeutic outcome expected from glucagon therapy is elimination of symptoms associated with hypoglycemia.

❖ NURSING IMPLICATIONS FOR GLUCAGON

■ Premedication Assessment

1. Confirm patient unresponsiveness before administration. If patient is conscious, oral antihypoglycemic therapy is usually more appropriate.
2. Hypoglycemia is a medical emergency. If suspected, it should be treated by authorized personnel as soon as possible.

■ Availability

Subcutaneous, IM, IV: 1-mg vials.

■ Dosage and Administration

Adult: Subcutaneous, IM, IV: Administer 1 mg. A response should be observed within 5 to 20 minutes. If response is minimal, one or two additional doses may be administered. If the patient is slow to arouse, consider administering glucose by the IV route.

■ Common and Serious Adverse Effects

Gastrointestinal

Nausea, vomiting. These adverse effects may also occur with hypoglycemia. Take precautions to prevent aspiration of vomitus.

■ Drug Interactions

Warfarin. Glucagon may potentiate the anticoagulant effects of warfarin if used for several days. Monitor the patient's international normalized ratio and reduce the dosage of warfarin accordingly.

Get Ready for the NCLEX® Examination!

Key Points

- Diabetes mellitus is a complex group of chronic diseases that is associated with both short- and long-term complications. The long-term objective of control of the disease must involve mechanisms to stop the progression of the complications of the disease.
- Patient education and reinforcement are extremely important to successful therapy. Major determinants to

success are the patient's taking responsibility for a balanced diet, insulin or oral hypoglycemic therapy, routine exercise, and good hygiene.
- The nurse plays a critical role as a health educator by discussing treatment options, planning lifestyle changes, counseling before discharge, and reinforcing key points during office visits. Best results are attained when the patient, family, and nurse work together in developing the care plan.

Additional Learning Resources

SG Go to your Study Guide for additional Review Questions for the NCLEX® Examination, Critical Thinking Clinical Situations, and other learning activities to help you master this chapter content.

evolve Go to your Evolve website (http://evolve.elsevier.com/Clayton) for additional online resources.

Review Questions for the NCLEX® Examination

1. The nurse is educating a new diabetic patient on how to manage dietary requirements and prevent hypoglycemia. The patient needed further teaching after he stated the following:
   1. "If I increase my carbohydrate intake, I will need to adjust my daily insulin dose."
   2. "So as I understand it, when I increase my protein intake, I can decrease my physical activity without affecting my blood sugar."
   3. "When I take a beta blocker with insulin, it can cause my blood sugar to drop."
   4. "If I take insulin and do not eat enough carbohydrates, I could become hypoglycemic."

2. After learning the symptoms of hypoglycemia, a patient performing teach-back to the nurse included all of the following in the discussion. (Select all that apply.)
   1. Hunger
   2. Rapid shallow respirations
   3. Nausea, vomiting, and abdominal pain
   4. Sweating
   5. Weakness and blurred vision

3. These types of insulin are the rapid-acting types. (Select all that apply.)
   1. Lispro
   2. Humulin R
   3. Glargine
   4. Glulisine
   5. Aspart

4. A patient who received her morning insulin at breakfast started to complain around noon about feeling shaky, off balance, sweaty, and could not focus. The nurse suspected that the patient was experiencing:
   1. lactic acidosis.
   2. kidney failure.
   3. hyperglycemia.
   4. hypoglycemia.

5. During a clinic visit 3 months following a diagnosis of type 2 diabetes, a patient reports following the reduced-calorie diet without any weight loss. The patient has also neglected to bring a record of glucose monitoring results. The best indicator of this patient's control of diabetes since the initial diagnosis and instruction is apparent using this laboratory value.
   1. Fasting glucose level
   2. Potassium level
   3. A1$_C$ level
   4. Urine ketones

6. A nurse is administering insulin subcutaneously to a patient. List in order the actions the nurse will take.
   1. Draw up insulin
   2. Document the medication
   3. Inject insulin
   4. Check the order
   5. Verify the correct patient

7. A newly diagnosed diabetic patient asks the nurse how long it takes for insulin to "kick in." The best response by the nurse would be:
   1. "Depending on the type of insulin you receive, it can take as long as 2 hours and as short as 15 minutes."
   2. "Insulin lasts as long as there is glucose circulating in your system."
   3. "The half-life of insulin is rather short, which is why you need to take it so frequently."
   4. "Insulin is only effective when it is given before a meal and only lasts as long as it takes to digest the meal."

8. A patient asked the nurse how the antidiabetic drug pioglitazone works to lower his blood glucose. The best response by the nurse is:
   1. "This medication works by stimulating the release of insulin from beta cells in the pancreas."
   2. "Unfortunately, this medications works by an unknown mechanism of action."
   3. "This is one of the antidiabetic agents that work by increasing muscle and fat tissue sensitivity to allow more glucose to enter the cell in the presence of insulin."
   4. "This medication works by affecting certain enzymes used in the digestion of sugars, which results in delayed glucose absorption."

9. The nurse is educating a patient who was admitted with peripheral edema and acute kidney injury. After discussing the complications of diabetes, the patient was able to correctly identify examples of macrovascular complications, which include: (Select all that apply.)
   1. stroke.
   2. kidney disease.
   3. nonhealing ulcers.
   4. retinopathy.
   5. myocardial infarction.

Drugs Used to Treat Thyroid Disease

Objectives

1. Describe the function of the thyroid gland.
2. Identify the two classes of drugs used to treat thyroid disease.
3. Describe the signs, symptoms, treatment and nursing interventions associated with hypothyroidism and identify the drug of choice for hypothyroidism.
4. Describe the signs, symptoms, treatments, and nursing interventions associated with hyperthyroidism.
5. Discuss the drug interactions associated with thyroid hormones and antithyroid medicines.
6. Cite the actions of propylthiouracil on the synthesis of T_3 and T_4.

Key Terms

thyroid-stimulating hormone (TSH) (THĪ-royd STĬM-yū-lā-tĭng HŌR-mōn) (p. 571)

triiodothyronine (T_3) (trī-ī-ō-dō-THĪ-rō-nēn) (p. 571)

thyroxine (T_4) (thī-RŎKS-ēn) (p. 571)

hypothyroidism (hī-pō-THĪ-royd-ĭzm) (p. 571)

myxedema (mĭk-sĕ-DĒ-mă) (p. 571)

cretinism (KRĒ-tĭn-ĭzm) (p. 571)

hyperthyroidism (hī-pĕr-THĪ-royd-ĭzm) (p. 572)

thyrotoxicosis (thī-rō-tŏk-sĭ-KŌ-sĭs) (p. 572)

iodine-131 (^{131}I) (ī-ō-d īn) (p. 576)

THYROID GLAND

The thyroid gland is a large, reddish, ductless gland in front of and on either side of the trachea. It consists of two lateral lobes and a connecting isthmus and is roughly butterfly shaped. It is enclosed in a covering of areolar connective tissue. The thyroid is made up of numerous closed follicles containing colloid matter and is surrounded by a vascular network. This gland is one of the most richly vascularized tissues in the body. It can be palpated by placing fingers on either side of the trachea and asking the patient to swallow (Figure 36-1).

As with other endocrine glands, thyroid gland function is regulated by the hypothalamus and the anterior pituitary gland. The hypothalamus secretes thyrotropin-releasing hormone (TRH), which stimulates the anterior pituitary gland to release thyroid-stimulating hormone (TSH). Thyroid-stimulating hormone stimulates the thyroid gland to release its hormones, triiodothyronine (T_3) and thyroxine (T_4).

The thyroid hormones regulate general body metabolism. Imbalance in thyroid hormone production may also interfere with the following body functions: growth and maturation; carbohydrate, protein, and lipid metabolism; thermal regulation; cardiovascular function; lactation; and reproduction.

THYROID DISEASES

Hypothyroidism is the result of inadequate thyroid hormone production. Myxedema is hypothyroidism that occurs during adult life. The onset of symptoms is usually mild and vague. Patients develop slowness in motion, speech, and mental processes. They often develop more lethargic, sedentary habits; have decreased appetites; gain weight; are constipated; cannot tolerate cold; become weak; and fatigue easily. The body temperature may be subnormal; the skin becomes dry, coarse, and thickened; and the face appears puffy. Patients often have decreased blood pressure and heart rate, elevated cholesterol levels, and develop anemia. These patients have an increased susceptibility to infection and are sensitive to small doses of sedative-hypnotics, anesthetics, and narcotics. Myxedema may be caused by excessive use of antithyroid drugs used to treat hyperthyroidism, radiation exposure, thyroid surgery, acute viral thyroiditis, or chronic thyroiditis.

Congenital hypothyroidism occurs when a child is born without a thyroid gland or one that is hypoactive. The historic name of this disease is cretinism. Fortunately, this disorder is becoming rare because most states require diagnostic testing of the newborn for hypothyroidism.

FIGURE 36-1 Palpation of the thyroid gland. (From Thompson JM, Wilson SF: *Health assessment for nursing practice*, St. Louis, Mosby, 1996.)

Although the symptoms of hypothyroidism in both infants and adults are for the most part classical, the final diagnosis is usually not made until diagnostic tests have been completed. These tests include determining serum levels of circulating T_3 and T_4 hormones. If the levels are low, the patient is considered to be hypothyroid. Further diagnostic testing is required to determine the cause of thyroid hypofunction.

Hyperthyroidism is caused by excess production of thyroid hormones. Disorders that may cause hyperactivity of the thyroid gland are Graves' disease, nodular goiter, thyroiditis, thyroid carcinoma, overdoses of thyroid hormones, and tumors of the pituitary gland.

The clinical manifestations of hyperthyroidism are rapid bounding pulse (even during sleep), cardiac enlargement, palpitations, and dysrhythmias. Patients are nervous and easily agitated. They develop tremors, a low-grade fever, and weight loss, despite an increased appetite. Hyperactive reflexes and insomnia are also usually present. Patients are intolerant of heat; the skin is warm, flushed, and moist, with increased sweating; and edema of the tissues around the eyeballs produces characteristic eye changes, including exophthalmos. Patients develop amenorrhea; dyspnea with minor exertion; hoarse, rapid speech; and an increased susceptibility to infection. Elevated circulating thyroid hormone levels easily diagnose hyperthyroidism. Further diagnostic studies are required to determine the cause.

Excessive formation of thyroid hormones and their secretion into the circulatory system causes hyperthyroidism, also known as *thyrotoxicosis*. Symptoms include increased metabolic rate, increased pulse rate (to perhaps 140 beats/min), increased body temperature, restlessness, nervousness, anxiety, sweating, muscle weakness and tremors, and a sensation of feeling too warm. This condition is treated with antithyroid drugs or surgical removal of the thyroid gland.

TREATMENT OF THYROID DISEASES

The primary goal of therapy for hyperthyroidism and hypothyroidism is to return the patient to a normal thyroid (euthyroid) state. Hypothyroidism can be treated successfully by replacement of thyroid hormones (see monographs on individual agents). After therapy is initiated, the dosage of thyroid hormone is adjusted until serum levels of the thyroid hormones are within the normal range.

Three types of treatment can be used to reduce the hyperthyroid state—subtotal thyroidectomy, radioactive iodine, and antithyroid medications. Until treatment is under way, the patient requires nutritional and psychological support.

 Life Span Considerations
Treatment of Hypothyroid State

During initial treatment of the hypothyroid state in the older adult patient, be alert for and report increased frequency of angina or symptoms of heart failure.

DRUG THERAPY FOR THYROID DISEASES

Two general classes of drugs are used to treat thyroid disorders: (1) those used to replace thyroid hormones in patients whose thyroid glandular function is inadequate to meet metabolic requirements (hypothyroidism); and (2) antithyroid agents used to suppress synthesis of thyroid hormones (hyperthyroidism). Thyroid hormone replacements available are levothyroxine (T_4), liothyronine (T_3), liotrix, and thyroid USP. Antithyroid drugs interfere with the formation or release of the hormones produced by the thyroid gland. Antithyroid agents include radioactive iodine, propylthiouracil, and methimazole.

❖ NURSING IMPLICATIONS FOR PATIENTS WITH THYROID DISORDERS

Hypothyroidism and hyperthyroidism are treated primarily on an outpatient basis unless surgery is indicated or complications occur. Nurses must be able to offer guidance to the patients requiring treatment on an inpatient or ambulatory basis. In general, body processes are slowed with hypothyroidism and accelerated with hyperthyroidism.

▪ Assessment

Take a history of treatment prescribed for hypothyroidism or hyperthyroidism (e.g., surgery, iodine-131, or hormone replacement). Ask for specific information regarding treatment for any cardiac disease or adrenal insufficiency.

Medications. Request a list of all prescribed and over-the-counter medications being taken. Ask if any of the prescribed medications are taken on a regular basis. If not taken regularly, what factors have caused the patient to decrease administration?

Description of Current Symptoms. Ask the patient to explain symptoms experienced and what changes in functioning have occurred over the past 2 to 3 months.

Focused Assessment. Perform a focused assessment of the body systems generally affected by hypothyroid or hyperthyroid states:

- Implement monitoring parameters for vital signs, intake and output, daily weights, and mental status checks. Schedule regular assessment of intake and output, vital signs, mental status, and daily weights on the Kardex or computer.

- *Cardiovascular:* Take current vital signs, including an apical pulse. Note bradycardia or tachycardia and any alterations in rhythm and pulsations (e.g., bounding or thready), subnormal or elevated temperature, and hypertension. Monitor for cardiac symptoms (e.g., heart failure). Ask whether the pulse rate is decreased or elevated on awakening, before any stimulus. Does the patient experience any palpitations or a feeling that the pulse is rapid and bounding? Record heart sounds and any abnormal characteristics heard (or have a qualified nurse perform this).

- *Respiratory:* Does the patient experience dyspnea? Is it made worse by mild exertion?

- *Gastrointestinal:* Measure the person's height and weight. Monitor the pattern of bowel elimination and give as-needed (PRN) medications prescribed for diarrhea or constipation. Ask for a history of increase or decrease in weight over the past 3 months. Has there been a change in appetite? Does the individual experience nausea and vomiting? What have the characteristics of the stools been over the past several months—constipation, diarrhea or normal? Check and record bowel sounds.

- *Integumentary:* Note the temperature, texture, and condition of the skin and the characteristics of the hair and nails. Does the patient complain of intolerance to heat or cold?

- *Musculoskeletal:* What activity level is maintained? Does the person feel or act sluggish or hyperactive? Is the pattern of activity a change from the recent past? If so, when did this become apparent? Is there muscle weakness, wasting, or discomfort? Is dependent edema present?

- *Neurologic:* What is the patient's mental status—is the patient oriented to time, date, and place? What is the degree of alertness and pace of responsiveness (e.g., sluggish and slow in contrast with being quick or fast paced). Is the individual depressed, stuporous, or hyperactive? Has the individual or family and significant others noticed any change in personality in the recent past? Has the individual had tremors of hands, eyelids, or tongue? Has the individual experienced insomnia?

- *Sensory:* What is the condition of the eyes? Do the eyelids retract, or is exophthalmos present?

- *Reproductive:* Obtain a history of changes in the pattern of menses and libido.

- *Immunologic:* Has the individual had any recent infections? What types of infections and at what frequency has the patient had infections over the last year?

Laboratory and Diagnostic Studies and Surgery. Review laboratory and diagnostic studies available on the patient's record associated with thyroid disorders such as total thyroxine (TT_4) and total triiodothyronine (TT_3), free thyroxine (FT_4) and free triiodothyronine (FT_3) tests, TSH levels, TRH stimulation test, thyroid autoantibodies, thyroglobulin, calcitonin assay, ultrasound, fine-needle biopsy, radioactive iodine uptake, electrocardiography, and thyroid scan. If surgery is scheduled for hyperthyroidism, schedule routine postoperation vital signs, and order a tracheostomy set for the bedside. Indicate on the care plan and/or computer to check dressings for bleeding, perform respiratory assessments, perform voice checks for hoarseness, and monitor for development of tetany for the first 24 to 48 hours, as ordered by the healthcare provider. Gather calcium gluconate and supplies needed for IV administration, and have them ready for use.

■ **Implementation**

Environment

- For the hyperthyroid individual, plan to provide a cool, quiet, structured environment because the patient lacks the ability to respond to change and anxiety-producing situations and has intolerance to heat.

- For the hypothyroid individual, plan to provide a warm, quiet, structured environment that supports the patient's needs. Provide support and give directions slowly and with patience because the individual may have difficulty processing the information. Incorporate the family into the provision of care, as appropriate.

Nutrition

- *Hyperthyroid*: Order the prescribed diet, usually a high-calorie diet of 4000 to 5000 calories per day with balanced nutrients. Mark the Kardex or enter data into the computer specifying no caffeine products (e.g., coffee, tea, colas) or tobacco. If diarrhea is present, mark the Kardex or enter data into the computer to check trays for any foods with a laxative or stimulating effect such as bran products, fruits, and fresh vegetables.

- *Hypothyroid*: Order the prescribed diet, usually a low-calorie diet with increased bulk to alleviate constipation. Encourage adequate fluid intake, unless comorbidities prohibit it. Encourage the patient to comply with dietary orders.

Psychosocial Care

- Mark the Kardex or enter data into the computer to monitor the mental status at least every shift.

- Plan to incorporate the family into the health teaching plan because the patient may be unable to understand or implement all facets of the therapeutic regimen.

Activity and Exercise. Enter data into the computer with the prescribed level of activity ordered by the healthcare provider. Institute safety precautions for individuals with muscle weakness, wasting, or pain that would place them at risk for injury.

Medications. Give prescribed medications and monitor for response to therapy. Transcribe orders to the medication profile or enter data into the computer. Thyroid medications usually are scheduled early in the day to prevent insomnia.

■ **Patient Education**
Medications
- Stress the need for lifelong administration of medications for the treatment of hypothyroidism and the need for periodic laboratory studies and evaluation by the healthcare provider.
- Stress that several medications interact with thyroid drugs so it is important to inform any prescribing healthcare provider of the thyroid disease and the medications being taken.
- Patients scheduled for outpatient diagnostics must receive detailed written instructions regarding the prescribed medications to be taken in preparation for testing.
- The patient and, as appropriate, family or significant others must understand the anticipated therapeutic response sought from prescribed medications. Teach specific indications of a satisfactory response to pharmacologic therapy. Stress the need to contact the healthcare provider if signs of an excess or deficit in dosage occur. Ensure that the individual can monitor the resting pulse.
Environment
- Explain the need for a cool environment for a patient with hyperthyroidism or a warm environment for the person with hypothyroidism.
- Involve the family and significant others in identifying an appropriate home environment that will support the individual's needs until the preillness status has been reached.
Nutrition
- In patients with diarrhea secondary to hyperthyroidism, explain the need for a high-calorie diet with reduced roughage.
- Explain the need for a low-calorie diet with increased roughage to the individual with hypothyroidism. Encourage patients with constipation to drink eight to ten 8-ounce glasses of water and add roughage to the diet each day.
- As the patient returns to a more normal thyroid function through medication, the caloric requirements of the diet will also change.
Psychosocial. The patient may have had a major personality change, may be depressed, or (at the other end of the spectrum) may be hyperactive. Explain these symptoms to the family and involve them in examining potential interventions that can be used in

the home environment until the individual returns to the preillness level of functioning.
Activity and Exercise
- Provide for patient safety during ambulation if muscle weakness, wasting, or discomfort is present. Discuss measures needed to provide for patient safety with the family and significant others.
- As the patient returns to a more normal thyroid function through medication, the activity level should change. Encourage moderate exercise.
Fostering Health Maintenance
- Throughout the course of treatment, discuss information about the medication and how it will benefit the patient. Recognize that nonadherence with lifelong treatment, when prescribed, may occur, and stress positive outcomes that result from regular medication adherence.
- Provide the patient and significant others with important information contained in the specific drug monograph for the medications prescribed. Additional health teaching and nursing interventions for the common and serious adverse effects are described in the drug monographs.
- Seek cooperation and understanding of the following points so that medication adherence is increased: name of medication; dosage, route, and times of administration; and common and serious adverse effects.
- When laboratory studies for thyroid function are scheduled, thyroid preparations may be discontinued for one or more days in advance of the tests. Always consult the prescriber for detailed instructions.
Patient Self-Assessment. Enlist the patient's aid in developing and maintaining a written record (see Patient Self-Assessment Forms for Thyroid Medications and Antithyroid Medications on the Evolve website). Complete the Pre-medication Data column for use as a baseline to track response to drug therapy. Ensure that the patient understands how to use the form, and instruct the patient to bring the completed form to follow-up visits. During follow-up visits, focus on issues that will foster adherence with the therapeutic interventions prescribed.

DRUG CLASS: THYROID REPLACEMENT HORMONES
ACTIONS

Thyroid hormones are either hormones extracted from animal thyroid glands or are synthetically manufactured to be equivalent to natural thyroid hormones. Triiodothyronine (T_3) and thyroxine (T_4) are normally secreted from the properly functioning thyroid gland. T_4 is partially metabolized to T_3, so therapy with thyroxine provides physiologic replacement of both hormones.

USES

The primary goal of thyroid hormone therapy is to return the patient to a normal thyroid (euthyroid) state. Several forms of thyroid hormone replacement are available from natural and synthetic sources.

Synthetic levothyroxine (T_4) is now considered the drug of choice for hormone replacement in hypothyroidism. All the U.S. Food and Drug Administration (FDA)–approved brands of T_4 are not bioequivalent. There are subtle differences in their composition. The bioavailability of a given brand at a given time after ingestion might be different. That's why endocrinologists recommend that once a brand is started, the patient should stick with the same brand. Changing brands may change the dose slightly, which in turn may change how the patient feels.

Liothyronine is a synthetic form of the natural thyroid hormone T_3. Its onset of action is more rapid than that of levothyroxine, and it is used occasionally as a thyroid hormone replacement when prompt action is necessary. It is not recommended for patients with cardiovascular disease unless a rapid onset of activity is deemed essential.

Liotrix is a synthetic mixture of levothyroxine and liothyronine in a ratio of 4:1, respectively. A few endocrinologists prefer this combination because of the standardized content of the two hormones that results in consistent laboratory test results, which is more in agreement with the patient's clinical response.

Thyroid USP (desiccated thyroid) is derived from pig, beef, and sheep thyroid glands. Thyroid USP is the oldest thyroid hormone replacement available and the least expensive. Because of its lack of purity, uniformity, and stability, however, it is generally not the drug of choice for the initiation of thyroid replacement therapy.

THERAPEUTIC OUTCOME

The primary therapeutic outcome expected from thyroid hormone replacement therapy is return of the patient to a euthyroid metabolic state.

❖ NURSING IMPLICATIONS FOR THYROID HORMONE REPLACEMENT THERAPY

■ Premedication Assessment

1. Record baseline vital signs, including apical pulse, weight, and bowel elimination patterns before initiating therapy. Establish a once-daily schedule in which these assessments are retaken. Assess for patterns that may indicate early signs of hyperthyroidism (e.g., weight loss, nervousness, diaphoresis, muscle cramps, palpitations, angina pectoris).
2. Ensure that laboratory studies (e.g., thyroid hormone levels) have been completed before administration of the medication.

■ Availability

See Table 36-1.

■ Dosage and Administration

Adult: PO: Therapy may be initiated in low dosages of levothyroxine, such as 0.05 to 0.1 mg daily. Dosages are gradually increased over the next few weeks to an average daily maintenance dosage of 0.1 to 0.2 mg. The dose should be taken on an empty stomach at least 45 minutes before ingestion of food. Most patients take it immediately upon arising, 45 minutes before breakfast.

Table 36-1   Thyroid Hormones

GENERIC NAME	BRAND NAME	AVAILABILITY	COMPOSITION	DOSAGE RANGE
levothyroxine ⇄ *Do not confuse levothyroxine with Lanoxin or leucovorin.*	Synthroid ⇄ *Do not confuse Synthroid with Symmetrel.* Levoxyl ⇄ *Do not confuse Levoxyl with Lanoxin or Luvox.*	Tablets/capsules: 25, 50, 75, 88, 100, 112, 125, 137, 150, 175, 200, 300 mcg Injection: 100, 200, 500 mcg/10-mL vial	L-thyroxine (L-T_4)	PO: Initial: 25-50 mcg daily Maintenance: 100-200 mcg daily
liothyronine	Cytomel	Tablets: 5, 25, 50 mcg	liothyronine (T_3)	PO: Initial: 25 mcg daily
	Triostat	Injection: 10 mcg/mL in 1-mL vials	—	Maintenance: 25-75 mcg daily
liotrix	Thyrolar	Tablets: 15-, 30-, 60-, 120-, 180-mg thyroid equivalents	T_4:T_3 = 4:1	PO: Maintenance: 60-180 mg thyroid equivalents daily
thyroid USP	Armour Thyroid	Tablets: 15, 30, 60, 90, 120, 180, 240, 300 mg	Unpredictable T_4:T_3 ratio	PO: Maintenance: 60-180 mg daily

Medication Safety Alert

The age of the patient, severity of hypothyroidism, and other concurrent medical conditions determine the initial dosage and the interval of time necessary before increasing the dosage. Hypothyroid patients are sensitive to replacement of thyroid hormones. Monitor patients closely for adverse effects.

■ **Common and Serious Adverse Effects**
Endocrine
Signs of hyperthyroidism. Adverse effects of thyroid replacement preparations are dose related and may occur 1 to 3 weeks after changes in therapy have been initiated. Symptoms of adverse effects are tachycardia, anxiety, weight loss, abdominal cramping and diarrhea, cardiac palpitations, dysrhythmias, angina pectoris, fever, and intolerance to heat. Symptoms may require a reduction or discontinuation of therapy. Patients may require up to a month without medication for toxic effects to fully dissipate. Therapy must be restarted at lower dosages after symptoms have stopped.

■ **Drug Interactions**
Warfarin. Patients with hypothyroidism require increased dosage of anticoagulants. If thyroid replacement therapy is initiated while the patient is receiving warfarin therapy, the patient should have frequent prothrombin time (international normalized ratio [INR]) determinations and should be counseled to observe closely for the development of petechiae, ecchymoses, nosebleeds, bleeding gums, dark tarry stools, and bright red or coffee-ground emesis. The dosage of warfarin may have to be reduced by one third to one half over the next 1 to 4 weeks.

Digoxin. Patients with hypothyroidism require a decreased dosage of digoxin. If thyroid replacement therapy is started while the patient is receiving digoxin, a gradual increase in the digoxin will also be necessary to maintain adequate therapeutic activity.

Estrogens. Patients who have no thyroid function and who start estrogen therapy may require an increase in dosage of the thyroid hormone. Estrogens increase thyroid-binding globulin levels, which reduce the level of circulating free T_4. The total level of T_4 is normal or increased. Do not adjust the thyroid hormone dosage until the patient shows clinical signs of hypothyroidism.

Cholestyramine. To prevent binding of thyroid hormones by cholestyramine, administer doses at least 4 hours apart.

Hyperglycemia. Patients with diabetes should be monitored for the development of hyperglycemia, particularly during the early weeks of therapy. Assess regularly for hyperglycemia or glycosuria and report if it occurs with any frequency. Patients receiving oral hypoglycemic agents or insulin may require an adjustment in dosage.

DRUG CLASS: ANTITHYROID MEDICATIONS

iodine-131 (^{131}I) (Ī-ō-dīn–WŬN THŬR-tē WŬN)

ACTIONS

The synthesis of thyroid hormones and their maintenance in the bloodstream in adequate amounts depend on sufficient iodine intake through food and water. Iodine is converted to iodide and stored in the thyroid gland before reaching the circulation.

Iodine-131 (^{131}I) is a radioactive isotope of iodine. When administered, it is absorbed into the thyroid gland in high concentrations. The liberated radioactive isotope destroys the hyperactive thyroid tissue, with essentially no damage to other tissues in the body.

USES

Radioactive iodine is used most commonly for treating hyperthyroidism in the following individuals: older patients who are beyond the childbearing years, those with severe complicating diseases (e.g., heart disease), those with recurrent hyperthyroidism after previous thyroid surgery, those who are poor surgical risks, and those who have unusually small thyroid glands.

It often takes 3 to 6 months after a dose of radioactive iodine to fully assess the benefits gained. Normal thyroid function occurs in about 60% of patients after one dose; the remaining patients require two or more doses. If more than one dose is required, an interval of at least 3 months between doses is required.

THERAPEUTIC OUTCOME

The primary therapeutic outcome expected from radioactive iodine is a return to a normal thyroid state.

❖ **NURSING IMPLICATIONS FOR RADIOACTIVE IODINE**
■ **Premedication Assessment**
1. Review policy for both institutional personnel and patients regarding precautions, storage, handling, administration, and disposal of radioactive substances.
2. Have all supplies immediately available in case of a spill.
3. Have all supplies needed according to institutional procedure to dispose of patient's waste, such as urine and feces, because it will be a radioactive biohazard.

■ **Availability**
Each dose is prepared for an individual patient from a nuclear pharmacy.

■ **Administration**
Administration of radioactive iodine preparation seems simple—it is added to water and swallowed. It

has no color or taste. The radiation, however, is extremely dangerous.

- Minimize exposure as much as possible. Maintain hazardous medication precautions according to the institution's policy. Wear latex gloves whenever administering radioactive iodine or disposing of the patient's urine and feces.
- If the radioactive iodine or the patient's urine or feces spills, follow institutional policy. In general, collect the clothing, bedding, bedpan, urinal, and any other contaminated materials and place them in special containers for radioactive waste disposal.
- *Avoid spills! Report any accidental contamination at once to the supervisor, and follow directions for the institution's contamination clean-up technique, and then complete an incident report.*

■ Common and Serious Adverse Effects
Endocrine

Tenderness in the thyroid gland. Adverse effects include radioactive thyroiditis, which causes tenderness over the thyroid area and occurs during the first few days or few weeks after radioactive iodine therapy.

Hyperthyroidism. A return of symptoms of hyperthyroidism occurs in about 40% of patients who have received one dose of radioactive iodine. Additional doses may be required.

Hypothyroidism. Some patients who receive radioactive iodine develop hypothyroidism, which requires thyroid hormone replacement therapy.

■ Drug Interactions
Lithium Carbonate. Lithium and iodine may cause synergistic hypothyroid activity. Concurrent use may result in hypothyroidism. Monitor patients for both hypothyroidism and bipolar disorder.

---

propylthiouracil (PRŌ-pĭl-thī-ō-YŪ-ră-sĭl)
  ⇄ *Do not confuse propylthiouracil with Purinethol.*
methimazole (mĕ-THĬM-ă-zōl)
  ⇄ *Do not confuse methimazole with methazolamide.*
  Tapazole (TĂP-ă-zōl)

ACTIONS

Propylthiouracil and methimazole are antithyroid agents that act by blocking synthesis of T_3 and T_4 in the thyroid gland. They do not destroy any T_3 or T_4 already produced, so there is usually a latent period of a few days to 3 weeks before symptoms improve once therapy has been started.

USES

Propylthiouracil and methimazole may be used for long-term treatment of hyperthyroidism or for short-term treatment before subtotal thyroidectomy. Therapy for long-term use is often continued for 1 to 2 years to control symptoms. After discontinuation, some patients gradually return to the hyperthyroid state, and antithyroid therapy must be reinitiated.

The FDA suggests that because of potential hepatotoxicity, it may be appropriate to reserve the use of propylthiouracil for those who cannot tolerate other treatments such as methimazole, radioactive iodine, or surgery. In addition, because of the potential for birth defects that have been observed with the use of methimazole in pregnant women during the first trimester, propylthiouracil may be the treatment of choice during and just before the first trimester of pregnancy.

THERAPEUTIC OUTCOME

The primary therapeutic outcome expected from propylthiouracil or methimazole is a gradual return to normal thyroid metabolic function.

❖ NURSING IMPLICATIONS FOR PROPYLTHIOURACIL AND METHIMAZOLE

■ Premedication Assessment
1. Record baseline vital signs, weight, and bowel elimination patterns before initiating therapy. Establish an alternate-day schedule in which these assessments are retaken. Assess for patterns that may indicate early signs of hypothyroidism.
2. Ensure that laboratory studies (e.g., complete blood count with differential; thyroid hormone, TSH, blood urea nitrogen [BUN], serum creatinine, liver enzyme levels) have been completed before administering the medication.

■ Availability
PO: Propylthiouracil: 50-mg tablets. Methimazole: 5- and 10-mg tablets.

■ Dosage and Administration
Adult
- Propylthiouracil: *PO:* Initially, 100 to 150 mg every 6 to 8 hours. Dosage ranges up to 900 mg daily. The maintenance dosage is 50 mg two or three times daily.
- Methimazole: *PO:* Initially, 5 to 20 mg every 8 hours. Daily maintenance dosage is 5 to 15 mg.

■ Common and Serious Adverse Effects
Integumentary

Purpuric maculopapular rash. The most common reaction (in 5% of all patients) that occurs with propylthiouracil therapy is a purpuric maculopapular skin eruption. This skin eruption often occurs during the first 2 weeks of therapy and usually resolves spontaneously without treatment. If pruritus becomes severe, a change to methimazole and the use of short-term oral steroids may be necessary. Cross-sensitivity is uncommon. These adverse effects are usually mild and tend to resolve with continued therapy. Encourage the patient not to discontinue therapy without first consulting the healthcare provider. Other adverse reactions include headaches, salivary gland and lymph node enlargement, and loss of taste.

Immunologic

Bone marrow suppression, lymph node enlargement. Routine laboratory studies (e.g., red blood cell [RBC], white blood cell [WBC], differential counts) should be scheduled. Stress the importance of the patient's returning for this laboratory work. Monitor the patient for the development of a sore throat, fever, purpura, jaundice, or excessive progressive weakness.

Gastrointestinal

Hepatotoxicity. The symptoms of hepatotoxicity are anorexia, nausea, vomiting, jaundice, hepatomegaly, splenomegaly, and abnormal liver function (e.g., elevated bilirubin, aspartate aminotransferase [AST], alanine aminotransferase [ALT], gamma-glutamyl transferase [GGT], and alkaline phosphatase levels; increased prothrombin time [INR]).

Renal

Nephrotoxicity. Monitor urinalyses and kidney function tests for abnormal results. Report increased BUN and creatinine levels, decreased urine output or decreased specific gravity (despite amount of fluid intake), casts or protein in the urine, frank blood or smoke-colored urine, or RBCs in excess of 0 to 3 per high-power field on the urinalysis report.

▪ Drug Interactions

Warfarin. Patients with hyperthyroidism require reduced dosage of anticoagulants. If antithyroid therapy is initiated while the patient is receiving warfarin therapy, the patient should have frequent prothrombin time (INR) determinations and be counseled to observe closely for the development of petechiae, ecchymoses, nosebleeds, bleeding gums, dark tarry stools, and bright red or coffee-ground emesis. The dosage of warfarin may have to be increased over the next 1 to 4 weeks.

Digoxin. Patients with hyperthyroidism require an increased dosage of digoxin. If antithyroid replacement therapy is started while the patient is receiving digoxin, a gradual reduction in the digoxin will be necessary to prevent signs of toxicity. Monitor for the development of digoxin toxicity.

Get Ready for the NCLEX® Examination!

Key Points

- Thyroid disease can be manifested as hyperthyroidism or hypothyroidism, depending on the amount of circulating thyroid hormone. These are relatively common disorders that are easily treated.
- Most therapies for hypothyroidism require lifetime treatment to maintain normal thyroid function.
- Nurses can play a significant role in education and reinforcement of the treatment plan. Best results are attained when the patient, family, significant other(s), and nurse work together in reinforcing the care plan.

Additional Learning Resources

Review Questions for the NCLEX® Examination

1. The thyroid gland functions to:
   1. regulate the metabolism of carbohydrates and proteins.
   2. release TSH.
   3. release T_3 and T_4.
   4. regulate body temperature.

2. A patient receiving levothyroxine (Synthroid) is monitored for which signs and symptoms of overdose?
   1. Bradycardia, weight gain
   2. Cold intolerance, bradycardia
   3. Palpitations, tachycardia, heat intolerance
   4. Sluggish, slow speech; increasing confusion

3. A patient comes in to the clinic complaining of weight gain even though his appetite is poor, he is feeling fatigued, and he has intolerance to cold. The nurse anticipates that the patient may be diagnosed with:
   1. hyperthyroidism.
   2. hypothyroidism.
   3. cretinism.
   4. thyrotoxicosis.

4. The thyroid hormones regulate general body metabolism such as: *(Select all that apply.)*
   1. temperature regulation.
   2. growth and maturation.
   3. reproduction.
   4. stimulating the release of TSH.
   5. maintaining sleep cycles.

5. Patients with hyperthyroidism present with the following symptoms. *(Select all that apply.)*
   1. Palpitations
   2. Bradycardia
   3. Heat intolerance
   4. Tachycardia
   5. Weight gain

6. A patient with hyperthyroidism has been prescribed propylthiouracil (Propacil), which works by:
   1. converting iodine to active iodine.
   2. blocking synthesis of T_3 and T_4 in the thyroid gland.
   3. destroying T_3 and T_4.
   4. being a synthetic form of thyroid.

7. Patients treated for hypothyroidism with levothyroxine require careful management of warfarin to prevent bleeding. This management includes: *(Select all that apply.)*
   1. frequent INR checks.
   2. increasing the dose of warfarin slowly over 1 to 4 weeks.
   3. observing for nosebleeds and petechiae.
   4. frequent assessment of TSH levels.
   5. reducing the dose of warfarin slowly over 1 to 4 weeks.

Objectives

1. Discuss the normal actions of mineralocorticoids and glucocorticoids in the body.
2. Cite the disease states caused by hyposecretion of the adrenal gland.
3. Identify the baseline assessments needed for a patient receiving corticosteroids.
4. Discuss the clinical uses and potential adverse effects associated with corticosteroids.

Key Terms

corticosteroids (kōr-tĭ-kō-STĔR-ōydz) (p. 580)
mineralocorticoids (mĭn-ĕr-ăl-ō-KŌR-tĭ-kōydz) (p. 580)

glucocorticoids (glū-kō-KŌR-tĭ-kōydz) (p. 580)
cortisol (KŌR-tĭ-sōl) (p. 584)

CORTICOSTEROIDS

Corticosteroids are hormones secreted by the adrenal cortex of the adrenal gland. Corticosteroids are divided into two categories based on structure and biologic activity. The mineralocorticoids (fludrocortisone and aldosterone) maintain fluid and electrolyte balance and are used to treat adrenal insufficiency caused by hypopituitarism or Addison's disease. The glucocorticoids (e.g., cortisone, hydrocortisone, prednisone) regulate carbohydrate, protein, and fat metabolism. Glucocorticoids have antiinflammatory, antiallergic, and immunosuppressant activity. See Drug Class: Glucocorticoids below.

❖ NURSING IMPLICATIONS FOR CORTICOSTEROID THERAPY

■ Assessment

The minimum assessment data for a patient receiving corticosteroids include baseline weight, blood pressure, and results of electrolyte and glucose studies. Monitoring all aspects of intake, output, diet, electrolyte balance, and state of hydration is important to the long-term success of corticosteroid therapy. Although many of the parameters used for assessment may initially be normal, it is important that a baseline for these parameters be established so that they may be used to monitor steroid therapy.

- Ask the patient to describe the current problems that initiated this visit or admission.
- How long have the symptoms been present?
- Is this a recurrent problem? If so, how has it been treated?
- If an infectious process is suspected, determine when the patient was last tested for tuberculosis.

History of Pain Experience. See Chapter 19, Drugs Used for Pain Management, Nursing Implications for Pain Management, Assessment, History of Pain Experience.

Medication Use. Obtain a detailed history of all prescribed and over-the-counter medications (including herbal medicines). Ask if the patient understands why each is being taken. Ask specifically whether corticosteroids have been taken within the past year and for what purpose. Tactfully determine if the prescribed medications are being taken regularly and if not, why not.

Physical Assessment

- *Blood pressure:* Take a baseline blood pressure reading in the sitting, lying, and standing positions. Because patients receiving corticosteroids accumulate fluid and gain weight, hypertension may develop.
- *Temperature:* Record temperature daily, and monitor more frequently if elevated. Patients receiving corticosteroids are more susceptible to infection, and fever is often an early indicator of infection. Glucocorticoids, however, sometimes suppress a febrile response to infection.
- *Weight and fat distribution:* Obtain the patient's weight on admission and use as a baseline in assessing therapy. Because patients receiving corticosteroids have a tendency to accumulate fluid and gain weight, the daily weight is an important tool in assessing ongoing therapy. Observe any changes in the distribution of fat and any muscle weakness or muscle wasting.
- *Pulse:* Record rate, quality, and rhythm of pulse.
- *Heart and lung sounds:* Nurses with advanced skills can perform auscultation and percussion to note

Coping With Stress

- Patients receiving high doses of corticosteroids do not tolerate stress well. Patients should be instructed to notify the healthcare provider before exposure to additional stress, such as dental procedures. If a patient sustains an accidental injury or sudden emotional stress, the attending healthcare provider should be told that the patient is receiving steroid therapy. An additional steroid dose may be needed to support the patient through a stressful situation.
- Explore the mechanisms that the person uses to cope with stress. Discuss how the patient is adapting to the needed lifestyle changes to manage the disease process. Address depression issues, if present.

Avoidance of Infections. Advise the patient to avoid crowds or people known to have infections. Report even minor signs of an infection (e.g., general malaise, sore throat, low-grade fever) to the physician.

Nutritional Status

- Assist the patient in developing a specific schedule for spacing daily fluid intake and planning sodium restrictions, as prescribed by the physician.
- If weight gain is a specific problem (not related to fluid accumulation), plan for calorie restrictions and spacing of daily intake.
- If a high-potassium diet is prescribed, help the patient become familiar with foods that should be consumed. Teach the signs and symptoms of potassium deficiency or excess, depending on medications prescribed.
- Further dietary needs may include increases in vitamin D and calcium.
- Fluid restrictions may be imposed; discuss specific ways to manage these limitations.

Activity and Exercise

- Participation in regular exercise is essential. The patient may resume activities of daily living within the boundaries set by the healthcare provider. Encourage activities such as regular and moderate exercise, meal preparation, resumption of usual sexual activity, and social interactions. Help the patient plan for appropriate alterations, depending on the disease process and degree of impairment.
- Encourage weight-bearing measures to prevent calcium loss. Active and passive range-of-motion exercises maintain mobility and joint and muscle integrity.
- Individuals unable to attain the degree of activity anticipated as a result of drug therapy may become frustrated. Allow for verbalization of feelings, and then implement actions appropriate to the circumstances.

Fostering Health Maintenance

- Throughout the course of treatment, discuss medication information and how the medication will benefit the patient.

- Drug therapy is one component of the treatment of illnesses for which steroids are prescribed; it is critical that the medications be taken as prescribed. Ensure that the patient understands the entire medication regimen, including the importance of not adjusting the dosage without healthcare provider approval. If corticosteroid therapy is to be discontinued, a tapering schedule is used. Stress the importance of not withdrawing the prescribed medication suddenly.
- Patients on steroid therapy should carry identification cards or a bracelet with the name of the healthcare provider to contact in an emergency, as well as the drug name, dosage, and frequency of use. Emphasize situations requiring healthcare provider consultation for drug dosage adjustments (e.g., stress, dental procedures, infection).
- Provide the patient and significant others with the important information contained in the specific drug monograph for the drugs prescribed. Additional health teaching and nursing interventions for common and serious adverse effects are in each drug monograph.
- Seek the patient's cooperation and understanding of the following points to increase medication adherence: name of medication; dosage, route, and times of administration; and common and serious adverse effects.

Patient Self-Assessment. Enlist the patient's aid in developing and maintaining a written record of monitoring parameters (e.g., pulse rate, blood pressure, body weight, edema, exercise tolerance, pain relief). (See the Patient Self-Assessment Form for Corticosteroids on the Evolve website.) Instruct the patient to ⓔ take this written record to follow-up visits.

DRUG CLASS: MINERALOCORTICOIDS

fludrocortisone (flū-drō-KOR-tǐ-sōn)

ACTIONS

Fludrocortisone is an adrenal corticosteroid with potent mineralocorticoid and glucocorticoid effects. It affects fluid and electrolyte balance by acting on the distal renal tubules, causing sodium and water retention and potassium and hydrogen excretion.

USES

Fludrocortisone is used in combination with glucocorticoids to replace mineralocorticoid activity in patients who suffer from adrenocortical insufficiency (Addison's disease) and to treat salt-losing adrenogenital syndrome.

THERAPEUTIC OUTCOMES

The primary therapeutic outcomes expected from fludrocortisone therapy are as follows.

1. Control of blood pressure
2. Restoration of fluid and electrolyte balance

❖ NURSING IMPLICATIONS FOR FLUDROCORTISONE

■ Premedication Assessment

1. Check the electrolyte reports for early indications of electrolyte imbalance.
2. Keep accurate records of intake and output, daily weights, and vital signs.
3. Ask the patient about any signs of infection (e.g., sore throat, fever, malaise, nausea, vomiting). Corticosteroid therapy can mask symptoms of infection.
4. Perform a baseline assessment of the patient's degree of alertness; orientation to name, place, and time; and rationality of responses.
5. Ask the patient about previous treatment for an ulcer, heartburn, or stomach pain. Testing stools for occult blood should be done periodically.

■ Availability
PO: 0.1-mg tablets.

■ Dosage and Administration
Adult: PO: 0.1 mg daily. Dosage may be adjusted as needed. Cortisone or hydrocortisone also is usually administered to provide additional glucocorticoid effect. Because fludrocortisone is a natural hormone, adverse effects reflect fludrocortisone excess, such as sodium accumulation and potassium depletion.

■ Common Adverse Effects, Serious Adverse Effects, and Drug Interactions
See equivalent section under Drug Class: Glucocorticoids below.

DRUG CLASS: GLUCOCORTICOIDS

ACTIONS

The major glucocorticoid of the adrenal cortex is **cortisol.** The hypothalamic-pituitary axis regulates the secretion of cortisol by increasing or decreasing the output of corticotropin-releasing factor (CRF) from the hypothalamus. Corticotropin-releasing factor stimulates the release of adrenocorticotropic hormone (ACTH) from the pituitary gland; ACTH then stimulates the adrenal cortex to secrete cortisol. As serum levels of cortisol increase, the amount of CRF secreted by the hypothalamus is decreased, resulting in diminished secretion of cortisol from the adrenal cortex.

USES

Glucocorticoids are usually given because of their anti-inflammatory and antiallergenic properties. They do not cure disease, but they relieve the symptoms of tissue inflammation. When glucocorticoids are used to control rheumatoid arthritis, symptom relief is noted within a few days. Joint and muscle stiffness, muscle tenderness and weakness, joint swelling, and soreness are significantly reduced. However, it is important to assess the patient's predrug activity level because pain relief may lead to overuse of the diseased joints. Appetite, weight, and energy levels are increased; fever is reduced; and sedimentation rates are reduced or return to normal. Anatomic changes and joint deformities already present remain unchanged. Symptoms usually return shortly after glucocorticoid withdrawal.

Glucocorticoids are also effective for immunosuppression in the treatment of certain cancers, organ transplantation, autoimmune diseases (e.g., lupus erythematosus, dermatomyositis, rheumatoid arthritis), relief of allergic manifestations (e.g., serum sickness, severe hay fever, status asthmaticus), and treatment of shock. They also may be used to treat nausea and vomiting secondary to chemotherapy (see Chapter 33).

THERAPEUTIC OUTCOMES

The primary therapeutic outcomes expected from glucocorticoid therapy are as follows:
1. Reduced pain and inflammation
2. Minimized shock syndrome and faster recovery
3. Reduced nausea and vomiting associated with chemotherapy

❖ NURSING IMPLICATIONS FOR GLUCOCORTICOIDS

■ Premedication Assessment

1. Check the electrolyte and glucose reports for early indications of electrolyte imbalance or hyperglycemia.
2. Keep accurate records of intake and output, daily weights, and vital signs.
3. Ask the patient about any signs of infection (e.g., sore throat, fever, malaise, nausea, vomiting). Corticosteroid therapy can mask symptoms of infection.
4. Perform a baseline assessment of the patient's degree of alertness; orientation to name, place, and time; and rationality of responses.
5. Ask the patient about previous treatment for an ulcer, heartburn, or stomach pain. Testing stools for occult blood should be done periodically.

■ Availability, Dosage, and Administration
See Table 37-1.

When a therapeutic dosage is administered for 2 weeks or longer, it must be assumed that the internal production of corticosteroids is suppressed. General guidelines are that if a patient has received prednisone 2 mg/kg/day or less, or 20 mg/day for 14 days or less, the patient does not need to be tapered off the corticosteroid. Abrupt discontinuation of glucocorticoids may result in adrenal insufficiency if higher dosages are being received. Therapy should be withdrawn gradually (often called a *steroid taper*). The time required to decrease glucocorticoids depends on the

Table 37-1 Corticosteroid Preparations*

GENERIC NAME	BRAND NAME	DOSAGE FORMS
alclometasone	Aclovate	Cream, ointment
amcinonide	—	Cream, ointment, lotion
betamethasone	Celestone, Luxiq	Tablets, syrup, injection, cream, ointment, lotion, aerosol, gel, foam, powder, solution
budesonide	Entocort EC, Pulmicort	Oral extended-release capsule, inhalation, intranasal
clobetasol	Temovate, Clobex, Olux	Cream, scalp application, lotion, gel, foam
clocortolone	Cloderm	Cream
cortisone	Cortisone	Tablets
desonide	DesOwen, Verdeso, LoKara	Cream, ointment, lotion, foam
desoximetasone	Topicort	Cream, ointment, gel, liquid
dexamethasone	Maxidex, Baycadron	Cream, aerosol, injection, tablets, elixir, solution
diflorasone	ApexiCon	Cream, ointment
fludrocortisones		Tablets
fluocinolone	Capex, Derma-Smoothe/FS Body, Synalar	Cream, ointment, solution, shampoo, oil
fluocinonide ⇄ Do not confuse fluocinonide with fluorouracil.	Vanos	Cream, ointment, gel, solution
flurandrenolide	Cordran	Cream, ointment, tape, lotion
fluticasone	Cutivate	Cream, ointment, lotion, inhalation
halcinonide	Halog	Cream, ointment
halobetasol	Ultravate	Cream, ointment
hydrocortisone ⇄ Do not confuse hydrocortisone with hydralazine or hydrocodone.	Cortef ⇄ Do not confuse Cortef with Lortab. Solu-Cortef, Hydrocortone	Cream, ointment, tablets, enema, gel, lotion, suppositories, foam, injection, oral suspension, spray
methylprednisolone ⇄ Do not confuse methylprednisolone with medroxyprogesterone.	Solu-Medrol, Depo-Medrol, Medrol	Tablets, injection, powder, suspension
mometasone	Elocon, Asmanex, Nasonex	Cream, ointment, lotion, spray, inhalant, solution
prednicarbate	Dermatop	Cream, ointment
prednisolone	Prelone, Pred Mild, Pred Forte, Veripred 20, Pediapred	Tablets, syrup, suspension, solution
prednisone ⇄ Do not confuse prednisone with potassium, Prilosec, primidone, or pseudoephedrine.	—	Tablets, solution, liquid concentrate
triamcinolone	Kenalog, Nasacort HFA, Azmacort, Triderm	Cream, ointment, lotion, injection, tablets, syrup, aerosol, paste, inhalant, spray

*Ophthalmic products, Chapter 42; nasal inhalation products, Chapter 29.

duration of treatment, dosage amount, mode of administration, and glucocorticoid being used.

- *Abrupt discontinuation:* Patients who have received corticosteroids for at least 2 weeks must not abruptly discontinue therapy. Symptoms of abrupt discontinuation include fever, malaise, fatigue, weakness, anorexia, nausea, orthostatic dizziness, hypotension, fainting, dyspnea, hypoglycemia, muscle and joint pain, and possible exacerbation of the disease process.

- *Application:* Topical corticosteroids are applied as directed by the manufacturer. Specific instructions regarding use of an occlusive dressing should be clarified before application.
- *Alternate-day therapy:* Alternate-day therapy may be used to treat chronic conditions. Corticosteroids are usually given between 6 and 9 AM on alternate days to minimize suppression of normal adrenal function. Administer with meals to minimize gastric irritation.
- *Pediatric patients:* The correct dosage for a child is usually based on the disease being treated rather than the patient's weight. Monitoring of skeletal growth may be required in children if prolonged therapy is required.

⚠ Medication Safety Alert

Glucocorticoids are potent agents that produce many undesirable adverse effects as well as therapeutic benefits. Unless immediate life-threatening conditions exist, other therapeutic methods should be exhausted before corticosteroid therapy is initiated. Many of the adverse effects of the steroids are related to dosage and duration of therapy. These drugs must be used with caution in patients with diabetes mellitus, heart failure, hypertension, peptic ulcer disease, mental disturbance, immunocompromise, and suspected infections.

■ Common and Serious Adverse Effects
Fluid and Electrolyte Disturbances
Electrolyte imbalance, fluid accumulation. The electrolytes most commonly altered are potassium (K^+), sodium (Na^+), and chloride (Cl^-). Hypokalemia is most likely to occur. Many symptoms associated with altered fluid and electrolyte balance are subtle and interspersed with general symptoms of drug toxicity or the disease process itself. Obtain data about changes in the patient's mental status (alertness, orientation, and confusion), muscle strength, muscle cramps, tremors, nausea, and general appearance (drowsy, anxious, or lethargic). Always check the electrolyte reports for early indications of electrolyte imbalance. Keep accurate records of intake and output, daily weights, blood glucose, and vital signs.

Immune System
Susceptibility to infection. Always question the patient before initiation of therapy about any signs and symptoms of possible infection. Corticosteroid therapy often masks symptoms of infection. Monitor the patient for signs of infection, such as sore throat, fever, malaise, nausea, and vomiting. Encourage the patient to avoid exposure to infections.

Psychological
Behavioral changes. Psychotic behaviors are more likely to occur in patients with previous histories of mental instability. Perform a baseline assessment of the patient's degree of alertness; orientation to name, place, and time; and rationality of responses *before* initiating therapy. Make regularly scheduled mental status evaluations, and compare the findings. Report the development of alterations.

Metabolic
Hyperglycemia. Patients with prediabetes or diabetes must be monitored for the development of hyperglycemia, particularly during early weeks of therapy. Assess regularly for hyperglycemia and report any abnormal findings. Patients receiving oral hypoglycemic agents or insulin may require an adjustment in dosage.

Gastrointestinal
Peptic ulcer formation. Before initiating therapy, ask the patient about any previous treatment for an ulcer, heartburn, or stomach pain. Periodic testing of stools for occult blood may be ordered. Antacids may also be recommended by the prescriber to minimize gastric symptoms.

Integumentary
Delayed wound healing. Patients who have recently had surgery must have their surgical sites monitored closely for signs of dehiscence. Teach surgical patients to splint the wounds while coughing and breathing deeply. Inspect surgical sites and report statements such as, "When I coughed, I felt something pop."

Sensory
Visual disturbances. Visual disturbances noted by patients on long-term therapy must be reported. Glucocorticoid therapy may produce cataracts.

Musculoskeletal
Osteoporosis. Long-term glucocorticoid therapy may produce osteoporosis.

■ Drug Interactions
Diuretics (e.g., Furosemide, Bumetanide, Thiazides). Corticosteroids may enhance the loss of potassium. Check potassium levels and monitor the patient more closely for hypokalemia when these agents are used concurrently. Many symptoms of altered fluid and electrolyte balance are subtle and interspersed with general symptoms of drug toxicity or the disease process itself.

Gather data about changes in the patient's mental status (alertness, orientation, and confusion), muscle strength, muscle cramps, tremors, nausea, and general appearance (drowsy, anxious, and lethargic). Always check the electrolyte reports for early indications of electrolyte imbalance. Keep accurate records of intake and output, daily weights, and vital signs.

Warfarin. Steroids may enhance or decrease the anticoagulant effects of warfarin. Observe for the development of petechiae, ecchymoses, nosebleeds, bleeding gums, dark tarry stools, and bright red or coffee-ground emesis. Monitor the prothrombin time (international normalized ratio), and adjust the dosage of warfarin if necessary. Because of the ulcerogenic potential of steroids, close observation of patients taking anticoagulants is necessary to reduce the possibility of hemorrhage.

Hyperglycemia. Patients with prediabetes or diabetes must be monitored for the development of hyperglycemia, particularly during the early weeks of therapy. Assess regularly for hyperglycemia and report any frequent occurrences. Patients receiving oral hypoglycemic agents or insulin may require an adjustment in dosage.

Rifampin. Rifampin may enhance the metabolism of corticosteroids, thus reducing therapeutic effect. Monitor for diminished therapeutic effect, and increase the corticosteroid dose if necessary.

Get Ready for the NCLEX® Examination!

Key Points

- Corticosteroids are potent agents that produce many therapeutic benefits as well as undesirable adverse effects.
- Many of the adverse effects of the steroids are related to dosage and duration of therapy. These drugs must be used with caution in patients with diabetes mellitus, heart failure, hypertension, peptic ulcer disease, mental disturbance, and suspected infections.
- Nurses can play a significant role in helping patients monitor therapy and can assist them in seeking medical attention at the earliest signs of impending trouble.

Additional Learning Resources

SG Go to your Study Guide for additional Review Questions for the NCLEX® Examination, Critical Thinking Clinical Situations, and other learning activities to help you master this chapter content.

evolve Go to your Evolve website (http://evolve.elsevier.com/Clayton) for additional online resources.

Review Questions for the NCLEX® Examination

1. Mineralocorticoids have the following actions in the body and are used to:
   1. regulate serum glucose levels.
   2. maintain fluid and electrolyte balance.
   3. treat hyperpituitarism.
   4. regulate body temperature.

2. Glucocorticoids regulate carbohydrate, protein, and fat metabolism and have the following properties. *(Select all that apply.)*
   1. Antiinflammatory
   2. Antiallergenic
   3. Immunosuppressant
   4. Antihypertensive
   5. Antipyretic

3. The nurse is explaining to the patient the reason for corticosteroids to be prescribed for rheumatoid arthritis. During the teach-back session, this response by the patient indicates that further teaching is needed:
   1. "I know that I can't overdo activity, even though I may be feeling less pain with the prednisone."
   2. "When I take this drug, I can gain water weight, so I need to weigh myself every day."
   3. "I should let my doctor know if I get a sore throat, fever, and start to feel crummy."
   4. "I know that this drug will cure my arthritis."

4. Patients receiving a corticosteroid should be questioned regarding any history of these disorders.
   1. Gastric ulcers
   2. Blood dyscrasias
   3. Heart disease
   4. Respiratory disease

5. These two types of electrolyte imbalances are most likely to be caused by corticosteroids.
   1. Hyperkalemia and hyponatremia
   2. Hypokalemia and hypernatremia
   3. Hypercalcemia and hypermagnesemia
   4. Hypocalcemia and hypomagnesemia

6. A 35-year-old prediabetic patient was prescribed prednisone 20 mg daily. The nurse knows that this may induce which condition?
   1. Hypoglycemia
   2. Hyperglycemia
   3. Insulin resistance
   4. No effects

7. Steroid replacement therapy needs to be gradually discontinued in small increments because:
   1. this will maintain a more normal body rhythm.
   2. this will lessen the risk of adverse effects.
   3. this will ensure that the patient's adrenal glands are able to start secreting steroids appropriately.
   4. this will decrease the risk of electrolyte imbalance.

Objectives

1. Describe gonads and their function.
2. Discuss the body changes that can be anticipated with the administration of androgens, estrogens, or progesterone.
3. Identify the uses of estrogens and progestins.
4. Compare the adverse effects seen with the use of estrogen hormones with those seen with androgens.

Key Terms

gonads (GŌ-nădz) (p. 588)
testosterone (tĕs-tŎS-tĕr-ōn) (p. 588)
androgens (ĂN-drō-jĕnz) (p. 588)

ovaries (Ō-văr-ēz) (p. 588)
estrogen (ĔS-trō-jĕn) (p. 588)
progesterone (prō-JĔS-tĕr-ōn) (p. 588)

THE GONADS AND GONADAL HORMONES

The **gonads** are the reproductive glands—the testes of the male and the ovaries of the female. In addition to producing sperm, the testes produce **testosterone**, the male sex hormone. Testosterone controls the development of the male sex organs and influences characteristics such as voice, hair distribution, and male body form. **Androgens** are other steroid hormones that produce masculinizing effects.

The **ovaries** produce estrogen and progesterone. These are hormones that stimulate maturation of the female sex organs. They influence breast development, voice quality, and the broader pelvis of the female body form. Menstruation is established because of the hormone production of the ovaries. **Estrogen** is responsible for most of these changes. **Progesterone** is thought to be associated mainly with body changes that favor the implantation of the fertilized ovum, continuation of pregnancy, and preparation of the breasts for lactation.

❖ NURSING IMPLICATIONS FOR GONADAL HORMONES

■ Assessment

History. Ask the patient to describe the current problem that initiated this visit. How long have the symptoms been present? Is this a recurrent problem? If so, how was it treated?

Reproductive. Ask the patient to describe the following, as appropriate: age of menarche; usual pattern of menses (i.e., duration, number of pads used, last menstrual period); number of pregnancies, live births, miscarriages, and abortions; vaginal discharges, itching, infections, and how treated; and breast self-examination routine (if not being performed regularly, explain the correct procedure). Male patients should be asked whether testicular self-examinations are performed (if not being performed regularly, explain the correct procedure). As appropriate, obtain information regarding impotence, sterility, or alterations in libido.

Prior illnesses. Any indication of hypertension, heart or liver disease, thromboembolic disorders, or cancer of the reproductive organs is of particular concern.

Medication. Obtain a detailed history of all prescribed medications, including oral contraceptives; over-the-counter medications, including herbal medicines (e.g., dong quai, black cohosh); and any street drugs (e.g., "muscle-building" steroids). Ask if the patient understands why each is being taken. Tactfully determine if the prescribed medications are being taken regularly and, if not, why not?

Smoking. Does the person smoke?

Physical Examination

- A complete physical examination is usually done as part of the preliminary workup before treatment of any disorders using gonadal hormones. With children and adolescent patients, include questions to collect data regarding growth and development (note in particular the development of long bones), changes in hair growth and distribution, and size of the genitalia.

- Record basic patient data: height, weight, and vital signs. Blood pressure readings are of particular concern so that recordings on future visits can be evaluated for any change.

- Collect urine for urinalysis and blood samples for hemoglobin, hematocrit, measurement of gonadotropic hormones, and other laboratory studies deemed appropriate by the healthcare provider. Usually, patients with family histories of diabetes mellitus should be tested for hyperglycemia before starting gonadal hormone therapy.
- The physical examination for a female patient should include a breast examination and a pelvic examination, including a Papanicolaou (Pap) test. Observe the distribution of body hair and the presence of scars. Stress the need for periodic physical examinations while receiving gonadal hormones.

Psychosocial. Patients requiring androgen therapy may need to be encouraged to discuss feelings relating to sexuality, sterility, or altered libido.

 Life Span Considerations

Diabetes Mellitus

Patients with diabetes mellitus who receive gonadal hormones may experience alterations in the blood glucose levels. Parameters should be established and a written record for glucose monitoring maintained for reporting to the physician or healthcare provider.

Most gonadal hormones are prescribed to patients for prolonged self-administration. Therefore planning should stress patient education specific to the type of gonadal hormone prescribed and its intended actions, including monitoring of common and serious adverse effects. Ensure that the patient understands the dosage and specific time schedule for administration of the prescribed medication.

▪ Implementation

Obtain baseline data for subsequent evaluation of therapeutic response to therapy (e.g., weight, vital signs, and blood pressure in sitting, lying, and standing positions). Assist with the physical examination.

▪ Patient Education

Expectations of Therapy. Discuss the expectations of therapy with the patient (e.g., degree of pain relief, frequency of use of therapy, relief of menopausal symptoms, sexual maturation, regulation of menstrual cycle, sexual activity, maintenance of mobility, activities of daily living and/or work).

Smoking. Explain the risks of continuing to smoke, especially when the patient is receiving estrogen or progestin therapy. (The incidence of fatal heart attacks, thromboembolic disorders, and stroke is increased for women older than 35 years.) Provide smoking cessation education.

Physical Examination. Stress the need for regular periodic medical examinations and laboratory studies.

Fostering Health Maintenance. Discuss medication information and how it will benefit the course of treatment to produce an optimal response. Seek cooperation and understanding of the following points so that medication adherence is increased: name of medication; dosage, route, and times of administration; and common and serious adverse effects. If estrogen has been prescribed for the purpose of delaying the advancement of osteoporosis, stress the importance of adhering to the regimen to achieve the maximum effect.

Patient Self-Assessment. Plan to teach the individual to monitor vital signs and weight daily. Enlist the patient's aid in developing and maintaining a written record of monitoring parameters (e.g., blood pressure, pulse, daily weight, degree of pain relief, menstrual cycle information, breakthrough bleeding, nausea, vomiting, cramps, breast tenderness, hirsutism, gynecomastia, masculinization, hoarseness, headaches, sexual stimulation). (See Appendix B: Template for Developing a Written Record for Patients to Monitor Their Own Therapy.) Complete the Premedication Data column for use as a baseline to track response to drug therapy. Ensure that the patient understands how to use the form, and instruct the patient to take the completed form to follow-up visits. During follow-up visits, focus on issues that will foster adherence to the therapeutic interventions prescribed.

DRUG THERAPY WITH GONADAL HORMONES

DRUG CLASS: ESTROGENS

ACTIONS

The natural estrogenic hormone released from the ovaries is composed of several closely related chemical compounds—estradiol, estrone, and estriol. The most potent is estradiol. It is metabolized to estrone, which is half as potent. Estrone is further metabolized to estriol, which is considerably less potent. Estrogens are responsible for development of the sex organs during growth in utero and for maturation at puberty. They are also responsible for characteristics such as growth of hair, texture of skin, and distribution of body fat. Estrogens affect the release of pituitary gonadotropins; cause capillary dilation, fluid retention, and protein metabolism; and inhibit ovulation and postpartum breast engorgement.

USES

Estrogen products are used for relief of hot flash symptoms of menopause; for contraception; for hormone replacement therapy after an oophorectomy, in conjunction with appropriate diet, calcium, and physical therapy for the treatment of osteoporosis; for treatment of severe acne in females; and to slow the disease progress (and minimize discomfort) in patients with advanced prostatic cancer and certain types of breast cancer.

Postmenopausal women with an intact uterus are at an increased risk of developing endometrial cancer with the use of estrogens alone. If estrogen therapy is indicated, it should be accompanied by progestin therapy to reduce the risk of endometrial cancer. There is no evidence that "natural" estrogens are more or less hazardous than "synthetic" estrogens at equiestrogenic dosages.

Results of a controlled study, the Women's Health Initiative (WHI), have indicated that hormone replacement therapy is associated with a small increase in the risk of coronary heart disease (CHD) (Rossouw et al, 2002). Follow-up studies reaffirm that hormone therapy is effective for relief of vasomotor symptoms associated with menopause, and that the risk of CHD tended to be reduced in women close to menopause compared with increased risk in women more distant from menopause. Based on WHI data, use of hormone replacement therapy for fewer than 5 years is a reasonable option for relief of moderate to severe vasomotor symptoms. However, prior to initiation of therapy, the patient should have a baseline risk assessment (family history of CHD, age, body weight, diabetes, smoking) and then should be monitored annually. Long-term use of hormone replacement therapy is not recommended due to the risk of stroke, venous thromboembolism, and breast cancer that has been documented in studies completed since 2002 (Rossouw, 2013).

THERAPEUTIC OUTCOMES

The primary therapeutic outcomes expected from estrogen therapy are as follows:
1. Contraception (see Chapter 40)
2. Hormonal balance
3. Prevention of osteoporosis
4. Palliative treatment of prostate and breast cancer
5. Treatment of severe acne in females

❖ NURSING IMPLICATIONS FOR ESTROGEN THERAPY

▪ Premedication Assessment
1. Determine whether the patient is pregnant before starting estrogen therapy; hold the medication and consult the prescriber if there is a possibility of pregnancy.
2. Obtain baseline weight and vital signs, especially accurate blood pressure readings.
3. Ask whether the individual has a history of thromboembolic disorders or cancer of the reproductive organs; if so, hold medication and contact the healthcare provider.

▪ Availability, Dosage, and Administration
See Table 38-1.

 Medication Safety Alert

The use of estrogens during early pregnancy is contraindicated. Serious birth defects have been reported, and it has been found that the female offspring have an increased risk of developing vaginal or cervical cancer later in life.

▪ Common Adverse Effects
Neurologic

Headache, migraine, dizziness, insomnia, anxiety, nervousness, emotional lability. These symptoms tend to be mild and resolve with continued therapy. If they do not resolve or become particularly bothersome, the patient should consult the prescriber.

Endocrine

Weight gain, edema, breast tenderness, nausea. These symptoms tend to be mild and resolve with continued therapy. If they do not resolve or become particularly bothersome, the patient should consult the prescriber.

▪ Serious Adverse Effects
The following are all complications associated with estrogen therapy. It is extremely important that the patient be evaluated by her healthcare provider for any of the following symptoms or other symptoms that the patient recognizes to be of concern.

Cardiovascular. Hypertension, thrombophlebitis, and thromboembolism.

Metabolic. Hyperglycemia.

Gynecologic. Breakthrough bleeding; long-term exposure to estrogens can increase the risks of breast, endometrial, and vaginal cancers in women. Too much estrogen aggravates endometriosis, a painful growth of the uterine lining outside the uterus, whereas too little estrogen weakens bones (osteoporosis).

▪ Drug Interactions
Warfarin. This medication may diminish the anticoagulant effects of warfarin. Monitor the prothrombin time (international normalized ratio [INR]) and increase the dosage of warfarin if necessary.

Phenytoin. Estrogens may inhibit the metabolism of phenytoin, resulting in phenytoin toxicity. Monitor patients with concurrent therapy for signs of phenytoin toxicity (e.g., nystagmus, sedation, lethargy). Serum levels may be ordered, and a reduced dosage of phenytoin may be required.

Thyroid Hormones. Patients who have no thyroid function and who start estrogen therapy may require an increase in thyroid hormone dosage. Estrogens increase thyroid-binding globulin levels, which reduce the level of circulating free thyroxine (T_4). The total level of T_4 is normal or increased. Do not adjust the thyroid dosage until the patient shows clinical signs of hypothyroidism.

DRUG CLASS: PROGESTINS
ACTIONS

Progesterone and its derivatives (the progestins) inhibit the secretion of pituitary gonadotropins, preventing maturation of ovarian follicles and thus inhibiting ovulation.

Table 38-1 Estrogens

GENERIC NAME	BRAND NAME	AVAILABILITY	USES	DOSAGE RANGE
conjugated estrogen	Premarin ⇄ Do not confuse Premarin with Prevacid. C.E.S. ♣	Tablets: 0.3, 0.45, 0.625, 0.9, 1.25 mg IV: 25 mg in 5-mL vial Cream: 0.625 mg/g	Menopause, atopic vaginitis Female hypogonadism Ovarian failure or postoophorectomy Osteoporosis Breast carcinoma Prostatic carcinoma	PO: 0.3-1.25 mg daily cyclically* Intravaginal cream: 0.5-2 g intravaginally daily cyclically* PO: 0.3-0.625 mg daily for 20 days, followed by 10 days off PO: 1.25 mg daily for 21 days, followed by 7-10 days off PO: 0.3-0.625 mg daily cyclically* PO: 10 mg three times daily for at least 3 mo PO: 1.25-2.5 mg three times daily
esterified estrogen	Menest	Tablets: 0.3, 0.625, 1.25, 2.5 mg	Menopause, atropic vaginitis Female hypogonadism, postoophorectomy, ovarian failure Breast carcinoma Prostatic carcinoma	PO: 0.3-1.25 mg daily cyclically* PO: 1.25-7.5 mg daily cyclically* PO: 10 mg three times daily PO: 1.25-2.5 mg three times daily

estradiol ⇄ Do not confuse estradiol with Risperdal.	Estrace ⇄ Do not confuse Estrace with Evista.	Tablets: 0.5, 1, 2 mg
		Injections:
		  Cypionate in oil:
		    5 mg/mL
		  Valerate in oil:
		    10, 20, 40 mg/mL
		Cream, vaginal:
		    0.1 mg/g
			Menopause, atropic vaginitis, hypogonadism, postoophorectomy, ovarian failure
			Prostatic carcinoma
			
			Breast carcinoma
				PO: 1-2 mg daily or cyclically*
				IM: Cypionate: 1-5 mg q3-4 wk
				Valerate: 10-20 mg q4 wk
				
				PO: 1-2 mg three times daily
				IM: Valerate 30 mg q1-2 wk
				PO: 10 mg three times daily for at least 3 mo

	Vivelle,† Alora, Climara, Estraderm, Menostar, Vivelle-Dot	Transdermal patch: 0.025, 0.038, 0.05, 0.06, 0.075, 0.1 mg	Menopause, female hypogonadism, primary ovarian failure, atropic vaginitis, postoophorectomy, osteoporosis prevention	Transdermal system†: patch should be placed on clean, dry area of skin on trunk (usually abdomen or buttock) twice weekly on cyclic schedule†; rotate application site; interval of 1 wk between uses of same site
	Divigel	Transdermal gel: 0.25 mg/0.25 g; 0.5 mg/0.5 g; 1 mg/g	Menopause	0.25 g applied once daily; 0.25 to 1 g daily based on symptoms
	Elestrin	Transdermal gel: 0.52 mg/0.87 g	Menopause	0.87 g applied once daily; 0.87 to 1.7 g daily based on symptoms
	EstroGel	Topical gel: 0.06% in pump	Menopause, vaginal atrophy	Topical: apply contents of one pump daily to one arm, spreading from wrist to upper arm on all sides; allow to dry; wash hands with soap and water; if uterus intact, progestin should also be taken to prevent endometrial cancer; alcohol gel is flammable until dry so avoid fire, flame, or smoking until dry
	Evamist	Transdermal spray: 1.53 mg/spray	Menopause	Topical: 1 spray once every morning May apply 1-3 sprays daily based on symptoms
estropipate	—	Tablets: 0.75, 1.5, 3 mg	Menopause, atropic vaginitis Female hypogonadism, postoophorectomy, ovarian failure Osteoporosis prevention	PO: 0.75-6 mg daily cyclically* PO: 1.25-9 mg daily cyclically* PO: 0.75 mg daily cyclically*

♣ Available in Canada.
*Cyclically = 3 weeks of daily estrogen followed by 1 week off.
†Alora, Estraderm, Vivelle, and Vivelle-Dot are applied twice weekly. Climara and Menostar are applied once weekly.

USES

Progestins are used primarily to treat secondary amenorrhea, breakthrough uterine bleeding, and endometriosis, but they may also be used in combination with estrogens as contraceptives (see Chapter 40).

THERAPEUTIC OUTCOMES

The primary therapeutic outcomes expected from progestin therapy are as follows:
1. Contraception
2. Relief of symptoms of endometriosis
3. Hormonal balance to relieve amenorrhea or abnormal uterine bleeding

❖ NURSING IMPLICATIONS FOR PROGESTINS

■ Premedication Assessment

1. Determine whether the patient is pregnant before starting progestin therapy; hold the medication and consult the healthcare provider if there is a possibility of pregnancy.
2. Obtain baseline weight and vital signs, especially accurate blood pressure readings.
3. Ask whether the individual has a history of thromboembolic disorders or cancer of the reproductive organs; if so, withhold medication and contact the healthcare provider.

■ Availability, Dosage, and Administration
See Table 38-2.

Medication Safety Alert

The use of progestins in early pregnancy has been associated with birth defects. If pregnancy is suspected, the healthcare provider should be consulted immediately.

■ Common Adverse Effects

These symptoms tend to be mild and resolve with continued therapy. If they do not resolve or become particularly bothersome, instruct the patient to consult the healthcare provider.

Endocrine. Weight gain, edema, tiredness, oily scalp, acne.

Gastrointestinal. Nausea, vomiting, diarrhea.

■ Serious Adverse Effects

The following are all complications associated with progestin therapy. It is extremely important that the patient be evaluated by the healthcare provider to consider therapeutic alternatives.

Gynecologic

Breakthrough bleeding, amenorrhea, breast enlargement, teratogenicity. Because of the possibility of birth defects, a healthcare provider should be consulted immediately.

Neurologic. Continuing headache, depression.

Gastrointestinal. Cholestatic jaundice.

Table 38-2   Progestins

GENERIC NAME	BRAND NAME	AVAILABILITY	USES	DOSAGE RANGE
medroxyprogesterone ⇄ *Do not confuse medroxyprogesterone with methylprednisolone.*	Provera ⇄ *Do not confuse Provera with Covera, Premarin, or Parlodel.*	Tablets: 2.5, 5, 10 mg	Secondary amenorrhea Abnormal uterine bleeding	PO: 5-10 mg daily for 5-10 days PO: 5-10 mg daily for 5-10 days, beginning on day 16 or 21 of menstrual cycle
norethindrone	Aygestin	Tablets: 5 mg	Amenorrhea, abnormal uterine bleeding	PO: 2.5-10 mg starting on day 20 and ending on day 25 of menstrual cycle
			Endometriosis	PO: 5 mg for 2 wk; increase in increments of 2.5 mg/day q2 wk until 15 mg/day is reached
progesterone	Progesterone	Tablets, capsules: 100, 200 mg Injection: 50 mg/mL Vaginal gel: 4%, 8% Vaginal suppositories: 25, 50, 100, 200, 400 mg	Amenorrhea, endometrial hyperplasia, functional uterine bleeding	PO: 200 mg at bedtime for 12 days sequentially per 28-day cycle for postmenopausal women with a uterus who receive daily conjugated estrogens IM: 5-10 mg for 6-8 consecutive days

- **Drug Interactions**

Rifampin. Rifampin may enhance the metabolism of norethindrone. The dosage of norethindrone may need to be increased to provide therapeutic benefit.

DRUG CLASS: ANDROGENS

ACTIONS

The dominant male sex hormone is testosterone. It is the primary natural androgen produced by the testicles. Androgens are responsible for the normal growth and development of male sex organs and for maintenance of secondary sex characteristics. These effects include the growth and maturation of the prostate, seminal vesicles, penis, and scrotum; the development of male hair distribution; laryngeal enlargement (Adam's apple); vocal cord thickening; alterations in body musculature; and fat distribution.

USES

Androgens are used to treat hypogonadism and androgen deficiency, as well as for palliation of breast cancer in postmenopausal women with certain cell types of cancer. When androgens are used for palliation of cancer in women, they suppress cancer cell growth. In addition, androgens may be used to treat wasting syndrome associated with acquired immune deficiency.

THERAPEUTIC OUTCOMES

The primary therapeutic outcomes expected from androgen therapy are as follows:
1. Restoration of hormonal balance in androgen deficiency
2. Reduced discomfort associated with breast cancer
3. Increased muscle mass

❖ NURSING IMPLICATIONS FOR ANDROGENS

- **Premedication Assessment**
1. Obtain baseline vital signs and weight, and assess mental status.
2. Check baseline electrolyte values; report abnormal findings. Be especially alert for hypercalcemia.
3. Identify baseline glucose levels for those initiating androgen therapy who are taking insulin or oral hypoglycemic agents, because the use of androgens may cause hypoglycemia.

- **Availability, Dosage, and Administration**
See Table 38-3.

- **Common Adverse Effects**
Gastrointestinal
Gastric irritation. If gastric irritation occurs, administer drug with food or milk. If symptoms persist or increase in severity, report for healthcare provider evaluation.

- **Serious Adverse Effects**
Metabolic
Electrolyte imbalance, edema. The most commonly altered electrolytes are potassium (K^+), sodium (Na^+), and chloride (Cl^-). Hyperkalemia is most likely to occur. Many symptoms associated with altered fluid and electrolyte balance are subtle and interspersed with general symptoms of drug toxicity or the disease process itself. Gather data about changes in the patient's mental status (e.g., alertness, orientation, confusion), muscle strength, muscle cramps, tremors, nausea, and general appearance (e.g., drowsy, anxious, lethargic). Always check the electrolyte reports for early indications of electrolyte imbalance. Keep accurate records of intake and output, daily weights, and vital signs. Patients should report weight gains of more than 2 pounds per week. Diuretic therapy, with or without dietary reduction of salt, may be prescribed if edema is significant.

Hypercalcemia. In immobilized patients and patients with breast cancer, androgen therapy may cause hypercalcemia. Monitor patients for nausea, vomiting, constipation, poor muscle tone, and lethargy. These are indications of hypercalcemia and are indications for discontinuation of androgen therapy. Force fluids to minimize the possibility of renal calculi. Encourage the patient to drink eight to twelve 8-ounce glasses of water daily. The patient should perform weight-bearing and active and passive exercises to the degree tolerated to minimize loss of calcium from bones.

Endocrine
Masculinization. Women receiving high doses of androgens may develop signs of masculinization. Women should be monitored for signs of masculinization (e.g., deepening of the voice, hoarseness, growth of facial hair, clitoral enlargement, and menstrual irregularities) during androgen therapy. The drug should usually be discontinued when mild masculinization is evident because some adverse androgenic effects (e.g., voice changes) may not reverse with discontinuation of therapy. In consultation with the healthcare provider, the woman may decide that some masculinization is acceptable during treatment for breast cancer. Help patients adjust to a possible change in self-image or self-esteem caused by the effects of masculinization.

Males should be carefully monitored for the development of gynecomastia, priapism, or excessive sexual stimulation. These are indications of androgen overdose.

Gastrointestinal
Hepatotoxicity. The symptoms of hepatotoxicity include anorexia, nausea, vomiting, jaundice, hepatomegaly, splenomegaly, and abnormal liver function test (e.g., elevated bilirubin, aspartate aminotransferase [AST], alanine aminotransferase [ALT], gamma-glutamyl transferase [GGT], alkaline phosphatase levels; increased prothrombin time).

Table 38-3 Androgens

GENERIC NAME	BRAND NAME	AVAILABILITY	USES	DOSAGE RANGE
Short-Acting Agents				
testosterone gel	AndroGel, Testim	Topical gel: 1%	Hypogonadism	Topical: open one or more hormone packets (depending on dosage); squeeze entire contents onto palm of hand; apply to clean, dry, intact skin of shoulders, upper arms, and abdomen; allow to dry prior to dressing; wash hands with soap and water; do not apply to genitals
testosterone USP in gel base	Androderm Transdermal System	Transdermal patch: 2, 4 mg	Androgen deficiency	Transdermal system: one to three patches applied to skin on hips, abdomen, thighs, or buttocks nightly for 24 hr; replace q24 h; do not apply to scrotum
Long-Acting Agents				
testosterone pellets	Testopel	Pellets: 75 mg	Hypogonadism; delayed puberty	Subcutaneous: two to six pellets implanted subcutaneously q3-6 mo
testosterone enanthate	Delatestryl	IM: 200 mg/mL	Eunuchism, androgen deficiency Oligospermia	IM: 50-400 mg q2-4 wk IM: 100-200 mg q4-6 wk
testosterone cypionate		IM: 100, 200 mg/mL	As for testosterone enanthate	As for testosterone enanthate
Oral Products				
testosterone	Striant	Buccal system: 30 mg	Hypogonadism	PO: One buccal system applied to gum above incisor tooth q12 h; alternate with opposite side for each new dose; when applying, hold rounded surface against gum for 30 sec to ensure adhesion; do not chew or swallow
methyltestosterone	Methitest, Testred	Tablets: 10 mg Capsules: 10 mg	Eunuchism Cryptorchidism Breast carcinoma	PO: 10-50 mg daily PO: 10 mg three times daily PO: 50-200 mg daily, in 1-4 doses
fluoxymesterone	Androxy	Tablets: 10 mg	Male hypogonadism Female breast carcinoma	PO: 2-20 mg daily, divided. PO: 10-40 mg daily, divided

Life Span Considerations

Androgens

Male children receiving androgens must have the effects of the drug on long bones monitored by periodic radiographs of long bones. Usually, radiographs of long bones are obtained every 3 to 6 months to check the status of the epiphyseal line. Androgens may prematurely close the epiphyseal line, preventing bone elongation.

■ Drug Interactions

Warfarin. Androgens may enhance the anticoagulant effects of warfarin. Observe for the development of petechiae, ecchymoses, nosebleeds, bleeding gums, dark tarry stools, and bright red or coffee-ground emesis. Monitor the prothrombin time (INR), and reduce the dosage of warfarin if necessary.

Oral Antidiabetic Agents, Insulin. Monitor for hypoglycemia: headache, weakness, decreased coordination, general apprehension, diaphoresis, hunger, and blurred or double vision. The dosage of the hypoglycemic agent or insulin may need to be reduced. Notify the healthcare provider if any of these symptoms appear.

Corticosteroids. Concurrent use may increase the possibility of electrolyte imbalance and fluid retention. See earlier in this chapter for monitoring parameters.

Get Ready for the NCLEX® Examination!

Key Points

- The gonadal hormones are necessary for the body to grow and mature into the adult form and for reproduction.
- Male and female gonads secrete hormones. The male testes secrete predominantly androgens, and the female ovaries secrete primarily estrogens and progesterone.
- These hormones are responsible for the shape and secondary sex characteristics associated with the male and female body forms.

Additional Learning Resources

SG Go to your Study Guide for additional Review Questions for the NCLEX® Examination, Critical Thinking Clinical Situations, and other learning activities to help you master this chapter content.

evolve Go to your Evolve website (http://evolve .elsevier.com/Clayton) for additional online resources.

Review Questions for the NCLEX® Examination

1. The reproductive glands of both sexes produce hormones that control the development and maturation of the sex organs. These hormones are: *(Select all that apply.)*
   1. testosterone.
   2. cortisol.
   3. progesterone.
   4. luteinizing hormone.
   5. estrogen.

2. Androgens, when given to a patient with breast cancer, may result in the development of these adverse effects. *(Select all that apply.)*
   1. Hypertension
   2. Weight gain and edema
   3. Masculinization
   4. Hypercalcemia
   5. Hyperglycemia

3. Estrogens are given to women for the following therapeutic outcomes. *(Select all that apply.)*
   1. Hormonal balance
   2. Prevention of osteoporosis
   3. Relief of headaches and insomnia
   4. Treatment of severe acne
   5. Prevention of coronary artery disease

4. When women take androgens for treatment of discomfort associated with breast cancer, symptoms of masculinization can occur, which include: *(Select all that apply.)*
   1. growth of long bones.
   2. deeper voice quality.
   3. growth of facial hair.
   4. irregular menses.
   5. shrinking breast tissue.

5. Progestin is used to treat the following conditions in women. *(Select all that apply.)*
   1. Prevent ovulation for contraceptive use
   2. Breakthrough uterine bleeding
   3. Relief of symptoms of endometriosis
   4. Treat breast cancer symptoms
   5. Hypogonadism

Drugs Used in Obstetrics

Objectives

1. Identify appropriate nursing assessments during normal labor and delivery.
2. Discuss potential complications of preterm labor and when uterine relaxants and magnesium sulfate are used.
3. Describe when uterine stimulants are administered for induction of labor, augmentation of labor, and postpartum atony and hemorrhage.
4. State the actions of clomiphene citrate and the primary use.
5. Identify the action and proper timing of the administration of Rho(D) immune globulin.
6. Cite education needed for care of the neonate, including erythromycin ophthalmic ointment and phytonadione administration.

Key Terms

pregnancy hypertension disorders (PRĔG-nĕn-sē hĭ-pĕr-TĔN-shŭn) (p. 598)
lochia (LŌ-kē-ă) (p. 599)
precipitous labor and delivery (prē-SĬP-ĭ-tŭs LĀ-bŭr) (p. 606)

augmentation (ŏg-mĕn-TĀ-shŭn) (p. 606)
dysfunctional labor (dĭs-FŬNK-shŭn-ăl LĀ-bŭr) (p. 606)

OBSTETRICS

Obstetrics is the field of healthcare practice associated with pregnancy, the health of the mother and the child, and the process of birth. The current culture is to have mothers who are expecting to deliver a child to be admitted to a hospital or birthing center and have the baby under controlled conditions. The labor and delivery process is unpredictable to some extent, and having trained clinicians present during the birth provides a sense of control. Nurses working in obstetrics are trained in assessment of the mother during the trimesters of fetal growth and the baby upon delivery.

❖ NURSING IMPLICATIONS FOR OBSTETRICS

▪ Assessment

Prenatal Assessment. Obtain basic historical information about the woman and family concerning acute or chronic conditions, surgeries, and deaths.

- Has the patient been treated for kidney or bladder problems; high blood pressure; heart disease; rheumatic fever; hypothyroidism or hyperthyroidism; diabetes mellitus; allergies to any foods, drugs, or environmental substances; or sexually transmitted infections (STIs)?

- Has the patient been exposed to any communicable diseases since becoming pregnant?
- Has the patient received blood or blood products?
- Does the patient smoke or use any substances of abuse (e.g., illicit drugs, alcohol)?

If the woman answers yes to any of these questions, find out which healthcare provider made the diagnosis, when the condition occurred, and how the condition was treated. Request the approximate date of the last Papanicolaou (Pap) test and results.

Gather data about menstrual pattern (e.g., age of initial onset, duration and frequency of monthly periods, date of last full menstrual cycle, any bleeding since the last full menstrual period) and contraceptive use (e.g., condoms, foam, diaphragm, sponge, oral contraceptives, intrauterine devices).

Take an obstetric history. Ask the woman if she has had any previous live births, stillbirths, or spontaneous or therapeutic abortions. If any of the deliveries were premature, obtain additional information about the infant's gestational age, survival of the child, suspected causes of prematurity, and infections. Ask whether any of the births required a cesarean delivery. If yes, ask why. Ask if Rho(D) immune globulin (RhoGAM) has been given for Rh factor incompatibility.

Nutritional history

- What is the patient's usual or prepregnant weight? How much weight has she gained or lost in the past 3 months?
- What are the woman's favorite foods? Are there any foods that she avoids? How often does she eat? What has she eaten in the past 3 days? Does she normally take daily vitamins, minerals, or herbal products?
- Are there any cultural food practices to be maintained during the pregnancy?

Elimination pattern

- What is the patient's elimination pattern?
- How often does she have bowel movements?
- What is the stool consistency and color?
- Is there any bleeding?
- Are laxatives ever needed? If so, how often?

Psychosocial cultural history

- Determine how the woman feels about this pregnancy (e.g., excited, nervous, or if the baby is not intended).
- Determine cultural patterns regarding prenatal care (e.g., language spoken, activities that she cannot do while pregnant, whether she prefers a female caregiver). Ask the pregnant woman what specific cultural practices she would like to follow during the pregnancy.
- Who makes up her support group: husband, boyfriend, friends, partner, family, tribal healer?
- Ask about her employment status and what type of work she performs.
- Determine the woman's level of education, economic status, and general interest in learning more about effective management of the pregnancy. Will referral to social services agencies be necessary?

Medication history. Ask the woman if she takes any prescribed medications, over-the-counter (OTC) medications, or herbal remedies. If she is not currently taking any medications, ask whether she has taken any over the past 6 months. Determine which have been prescribed and for what purpose.

Determine the use of alcohol and street or recreational drugs of any type, including what, how much, and how frequently.

Physical examination. Assist the woman to undress and prepare for examination, including a pelvic examination and Pap smear.

- *Height and weight:* Record height and weight. (See an obstetric textbook for a detailed guide to all aspects of a prenatal visit and the initial assessments performed.)
- *Hypertension:* Take the blood pressure. Ask if any treatment has been given for high blood pressure. If so, inquire about the onset, treatment, and degree of control achieved.
- *Heart rate:* At prenatal visits, count the pulse for 1 full minute. Report irregularities in rate, rhythm, or volume. On subsequent visits, anticipate an increase in rate of approximately 10 beats/min during the course of the pregnancy.
- *Respirations:* Record the rate of respirations. As the pregnancy progresses, observe for hyperventilation and thoracic breathing.
- *Temperature:* If the temperature is elevated, ask about any signs of infection or exposure to people with known communicable diseases.
- *Laboratory and diagnostic studies:* Obtain a urine specimen using the clean-catch method.
- *Blood tests:* Testing for complete blood count (CBC), hemoglobin, hematocrit, hemoglobin electrophoresis, rubella titer, Rh factor, and STIs (e.g., syphilis, gonorrhea, chlamydia) may be ordered at this initial visit. These may include antibody, sickle cell, and thalassemia screens; folic acid level; and, as appropriate, purified protein derivative, human immunodeficiency virus (HIV), hepatitis B screen, and toxicology screen. With a history of diabetes, hypertension, or renal disease, additional laboratory testing may be ordered (e.g., 1-hour glucose tolerance, creatinine clearance, total protein excretion).

Assessment During First, Second, and Third Trimesters. Assessment done at routine visits during the pregnancy includes weight; measurement of blood pressure, pulse, and respirations; and examination of the abdomen, with measurement of fundal height and fetal heart sounds. Any problems or concerns should be discussed. Hemoglobin and hematocrit may be periodically rechecked.

The pregnant woman who is not experiencing complications is usually examined monthly for the first 6 months, every 2 weeks in the seventh and eighth months, and weekly during the last month. Vaginal examinations are usually performed on the initial visit and are not repeated until 2 to 3 weeks before the estimated date of delivery or estimated date of birth, or due date, at which time the cervical status, degree of engagement, and fetal presentation are evaluated. A sonogram may be obtained in early pregnancy.

Assessment of the Pregnant Patient at Risk. Assess for signs and symptoms of potential obstetric complications (see an obstetrics text for further details of each complication): infection, hyperemesis gravidarum, abortion, preterm labor, premature rupture of membranes (PROM), gestational diabetes, preeclampsia, HELLP (*h*emolysis, *e*levated *l*iver enzymes, and *l*ow *p*latelet count) syndrome, and intrauterine fetal death.

- *Infection:* Record the patient's temperature. Report any elevations to the healthcare provider immediately for further evaluation. As appropriate, obtain urine for urinalysis.
- *Hyperemesis gravidarum:* Obtain details of persistent, severe vomiting.
- *Early pregnancy loss, placental separation, abortion:* Assess for signs of bleeding. Gather specific

information about the onset, duration, volume (number of pads used), and color and report any clots or tissue.

- Ask the patient to describe any pain experienced using a scale of 0 to 10. Has she had any backache or pelvic cramping, sharp abdominal pain, faintness, or pain in the shoulder area?
- Vital signs should be taken and compared with baseline data whenever bleeding is suspected. Assess for development of shock—restlessness, perspiration, pallor, clammy skin, dyspnea, tachycardia, and blood pressure changes. Record fetal heart tones at regular intervals.
- *Preterm labor:* Preterm labor is defined as:
  - Labor occurring after 20 and before 37 completed weeks of gestation *plus*
  - Clinically documented uterine contractions (4/20 minutes or 6/60 minutes) *plus*
  - Ruptured membranes *or*
  - Intact membranes and cervical dilation greater than 2 cm *or*
  - Intact membranes and cervical effacement greater than 80% *or*
  - Intact membranes and cervical change during observation.

These can be measured by changes in dilation or effacement, or by changes in cervical length measured clinically, or by ultrasound.

A fetal fibronectin test (FFN) may be ordered to assess the presence of preterm labor in patients whose presenting symptoms are questionable so that early intervention (e.g., tocolytic therapy, corticosteroids, transport to a tertiary center) can be initiated when indicated or, if negative, unnecessary interventions can be avoided. This test is for women with intact membranes and cervical dilation of less than 3 cm. This test may detect the probability of preterm labor from 24 to 34 weeks' gestation. If the test is negative, the patient is unlikely to experience preterm delivery in the next 7 to 14 days (Figure 39-1). Home uterine activity monitoring using a tocodynamometer may be used to detect excessive uterine contractions.

- *Premature rupture of membranes:* Assess for and obtain specifics of any signs of leakage of amniotic fluid from the vagina.
- *Gestational diabetes:* Review urinalysis reports for glycosuria. Review history of symptoms, especially during previous pregnancies. Review 1- and 3-hour glucose tolerance blood test results.
- *Pregnancy hypertension disorders:* Assess for and report sudden hypertension (an elevation of systolic pressure 30 mm Hg or more above prior readings, systolic blood pressure of 140 mm Hg or more, or diastolic pressure of 90 mm Hg or more). **Pregnancy hypertension disorders** include preeclampsia (elevated blood pressure; proteinuria due to hypoperfusion secondary to a vasospastic process that affects the fetus, the placenta, and maternal organs

and vasculature) and eclampsia (convulsions accompanying preeclampsia).

- Assess for edema of any body parts (e.g., fingers, hands, face, legs, ankles). Assess hydration status, and, in particular, obtain daily weights.

Life Span Considerations

The status of the fetus may be assessed by fetal movement counts, contraction stress testing, biophysical profile, and ultrasonography for placental placement and measurement of maturity indicators. Amniocentesis may be performed to assess fetal lung maturity and detect fetal disorders.

Review laboratory reports for indications of abnormal electrolytes, elevated uric acid or hematocrit levels, thrombocytopenia, and the presence of red blood cells (RBCs) and protein in the urine.

- Assess for signs and symptoms of seizure activity.
- Monitor fetal heart rate and movements.
- Assess for start of labor or signs of other complications, such as pulmonary edema, disseminated intravascular coagulation (DIC), heart failure, abruptio placentae, or cerebral hemorrhage.

When giving magnesium sulfate for preeclampsia, assess deep tendon reflexes, respiratory status (report depression), sedation level, intake and output, seizure precautions, and cardiac status. (Always have calcium gluconate, the antidote for magnesium sulfate, available.)

Assessment During Normal Labor and Delivery

History of pregnancy. On admission to the hospital, obtain the following information:

- Name and age
- Obstetric history (gravida, para, abortions, fetal deaths, birth weight of previous children, and complications during previous deliveries)
- Estimated due date, estimated gestational age, and day of last menstrual period
- Prenatal care (type and amount, any significant problems)
- Prenatal education (type and extent of childbirth preparation)
- Plan for infant feeding
- Status of membranes (intact, ruptured, time ruptured, amount, and color of fluid that escaped)
- Status of labor (time of onset of contractions, frequency, duration and intensity, how patient is coping with contractions)
- Time of last meal

Physical examination. The physical examination should include the following:

- Height, weight, vital signs (temperature, blood pressure, pulse, and respirations)
- State of hydration, including presence of edema
- Size and contour of abdomen and fundus
- Frequency of contractions
- Fetal heart rate

The progestin-only pills, or minipills, represent a common form of oral contraceptive therapy. Many adverse effects of combination-type contraceptives are caused by the estrogen component of the tablet. For those women particularly susceptible to adverse effects of estrogen therapy, the minipill provides an alternative. Women who might prefer the minipill are those with a history of migraine headaches, hypertension, mental depression, weight gain, and breast tenderness and those who want to breastfeed postpartum. The minipill is not without its disadvantages, however. Between 30% and 40% of women taking the minipill continue to ovulate. **Dysmenorrhea,** manifested by irregular periods, infrequent periods, and spotting between periods, is common in women taking the minipill. Birth control is maintained by progestin activity on cervical mucus, uterine and fallopian transport, and implantation. There is a slightly higher incidence of both uterine and tubal pregnancies.

New dosage forms for oral contraceptives have become available that are known as extended- and continuous-cycle oral contraceptives. These new monophasic combination oral contraceptives are given in the following regimens: 24 days, followed by placebo for 4 days (24/4; e.g., Yaz, Loestrin 24 Fe, Gianvi); 84 days, followed by placebo for 7 days (84/7; e.g., Jolessa, Quasense, Introvale); or continuously (without placebo; Amethyst). A primary purpose for these contraceptive products is to shorten the duration of menses, decreasing the frequency to four times per year, or completely eliminating menses. With sustained hormone use, there is greater suppression of endometrial growth, reducing pregnancy risk, and a lighter period, if any, lasting about 2 days during the 7 days off the active tablets (84/7 regimen). Other advantages to these products, in addition to fewer periods, is a lower cumulative dose of hormones taken compared with oral contraceptives cycled monthly, and the alleviation of symptoms of coexisting medical conditions that may be exacerbated during menses, e.g., anemia.

Clinical trials indicate that extended- and continuous-cycle oral contraceptives are as effective in preventing pregnancy as monthly oral contraceptives. The new products have similar adverse effect profiles; the only significantly different adverse effect compared with monthly oral contraceptives is a change in bleeding pattern. These oral contraceptives are associated with more breakthrough bleeding and spotting than the monthly oral contraceptive pills.

Cigarette smoking increases the risk of serious adverse cardiovascular effects (e.g., blood clots) in persons who both smoke and use combination oral contraceptives. This risk increases with age and heavy smoking (at least 15 cigarettes daily), and is quite significant in women older than 35 years. Women who use oral contraceptives are strongly encouraged not to smoke.

THERAPEUTIC OUTCOME

The primary therapeutic outcome associated with oral contraceptive therapy is prevention of pregnancy.

❖ NURSING IMPLICATIONS FOR ORAL CONTRACEPTIVES

■ Premedication Assessment

1. Review the medical history. If there is a history of obesity, smoking, hypertension, gallbladder disease, diabetes mellitus, severe varicose veins, seizure disorders, oligomenorrhea or amenorrhea, rheumatic heart disease, thromboembolic disease, stroke, malignancy of breast or the reproductive system, renal or liver disease, severe mental depression, suspected pregnancy, or repeated contraceptive failure, consult with a healthcare provider before dispensing birth control pills.
2. Take a baseline body weight measurement, along with blood pressure measurement in the supine and sitting positions.
3. Ensure that a pregnancy test has been given and that the patient is not pregnant.

■ Availability

See Tables 40-2, 40-3, 40-4, and 40-5 and Box 40-3.

■ Dosage and Administration

The estrogenic component of the combination-type pills is responsible for most of the adverse effects associated with therapy. The U.S. Food and Drug Administration (FDA) has recommended that therapy be initiated with a product containing a low dose of estrogen. Adverse effects must be reviewed in relation to individual case histories, but many healthcare providers initiate therapy with products similar to Norinyl 1 + 50 or Ortho-Novum 1/50. Therapy, and therefore products, may be adjusted based on the incidence and type of adverse effects.

Before Initiating Therapy. The patient should have a complete physical examination that includes blood pressure, body weight, pelvic and breast examinations, Pap smear, urinalysis, and hemoglobin or hematocrit.

Instructions for Using Combination Oral Contraceptives. Start the first pill on the first Sunday after period begins. Take one pill daily, at the same time, until the pack is gone. If using a 21-day pack, wait 1 week and restart on the next Sunday. If using a 28-day pack, start a new pack the day after finishing the last pack. Full protection by the pill during the first month may not occur, so the use of an additional form of birth control (condoms, foam) during the first month is advised. If the product prescribed also contains an iron supplement, be sure to take the 7 inert tablets monthly. The iron supplement is in the 7 inert tablets, not the 21 tablets containing hormones. (Many women skip the inert tablets each month, thinking that they have no benefit.)

- *Missed pills:* Take the pill as soon as a missed pill is remembered; take the next pill at the regularly scheduled time. If two pills are missed, take two pills as soon as remembered and two pills the next day. Spotting may occur when two pills are missed. Use another form of birth control (condoms, foam) until the pack of pills is finished. If *three or more pills* are missed, start using another form of birth control immediately. Start a new pack of pills on the next Sunday even if menstruating. Discard the old pack of pills. Use other forms of birth control through the next month after missing three or more pills.
- *Missed pills and skipped periods:* Return to healthcare provider for a pregnancy test.
- *Skipping one period but not missing a pill:* It is not uncommon for a woman to miss a period occasionally when on the pill. Start the next pack on the appropriate Sunday.
- *Spotting for two or more cycles:* See the healthcare provider. A dosage adjustment may be necessary.
- *Periodic examinations:* A yearly examination should include blood pressure tests, pelvic examination, urinalysis, breast examination, and Pap smear.
- *Discontinuing the pill for conception:* Because of a possibility of birth defects, the pill should be discontinued 3 months before attempting pregnancy. Use other methods of contraception for these 3 months.
- *Duration of oral contraceptive therapy:* Many healthcare providers prefer to have patients discontinue the pill for 3 of every 28 months. This allows the body to return to a normal cycle. Be sure to use other forms of contraception during this time. Long-term use (3 or more years) must be determined on an individual basis.
- *Serious adverse effects to be reported as soon as possible:* Severe headaches, dizziness, blurred vision, leg pain, shortness of breath, chest pain, and acute abdominal pain. Although these adverse effects are usually of minor consequence, a more serious condition must be ruled out.

NOTE: When being seen by a healthcare provider or a dentist for other reasons, be sure to mention taking oral contraceptives.

Instructions for Using the Minipill. Start using the minipill on the first day of menstruation. Take one tablet daily, every day, regardless of when the next period is. Tablets should be taken at approximately the same time every day.

- *Missed pills:* If one pill is missed, take it as soon as remembered, and take the next pill at the regularly scheduled time. Use another form of birth control until the next period. If two pills are missed, take one of the missed pills immediately and take the regularly scheduled pill for that day on time. The next day, take the regularly scheduled pill and the other missed pill. Use another method of birth control until the next period.

- *Missed periods:* Some women note changes in the time as well as duration of their periods while using minipills. This is to be expected. If menses is every 28 to 30 days, ovulation may still be occurring. For maximal safety, use alternative forms of contraception on days 10 through 18. If irregular bleeding occurs every 25 to 45 days, ovulation is probably not regular. If all tablets are taken correctly but no period has resulted for more than 60 days, speak to the healthcare provider about a pregnancy test.
- NOTE: Report sudden, severe abdominal pain, with or without nausea and vomiting, to the healthcare provider immediately. There is a higher incidence of ectopic pregnancy with the minipill because it does not inhibit ovulation in all women.
- *Serious adverse effects to be reported as soon as possible:* Severe headaches, dizziness, blurred vision, leg pain, shortness of breath, chest pain, and acute abdominal pain. Although these adverse effects are usually of minor consequence, a more serious condition must be ruled out.
- *Duration of oral contraceptive therapy:* Many healthcare providers prefer to have their patients discontinue the pill for 3 of every 28 months. This allows the body to return to a normal cycle. Be sure to use other forms of contraception during this time. Long-term use (3 or more years) must be determined on an individual basis.
- *Discontinuing the pill for conception:* Because of a possibility of birth defects, discontinue the pill 3 months before attempting pregnancy. Use other methods of contraception for these 3 months.

■ Common Adverse Effects

These are the most common adverse effects of hormonal contraceptive therapy. If these symptoms are not resolved after 3 months of therapy, the woman should return to her healthcare provider for reevaluation and a possible change in prescription.

Gastrointestinal. Nausea.

Gynecologic, Hormonal. Weight gain, spotting, changed menstrual flow, missed periods, chloasma.

Psychological, Neurologic. Depression, mood changes, headaches.

■ Serious Adverse Effects

The following symptoms represent the development of secondary disorders. Examination, a change in oral contraceptive, and possible treatment with other medications may be necessary.

Gynecologic. Vaginal discharge, breakthrough bleeding, yeast infection.

Neurologic

Blurred vision, severe headaches, dizziness. Report as soon as possible. These adverse effects are usually of minor consequence, but they may be early indications of serious adverse effects.

Cardiovascular

Leg pain, chest pain, shortness of breath. Report as soon as possible; these may be early indications of serious adverse effects.

Gastrointestinal

Acute abdominal pain. Report as soon as possible; this may be an early indication of serious adverse effects.

■ Drug Interactions

Drugs That Reduce Therapeutic Effects

- Barbiturates, carbamazepine, oxcarbazepine, felbamate, phenytoin, primidone, topiramate, St. John's wort, and the antiviral protease inhibitors (e.g., saquinavir, ritonavir, indinavir, nelfinavir, amprenavir) may increase the rate of metabolism of the oral contraceptive hormones in the liver, possibly decreasing their contraceptive effect. An alternative or additional form of birth control is advisable during concurrent use.

- Antibacterial agents (e.g., penicillins, tetracyclines, rifampin, isoniazid, griseofulvin) apparently alter metabolism of hormones in the gut, making the contraceptive less effective. An alternative or additional form of birth control is advisable during concurrent use.

 Herbal Interactions

St. John's Wort

St. John's wort may increase the liver's metabolism of oral contraceptive hormones, possibly resulting in decreased contraceptive effect. An alternative or additional form of birth control is advisable during concurrent use.

Drugs That Enhance Therapeutic and Toxic Effects. Itraconazole and ketoconazole may inhibit the metabolism of oral contraceptives. Menstrual irregularities also may be noted. Adjustment of hormone dosage may be necessary.

Warfarin. Oral contraceptives may diminish or enhance the anticoagulant effects of warfarin. Monitor the prothrombin time and the international normalized ratio, and adjust the dosage of warfarin if necessary.

Phenytoin. Monitor patients with concurrent therapy for signs of breakthrough seizures or phenytoin toxicity—nystagmus, sedation, and lethargy. Serum levels may be ordered, and a change in dosage of phenytoin may be required.

Thyroid Hormones. Patients who have no thyroid function and who start estrogen therapy may require an increase in thyroid hormone dosage. Estrogens increase thyroid-binding globulin levels, which reduce the level of circulating free thyroxine (T_4). The total level of T_4 is either normal or increased. Do not adjust the thyroid hormone dosage until the patient shows clinical signs of hypothyroidism.

Benzodiazepines. Oral contraceptives appear to have a variable effect on the metabolism of benzodiazepines. Those that have reduced metabolism with an increase in therapeutic response and toxic effect are alprazolam, clorazepate, chlordiazepoxide, diazepam, flurazepam, halazepam, and prazepam. Benzodiazepines that have enhanced metabolism and reduced therapeutic activity when taken with oral contraceptives are lorazepam, oxazepam, and temazepam. Adjust the dosage of benzodiazepine accordingly.

DRUG CLASS: TRANSDERMAL CONTRACEPTIVES

norelgestromin–ethinyl estradiol transdermal system (nōr-ĕl-JĚS-trō-mĭn)
   Ortho Evra, Xulane (ŌR-thō ĔV-ră, ZŪ-lān)

ACTIONS

Ethinyl estradiol, an estrogen, and norelgestromin, a progestin, work together as a contraceptive by inhibiting ovulation. Estrogens block pituitary release of FSH, preventing the ovaries from developing a follicle that releases an ovum. Progestins inhibit pituitary release of LH, the hormone responsible for releasing an ovum from a follicle. Other mechanisms play a contributory role in preventing conception. Estrogens and progestins alter cervical mucus by making it thick and viscous, inhibiting sperm migration. Hormones also change the endometrial wall, impairing implantation of the fertilized ovum.

USES

The transdermal contraceptive system works very much like the combination oral contraceptives, except that the estrogen and progestin hormones are in a transdermal patch dosage form that is applied weekly for 3 weeks. During the fourth week of the menstrual cycle, no patch is worn, and withdrawal bleeding (menses) should begin.

In November 2005, the FDA issued a cautionary note about concern for greater exposure to estrogens from the patch compared with taking a similar oral contraceptive tablet product. In general, increased estrogen exposure increases the risk of blood clots. Although the FDA believes that the transdermal contraceptive system is a safe and effective method of contraception, the FDA encourages women to discuss the issue with their healthcare provider, particularly if they are at higher risk for cardiovascular diseases based on the presence of hypertension, obesity, diabetes, smoking, and/or age.

Cigarette smoking increases the risk of serious adverse cardiovascular effects (e.g., blood clots) in those who both smoke and use combination contraceptives. This risk increases with age and heavy smoking (at least 15 cigarettes per day) and is significant in women older than 35 years. Women who use combination contraceptives such as the transdermal patch are strongly encouraged not to smoke.

THERAPEUTIC OUTCOME

The primary therapeutic outcome associated with transdermal contraceptive therapy is prevention of pregnancy.

❖ NURSING IMPLICATIONS FOR TRANSDERMAL CONTRACEPTIVES

▪ Premedication Assessment

1. Review the medical history. If there is a history of hypertension, gallbladder disease, diabetes mellitus, severe varicose veins, seizure disorders, oligomenorrhea or amenorrhea, rheumatic heart disease, thromboembolic disease, stroke, malignancy of breast or the reproductive system, renal or liver disease, severe mental depression, suspected pregnancy, or repeated contraceptive failure, or if the patient smokes, consult with the healthcare provider before dispensing birth control patches.
2. Take a baseline blood pressure in the supine and sitting positions.
3. Ensure that a pregnancy test has been given and that the patient is not pregnant.

▪ Availability

Transdermal patch: 6 mg norelgestromin and 0.75 mg ethinyl estradiol per patch. The patch releases 150 mcg of norelgestromin and 20 mcg of ethinyl estradiol per 24 hours.

▪ Implementation

Before Initiating Therapy. The patient should have a complete physical examination that includes blood pressure, pelvic and breast examinations, Pap smear, urinalysis, and hemoglobin or hematocrit. A pregnancy test should be performed on sexually active female patients.

Instructions for Using Transdermal Contraceptives. A new patch should be applied on the same day of the week. This day is known as "patch change day." The patch should be applied to clean, dry, intact, healthy skin on the buttock, abdomen, upper outer arm, or upper torso in a place where it will not be rubbed by tight clothing. Patches should not be placed on red irritated skin or on the breasts. Patches should not be cut. Topical products such as makeup, powder, lotions, or creams should not be applied to the skin or to the patch area because the patch may not adhere properly and absorption of the hormones may be impaired.

Select one of the following methods:

- *First day start:* Apply the first patch during the first 24 hours of the menstrual period. Note on a calendar the day of the week as a reminder of patch change day. If the patch is started after the first 24 hours of the menstrual cycle, a nonhormonal backup contraceptive (condoms, spermicidal foam, diaphragm) should be used concurrently for the first 7 consecutive days of the first cycle.
- *Sunday start:* Start the first patch on the first Sunday after menses begins. A nonhormonal backup contraceptive (condoms, spermicidal foam, diaphragm) should be used concurrently for the first 7 consecutive days of the first cycle.

> ## ⓘ Medication Safety Alert
>
> When removing the patch, dispose of it properly. Fold the used patch over on itself and place in a sturdy container, preferably with a child-resistant cap, and discard in a waste receptacle out of reach of children and pets. It still contains active hormone residual. Do not flush down the toilet.

If a patch is partially or completely detached:

- *For less than 24 hours:* Try to reapply the patch in the same place or replace it with a new patch immediately. No backup contraception is necessary. Patch change day will remain the same. Do not try to reapply the patch if the adhesive will not adhere to the skin. Do not use other adhesives or tape to hold a patch in place. Apply a new patch in a different location.
- *For more than 24 hours or if not sure how long since detachment:* Because there may be a lack of protection from pregnancy, stop the current contraceptive cycle and start a new cycle immediately by applying a new patch. This is a "new day 1" and a new patch change day. A nonhormonal backup contraceptive (condoms, spermicidal foam, diaphragm) should be used concurrently for the first 7 consecutive days of the new cycle.

If a woman forgets to change the patch:

- *At the start of any patch cycle (week 1/day 1):* There may be a lack of protection from pregnancy. Apply the new patch as soon as it is remembered. This is a new day 1 and a new patch change day. A nonhormonal backup contraceptive (condoms, spermicidal foam, diaphragm) should be used concurrently for the first 7 consecutive days of the new cycle.
- In the middle of the patch cycle (week 2/day 8 or week 3/day 15):
  - *For up to 48 hours:* Apply a new patch immediately. The next patch should be applied on the usual patch change day. No backup contraception is needed.
  - *For more than 48 hours:* Because there may be a lack of protection from pregnancy, stop the current contraceptive cycle and start a new 4-week cycle immediately by applying a new patch. This is a new day 1 and a new patch change day. A nonhormonal backup contraceptive (condoms, spermicidal foam, diaphragm) should be used concurrently for the first 7 consecutive days of the new cycle.

- *At the end of the patch cycle (week 4/day 22):* The patch should be removed as soon as the woman remembers to remove it. The new cycle should be started on the usual patch change day, which is the day after day 28. No backup contraception is needed.
- *Switching from oral contraceptives to the patches:* Apply a patch on the first day of the menses. If there is no withdrawal bleeding within 5 days of the last active hormone tablet (after day 21), a pregnancy test should be completed to ensure that there is no pregnancy before the patch is started.

Missed patches and skipped periods:

- Return to the healthcare provider for a pregnancy test.
- *Skipping one period but not missing a patch:* It is not uncommon for a woman to occasionally miss a period when receiving hormone therapy. Start the next cycle on the same patch change day. If two consecutive periods are missed, a pregnancy test is in order. Contraceptive therapy should be discontinued if pregnancy is confirmed.
- *Spotting for two or more cycles:* See the healthcare provider to have other causes of bleeding assessed.
  - *Periodic examinations:* A yearly examination should include blood pressure tests, pelvic examination, urinalysis, breast examination, and Pap smear.
  - *Serious adverse effects to be reported as soon as possible:* Severe headaches, dizziness, blurred vision, leg pain, shortness of breath, chest pain, and acute abdominal pain. Although these adverse effects are usually of minor consequence, absence of serious adverse effects such as thromboembolism or ectopic pregnancy must be confirmed.

NOTE: When being seen by a healthcare provider or a dentist for other reasons, be sure to mention that hormonal contraceptives are being taken.

▪ Common and Serious Adverse Effects

See adverse effects of oral contraceptives (p. 626).

▪ Drug Interactions

See drug interactions for oral contraceptives.

DRUG CLASS: INTRAVAGINAL HORMONAL CONTRACEPTIVE

---

etonogestrel–ethinyl estradiol vaginal ring
(ē-tŏn-ō-GĔS-trĕl—ĔTH-ĭ-nĕl ĕs-TRĂ-dē-ŏl VĂ-gĭ-năl RĬNG)
  NuvaRing (NŪ-vă-rĭng)

ACTIONS

Ethinyl estradiol, an estrogen, and etonogestrel, a progestin, work together as a contraceptive by inhibiting ovulation. Estrogens block pituitary release of FSH, preventing the ovaries from developing a follicle that releases an ovum. Progestins inhibit pituitary release of LH, the hormone responsible for releasing an ovum from a follicle. Other mechanisms play a contributory role in preventing conception. Estrogens and progestins alter cervical mucus by making it thick and viscous, inhibiting sperm migration. Hormones also change the endometrial wall, impairing implantation of the fertilized ovum.

USES

The NuvaRing vaginal ring works very much like the combination oral contraceptives, except that the estrogen and progestin hormones are in a plastic ring dosage form that the woman inserts into her vagina for 3 weeks. The ring is removed for a 1-week break, during which withdrawal bleeding (menses) should begin.

Cigarette smoking increases the risk of serious adverse cardiovascular effects (e.g., blood clots) in persons who both smoke and use combination contraceptives. This risk increases with age and heavy smoking (at least 15 cigarettes per day) and is quite significant in women older than 35 years. Women who use hormone contraceptives are strongly encouraged not to smoke.

THERAPEUTIC OUTCOME

The primary therapeutic outcome associated with intravaginal hormone contraceptive therapy is prevention of pregnancy.

❖ NURSING IMPLICATIONS FOR INTRAVAGINAL HORMONAL CONTRACEPTIVE

▪ Premedication Assessment

1. Review the medical history. If there is a history of hypertension, gallbladder disease, diabetes mellitus, severe varicose veins, seizure disorders, oligomenorrhea or amenorrhea, rheumatic heart disease, thromboembolic disease, stroke, malignancy of breast or the reproductive system, renal or liver disease, severe mental depression, suspected pregnancy, or repeated contraceptive failure, or if the patient smokes, consult with the healthcare provider before dispensing the birth control ring.
2. Take a baseline blood pressure in the supine and sitting positions.
3. Ensure that a pregnancy test has been given and that the patient is not pregnant.

▪ Availability

NuvaRing releases 0.12 mg etonogestrel and 0.015 mg ethinyl estradiol per day.

▪ Implementation

Before Initiating Therapy. The patient should have a complete physical examination that includes blood pressure, pelvic and breast examinations, Pap smear, urinalysis, and hemoglobin or hematocrit.

Instructions for Using the Intravaginal Hormonal Contraceptive

- *Insertion:* Selecting a comfortable position, compress the ring and insert into the vagina. The exact position inside the vagina is not critical for its function. Insert on the appropriate day, as described later, and leave in place for 3 consecutive weeks.
- *Removal:* Remove the ring 3 weeks later on the same day of the week as it was inserted and at about the same time. Remove by hooking the index finger under the forward rim or by grasping the rim between the index and middle fingers and pulling it out. Place the used ring in the foil pouch and discard in a waste receptacle out of reach of children and pets. It still contains active hormone residual. Do not flush down the toilet.

Select one of the following methods to start contraception:

- *If no hormonal contraceptive was in use in the past month:* Counting the first day of menstruation as day 1, insert the contraceptive ring on or prior to day 5 of the cycle, even if menses is continuing. Note on a calendar the day of the week as a reminder of the removal day 3 weeks later. A nonhormonal backup contraceptive (e.g., condoms, spermicidal foam, diaphragm) should be used concurrently for the first 7 consecutive days of continuous ring use.
- *Switching from a combination oral contraceptive:* Insert the ring any time within 7 days after the last active combined oral contraceptive tablet and no later than the day that a new cycle of pills would have been started. No backup contraception is necessary.
- *Switching from a progestin-only minipill:* Insert the ring the following day after discontinuing the minipill. A nonhormonal backup contraceptive (e.g., condoms, spermicidal foam, diaphragm) should be used concurrently for the first 7 consecutive days of continuous ring use.

If the ring is expelled or removed, or there is a prolonged ring-free interval during the active 3 weeks:

- *For less than 3 hours:* Rinse the ring in cool or lukewarm (not hot) water and reinsert as soon as possible.
- *For longer than 3 hours or if not sure how long since expelled:* If the ring has been out for longer than 3 hours, there may be a lack of protection from pregnancy. Reinsert the ring, but use a nonhormonal backup contraceptive (e.g., condoms, spermicidal foam, diaphragm) for the next 7 consecutive days of continuous ring use.

If a woman forgets to change the ring:

- *If left in place for up to 1 extra week (4 weeks total):* Remove it and insert a new ring after a 1-week ring-free interval. Use a nonhormonal backup contraceptive (e.g., condoms, spermicidal foam, diaphragm) for the next 7 consecutive days of continuous ring use.
- *If left in place for more than 4 weeks:* Remove the ring. Rule out pregnancy. Insert a new ring after a 1-week ring-free interval if not pregnant. Use a nonhormonal backup contraceptive (e.g., condoms, spermicidal foam, diaphragm) for the next 7 consecutive days of continuous ring use.

Other important points:

- *Missing one period but being adherent to the program:* It is not uncommon for a woman to occasionally miss a period when receiving hormone therapy. Start the next cycle on the same insertion day (i.e., on the 29th day). If two consecutive periods are missed, a pregnancy test is in order. Contraceptive therapy should be discontinued if pregnancy is confirmed.
- *Missed one period and the ring was out for more than 3 hours or was left in for more than 4 weeks:* Return to the healthcare provider for a pregnancy test.
- *Spotting for two or more cycles:* See the healthcare provider to have other causes of bleeding assessed.
- *Periodic examinations:* A yearly examination should include blood pressure tests, pelvic examination, urinalysis, breast examination, and Pap smear.
- *Serious adverse effects to be reported as soon as possible:* Severe headaches, dizziness, blurred vision, leg pain, shortness of breath, chest pain, and acute abdominal pain. Although these adverse effects are usually of minor consequence, absence of serious adverse effects such as thromboembolism or ectopic pregnancy must be confirmed.

NOTE: When being seen by a healthcare provider or a dentist for other reasons, be sure to mention that hormonal contraceptives are being taken.

■ **Common and Serious Adverse Effects**
See Adverse Effects for Oral Contraceptives on p. 626.

■ **Drug Interactions**
See Drug Interactions for Oral Contraceptives on p. 627.

DRUG THERAPY FOR BENIGN PROSTATIC HYPERPLASIA

The prostate gland functions as part of the male reproductive system. It is a firm organ, weighing about 20 g, the size of a walnut. It is located at the base of the urinary bladder and completely surrounds the proximal urethra. As part of the male reproductive system, it produces a fluid during ejaculation that mixes with sperm from the testes and fluid from the seminal vesicles to form semen. The gland may also protect against urinary tract infections through secretion of prostatic antibacterial factor. Two other chemicals secreted by the prostate gland are acid phosphatase and prostate specific antigen (PSA) an elevated PSA level may indicate the presence of cancer.

Enlargement of the prostate gland as men age is an almost universal phenomenon. A condition called *enlarged prostate, prostatism,* or *benign prostate hyperplasia (BPH)* is common later in life, affecting more than 50% of men in their 60s and as many as 90% in their 70s and 80s. Many men with BPH will need some type of treatment. Although an enlarged prostate is an apparently normal part of aging, problems with urination that often accompany this enlargement are not normal.

Benign prostate hyperplasia is much more common than prostate cancer; however, an enlarged prostate gland can be caused by prostate cancer. Because the signs of enlarged prostate are often the same as the signs and symptoms of prostate cancer, it is important to obtain a healthcare provider's opinion so that the proper diagnosis can be made. The healthcare provider may also need to rule out prostate infection and other possible causes of the patient's symptoms.

The pathogenesis of BPH is not well understood, but it appears to involve the presence of increasing levels of dihydrotestosterone (DHT), either caused by a slow increase in production, reduced metabolism, or both, which stimulates the growth of new prostate cells. Dihydrotestosterone is formed in the prostate gland from testosterone produced in the testes. The conversion of testosterone to DHT is catalyzed by the enzyme 5-alpha reductase.

The symptoms of BPH are highly variable and patient specific, and are divided into two categories: obstructive and irritative (Box 40-4). Obstructive symptoms result directly from narrowing of the bladder neck and urethra. Irritative symptoms result from incomplete bladder emptying or urinary tract infection secondary to prostatic obstruction. As the prostate gland enlarges, it compresses the urethra, partially or completely obstructing urine flow from the bladder. Over time, symptoms become progressively worse, requiring medical attention. When necessary, the hyperplastic tissue may be removed surgically to reduce the urinary obstruction. Transurethral resection or laser therapy may be used to treat glands smaller than 60 g, whereas larger glands are removed surgically (prostatectomy). Intermittent catheterization several times daily or placement of a permanent indwelling catheter may be used if the patient is not a candidate for surgery.

Benign prostate hyperplasia may also be treated successfully with medicines. Alpha-1 adrenergic blocking agents (e.g., doxazosin, terazosin) are also used to treat hypertension (see Chapter 22), and alfuzosin or tamsulosin is used to relax the smooth muscle of the bladder and prostate. Antiandrogen agents, such as finasteride and dutasteride, selectively block androgens at the prostate cellular level and cause the prostate gland to shrink. Studies indicate that a combination of an alpha blocker with a 5-alpha reductase inhibitor is more effective in slowing the progression of BPH than either agent alone.

DRUG CLASS: ALPHA-1 ADRENERGIC BLOCKING AGENTS

ACTIONS

Alpha-1A blocking agents have selectivity for the alpha-1A receptor subtype found on the prostate gland. Approximately 70% of the alpha-1 receptors in the human prostate are of the alpha-1A subtype. Alfuzosin, silodosin, and tamsulosin are alpha-1A–specific adrenergic blocking agents, whereas doxazosin and terazosin are nonspecific alpha-1 blocking agents. These agents block alpha-1 receptors on the prostate gland and certain areas of the bladder neck, causing muscle relaxation, allowing greater urinary outflow in men with an enlarged prostate gland. Alpha-1 blocking agents do not reduce prostate size or inhibit testosterone synthesis like the 5-alpha-reductase inhibitors, nor do they affect PSA levels.

USES

Alpha-1 blocking agents are used to reduce mild to moderate urinary obstruction manifestations (e.g., hesitancy, terminal urine dribbling, interrupted stream, impaired size and force of stream, sensation of incomplete bladder emptying) in men with BPH. They produce a 20% to 30% increase in urine flow rate in up to 50% of men with urinary symptoms. Symptoms show improvement after 1 week of therapy, but 2 to 3 months of continued therapy is required to assess full effect. Alpha-1A–specific drugs (i.e., alfuzosin, tamsulosin, silodosin) are not used to treat hypertension.

THERAPEUTIC OUTCOMES

The primary therapeutic outcomes expected from alpha-1 blocker therapy are reduced symptoms and improvement in urine flow associated with prostate gland enlargement.

Box **40-4**	Symptoms of Benign Prostatic Hyperplasia

OBSTRUCTIVE
- Reduced force of urinary stream
- Resistance to initiate voiding
- Prolonged dribbling after urination
- Sensation of incomplete bladder emptying
- Decreased or interrupted stream
- Double voiding
- Strain or push to urinate

IRRITATIVE
- Increased frequency
- Nocturia
- Difficult or painful urination (dysuria)
- Sudden urgency
- Urge incontinence

❖ NURSING IMPLICATIONS FOR ALPHA-1 BLOCKING AGENTS

▪ Premedication Assessment
1. Obtain baseline blood pressure readings in supine and standing positions.
2. Check if the patient has a history of severe cerebral or coronary arteriosclerosis, gastritis, or peptic ulcer disease. (Reduction of blood pressure may diminish blood flow to these regions, causing therapy to worsen the condition.)

▪ Availability, Dosage, and Administration
See Table 40-6.

⚠ Medication Safety Alert

The initial doses of the alpha-1 blocking agents may cause dizziness (6% to 7%) and hypotension with tachycardia and fainting (<0.5%) in patients starting therapy. This effect may be minimized by giving the first doses with food. Patients should be warned that this adverse effect might occur, it is transient, and they should lie down immediately if symptoms develop.

▪ Common Adverse Effects
Neurologic
Drowsiness, headache, dizziness, weakness, lethargy. Tell the patient that these adverse effects may occur but tend to be self-limiting. The patient should not stop taking the medication and should consult the healthcare provider if the problem becomes unacceptable.

Cardiovascular
Dizziness, tachycardia, fainting. Dizziness may occur in more than 2% of patients, and orthostatic hypotension occurs in less than 0.5% of patients when therapy is initiated. Symptoms develop 15 to 90 minutes after the first dose is taken. To decrease the incidence, administer the first dose with food. Instruct the patient to lie down immediately if these symptoms occur. Provide for the patient's safety.

▪ Drug Interactions
Drugs That Enhance Therapeutic and Toxic Effects. Diuretics, cimetidine, tranquilizers, alcohol, barbiturates, antihistamines, beta-adrenergic blocking agents (e.g., propranolol, atenolol), and other antihypertensive agents should not be used with alfuzosin. Monitor the blood pressure response to the cumulative effects of antihypertensive agents. Take the patient's blood pressure in supine and erect positions.

Ketoconazole, itraconazole, ritonavir, diltiazem, and other potent CYP3A4 inhibitors inhibit the metabolism of alfuzosin and should not be used concurrently with alfuzosin.

Monitor for an increase in severity of adverse side effects such as sedation, hypotension, and bradycardia or tachycardia.

Avanafil, Sildenafil, Tadalafil, Vardenafil. These drugs are used to treat erectile dysfunction. They may aggravate hypotensive effects of doxazosin and terazosin, causing dizziness and tachycardia. Adjust by reducing the dose of the drugs used to treat erectile dysfunction.

DRUG CLASS: ANTIANDROGEN AGENTS

dutasteride (dŭ-TĂS-tĕr-īd)
Avodart (ĂV-ō-dărt)

 Table 40-6   Alpha-1 Blocking Agents Used for Benign Prostatic Hyperplasia

GENERIC NAME	BRAND NAME	AVAILABILITY	DOSAGE
alfuzosin	Uroxatral	Tablets, extended-release (24 hr): 10 mg	PO: 10 mg daily to be taken immediately after the same meal each day Tablets should not be crushed or chewed
doxazosin	Cardura Cardura XL	Tablets: 1, 2, 4, 8 mg Tablets, extended-release, (24 hr): 4, 8 mg	PO: 1-8 mg once daily
silodosin	Rapaflo	Capsules: 4, 8 mg	PO: 8 mg daily; 4 mg daily for patients with renal impairment
tamsulosin	Flomax	Capsules: 0.4 mg	PO: 0.4 mg daily, taken approximately 30 min following the same meal each day If symptoms are not adequately controlled after 2 to 4 wk of therapy, the dose may be increased to 0.8 mg once daily If administration is discontinued or interrupted for several days, at either the 0.4- or 0.8-mg dose, start therapy again with the 0.4-mg once-daily dose
terazosin	—	Capsules: 1, 2, 5, 10 mg	PO: Initial: 1 mg daily at bedtime Increase stepwise to 2 mg, 5 mg, or 10 mg daily to achieve desired response of symptoms and flow rate Maximum dose is 20 mg divided twice daily

ACTIONS

Dutasteride is an androgen hormone inhibitor that acts by inhibiting the enzyme 5-alpha reductase. The conversion of testosterone to DHT is catalyzed by 5-alpha reductase types 1 and 2. Reduction in DHT levels reduces the hyperplastic cell growth associated with prostatic hyperplasia.

USES

Dutasteride inhibits 5-alpha reductase types 1 and 2. It is used to treat the symptoms associated with BPH, reduce the risks associated with urinary retention, and minimize the need for surgery associated with BPH. More than 6 to 12 months of treatment may be necessary to assess whether a therapeutic response has been achieved. Patients who respond to therapy have fewer symptoms associated with partial obstruction, improved urinary flow rates, and a smaller prostate gland. Dutasteride is not approved by the FDA to treat male pattern baldness.

THERAPEUTIC OUTCOMES

The primary therapeutic outcomes expected from dutasteride therapy are as follows:
- Reduced symptoms and improvement in urine flow associated with prostatic enlargement
- Reduced need for surgery for BPH

❖ NURSING IMPLICATIONS FOR DUTASTERIDE

▪ Premedication Assessment

Obtain a baseline PSA blood level. Dutasteride causes a decrease in serum PSA levels by about 50% in patients with BPH, even in the presence of prostate cancer. Any sustained increase in PSA levels while a patient is receiving dutasteride should be investigated, including consideration of prostate cancer and noncompliance with therapy.

▪ Availability

Capsules: 0.5 mg.

▪ Dosage and Administration

PO: 0.5 mg once daily, with or without food.

 Medication Safety Alert

Dutasteride is absorbed through human skin. A woman who is pregnant or who may become pregnant should not handle crushed or broken dutasteride capsules. Dutasteride is contraindicated in women who are or may become pregnant because it may cause abnormalities of the external genitalia of a male fetus of a pregnant woman who has received dutasteride.

Men treated with dutasteride should not donate blood until at least 6 months after stopping therapy to avoid introducing the drug to a pregnant woman.

▪ Common Adverse Effects

Reproductive

Impotence, decreased libido, decreased volume of ejaculate. These adverse effects appear in small numbers of men receiving higher doses of dutasteride. Tell the patient that these adverse effects may occur but tend to be self-limiting. The incidence of impotence, decreased libido, and ejaculation disorder decreases with increasing duration of treatment. Decreased volume of ejaculate does not appear to interfere with normal sexual function. The patient should not stop taking the medication and should consult his healthcare provider if the problem becomes unacceptable.

▪ Drug Interactions

Drugs That Enhance Toxic Effects. Ketoconazole, itraconazole, ritonavir, diltiazem, verapamil, cimetidine, ciprofloxacin, and troleandomycin inhibit the metabolism of dutasteride. Dutasteride should be given with extreme caution to men taking any of these medications.

---

finasteride (fĭn-ĂS-tĕr-īd)
 Proscar (PRŌ-skăr), **Propecia** (prō-PĒ-shē-ă)

ACTIONS

Finasteride is an androgen hormone inhibitor that acts by inhibiting the enzyme 5-alpha reductase. The conversion of testosterone to DHT is catalyzed by 5-alpha reductase. Reduction in DHT levels reduces the hyperplastic cell growth associated with prostatic hyperplasia. Elevated DHT levels also induce androgenetic alopecia, more commonly known as *male pattern baldness* (vertex and anterior midscalp).

USES

Finasteride inhibits 5-alpha reductase, type 2. Finasteride (Proscar, 5 mg) is used to treat the symptoms associated with BPH, to reduce the risks associated with urinary retention, and minimize the need for surgery associated with BPH. More than 6 to 12 months of treatment may be necessary to assess whether a therapeutic response has been achieved. Patients who respond to therapy have fewer symptoms associated with partial obstruction, improved urinary flow rates, and a smaller prostate gland.

Finasteride (Propecia, 1 mg) is used to treat androgenetic alopecia. After at least 3 months of daily use, finasteride maintains hair count and stimulates new hair growth in those who respond. Continued use is necessary to sustain the results. With discontinuation of treatment, the effects are reversed within 1 year. Finasteride does not appear to affect nonscalp body hair.

THERAPEUTIC OUTCOMES

The primary therapeutic outcomes expected from finasteride therapy are as follows:

- Reduced symptoms and improvement in urine flow associated with prostatic enlargement
- Reversal of male pattern hair loss

❖ NURSING IMPLICATIONS FOR FINASTERIDE

▪ Premedication Assessment

Obtain a baseline PSA blood level. Finasteride causes a decrease in serum PSA levels by about 50% in patients with BPH, even in the presence of prostate cancer. Any sustained increase in PSA levels while receiving finasteride should be investigated, including consideration of prostate cancer and noncompliance with therapy.

▪ Availability

PO: Proscar tablets: 5 mg; Propecia tablets: 1 mg.

▪ Dosage and Administration

BPH: *PO:* 5 mg once daily, with or without food.

Androgenetic alopecia: *PO:* 1 mg once daily, with or without food.

 Medication Safety Alert

Finasteride is contraindicated in women who are or may become pregnant. Finasteride may cause abnormalities of the external genitalia of a male fetus of a pregnant woman who received the drug. A woman who is pregnant or who may become pregnant should not handle crushed or broken finasteride tablets. Tablets are coated and will prevent contact with the active ingredient during normal handling.

▪ Common Adverse Effects

Reproductive

Impotence, decreased libido, decreased volume of ejaculate. These adverse effects appear in small numbers of men receiving higher doses of finasteride. Tell the patient that these adverse effects may occur but tend to be self-limiting. The decreased volume of ejaculate does not appear to interfere with normal sexual function. The patient should not stop taking the medication and should consult his healthcare provider if the problem becomes unacceptable.

▪ Drug Interactions

No clinically significant drug interactions have been reported to date.

DRUG THERAPY FOR ERECTILE DYSFUNCTION

Erectile dysfunction (ED) is the consistent inability to achieve or maintain an erection sufficient for satisfactory sexual activity. There has been a significant increase in discussion about ED, sometimes called *impotency*, because of the availability and high efficacy of oral medicine used to treat certain types of cases of ED. The prevalence of ED increases with age, although it is not an inevitable outcome of aging. Approximately 5% of men experience the problem at the age of 40, and 15% to 25% of men age 65 years or older are affected.

Erectile dysfunction usually is the result of a combination of vascular, neurologic, and psychological factors. Vascular and neurogenic causes of ED increase with age. Risk factors include cigarette smoking, hyperlipidemia, hypertension, diabetes mellitus, coronary artery disease, and peripheral vascular disease. Other causes of ED are psychological (e.g., stress, depression, interpersonal relationships), damage to neurologic pathways (e.g., trauma from bicycle seats, prostatectomy, transurethral resection of the prostate, diabetes mellitus, alcohol abuse). A common cause of ED is the use of medicines for other medical conditions (Box 40-5). It is often difficult to determine whether ED is caused by medicines, the condition for which the medicine is used, or both.

The diagnosis of ED is based on a medical and sexual history, physical examination, and laboratory studies. An abrupt onset and intermittent pattern of difficulty achieving or maintaining an erection may suggest a psychological cause, whereas a gradual onset in ED is more likely the result of a vascular or neurologic cause. The cause of ED is usually multifactorial. A variety of treatments have been developed for ED, each with advantages and disadvantages—psychotherapy, intracavernosal injection with prostaglandins, intraurethral prostaglandin, vacuum constriction devices, vascular surgery, hormonal therapy, penile prostheses, and oral phosphodiesterase inhibitor therapy.

DRUG CLASS: PHOSPHODIESTERASE INHIBITORS

ACTIONS

Phosphodiesterase inhibitors are selective inhibitors of the phosphodiesterase type 5 (PDE5) enzyme. Research indicates that nitric oxide, a naturally occurring neurotransmitter found in nerve endings and endothelial cells, activates the enzyme guanylate cyclase, which converts guanosine triphosphate to cyclic guanosine monophosphate (cGMP) in smooth muscle cells. The increase in cGMP causes smooth muscle relaxation. In the corpus cavernosum of the penis, smooth muscle relaxation allows blood inflow to fill the many small sinusoidal spaces, resulting in an erection. In the corpus cavernosum, the enzyme PDE5 inactivates cGMP. The phosphodiesterase inhibitors enhance the relaxant effect of nitric oxide released in response to sexual stimulation by increasing cGMP concentration in the corpus cavernosum, resulting in smooth muscle relaxation and greater blood flow into the corpus cavernosum, which produces an erection.

Box 40-5 | Drugs That May Cause Erectile Dysfunction

ANTIHYPERTENSIVE AGENTS
- Thiazide diuretics (most common)
- Beta-adrenergic blocking agents (especially propranolol and nonselective agents; less so with beta-1 selective agents)
- Alpha-adrenergic blocking agents (e.g., prazosin, terazosin)
- Sympatholytic agents (e.g., clonidine, methyldopa, reserpine)
- Spironolactone (antiandrogen effect)

CENTRAL NERVOUS SYSTEM DEPRESSANTS
- Phenothiazine antipsychotic agents (e.g., fluphenazine, thioridazine)
- Butyrophenones (e.g., haloperidol)
- Monoamine oxidase inhibitors
- Tricyclic antidepressants
- Selective serotonin reuptake inhibitors (e.g., sertraline, paroxetine)
- Lithium

CARDIOVASCULAR AGENTS
- Digoxin (estrogen effect)
- Clofibrate
- Gemfibrozil

MISCELLANEOUS AGENTS
- Substances of abuse (e.g., smoking, alcohol, cocaine, marijuana)
- Chemotherapy agents (e.g., chlorambucil, cyclophosphamide, methotrexate)
- Anabolic steroids
- Estrogens
- Corticosteroids
- Cimetidine (antiandrogen effect)
- 5-alpha reductase inhibitors (finasteride, dutasteride)
- Interferon-α

Data from Koeneman KS, Mulhall JP, Goldstein I: Sexual health for the man at midlife: in-office workup, *Geriatrics* 52:76-86, 1997; Brock GB, Lue TF: Drug-induced male sexual dysfunction, an update, *Drug Saf* 8:414-426, 1993; McVary KT: Erectile dysfunction, *N Engl J Med* 357:2472-2481, 2007.

USES

Sildenafil was approved in 1998 as the first oral therapy to treat male ED. Three other products, vardenafil, tadalafil, and avanafil, have since been approved. Sexual stimulation is required for an erection because the phosphodiesterase inhibitors do not have a direct relaxant effect on the smooth muscle of the corpus cavernosum. In the absence of sexual stimulation, these agents have no pharmacologic effect. They are not an aphrodisiac; they do not increase sexual desire or sexual stimulation or affect the frequency of sexual intercourse. Sildenafil and vardenafil are taken at any point from 30 minutes to 4 hours before sexual activity. Avanafil is approved to be taken 15 minutes before sexual activity. Tadalafil also starts to work within 30 minutes, but may last for up to 36 hours. Tadalafil has also been approved as a once-daily dose that, when taken daily, may significantly reduce the onset of action, allowing more spontaneity in sexual relations. Tadalafil is also approved for the treatment of BPH.

Sexual stimulation is required with all four agents for erection. The erection lasts for an hour or so, although it is highly variable, based on continued sexual stimulation, attainment of orgasm, and the individual patient. The phosphodiesterase inhibitors should not be taken more often than once every 24 hours. The phosphodiesterase inhibitors have been tested in women to treat sexual dysfunction, but the results to date have been inconclusive, so phosphodiesterase inhibitors are not recommended for women.

Phosphodiesterase inhibitors are also finding a new therapeutic use in a rare lung condition known as *pulmonary arterial hypertension.* By similar mechanisms in lung tissue, compared with penile tissue as described earlier, phosphodiesterase inhibitors cause an increase in cGMP in pulmonary tissue, leading to relaxation of smooth muscle and vasodilation of the pulmonary arterial bed, reducing hypertension. Sildenafil has been approved for use in pulmonary arterial hypertension under the brand name Revatio.

THERAPEUTIC OUTCOME

The primary therapeutic outcome expected from phosphodiesterase inhibitor therapy is improved erectile function and overall sexual satisfaction in men with ED. Tadalafil may also be used to reduce symptoms and improvement in urinary flow associated with prostatic enlargement.

❖ NURSING IMPLICATIONS FOR PHOSPHODIESTERASE INHIBITORS

▪ Premedication Assessment

Obtain baseline vital signs and a history of recent use of medicines, including recreational drugs. Patients with cardiovascular disease should seek their healthcare provider's approval before starting phosphodiesterase inhibitor therapy.

▪ Availability, Dosage, and Administration

See Table 40-7. Phosphodiesterase inhibitors do not protect against STIs or pregnancy. Use of a condom and a spermicide containing nonoxynol-9 will help protect against some STIs and unwanted pregnancy. Phosphodiesterase inhibitors do not affect sperm count or motility and do not reduce fertility.

▪ Common Adverse Effects
Vascular

Headache, flushing of the face and neck. These adverse effects appear in small numbers of men receiving higher doses of phosphodiesterase inhibitors. Tell the patient that these adverse effects may occur but tend to be self-limiting. If they continue to be a problem, a reduced dosage may eliminate the adverse effects. The patient should consult his healthcare provider if the problem becomes unacceptable.

Table 40-7   Phosphodiesterase Inhibitors Used for Erectile Dysfunction

GENERIC NAME	BRAND NAME	AVAILABILITY (mg)	DOSAGE (mg)
avanafil	Stendra	Tablets: 50, 100, 200	Initial: 100 Maintenance: 50-100 Maximum: 200/24 hr
sildenafil	Viagra	Tablets: 25, 50, 100	Initial: 50 Maintenance: 25-50 Maximum: 100/24 hr
tadalafil*	Cialis	Tablets: 2.5, 5, 10, 20	Intermittent use: initial, 10 Maintenance: 5-10 Maximum: 20/24 hr Daily use: initial, 2.5; maximum for daily use, 5
vardenafil **Staxyn and Levitra are not interchangeable.**	Levitra	Tablets: 2.5, 5, 10, 20	Initial: 10; older than 65 yr, 5 Maintenance: 5-10 Maximum: 20/24 hr
	Staxyn	Tablet, dispersible: 10	Initial: 10 Maximum: 10; if dosage adjustment is needed, use Levitra

*Tadalafil is also approved for treatment of benign prostatic hyperplasia, 5 mg once daily.

Sensory

Color vision impairment. Mild, transient reversible impairment of blue or green color interpretation may occur. This is thought to be caused by inhibition of the PDE6 enzyme, which plays a role in phototransduction in the retina. If this continues to be problem, a reduced dosage may eliminate the adverse effect. Tell the patient to consult a healthcare provider if the problem becomes unacceptable.

■ Serious Adverse Effects

Cardiovascular

Hypotension, dizziness, angina. Patients with heart disease, angina, diabetes mellitus, and hypertension should seek their healthcare provider's approval before using phosphodiesterase inhibitors. Patients receiving nitroglycerin or isosorbide should not take phosphodiesterase inhibitors because of a potentially fatal interaction. If hypotension, dizziness, or angina develops, the patient should lie down, discontinuing sexual activity. **Do not take nitroglycerin for angina.** It may worsen the symptoms. Seek medical attention, as needed.

Sensory

Loss of vision. A small number of cases of sudden vision loss caused by nonarteritic ischemic optic neuropathy (NAION) have been reported. This is a condition in which blood flow is blocked to the optic nerve. People suffering sudden reduction in vision or vision loss should stop taking these medicines and seek medical attention quickly. Patients who are considering taking these medicines should inform their healthcare provider if they have ever had severe loss of vision, which might reflect a prior episode of NAION. At this time, it is not known whether these medicines for erectile dysfunction are the cause of the loss of vision or whether the problem is related to other medical conditions, such as high blood pressure, diabetes, or a combination of these problems.

Reproductive

Sustained erection. Priapism is an erection that will not go away. If an erection lasts more than 4 hours, medical attention should be sought quickly. Priapism must be treated as soon as possible or lasting damage can happen to the penis, including the inability to have erections.

■ Drug Interactions

Nitroglycerin Patches, Nitroglycerin Ointment, Amyl Nitrate. Nitrates increase the production of nitric oxide, potentially causing hypotension and arrhythmias. It is thought that nitrates inhaled for recreational use during sexual activity (e.g., butyl nitrate; amyl nitrate or nitrite, or "poppers") will have the same effect when combined with phosphodiesterase inhibitors. Nitrates from food sources do not react with phosphodiesterase inhibitors.

Cimetidine, Erythromycin, Ketoconazole, Itraconazole, Ritonavir, Indinavir, Saquinavir. These agents inhibit the metabolism of phosphodiesterase inhibitors, potentially causing an increased incidence of adverse effects such as flushing, hypotension, and dizziness. A lower dosage of the phosphodiesterase inhibitor may be necessary.

Alcohol. Alcohol and phosphodiesterase inhibitors are mild vasodilators. Excessive consumption of alcohol in combination with phosphodiesterase inhibitors may cause decreased blood pressure, dizziness, and orthostatic hypotension. Use caution when combining phosphodiesterase inhibitors and alcohol.

Alpha-Adrenergic Blocking Agents. Use of alpha-adrenergic blocking agents (e.g., terazosin, doxazosin, prazosin, tamsulosin, alfuzosin) and vardenafil or tadalafil is CONTRAINDICATED. Significant hypotension may result. Use with sildenafil is not contraindicated, but a lower dose of sildenafil may be required to prevent hypotension.

There are no recommendations for the use of avanafil and alpha-adrenergic blocking agents.

Rifampin. This drug may enhance the metabolism of sildenafil and tadalafil, reducing its duration of action. An increase in dosage or earlier sexual activity may resolve the problem.

Get Ready for the NCLEX® Examination!

Key Points

- There is a great need for counseling about contraception and about modes of transmission of STIs for all those who are sexually active. One age group that is frequently not receiving adequate counseling on safe sex practices is adolescents, many of whom are sexually active.
- Nurses must be leaders in encouraging people to report STIs and seek health care as soon as an STI is suspected.
- Nurses must be leaders in promoting health and wellness, encouraging men and women to complete annual physical examinations that could detect the early onset of disease.
- It is important for the consumer to be aware that hormonal contraceptives have reduced effectiveness when taken in combination with many other medications or when doses are missed, thus requiring an alternative form of contraception.
- Benign prostatic hyperplasia (BPH) and erectile dysfunction (ED) are the two most common male reproductive system conditions that are treated successfully with pharmacotherapy.

Additional Learning Resources

SG Go to your Study Guide for additional Review Questions for the NCLEX® Examination, Critical Thinking Clinical Situations, and other learning activities to help you master this chapter content.

evolve Go to your Evolve website (http://evolve .elsevier.com/Clayton) for additional online resources.

Review Questions for the NCLEX® Examination

1. The nurse educating a patient being treated for chlamydia about personal hygiene will include these statements during the discussion: *(Select all that apply.)*
   1. "It is advisable to urinate before and after intercourse and to clean your private area thoroughly."
   2. "Remember that oral contraceptives do not protect you against sexually transmitted infections, but condoms provide a physical barrier against STIs."
   3. "Since you have an infection, you need to have your partner tested and treated."
   4. "Now that you have an infection, it is not necessary to practice safe sex."
   5. "I know this information can be overwhelming, so we can go over the rest of this when you return for your check-up."

2. These oral contraceptives reduce the number of yearly menstrual periods from 13 to 4.
   1. Monophasic
   2. Biphasic
   3. Triphasic
   4. Quadriphasic

3. It is quite important to get a thorough history on a woman who wishes to start oral contraceptives because the increased estrogen exposure may increase the risk for developing:
   1. blood clots.
   2. kidney disease.
   3. leukorrhea.
   4. Chlamydia.

4. The nurse was giving instructions to a patient about the use of the minipill and realized after this statement that the patient needed further education:
   1. "I will need to use condoms for the first month while on the pill to provide birth control."
   2. "I know that if I get a bad headache, dizziness, or blurred vision, I will need to contact this clinic as soon as possible."
   3. "I know I should switch to some other form of birth control for 3 months before I try to get pregnant."
   4. "I think I can remember to take the pill every day, but if I do forget, I can simply skip it and wait until the next day to take the pill again."

5. The drugs that are approved for use to reduce the symptoms of benign prostatic hyperplasia include: *(Select all that apply.)*
   1. avanafil (Stendra).
   2. alfuzosin (Uroxatral).
   3. tamsulosin (Flomax).
   4. dutasteride (Avodart).
   5. finasteride (Proscar).

6. The nurse is completing a patient history on a man who presents with erectile dysfunction and is requesting a prescription for sildenafil (Viagra). These conditions, if present, require the healthcare provider's assessment and approval prior to starting sildenafil. *(Select all that apply.)*
   1. STIs
   2. Diabetes mellitus
   3. Gastritis or peptic ulcer disease
   4. Cardiovascular disease
   5. Asthma

Drugs Used to Treat Disorders of the Urinary System

http://evolve.elsevier.com/Clayton

Objectives

1. Explain the major actions of drugs used to treat disorders of the urinary tract.
2. Identify baseline data that the nurse should collect for comparison and evaluation of drug effectiveness.
3. Identify important nursing implementations associated with the drug therapy and treatment of diseases of the urinary system.
4. Identify the symptoms, treatment, and medication used for overactive bladder syndrome.

Key Terms

pyelonephritis (pī-ă-lō-nĕ-FRĬ-tĭs) (p. 638)
cystitis (sĭs-TĬ-tĭs) (p. 638)
prostatitis (prŏs-tă-TĬ-tĭs) (p. 638)
urethritis (yū-rĕ-THRĬ-tĭs) (p. 638)
acidification (ă-sĭd-ĭ-fĭ-KĀ-shŭn) (p. 641)
frequency (FRĒ-kwĕn-sē) (p. 644)
urgency (ĔR-jĕn-sē) (p. 644)
incontinence (ĭn-KŌN-tĭ-nĕns) (p. 644)

urge incontinence (ĔRJ ĭn-KŌN-tĭ-nĕns) (p. 644)
stress incontinence (p. 644)
overflow incontinence (p. 644)
nocturia (nŏk-TŪ-rē-ă) (p. 644)
overactive bladder (OAB) syndrome (ō-vĕr-ĂK-tĭv BLĂ-dĕr SĬN-drōm) (p. 644)
urinary antispasmodic agents (YĔR-ĭn-ăr-ē ăn-tī-spăz-MŎD-ĭk Ā-jĕnts) (p. 645)

URINARY TRACT INFECTIONS

Urinary tract infections (UTIs) are among the most common infectious diseases in humans, accounting for more than 11 million healthcare providers' office visits yearly. Urinary tract infections are second only to upper respiratory tract infections as a cause of morbidity from infection. Urinary tract infections encompass several different types of infection of local tissue: **pyelonephritis** (the kidneys), **cystitis** (the bladder), **prostatitis** (the prostate gland), and **urethritis** (the urethra).

The incidence of UTIs in women is approximately 10 times higher than in men. The urethra is shorter in females than it is in males, so bacteria have a shorter distance to travel to the bladder. Proximity of the urethral meatus to the vagina and rectum can also make it easier for bacteria to cause an infection. The incidence increases in women with age, so that by 60 years of age, up to 20% of women will have suffered from at least one UTI in their lives.

Gram-negative aerobic bacilli from the gastrointestinal tract cause most UTIs. *Escherichia coli* accounts for about 80% of noninstitutionally acquired uncomplicated UTIs. Other common infecting organisms are *Staphylococcus saprophyticus*, *Klebsiella pneumoniae*, *Enterobacter* species, *Proteus mirabilis*, and *Pseudomonas*

aeruginosa. Nosocomial UTIs and those associated with urinary tract pathologic abnormalities are considered to be complicated UTIs. The pathogens tend to be the same types of bacteria, but they are frequently more resistant to the antibiotics commonly used. This requires the use of more potent antibiotics for longer courses of therapy, placing the patient at a greater risk for complications secondary to drug therapy.

The use of an indwelling urinary catheter should be avoided if possible. When used, adherence to strict aseptic technique and attachment to a closed drainage system is necessary to reduce the rate of infection.

❖ NURSING IMPLICATIONS FOR URINARY SYSTEM DISEASE

The information the nurse gains through assessment of the patient's clinical signs and symptoms is important to the healthcare provider when analyzing data for diagnosis and for evaluation of the patient's response to prescribed treatment.

■ Assessment

History of Urinary Tract Symptoms

- Does the individual have a history of a congenital disorder of the urinary tract, sexually transmitted infections, recent delivery of a baby, prostatic disease, recent catheterization, urologic instrumentation or surgical procedure, renal calculi, gout, UTI, or bladder dysfunction of neurologic origin? Obtain details applicable to the patient's responses.

- Is there a problem with defecation? When was the last bowel movement?
History of Current Symptoms
- Has the individual had any chills, fever, general malaise, or a change in mental status? New confusion in an older patient may be the only sign of a UTI. Ask questions relating to personal hygiene practices and sexual intercourse to evaluate for the possibility of bacterial contamination as an underlying cause of cystitis. Has the person been catheterized or on prolonged bed rest for any reason?
- *Pattern of urination:* Ask the individual to describe the symptoms that affect his or her ability to void. What is the current urination pattern, and have there been recent changes? Such details as frequency, dysuria, incontinence, changes in the urine stream, hesitancy in starting to void, hematuria, nocturia (does he or she awaken at night with the desire to urinate and, if so, how many times does this occur during an average night?), and urgency are all of significance. Ask if he or she is able to sit through a 2-hour meeting or ride in a car for 2 hours without urinating. State the onset, course of progression of the symptoms, and any self-treatment that has been attempted and response achieved. Is there blood or pus in the urine? Is it difficult to postpone urination when the urge to urinate is felt? Is there incontinence (leaking) of urine? If so, when does this happen and what causes it? Does the incontinence occur when coughing, walking, running, lifting a heavy object, or if one is unable to reach a toilet immediately?
- *Pattern of pain:* Record the details of any pain the patient describes—frequency, intensity, duration, and location. Use a pain rating scale (0 to 10: 0 for no pain; 10 for severe pain). Pain associated with renal pathology usually occurs at the groin, back, flank, and suprapubic area, and on urination (dysuria). Does the pain radiate? If so, obtain details.
- *Intake and output:* Ask specifically about the individual's usual daily fluid intake. How frequently does the patient usually void? What is the amount of each voiding?

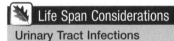 **Life Span Considerations**

Urinary Tract Infections

In children and men, UTIs may have a more serious cause than a case of cystitis. Therefore all UTIs must be thoroughly investigated to identify the underlying cause.

Medication History. Ask for a list of all prescribed over-the-counter medicines and herbal products being taken. Many pharmacologic agents (e.g., anti-

cholinergic agents, cholinergic agents, antihistamines, antihypertensives, chemotherapeutic agents, and immunosuppressants) can induce urinary retention or an altered urinary elimination pattern or urologic symptoms. Has the person recently been on medications to prevent or treat a UTI?
Nutritional History
- Has the individual been fasting for any prolonged period?
- How much alcoholic beverage has been consumed?
- Are vitamins, minerals, or other dietary supplements taken regularly?
- What kinds of fluids are taken daily: water, coffee, soft drinks, energy drinks?
- How many dairy, chocolate, spicy foods, or meat products are consumed daily?

Laboratory and Diagnostic Studies. Review diagnostic and laboratory reports (e.g., urinalysis, renal function tests, voiding evaluatory procedures, cystoscopy, and complete blood count [CBC] with differential, urine culture, and sensitivity results).

Urinalysis is a physical, chemical, and microscopic examination of the urine, and is the most routine test that the nurse encounters. The color, appearance (e.g., clear, foamy, turbid), and odor of the urine are noted, and the pH, protein, glucose, and ketones are determined with reagent dipsticks. Specific gravity is measured with a refractometer, and a microscopic examination of the urinary sediment is performed to detect the presence of red and white blood cells, bacteria, casts, and crystals. An understanding of the significant data that this basic test can reveal is imperative to monitoring the patient. Refer to Table 41-1 for a description of the data. See a general medical-surgical text for details of collecting urine samples correctly.

■ **Implementation**
- Individualize the care plan to address the type of urinary tract disorder (e.g., retention, incontinence, or cystitis).
- Administer medications prescribed and list on the medication administration record (MAR) or in the electronic medical record.
- Monitor laboratory studies (e.g., urinalysis, CBC with differential, and creatinine clearance).
- Mark dietary orders on the Kardex, or enter data into the computer; indicate the amount of fluid to be taken every shift to maintain an adequate intake.
- Mark the Kardex or enter data into the computer for daily weights and accurate intake and output as appropriate to diagnosis; indicate whether bladder training, Kegel exercises, or other measures should be taught and encouraged.
- Indicate the level of activity or exercise permitted.
- Perform focused assessment of symptoms (e.g., retention, urinary frequency, and pain).
- Monitor the pain level and provide appropriate supportive and pharmacologic interventions.

Table **41-1** Urinalysis

PROPERTY	NORMAL DATA	ABNORMAL DATA
Color, appearance	Straw, clear yellow, or amber	Dark smoky color, reddish, or brown may indicate blood; white or cloudy may indicate UTI or chyluria; dark yellow to amber may indicate dehydration; green, deep yellow, or brown may indicate liver or biliary disease; some drugs or food also alter urine color: red or red-brown foods (e.g., beets, rhubarb); reddish orange, phenazopyridine (Pyridium); dark yellow or brown, nitrofurantoin; blue, methylene blue; bright yellow, vitamin B complex; reddish orange, rifampin
Odor	Ammonialike on standing	Foul smell may indicate infection; dehydrated patient's urine is concentrated, with ammonia smell resulting from urea breakdown by bacteria; sweet or fruity odor associated with starvation or diabetic acidosis (ketoacidosis)
Protein	0 to trace	Foamy or frothy-appearing urine may indicate protein; proteinuria associated with kidney disease, toxemia of pregnancy; also found in leukemia, lupus erythematosus, cardiac disease
Glucose	0 to trace	Presence usually associated with diabetes mellitus or low renal threshold with glucose "spillage"; also seen at times of severe stress (e.g., major infection) or after high-carbohydrate intake
Ketones	0	Associated with dehydration, starvation, ketoacidosis, diet high in protein and low in carbohydrates
pH	4.5-8.0	pH <4.5 indicates metabolic acidosis, respiratory acidosis, diet high in meat protein and/or cranberries; medications can be prescribed to produce alkaline or acidic urine; pH >8.0 associated with bacteriuria (UTI from *Klebsiella* or *Proteus*), diet high in fruits and/or vegetables
Red blood cell count	0-3/high-power field (HPF)	Indicative of bleeding at some location in the urinary tract; infection, obstruction, calculi, renal failure, tumors, anticoagulants, excess aspirin, menstrual contamination
White blood cell count	0-5/HPF	Increase indicates infection somewhere in urinary tract; may also be associated with lupus nephritis, strenuous exercise
Casts	0	May indicate dehydration, possible infection within renal tubules, other types of renal disease
Bacteria	0	May indicate UTI or contaminated specimen collection
Specific gravity (sp gr)	1.003-1.029	Used as indicator of hydration (in absence of renal pathology); sp gr >1.018 is early sign of dehydration; sp gr <1.010 is "dilute urine" and may indicate fluid accumulation; fixed sp gr ≅1.010 may indicate renal disease; sp gr <1.005 may indicate diabetes insipidus, excess fluid intake, overhydration; sp gr >1.026 may indicate decreased fluid intake, vomiting, diarrhea, diabetes mellitus

UTI, Urinary tract infection.

- Administer prescribed medications; monitor response and adverse effects.
- Maintain adequate fluid intake and an accurate intake and output record. Instruct the patient to avoid foods known to be bladder irritants, such as spicy foods, citrus juices, alcohol, and caffeine.
- For inability to void, institute techniques to stimulate voiding (e.g., proper positioning to void, running water in sink, and pouring warm water over perineum).
- For incontinence, establish a regular toileting schedule, and initiate bladder-training measures as appropriate and as ordered. Start measures to prevent perineal irritation. Apply external urinary diversion devices as ordered, such as an external condom catheter. Use incontinent pads as needed. Keep the urinal or bedpan readily available.

- Facilitate modifications of the environment that promote regular, easy access to toilet facilities, and promote the patient's safety with features such as better lighting, ambulatory assistance equipment, clothing alterations, timed voiding, and toileting equipment, such as an elevated toilet seat or commode.
- Implement measures to maintain the individual's dignity and privacy and to prevent embarrassment when incontinence is present.
- Maintain the activity and exercise level prescribed.

■ **Patient Education**
For Incontinence

- Teach personal hygiene measures to keep the skin clean and dry and prevent perineal breakdown. Explore appliances and incontinence products available for personal use.

- Teach Kegel exercises and bladder training, and stress the importance of responding to the urge to void.

For Urinary Tract Infections

- Teach women the following measures to avoid future UTIs: avoid nylon underwear (use cotton) and tight, constrictive clothing in the perineal area; avoid frequent use of bubble bath; wash the perineal area immediately before and after sexual intercourse; and urinate immediately after intercourse.
- Teach women the proper method of wiping after defecation or urination (front to back) to prevent bacterial contamination. Explain the correct procedure for obtaining a clean-catch urine sample and the importance of having follow-up urine cultures collected as requested by the healthcare provider.
- Teach comfort measures, such as the use of a sitz bath.
- Stress the importance of adequate fluid intake and its effect of diluting the urine, decreasing bladder irritability and helping remove organisms present in the bladder. Define "adequate intake of fluid" to the individual in terms of the number and size of glasses of liquid to be consumed during the day.
- Explain the signs of improvement or worsening of the urinary condition appropriate to the individual's diagnosis. Emphasize symptoms that should be reported to the healthcare provider.

For Urinary Retention. Teach self-examination to assess for bladder distention, Credé's maneuver (manual compression of the bladder through pressure on the lower abdomen) to aid in emptying the bladder and, as appropriate, self-catheterization.

Medications

- For urinary retention, explain adverse effects to anticipate with the prescribed medications.
- For the urinary analgesic phenazopyridine hydrochloride, explain that the urine will be reddish orange. If discoloration of the skin or sclera occurs, contact the healthcare provider.
- For UTIs, instruct patients to take the medicines exactly as prescribed for the entire course of medication. Discontinuing the antimicrobial agent when the symptoms improve may result in another infection after approximately 2 weeks that will be resistant to antimicrobial treatment. See individual drug monographs for specific instructions relating to **acidification** of the urine and instructions on taking medications with food or milk to avoid gastric irritation.
- See individual drug monographs regarding treatment of acute attacks and how long before response can be anticipated. Stress the need for follow-up laboratory results to evaluate response to therapy.

Fostering Health Maintenance

- Discuss medication information and how it will benefit the course of treatment to produce an optimal response. Stress maintenance of adequate urine volume as a part of the overall treatment of urinary tract disorders.
- Seek cooperation and understanding of the following points so that medication adherence is increased: name of medication; dosage, route, and times of administration; and common and serious adverse effects. See individual drug monographs for additional teaching.

Patient Self-Assessment. Enlist the patient's aid in developing and maintaining a written record of monitoring parameters for urinary antimicrobial agents. (See the Patient Self-Assessment Form for Urinary Antibiotics on the Evolve website.) Complete the Premedication Data column for use as a baseline to track response to therapy. Ensure that the patient understands how to use the form, and instruct the patient to take the completed form to follow-up visits. During follow-up visits, focus on issues that will foster adherence with the therapeutic interventions prescribed.

DRUG THERAPY FOR URINARY TRACT INFECTIONS

DRUG CLASS: URINARY ANTIMICROBIAL AGENTS

ACTIONS

Urinary antimicrobial agents are substances that are secreted and concentrated in the urine in sufficient amounts to have an antiseptic effect on the urine and urinary tract.

USES

Selection of the product to be used is based on identification of the pathogens by Gram staining, or by urine culture in severe, recurrent, or chronic infections.

Fosfomycin, methenamine mandelate, and nitrofurantoin are used only for UTIs. Examples of other antibiotics that are also used to treat urinary infections are ampicillin, sulfisoxazole, cotrimoxazole, ciprofloxacin, levofloxacin, tetracycline, doxycycline, and gentamicin. These agents are effective in a variety of tissue infections against many different microorganisms. Because of their use in multiple organ systems, they are discussed in detail (with nursing processes) in Chapter 45.

Fluid intake should be encouraged so that there will be at least 2000 mL of urinary output daily. Duration of treatment depends on whether the infection is uncomplicated or complicated; acute, chronic, or recurrent; the pathogen being treated; the antimicrobial agent being used for treatment; and whether a follow-up culture can be collected to assess the success of the therapy.

DRUG CLASS: FOSFOMYCIN ANTIBIOTICS

fosfomycin (fŏs-fō-MĪ-sĭn)
  Monurol (MŎN-ĕr-ŏl)

ACTIONS

Fosfomycin is the first of a new class of fosfomycin antibiotics. Fosfomycins act by inhibiting bacterial cell wall synthesis and by reducing adherence of bacteria to epithelial cells of the urinary tract.

USES

Fosfomycin is the first antibiotic agent to be approved as a single-dose treatment for UTIs. It is used to treat uncomplicated acute cystitis in women caused by susceptible strains of *E. coli* and *Enterococcus faecalis*. It is not indicated for the treatment of kidney infections such as pyelonephritis.

THERAPEUTIC OUTCOME

The primary therapeutic outcome associated with fosfomycin therapy is resolution of the UTI.

❖ NURSING IMPLICATIONS FOR FOSFOMYCIN

▪ Premedication Assessment

1. Record voiding characteristics (e.g., frequency, amount, color, odor, and associated symptoms such as burning and pain) to serve as a baseline for monitoring therapy.
2. Assess for and record any existing gastrointestinal complaints before initiating therapy.
3. Record baseline vital signs.

▪ Availability

PO: Single-dose 3-g packets of fosfomycin granules.

▪ Dosage and Administration

Adult: PO: Pour the entire contents of a single-dose packet of fosfomycin into 90 to 120 mL (3 to 4 ounces) of water and stir to dissolve. Do not use hot water. Take immediately after dissolving in water. Fosfomycin may be taken with or without food. Do not take additional packets of medicine without approval from the healthcare provider. Additional adverse effects develop with multiple doses, but there is little therapeutic gain. Do not take in its dry form. Always mix fosfomycin with water before ingesting.

▪ Common Adverse Effects

Gastrointestinal

Nausea, diarrhea, abdominal cramps, flatulence. These adverse effects are usually mild and tend to resolve without need for therapy because only one dose of fosfomycin is administered.

▪ Serious Adverse Effects

Genitourinary

Perineal burning, dysuria. Burning with urination may be produced by the infection itself. Symptoms should improve in 2 to 3 days after taking fosfomycin; if not improved, the patient should contact his or her healthcare provider.

▪ Drug Interactions

Metoclopramide. Metoclopramide has been reported to lower the serum concentration and urinary excretion of fosfomycin by enhancing gastric motility. Other medicines that hasten gastrointestinal motility (e.g., cisapride) may produce a similar response.

DRUG CLASS: OTHER URINARY ANTIBACTERIAL AGENTS

methenamine mandelate (mĕth-ĔN-ă-mēn măn-DĔl-āt)

ACTIONS

Methenamine mandelate combines the action of methenamine and mandelic acid. Methenamine yields formaldehyde in the presence of an acidic urine. The formaldehyde released helps suppress the growth and multiplication of bacteria that may cause recurrent infection. Mandelic acid is present to help maintain the acidic urine. Ascorbic acid (vitamin C) also is often prescribed to help maintain the acidity of the urine.

USES

Methenamine mandelate is used only for patients susceptible to chronic, recurrent UTIs. It is not potent enough to be effective in patients suffering from a preexisting infection. The infection should be treated with antibiotics until the urine is sterile; methenamine should then be given to help prevent recurrence of the infection.

THERAPEUTIC OUTCOME

The primary therapeutic outcome associated with methenamine mandelate therapy is resolution of the UTI.

❖ NURSING IMPLICATIONS FOR METHENAMINE MANDELATE

▪ Premedication Assessment

1. Record voiding characteristics (e.g., frequency, amount, color, odor, and associated symptoms such as burning and pain) to serve as a baseline for monitoring therapy.
2. Check urine for acidification, give prescribed vitamin C, and recheck urine for acidification.
3. Record baseline vital signs.

▪ Availability

PO: 0.5- and 1-g tablets.

▪ Dosage and Administration

Adult

• *PO:* 1 g four times daily after meals and at bedtime. Gastrointestinal symptoms may be minimized by administering with meals. DO NOT crush the tablets! Crushing will allow the formation of form-aldehyde in the stomach, resulting in nausea and belching.

- pH testing: Perform urine testing for pH at regular intervals. Report values above 5.5.

■ Common Adverse Effects
Gastrointestinal

Nausea, vomiting, belching. These adverse effects are usually mild and tend to resolve with continued therapy. Encourage the patient not to discontinue therapy without first consulting his or her healthcare provider.

■ Serious Adverse Effects
Hypersensitivity

Hives, pruritus, rash. Report symptoms for further evaluation by the healthcare provider. Pruritus may be relieved by adding baking soda to the bath water.
Urinary

Bladder irritation, dysuria, frequency. Notify the healthcare provider of these symptoms because they may indicate the presence of another UTI.

■ Drug Interactions
Acetazolamide, Sodium Bicarbonate. Acetazolamide and sodium bicarbonate produce alkaline urine, preventing the conversion of methenamine to formaldehyde, thereby inactivating the medication.

---

nitrofurantoin (nī-trō-FŬR-ăn-tō-ĭn)
  Furadantin (fŭr-ă-DĂN-tĭn)
  Macrodantin (măk-rō-DĂN-tĭn)

ACTIONS

Nitrofurantoin is an antibiotic that acts by interfering with several bacterial enzyme systems.

USES

This antibiotic is not effective against microorganisms in the blood or in tissues outside the urinary tract. It is active against many gram-positive and gram-negative organisms, such as *S. faecalis*, *E. coli*, and *Proteus* species. It is not active against *P. aeruginosa* or *Serratia* species.

THERAPEUTIC OUTCOME

The primary therapeutic outcome associated with nitrofurantoin therapy is resolution of the UTI.

❖ NURSING IMPLICATIONS FOR NITROFURANTOIN
■ Premedication Assessment
1. Record voiding characteristics (e.g., frequency, amount, color, odor, and associated symptoms such as burning and pain) to serve as a baseline for monitoring therapy.
2. Assess for and record any gastrointestinal complaints present before initiating drug therapy.

3. When using nitrofurantoin, check for history of glucose-6-phosphate dehydrogenase deficiency; if present, withhold the drug and contact the healthcare provider.
4. To serve as a baseline, assess the patient for the presence of peripheral neuropathies before initiating therapy.
5. Record baseline vital signs.

■ Availability
PO: 25-, 50-, and 100-mg capsules; 25-mg/5 mL suspension.

■ Dosage and Administration
Adult: *PO:* 50 to 100 mg four times daily for a minimum of 3 days and a maximum of 14 days. Administer with food or milk to reduce gastrointestinal adverse effects. To maintain adequate urine concentrations, space the doses at even intervals around the clock.
  Pediatric: Do not administer to infants younger than 1 month of age. *PO:* 5 to 7 mg/kg/24 hr in four divided doses. *Suspension:* Store in a dark amber container away from bright light.

> **[!] Medication Safety Alert**
>
> Nitrofurantoin must be in the bladder in a sufficient concentration to be therapeutically effective. Nitrofurantoin therapy is *not* recommended for use in patients who have a creatinine clearance lower than 60 mL/min.

■ Common Adverse Effects
Gastrointestinal

Nausea, vomiting, anorexia. Administer with food or milk to reduce gastric irritation.
Urinary

Urine discoloration. Tell the patient that urine may be tinted rust brown to yellow and that this discoloration should not be a cause for alarm.

■ Serious Adverse Effects
Hypersensitivity, Immune System

Dyspnea, chills, fever, erythematous rash, pruritus. These symptoms are the early indications of an allergic reaction to nitrofurantoin. Acute reactions usually occur within 8 hours in previously sensitized individuals and within 7 to 10 days in patients who develop sensitivity during the course of therapy. Discontinue the drug and notify the healthcare provider.
Neurologic

Peripheral neuropathies. Nitrofurantoin may cause peripheral neuropathies, particularly in patients with renal impairment, anemia, diabetes, electrolyte imbalance, or vitamin B deficiency. Nitrofurantoin should be discontinued at the first sign of numbness or tingling in the extremities.
Inflammation, Immune System

Second infection. Inform the healthcare provider immediately if dysuria, pungent-smelling urine, or fever develop. These symptoms may be the early indication of a second infection by an organism resistant to nitrofurantoin.

■ Drug Interactions

Probenecid. Probenecid may inhibit the excretion of nitrofurantoin from the renal tubules. Monitor patients for the development of adverse effects of nitrofurantoin and for signs of incompletely treated UTI.

Eplerenone, Spironolactone. Nitrofurantoin may enhance the hyperkalemic effects of these two agents. Monitor serum potassium levels and for the development of dysrhythmias.

Antacids. Discourage the patient from taking products containing magnesium trisilicate (e.g., Gaviscon-2) concurrently with nitrofurantoin because the antacid may inhibit absorption of the nitrofurantoin.

DRUG THERAPY FOR OVERACTIVE BLADDER SYNDROME

Overactive bladder (OAB) syndrome, also known as *urge syndrome* and *urgency-frequency syndrome,* is a common problem thought to affect more than 33 million Americans annually; it affects 30% to 40% of those older than 75 years. Overactive bladder without urge incontinence is more common in men than in women. It is defined by the International Continence Society (ICS) as "urgency, with or without urge incontinence, usually with frequency and nocturia. These symptoms are thought to be due to detrusor muscle [of the bladder] overactivity, but can also be due to other urinary dysfunction. The diagnosis of OAB can be made if there is no proven infection or other obvious pathology."

The three primary symptoms of OAB syndrome are frequency, urgency, and urinary incontinence. **Frequency** is the need to void eight or more times daily. **Urgency,** the most common symptom associated with OAB, is a sudden, compelling desire to pass urine that is very difficult to ignore. **Incontinence** is the inability to control urine from passing from the bladder. Incontinence can be subdivided into urge incontinence, stress incontinence, and overflow incontinence. **Urge incontinence** is the involuntary leakage of urine accompanied or immediately preceded by urgency. **Stress incontinence** is the brief burst of incontinence brought on by exercise, running, lifting, sneezing, or coughing. Predisposing factors are age, pregnancy, childbirth, cognitive impairment, and obesity. **Overflow incontinence,** also known as *chronic urinary retention,* is urinary leakage resulting from an overfilled and distended bladder that is unable to empty, causing urine to leak from the distended bladder. This may be caused by the inability to feel the urge to urinate and the bladder never empties. This occurs in men with benign prostatic hyperplasia (BPH). **Nocturia** is the need to void at night. Nocturia usually accompanies urgency, with or without urge incontinence, and is the complaint that the individual has to wake at night one or more times to void.

Overactive bladder and incontinence are frequently but erroneously used interchangeably. **Overactive bladder (OAB) syndrome** is the need to urinate, with or without urge incontinence, and is usually accompanied by frequency during daytime and nighttime. About one third of OAB patients have urge incontinence, sometimes termed *OAB wet,* and two thirds have OAB without urge incontinence, or *OAB dry.* Stress incontinence is generally not associated with urgency, frequency, or nocturia, and therefore does not fit the definition of OAB. However, it is not uncommon for patients with OAB also to have stress incontinence. Proper diagnosis of the underlying condition is important because treatments are different.

In males, an overlapping and often confusing problem is BPH (see Chapter 40). Patients with BPH are also susceptible to frequent urination but, unlike OAB, BPH can cause hesitancy and decreased flow during urination. Many men have symptoms of OAB and BPH and can be treated for both at the same time.

Overactive bladder syndrome cannot be cured, but a variety of nonpharmacologic and pharmacologic treatments can be used to reduce the symptoms associated with the disease. The goals of therapy are to decrease frequency by increasing voided volume, decrease urgency, and reduce incidents of urinary urge incontinence. A diary to record the pattern and type of urinary leakage and frequency and volume of fluid consumption ("ins and outs") can be very helpful in developing an awareness of contributors and improvement or deterioration of symptoms over time. Lifestyle changes, such as spacing fluid consumption throughout the day instead of a large intake at one time; avoiding diureticlike stimulants, such as alcohol, caffeine and spicy foods; and avoiding fluid intake after 6:00 PM, can help with symptoms. Note "hidden" sources of caffeine such as Excedrin, Midol, Vanquish, and Anacin. Kegel exercises are recommended to strengthen external sphincter function and increase resistance when there is sudden urinary urgency. Bladder training—the patient is initially taught to void every hour on the hour, then asked to increase the duration between voids by 15 minutes each week—can help increase volume and control urgency. A combination of bladder training and Kegel exercises helps the patient regain bladder control, increasing voided volumes and the time interval between voids. Absorbent undergarment products are helpful in allowing social mobility and maintaining dry skin. They also help promote self-confidence and dignity.

The first line of pharmacologic treatment of OAB is anticholinergic agents. Anticholinergic agents with more selective action on the bladder are darifenacin, fesoterodine, oxybutynin, solifenacin, tolterodine, and trospium.

DRUG CLASS: ANTICHOLINERGIC AGENTS FOR OVERACTIVE BLADDER SYNDROME

ACTIONS

Anticholinergic agents, also known as *urinary antispasmodic agents*, block the cholinergic (muscarinic) receptors of the detrusor muscle of the bladder, causing relaxation. They decrease involuntary contractions of the detrusor muscle and improve bladder volume capacity.

USES

The anticholinergic agents are used to reduce the urgency and frequency of bladder contractions and delay the initial desire to void in patients with overactive bladder. Cholinergic receptors are found throughout the body, particularly in the salivary glands, eyes, colon, and brain. Thus inhibition of these receptors can lead to adverse effects, including dry mouth, blurred vision, constipation, confusion, and sedation. Each of these agents has some degree of selectivity for the cholinergic receptors in the bladder, but the agents are variable in whether they also block receptors in other parts of the body, leading to more adverse effects. They should not be used for patients with narrowangle glaucoma, myasthenia gravis, gastric retention, or bowel disease such as ulcerative colitis, or urinary retention caused by an obstructive uropathy such as prostatitis.

THERAPEUTIC OUTCOME

The primary therapeutic outcome expected from urinary anticholinergic agents is control of incontinence associated with OAB.

❖ NURSING IMPLICATIONS FOR URINARY ANTICHOLINERGIC AGENTS

▪ Premedication Assessment

1. Record voiding characteristics (e.g., frequency, amount, color, odor, associated symptoms such as burning and pain) to serve as a baseline for monitoring therapy.
2. Obtain baseline vital signs.

▪ Availability, Dosage, and Administration
See Table 41-2.

▪ Common Adverse Effects
Neurologic
Dry Mouth, urinary hesitancy, retention, sedation. These adverse effects are usually dosage related and respond to a reduction in dosage. Sedation often resolves with continued use. Instruct the patient to relieve dry mouth by sucking on ice chips or hard candy or by chewing gum.

Gastrointestinal
Constipation, bloating. Encourage balanced nutrition and inclusion of fresh fruits and vegetables for roughage and an adequate fluid intake to help alleviate this complication. If this approach is unsuccessful, suggest a stool softener or bulk-forming supplement. Avoid laxatives.

Sensory
Blurred vision. Caution patients not to drive or operate power equipment until they have adjusted to this adverse effect.

▪ Serious Adverse Effects
If any of the aforementioned adverse effects intensify, they should be reported to the prescriber for evaluation.

▪ Drug Interactions
Anticholinergic Agents. The concurrent use of the urinary anticholinergic agents with other anticholinergic agents may increase the frequency and severity of dry mouth, blurred vision, constipation, and other anticholinergic pharmacologic effects.

Fluoxetine, Erythromycin, Clarithromycin, Ketoconazole, Itraconazole, Miconazole, Vinblastine, Ritonavir, Nefazodone. These agents inhibit the metabolism of tolterodine, darifenacin, and solifenacin. It is recommended that dosages not be raised above the initial starting dosage in patients taking these medicines concurrently.

MISCELLANEOUS URINARY AGENTS

> **bethanechol chloride** (bĕth-ĂN-ĕ-kŏl)
> **Urecholine** (yŭr-ĕ-KŌL-ēn)

ACTIONS

Bethanechol is a parasympathetic nerve stimulant that causes contraction of the detrusor urinae muscle in the bladder, usually resulting in urination. It may also stimulate gastric motility, increase gastric tone, and restore impaired rhythmic peristalsis.

USES

Bethanechol is used in nonobstructive urinary retention, particularly in postoperative and postpartum patients to restore bladder tone and urination.

THERAPEUTIC OUTCOME

The primary therapeutic outcome associated with bethanechol therapy is restoration of bladder tone and urination.

❖ NURSING IMPLICATIONS FOR BETHANECHOL

▪ Premedication Assessment
1. Record voiding characteristics (e.g., frequency, amount, color, odor, and associated symptoms such

Table 41-2   Urinary Anticholinergic Agents

GENERIC NAME	BRAND NAME	AVAILABILITY	DOSAGE
darifenacin	Enablex ⇄ *Do not confuse Enablex with Enbrel.*	Tablets, extended release (24 hr): 7.5, 15 mg	Initial dose: 7.5 mg once daily Based on individual response, the dosage may be increased to 15 mg once daily as early as 2 wk after starting therapy May be taken without regard to food
oxybutynin ⇄ *Do not confuse oxybutynin with OxyContin.*	Ditropan ⇄ *Do not confuse Ditropan with diazepam, Diprivan, or Diovan.*	Tablets: 5 mg Syrup: 5 mg/5 mL	Initial dose: 5 mg (tablets or syrup) two or three times/day Maximum dose: 20 mg daily
	Ditropan XL	Extended-release tablets (24 hr): 5, 10, 15 mg	Initial dose: 5 mg once daily Dosage may be adjusted at weekly intervals in 5-mg increments Maximum dose: 30 mg daily May be administered with or without food and must be swallowed whole with the aid of liquids; do not crush or chew Pediatric (older than 5 yr): PO: 5 mg twice daily; maximum dose, 20 mg daily
	Gelnique	Topical gel: 10%	Apply the contents of one sachet once daily to clean, dry, intact skin on abdomen, thighs, or upper arms/shoulder Rotate site; do not apply to same site on consecutive days Wash hands after use Cover treated area with clothing after gel has dried to prevent transfer of medication to others Do not bathe, shower, or swim until 1 hr after gel is applied
	Oxytrol	Transdermal patch: 36 mg (3.9 mg/day release)	Initial dose: Apply one patch every 3 to 4 days to dry, intact skin on abdomen, hip, or buttock Select a new application site with each new patch to avoid reapplication to the same site within 7 days
fesoterodine	Toviaz	Extended-release tablets (24 hr): 4, 8 mg	4-8 mg daily; 4 mg daily for patients taking potent CYP3A4 inhibitors or with renal impairment
solifenacin	VESIcare	Tablets: 5, 10 mg	Initial dose: 5 mg once daily If well tolerated, dosage may be increased to 10 mg once daily May be taken without regard to food.
tolterodine ⇄ *Do not confuse tolterodine with tolcapone.*	Detrol ⇄ *Do not confuse Detrol with Datril.* Detrol LA	Tablets: 1, 2 mg Extended-release capsules (24 hr): 2, 4 mg	Initial dose: 1-2 mg twice daily based on individual response and tolerance Initial dose: 2-4 mg once daily taken with liquids and swallowed whole
trospium	Sanctura	Tablets: 20 mg	Initial dose: 20 mg twice a day at least 1 hr before meals on an empty stomach For patients with renal creatinine clearance <30 mL/min, recommended dose is 20 mg once daily at bedtime
	Sanctura XR	Extended-release capsules (24 hr): 60 mg	Initial dose: 60 mg daily in the morning; should be taken with water on an empty stomach at least 1 hr before food Not recommended for patients with renal impairment (CrCl <30 mL/min)

as burning and pain) to serve as a baseline for monitoring therapy.

2. Record any gastrointestinal symptoms present to serve as a baseline for monitoring therapy.

▪ Availability

PO: 5-, 10-, 25-, and 50-mg tablets.

▪ Dosage and Administration

Adult: PO: 10 to 50 mg two to four times daily. The maximum daily dosage is 120 mg. *Subcutaneous:* 2.5 to 5 mg. Atropine sulfate must be available to counteract serious adverse effects.

NOTE: If overdosage occurs, the pharmacologic actions of the drug can immediately be reversed by atropine.

▪ Common Adverse Effects

Vascular

Flushing of skin, headache. A pharmacologic property of the drug results in dilated blood vessels.

▪ Serious Adverse Effects

Gastrointestinal

Nausea, vomiting, sweating, colicky pain, abdominal cramps, diarrhea, belching, involuntary defecation. These effects are caused by a pharmacologic property of the drug. Consult the healthcare provider; a dosage adjustment may control these adverse effects. Provide support for the patient who develops diarrhea or involuntary defecation.

▪ Drug Interactions

Quinidine, Procainamide. Do not use these medications concurrently with bethanechol. The pharmacologic properties of these agents counteract those of bethanechol.

---

phenazopyridine hydrochloride
(fĕn-ā-zō-PĬR-ă-dēn)
Pyridium (pī-RĬD-ē-ŭm)

ACTIONS

Phenazopyridine is an agent that, as it is excreted through the urinary tract, produces a local anesthetic effect on the mucosa of the ureters and bladder. It acts within about 30 minutes after oral administration.

USES

Phenazopyridine relieves burning, pain, urgency, and frequency associated with UTIs. It also reduces bladder spasm, which relieves the resulting urinary retention and urgency. Phenazopyridine is also used for preoperative and postoperative surface analgesia in urologic surgical procedures and after diagnostic tests in which instrumentation is necessary. It is occasionally used to relieve the discomfort caused by an indwelling catheter.

THERAPEUTIC OUTCOME

The primary therapeutic outcome associated with phenazopyridine therapy is relief of burning, frequency, pain, and urgency associated with UTI.

❖ NURSING IMPLICATIONS FOR PHENAZOPYRIDINE

▪ Premedication Assessment

1. Record voiding characteristics (e.g., frequency, amount, color, odor, and associated symptoms such as burning and pain) to serve as a baseline for therapy.
2. Record skin color before initiating therapy.

▪ Availability

PO: 95-, 97.2-, 100-, and 200-mg tablets.

▪ Dosage and Administration

Adult: PO: 200 mg three times daily.
Pediatric (6 to 12 years of age): *PO:* 12 mg/kg/day in three divided doses for 2 days.

▪ Common Adverse Effects

Urinary

Reddish-orange urine discoloration. Be certain that the patient understands that the color of the urine will become reddish orange when this drug is used and that this discoloration is no cause for alarm.

▪ Serious Adverse Effects

Integumentary, Sensory

Yellow sclera or skin. The patient should report any yellowish tinge developing in the sclera (white portion) of the eye.

▪ Drug Interactions

Urine Colorimetric Procedures. Phenazopyridine interferes with colorimetric diagnostic tests performed on urine. Consult the hospital laboratory for alternative measures.

Get Ready for the NCLEX® Examination!

Key Points

- Urinary tract infections are some of the most common types of infections and are found in all patient care settings.
- For UTIs, instruct patients to take the medicines exactly as prescribed for the entire course of medication. Discontinuing the antimicrobial agent when the symptoms improve may result in another infection that may be resistant to antimicrobial treatment.
- The nurse can provide significant care by understanding and reporting the early symptoms associated with acute and chronic infections, and assisting patients who have difficulty with urinary retention and incontinence.

Additional Learning Resources

SG Go to your Study Guide for additional Review Questions for the NCLEX® Examination, Critical Thinking Clinical Situations, and other learning activities to help you master this chapter content.

evolve Go to your Evolve website (http://evolve.elsevier.com/Clayton) for additional online resources.

Review Questions for the NCLEX® Examination

1. The nurse is providing education to a patient who has been prescribed phenazopyridine hydrochloride (Pyridium). This common adverse effect is explained by the nurse to the patient:
   1. "You can expect some urinary retention with this drug."
   2. "Since it is common to get a dry mouth with this medication, you can suck on candy to counteract that effect."
   3. "Unfortunately, some patients experience colicky pain when taking this; please call us if that happens."
   4. "There is no cause for concern, but this drug will turn your urine a reddish-orange color."

2. Patients with cerebral palsy and known neurogenic bladder can expect this medication to be ordered:
   1. methenamine mandelate
   2. nitrofurantoin (Macrodantin)
   3. fosfomycin (Monurol)
   4. oxybutynin (Ditropan)

3. This drug yields formaldehyde in the presence of acidic urine:
   1. nitrofurantoin (Macrodantin)
   2. fesoterodine (Toviaz)
   3. methenamine mandelate
   4. probenecid (Benemid)

4. The nurse was teaching health promotion to a female patient with stress incontinence and realized that the patient needed further education after she made this statement:
   1. "I know that I need to keep my skin clean and dry and prevent skin breakdown so I don't get an infection."
   2. "I know that when I get the urge to urinate that it is okay to wait."
   3. "I understand that I can use some incontinence products so I am not embarrassed in public."
   4. "I will practice those Kegel exercises you taught me so that I have better control."

5. Anticholinergic agents will cause these side effects because of the many cholinergic receptors found throughout the body. *(Select all that apply.)*
   1. Dry mouth
   2. Blurred vision
   3. Constipation
   4. Urinary frequency
   5. Diarrhea

6. Bethanechol chloride (Urecholine) is used for the treatment of this disorder.
   1. Overactive bladder syndrome
   2. Acute cystitis
   3. Nonobstructive urinary retention
   4. Urinary tract infection

Drugs Used to Treat Glaucoma and Other Eye Disorders

Objectives

1. Describe the anatomy and physiology of the eye and the normal flow of aqueous humor.
2. Identify the changes in normal flow of aqueous humor caused by open-angle and closed-angle glaucoma.
3. Explain patient assessments needed for eye disorders.
4. Review the correct procedure for instilling eyedrops or eye ointments and discuss patient teaching needs for glaucoma medication use.

Key Terms

cornea (KŎR-nē-ă), (p. 649)
sclera (SKLĀR-ă), (p. 649)
iris (Ī-rĭs), (p. 649)
sphincter muscle (SFĬNK-tĕr MŬS-ŭl), (p. 649)
miosis (mī-Ō-sĭs), (p. 649)
dilator muscle (DĪ-lā-tŭr), (p. 649)
mydriasis (mī-DRĪ-ă-sĭs), (p. 649)
lens (LĔNZ), (p. 649)
near point (NĔR PŌYNT), (p. 649)

zonular fibers (ZŎN-yū-lăr), (p. 649)
cycloplegia (sī-klō-PLĒ-jē-ă), (p. 650)
lacrimal canaliculi (LĂ-krĭ-măl kăn-ă-LĬK-yū-lī), (p. 650)
intraocular pressure (IOP) (ĭn-tră-ŎK-yū-lăr), (p. 651)
closed-angle glaucoma (KLŌZD ĂN-gŭl glŏ-KŌ-mă), (p. 651)
open-angle glaucoma (ō-PĒN ĂN-gŭl glŏ-KŌ-mă), (p. 651)

ANATOMY AND PHYSIOLOGY OF THE EYE

The eyeball has three coats, or layers: the protective external, or corneoscleral coat; the nutritive middle vascular layer, called the *choroid*; and the light-sensitive inner layer, or retina (Figure 42-1).

The **cornea,** or outermost sheath of the anterior eyeball, is transparent so that light can enter the eye. The cornea has no blood vessels; it receives its nutrition from the aqueous humor and its oxygen supply by diffusion from the air and surrounding vascular structures. There is a thin layer of epithelial cells on the external surface of the cornea that is resistant to infection. An abraded cornea, however, is highly susceptible to infection. The cornea has sensory fibers, and any damage to the corneal epithelium will cause pain. Seriously injured corneal tissue is replaced by scar tissue that is usually not transparent. The **sclera** is the eye's white portion that is continuous with the cornea and is not transparent. The pupil is the center black portion of the eye, which is actually a hole in the iris that allows light to reach the retina.

The **iris** is a diaphragm that surrounds the pupil and gives the eye its color—blue, green, hazel, brown, or gray. The **sphincter muscle** within the iris encircles the pupil and is innervated by the parasympathetic nervous system. **Miosis** is contraction of the iris sphincter muscle, which causes the pupil to narrow. The **dilator muscle,** which runs radially from the pupillary margin to the iris periphery, is sympathetically innervated. **Mydriasis** is contraction of the dilator muscle and relaxation of the sphincter muscle, which causes the pupil to dilate (Figure 42-2).

Constriction of the pupil normally occurs with light or when the eye is focusing on nearby objects. Dilation of the pupil normally occurs in dim light or when the eye is focusing on distant objects.

The **lens** is a transparent gelatinous mass of fibers encased in an elastic capsule situated behind the iris. Its function is to ensure that the image on the retina is in sharp focus. It does this by changing shape (accommodation). This occurs readily in youth, but with age the lens becomes more rigid and the ability to focus close objects is lost. The **near point,** the closest point that can be seen clearly, recedes. With age, the lens may lose its transparency and become opaque, forming a cataract. Blindness can occur unless the cataract can be treated or surgically removed.

The lens has ligaments around its edge, called **zonular fibers,** which connect with the ciliary body. Tension on the zonular fibers helps change the shape of the lens. In the unaccommodated eye, the ciliary muscle is relaxed and the zonular fibers are taut. For

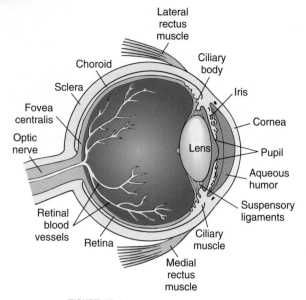

FIGURE 42-1 Cross-section of the eye.

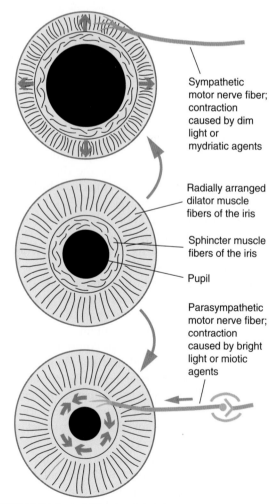

FIGURE 42-2 Effect of light or ophthalmic agents on the iris of the eye.

near vision, the ciliary muscle fibers contract, relaxing the pull on the ligaments and allowing the lens to become thick. Accommodation depends on two factors: (1) the ability of the lens to assume a more biconvex shape when tension on the ligaments is relaxed; and (2) ciliary muscle contraction. Paralysis of the ciliary muscle is termed *cycloplegia.* The ciliary muscle is innervated by parasympathetic nerve fibers.

The ciliary body secretes aqueous humor, which bathes and feeds the lens, posterior surface of the cornea, and iris. After it is formed, the fluid flows forward between the lens and the iris into the anterior chamber. It drains out of the eye through drainage channels located near the junction of the cornea and sclera into a meshwork that leads into Schlemm's canal and into the venous system of the eye.

Eyelids, eyelashes, tears, and blinking all protect the eye. There are about 200 eyelashes for each eye. The eyelashes cause a blink reflex whenever a foreign body touches them, closing the lids for a fraction of a second to prevent the foreign body from entering the eye. Blinking, which is bilateral, occurs every few seconds during waking hours. It keeps the corneal surface free from mucus and spreads the lacrimal fluid evenly over the cornea. Tears are secreted by lacrimal glands and contain lysozyme, a mucolytic lubrication for lid movements. They wash away foreign objects and form a thin film over the cornea, providing it with a good optical surface. Tear fluid is lost by drainage into two small ducts, the **lacrimal canaliculi,** at the inner corners of the eyelids and by evaporation.

GENERAL CONSIDERATIONS FOR TOPICAL OPHTHALMIC DRUG THERAPY

The most common route of administration for ophthalmic drugs is topical application. Advantages include convenience, simplicity, noninvasive nature, and the ability of the patient to self-administer. Topically administered medications do not penetrate adequately for use with posterior eye diseases, so topical administration is not used for such diseases as with the optic nerve or retina.

Proper administration is essential to optimal therapeutic response. The administration technique used often determines drug safety and efficacy (see Chapter 7, Figures 7-6 and 7-7).

- Based on the volume that the eye can retain, use of more than one drop per administration is questionable.
- If more than one drug is to be administered at about the same time, separate the administration of the different medications by at least 5 minutes. This ensures that the first medication is not washed away by the second, or that the second medication is not diluted by the first.
- Minimize systemic absorption of ophthalmic drops by compressing the tear duct at the inner canthus of

the eye for 3 to 5 minutes after instillation. This reduces the passage of medication via the nasolacrimal duct into areas of absorption, such as the nasal and pharyngeal mucosa.

- Eyecup use is discouraged because of the risk of contamination.
- Ophthalmic ointments may impede delivery of other ophthalmic drugs to the affected site by serving as a barrier to contact. Administer drops *before* applying ointments. Try not to administer drops for a few hours after the use of ointment. The ointment should be administered beginning at the inner canthus to the outer aspect of the eye.
- Ointments may blur vision during the waking hours. Use with caution in conditions in which visual clarity is critical (e.g., operating motor equipment, reading).
- Observe expiration dates closely. Do not use outdated medication.
- Solutions and ointments are frequently misused. Do not assume that patients know how to effectively use these agents.
- In an effort to enhance safety of ophthalmic medications, the ophthalmic medicine industry recommends the use of standard colors for drug labels and bottle caps (see the following chart). Ophthalmic drug labels include "For Ophthalmic Use." The nurse should become familiar with these colors and types of ophthalmic medications to help prevent inadvertently picking up and administering the wrong solution.

THERAPEUTIC CLASS	CAP AND LABEL COLOR
Antiinfectives	Brown or tan
Beta-adrenergic blocking agents	Yellow, blue, or both
Miotics	Green
Mydriatics and cycloplegics	Red
Nonsteroidal antiinflammatory agents	Gray

GLAUCOMA

Glaucoma is an eye disease characterized by abnormally elevated **intraocular pressure (IOP)**, which may result from excessive production of the aqueous humor or from diminished ocular fluid outflow. Increased pressure, if persistent and sufficiently elevated, may lead to permanent blindness. There are three major types of glaucoma: primary, secondary, and congenital. Primary includes **closed-angle glaucoma** (also known as narrow-angle glaucoma) and **open-angle glaucoma.** These are diagnosed by determination of the iridocorneal angle of the anterior chamber, where aqueous humor reabsorption takes place. Secondary glaucoma may result from previous eye disease or may occur after a cataract extraction and may require drug therapy for an indefinite period. Congenital glaucoma requires surgical treatment.

Open-angle glaucoma develops insidiously over the years as pathologic changes at the iridocorneal angle prevent the outflow of aqueous humor through the trabecular network to Schlemm's canal and into the veins of the eye (Figure 42-3). In cases of open-angle glaucoma, there is reduced outflow of aqueous humor through the trabecular network and Schlemm's canal because of resistance of the aqueous humor outflow; the iridocorneal angle is open (Figure 42-4).

Intraocular pressure builds up and, if not treated, will damage the optic disc. Initially, the patient has no symptoms, but over the years there is a gradual loss of peripheral vision. If untreated, total blindness may result.

Acute closed-angle glaucoma occurs when there is a sudden increase in IOP caused by a mechanical

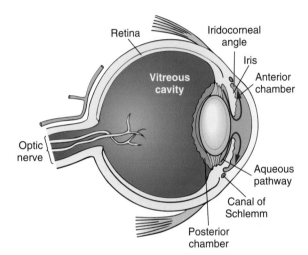

FIGURE 42-3 Anterior and posterior chambers of the eye. Arrows indicate the pathway of aqueous flow.

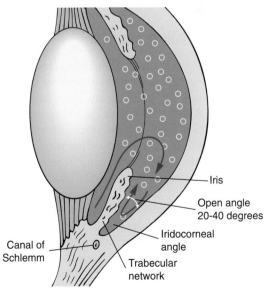

FIGURE 42-4 Open-angle glaucoma. Obstruction to the flow of the aqueous humor is caused by reduced outflow at Schlemm's canal in the trabecular network. There is no obstruction from closure of the iridocorneal angle.

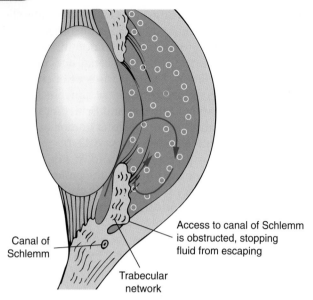

Canal of
Schlemm

Access to canal of Schlemm
is obstructed, stopping
fluid from escaping

Trabecular
network

FIGURE 42-5 Closed-angle glaucoma. Obstruction to the flow of
aqueous fluid, causing closed-angle glaucoma.

obstruction of the trabecular network in the iridocorneal angle (Figure 42-5). This occurs in patients who have narrow anterior chamber angles. Symptoms develop gradually and appear intermittently for short periods, especially when the pupil is dilated. (Dilation of the pupil pushes the iris against the trabecular meshwork, causing the obstruction.) Symptoms often reported are blurred vision, halos around white lights, frontal headache, and eye pain. Patients often associate the symptoms with stress or fatigue. An attack can also be precipitated by administration of a mydriatic agent, such as atropine or scopolamine, for eye examination.

DRUG THERAPY FOR GLAUCOMA

The treatment of open-angle glaucoma is maintenance of IOP at normal levels to prevent further blindness. Treatment options include surgery, laser surgery, and drug therapy. A beta-adrenergic blocking agent (e.g., timolol maleate) has become the initial drug of choice. Other agents that may also be used are prostaglandins (e.g., latanoprost), sympathomimetic agents (e.g., brimonidine) and carbonic anhydrase inhibitors (e.g., acetazolamide). The selection of the drug is determined to a great extent by the requirements of the individual patient and response to therapy.

Acute closed-angle glaucoma requires immediate treatment to reduce IOP. Intravenous mannitol, an osmotic diuretic, may be administered to draw aqueous humor from the eye. Topical corticosteroids may be used to reduce ocular inflammation. Other medications used to reduce formation of aqueous humor include beta blockers, prostaglandins, a sympathomi-

metic agent, or a carbonic anhydrase inhibitor. After IOP has been reduced, pilocarpine may be used to induce miosis, relieving the pressure of the iris against the trabecular network and allowing drainage of the aqueous humor. Analgesics and antiemetics may be administered if pain and vomiting persist. Surgery is then required to correct the abnormality.

❖ NURSING IMPLICATIONS FOR GLAUCOMA AND OTHER EYE DISORDERS

The nurse has an important role in educating the public and promoting safety measures to protect the eye from potential sources of injury. Healthcare professionals can participate in this role during their daily contacts with people in the community. The use of safety glasses in potentially hazardous situations, prevention of chemical burns from common household cleaning items or other agents at home or work, proper cleaning and wearing of contact lenses or glasses, and selection of safe toys and play activities for children are some areas about which the nurse can teach the public. These safety measures can significantly reduce the number of injuries that occur annually.

Nurses play an important role in detecting eye disorders and implementing treatment plans. An example of this is in patients with diabetes mellitus. Encourage annual, or more frequent, eye examinations to detect and prevent complications associated with the disease.

The primary delivery of eye care is through self-administration of drugs. One of the greatest challenges in the care of chronic eye disorders such as glaucoma is convincing the patient of the need for long-term treatment and adherence to the therapeutic regimen.

■ Assessment
Eye Examination
- When an eye injury has occurred, document visual acuity by screening vision with the Snellen chart. Comparison screenings should be performed at each subsequent visit.
- Observe for eyelid edema. It may be an indication of a systemic disease process or tumor. Report if present.
- Assess pupils for equality of size, roundness, and response to light. Report irregular contour, unequal size, or decreased response to light.
- Observe for and report nystagmus.
- Observe for any redness or drainage in the eyes.
- Observe for complete closure of the eyelid. This is essential for protection of the cornea. Patients who have received corneal anesthesia, have had fifth cranial nerve surgery, have exophthalmos, or are unconscious must have the cornea protected to prevent damage.
- Ask whether glasses or contact lenses are worn.
- Inspect the eye dressings and report immediately for evaluation if any drainage is observed. Never

remove the surgical dressing after surgery to inspect the eye.

History of Symptoms

- Ask the patient to describe the symptoms for which treatment is being sought. How do symptoms affect daily life? Do visual problems affect ability to read?
- Is there a family history of cataracts, glaucoma, or macular degeneration?
- Are activities limited in any way by any vision problem?
- Do any leisure activities have the potential for eye injury?
- Has the person had any noticeable pain, burning, foreign body sensation, blurred or halo vision, or loss of vision?
- Ask whether there is any difficulty in adjusting vision when going from a dark to a brightly lighted area or vice versa.
- Are colors clear and crisp, or do they lack clarity?
- Has there been an increase in tearing or discharge from the eye? If so, ask for details of appearance and amount of drainage.
- Has there been any recent nausea or vomiting?

Psychological. What type of response is the patient exhibiting to the disturbance in visual acuity? Is the patient withdrawing socially? Identify a support system available for at-home care and assistance. Plan a specific time to meet with the patient and significant others to discuss at-home care and community resources available if assistance is indicated.

Life Span Considerations

Diminished Visual Acuity

Diminished visual acuity affects most aspects of a person's life, so it is imperative to evaluate an individual's ability to perform the usual activities of daily living when visual impairment develops. Many medications used to treat other disorders can reduce visual acuity; this adverse effect should be anticipated and its consequences monitored. Every attempt must be made to help the patient adapt to the visual impairment and provide for personal safety.

Diagnostics. Ask the patient to describe what eye diagnostic procedures have been completed before admission (e.g., visual acuity measurement, tonometry, slit-lamp examination, visual fields). A tonometer is used to measure the IOP inside the eye to evaluate a patient's risk for glaucoma and to assess the success or failure of ongoing treatment. There are several types of tonometers available (e.g., applanation, Goldman, noncontact, ocular response analyzer), the use of which ranges from quick screening for increased intraocular pressure to very precise measurement of intraocular pressure. Most tonometers measure pressure in units of millimeters of mercury (mm Hg).

Medications. Ask for a list of all prescribed and over-the-counter medications and herbal products

being taken. Ask for details on medications, dosage, schedule, and degree of compliance. List all ordered medications on the medication administration record (MAR). If beta blockers are being taken, list the pulse and blood pressure on the MAR as a preassessment to administration of the ophthalmic drops. Mark the Kardex or enter data into the computer with parameters relating to the prevention of injury, the activity and exercise level permitted, and diet orders.

■ Implementation

- Perform assessments every shift consistent with the patient's status and diagnosis.
- Prepare the patient for eye examinations, diagnostics, or eye surgery.
- Administer cycloplegic and mydriatic medications prescribed for dilation of the eye before an eye examination or ophthalmic surgery.
- Administer miotic medication to produce constriction of the eye after eye examination or diagnostic procedures, as prescribed.
- Administer all ophthalmic medications prescribed while maintaining aseptic technique to prevent the transfer of infection from one eye to the other.
- Protect the cornea from damage during anesthesia or in an unconscious patient through the use of ophthalmic ointment or artificial tears to prevent corneal drying.
- Assist with diagnostic procedures (e.g., visual fields, tonometry, visual acuity).
- Take baseline vital signs.
- Institute appropriate comfort measures.
- If eye surgery has been performed (e.g., trabeculectomy), institute routine postoperative care measures. Position the patient as ordered, usually on the back or on the unoperated side. With the scleral buckling procedure, positioning orders may be extremely specific.
- Ensure that an eye patch and shield are applied properly to protect the eye from further injury.
- Explain and enforce activity and exercise restrictions. To prevent an increase in IOP, instruct the patient to avoid heavy lifting, straining on defecation, coughing, or bending and placing the head in a dependent position.
- A blind or disoriented patient or a patient with both eyes patched may experience effects of sensory deprivation.
- Always speak before touching a person with impaired vision.
- Check on the patient at frequent intervals; initiate conversations and regularly orient the patient to date, time, and place.
- If the patient is agitated, contact the prescriber; it may be necessary to obtain an order to remove one eye patch or sedate the patient.
- Provide emotional support.

Health Promotion

- Perform hand hygiene thoroughly each time the area is touched (before or after eye treatments or instillation of medications).
- Use only sterile medications or dressings on the eye.
- Wipe the eye from the inner canthus outward; discard the tissue used; perform hand hygiene before proceeding to the second eye.
- When an infection is present, prevent cross-contamination; always use a separate source of medication and dropper for each eye.
- Never touch the eyeball or face with the tip of the dropper or opening of the ointment container. Demonstrate the proper way to set the medication lid down so that the inside is not contaminated.
- When inserting or removing contact lenses, perform hand hygiene first and then follow the manufacturer's instructions regarding the cleansing and care of the lenses.
- Report any persistent redness or drainage from the eyes.

▪ Patient Education

After Eye Surgery

- Teach the patient and family proper hygiene and eye care techniques to ensure that medications, dressings, and/or surgical wounds are not contaminated during necessary eye care.
- Teach the patient and family about signs and symptoms of infections and when and how to report them to allow early recognition and treatment of possible infection.
- Instruct the patient to comply with postoperative restrictions on head positioning, bending, coughing, and the Valsalva maneuver to optimize visual outcomes and prevent increased IOP.
- Instruct the patient to instill the eye medications using aseptic techniques and to comply with the prescribed eye medication routine to prevent infection (see Figures 7-6 and 7-7). In general, using more than one drop per dose of medication does not improve response, but increases the frequency of adverse effects and the cost of therapy. Instruct the patient on how to block the nasolacrimal duct during instillation to minimize systemic effects.
- When using more than one medication, separate drop instillation of each agent by at least 5 minutes to provide optimal ocular contact for each medication.
- Instruct the patient to monitor pain and take prescribed pain medication as directed; report pain not relieved by prescribed medications.
- Instruct the patient about the importance of continued follow-up as recommended to maximize potential visual outcomes.

Disease or Disorder

- Reinforce the teaching of pertinent facts regarding the diagnosis and disease process.
- If the patient is being treated for glaucoma, stress the need for lifelong treatment and use of medications. Explain that adherence with the drug regimen can help prevent blindness.
- If an infectious process is present, teach personal hygiene measures to prevent introduction of an infection.

Visual Acuity

- Provide for patient safety.
- Assess whether diminished visual acuity will reduce the ability of the patient to perform his or her usual activities of daily living. Teach adaptation methods appropriate to the situation.
- Restrict the operation of tools or power equipment, as appropriate, to the degree of alteration present.

Medications

- Review the details of medication administration.
- Ensure that directions are printed in large, bold print that the individual can read.
- Have the patient store all medications in an area separate from other containers so that she or he cannot inadvertently put things other than medication in the eye.
- Have the person demonstrate the ability to self-administer the eye medications to ensure manual dexterity to perform the procedures.
- Keep an extra bottle of eye medications on hand, particularly those used to reduce IOP.

Fostering Health Maintenance

- Discuss medication information and how it will benefit the course of treatment (e.g., reduction of IOP, elimination of an infection).
- Seek cooperation and understanding of the following points so that medication compliance is increased: name of medication; dosage, route, and times of administration; and common and serious adverse effects. Verify ability to self-administer all medications. Additional health teaching is included in the individual drug monographs.
- Encourage the patient to discuss any adverse effects that the medications may produce with the healthcare provider to plan mutually for ways to minimize these effects or make adaptations rather than reduce the frequency or eliminate the use of the medications.

Patient Self-Assessment. Enlist the patient's aid in developing and maintaining a written record (see Patient Self-Assessment Form for Eye Medications on the Evolve website) of monitoring parameters (e.g., blood pressure and pulse with adrenergic and beta-adrenergic blocking agents, degree of visual disturbance, progression of impairment) and response to prescribed therapies for discussion with the physician. Encourage the patient to take this record to all follow-up visits.

Table 42-1   Carbonic Anhydrase Inhibitors

GENERIC NAME	BRAND NAME	AVAILABILITY	DOSAGE
acetazolamide	Diamox	Tablets: 125, 250 mg Capsules, extended release (12 hr): 500 mg Powder for injection: 500 mg	PO: 250 mg one to four times daily or 500 mg extended release twice daily
brinzolamide	Azopt	Ophthalmic solution: 1% in 10- and 15-mL dropper bottles	Intraocular: 1 drop in affected eye(s) three times daily If more than one ophthalmic agent is to be administered in the same eye, separate the administration by at least 10 min
dorzolamide	Trusopt	Ophthalmic solution: 2% in 10-mL dropper bottle	Intraocular: 1 drop in affected eye(s) three times daily If more than one ophthalmic agent is to be administered in the same eye, separate the administration by at least 10 min
methazolamide	Neptazane	Tablets: 25, 50 mg	PO: 50 to 100 mg, two or three times daily

DRUG CLASS: CARBONIC ANHYDRASE INHIBITORS

ACTIONS

These agents are inhibitors of the enzyme carbonic anhydrase. Inhibition of this enzyme results in a decrease in the production of aqueous humor, thus lowering IOP.

USES

These agents are used in conjunction with other treatments to control IOP in cases of intraocular hypertension and closed-angle and open-angle glaucoma. Dorzolamide has the advantage of intraocular administration, with less potential for systemic adverse effects.

THERAPEUTIC OUTCOME

The primary therapeutic outcome expected from carbonic anhydrase inhibitors is reduced IOP.

❖ NURSING IMPLICATIONS FOR CARBONIC ANHYDRASE INHIBITORS

- **Premedication Assessment**
1. Establish whether the patient is pregnant; if pregnancy is suspected, hold the medication and contact the healthcare provider.
2. Check for allergy to sulfonamide antibiotics; hold the medication and contact the healthcare provider if allergy is present.
3. Ensure that contact lenses have been removed before the instillation of dorzolamide drops.
4. Ensure that baseline electrolyte laboratory studies have been drawn as ordered.
5. Assess and record baseline weight, hydration data, vital signs, and mental status.
6. Record premedication IOP readings and visual acuity data.
7. Assess for signs of gastric symptoms before initiating drug therapy. If present, schedule medications for administration with milk or food.

- **Availability, Dosage, and Administration**

See Table 42-1.

Sulfonamides. Do not administer to patients allergic to sulfonamide antibiotics without healthcare provider approval. Observe closely for the development of hypersensitivity.

- **Common Adverse Effects**

Gastric Irritation. If gastric irritation occurs, administer the medication with food or milk. If symptoms persist or increase in severity, report to the healthcare provider for evaluation.

- **Serious Adverse Effects**

Hematologic

Electrolyte imbalance, dehydration. Although infrequent, treatment with carbonic anhydrase inhibitors may lead to excessive diuresis, resulting in water dehydration and electrolyte imbalance. The electrolytes most commonly altered are K^+, Na^+, and Cl^-. Hypokalemia is most likely to occur. Many symptoms associated with altered fluid and electrolyte balance are subtle and resemble general symptoms of drug toxicity or the disease process itself. Gather data about changes in the patient's mental status (e.g., alertness, orientation, confusion), muscle strength, muscle cramps, tremors, nausea, and general appearance (e.g., drowsy, anxious, lethargic). Always check the electrolyte reports for early indications of electrolyte imbalance. Keep accurate records of intake and output, daily weight, and vital signs.

Sulfonamide-like Reactions

Dermatologic, hematologic, neurologic reactions. Carbonic anhydrase inhibitors are sulfonamide derivatives and thus have the potential to cause adverse effects similar to those associated with sulfonamide antimicrobial therapy. These adverse effects, although rare, include dermatologic, hematologic, and neurologic reactions. (For further discussion see the section on sulfonamides in Chapter 45.)

Neurologic

Confusion. Perform a baseline assessment of the patient's degree of alertness and orientation to name, place, and time before initiating therapy. Make regularly scheduled subsequent mental status evaluations, and compare findings. Report changes in the patient's mental status.

Drowsiness. This adverse effect is usually mild and tends to resolve with continued therapy. Encourage the patient not to discontinue therapy without first consulting the healthcare provider. The patient who works with machinery, operates a motor vehicle, administers medications, or performs other duties that require mental alertness should not take these medications while working.

■ Drug Interactions

Quinidine. These diuretics may inhibit quinidine excretion. If the patient is also receiving quinidine, monitor closely for signs of quinidine toxicity (e.g., tinnitus, vertigo, headache, confusion, bradycardia, visual disturbances).

Digoxin. Patients receiving these diuretics may excrete excess potassium, which leads to hypokalemia. If the patient is also receiving digoxin, monitor closely for signs of digoxin toxicity (e.g., anorexia, nausea, fatigue, blurred or colored vision, bradycardia, dysrhythmias).

Corticosteroids (Prednisone, Others). Corticosteroids may enhance the loss of potassium. Check potassium levels and monitor more closely for hypokalemia when these two agents are used concurrently.

DRUG CLASS: CHOLINERGIC AGENTS

ACTIONS

Cholinergic agents produce strong contractions of the iris (miosis) and ciliary body musculature (accommodation).

USES

Cholinergic agents lower IOP in patients with glaucoma by widening the filtration angle, which permits outflow of aqueous humor. They also may be used to counter the effects of mydriatic and cycloplegic agents after surgery or ophthalmoscopic examination.

Cholinergic agents have several advantages: they are effective in many cases of chronic glaucoma, the adverse effects are less severe and occur less frequently than those of anticholinesterase agents, and they give better control of IOP with fewer fluctuations in pressure.

THERAPEUTIC OUTCOMES

The primary therapeutic outcomes expected from cholinergic agents are as follows:
1. Reduced IOP in patients with glaucoma
2. Reversal of the mydriasis and cycloplegia secondary to ophthalmic agents used in surgery or ophthalmic examination

❖ NURSING IMPLICATIONS FOR CHOLINERGIC AGENTS

■ Premedication Assessment
1. Obtain baseline vital signs.
2. Record premedication IOP readings and visual acuity data.

■ Availability, Dosage, and Administration
See Table 42-2.

■ Common Adverse Effects

Sensory

Reduced visual acuity. A common adverse effect of cholinergic agents is difficulty in adjusting quickly to changes in light intensity. Reduced visual acuity may be most notable at night, particularly in areas of poor lighting, as well as in older patients and those developing lens opacities. Advise patients to use caution while driving at night or performing hazardous tasks in poor light. Blurred vision can occur, particularly during the first 1 to 2 hours after instilling the medication. Be sure to keep eye medications separate from other solutions.

The ability to read for long periods is decreased because of impairment of near-vision accommodation. Provide for patient safety when visual impairment exists. In hospitals, orient to the hospital unit, furniture placement, and call light; place the bed in a low position. At home, do not move furniture or the individual's household or personal belongings.

Conjunctival Irritation, Erythema, Headache. These adverse effects are usually mild and tend to resolve with continued therapy. Encourage the patient not to discontinue therapy without first consulting the healthcare provider.

Pain, Discomfort. Because of pupillary constriction, an increase in pain or discomfort may occur, particularly in bright light. Stress the need for adherence and assure the patient that this adverse effect will diminish with continued use.

Neurologic

Headache. This adverse effect is usually mild and tends to resolve with continued therapy. Encourage the patient not to discontinue therapy without first consulting his or her healthcare provider.

■ Serious Adverse Effects

Systemic Adverse Effects. Rarely, a patient may develop signs of systemic toxicity manifested by

Table 42-2 Cholinergic Agents

GENERIC NAME	BRAND NAME	AVAILABILITY	DOSAGE	COMMENTS
acetylcholine chloride, intraocular	Miochol-E	20 mg in 2-mL vial for reconstitution making a 1:100 solution	0.5-2 mL instilled into the eye during surgery	Used only during surgery to produce complete miosis within seconds; duration of action is only a few minutes, so pilocarpine may be added to maintain miosis
carbachol, intraocular	Miostat	Solution: 0.01%	0.5 mL	Used only during surgery to produce complete miosis within 2-5 min
carbachol, topical	Isopto-Carbachol	Solution: 1.5%, 3%	1-2 drops into eye two or three times daily	Miotic action lasts 4-8 hr; may be particularly useful for patients resistant to pilocarpine
pilocarpine	Isopto-Carpine, Pilopine HS	Solution: 1%, 2%, 4% Gel: 4%	1-2 drops up to four times daily; 0.5%-4% solutions used most frequently Gel: 0.5-inch ribbon in the conjunctival sac at bedtime	Safest, most commonly used miotic for glaucoma; also used to reverse mydriasis after eye examination; onset is 10-30 min; lasts for 4-8 hr

diaphoresis, salivation, abdominal discomfort, diarrhea, bronchospasm, muscle tremors, hypotension, dysrhythmias, and/or bradycardia. These symptoms are indications of excessive administration. Report to the healthcare provider for dosage adjustment. The adverse effects themselves usually do not need to be treated because they will resolve by withholding cholinergic therapy. Prevent systemic effects by carefully blocking the inner canthus for 3 to 5 minutes after instilling the medication to prevent absorption via the nasolacrimal duct. During drug therapy, assess the blood pressure every shift, and report significant changes from the baseline data. If accidental overdose occurs during instillation, flush the affected eye with water or normal saline.

■ **Drug Interactions**

Carbamate and/or Organophosphate Insecticides and Pesticides. Gardeners, farmers, manufacturing employees, and others who are exposed to these pesticides and insecticides and who are receiving cholinergic agents should be warned of the added risk of systemic symptoms from absorption of these chemicals through the skin and respiratory tract. Respiratory masks, frequent washing, and clothing changes are advisable.

DRUG CLASS: ALPHA ADRENERGIC AGENTS

ACTIONS

Adrenergic agents have several uses in ophthalmology. Sympathomimetic agents cause pupil dilation, increased outflow of aqueous humor, vasoconstriction, relaxation of the ciliary muscle, and a decrease in the formation of aqueous humor.

USES

Adrenergic agents are used to lower IOP in open-angle glaucoma, relieve congestion and hyperemia, and produce mydriasis for ocular examinations. Use with caution in patients with hypertension, diabetes mellitus, hyperthyroidism, heart disease, arteriosclerosis, or long-standing bronchial asthma.

THERAPEUTIC OUTCOMES

The primary therapeutic outcomes expected from adrenergic agents are as follows:
1. Mydriasis for ophthalmic examination
2. Reduced IOP in open-angle glaucoma
3. Reduced redness of the eyes from irritation

❖ NURSING IMPLICATIONS FOR ALPHA ADRENERGIC AGENTS

■ **Premedication Assessment**
1. Obtain baseline vital signs, including blood pressure and pulse.
2. Record premedication IOP readings and visual acuity data.

■ **Availability, Dosage, and Administration**
See Table 42-3.

■ **Common Adverse Effects**
Sensory
Sensitivity to bright light. The mydriasis produced allows excessive amounts of light into the eyes, which causes the patient to squint. Sunglasses will help

Table 42-3   Alpha Adrenergic Agents

GENERIC NAME	BRAND NAME	AVAILABILITY	DOSAGE	COMMENTS
apraclonidine	Iopidine	0.5%, 1% solution	1 drop 1 hr before surgery and 1 drop immediately after surgery.	An alpha-2 adrenergic agent used to control IOP after laser surgery
brimonidine	Alphagan P	0.1%, 0.15%, 0.2% solution	1 drop q8h in affected eye(s)	An alpha-2 adrenergic agent used to lower IOP in open-angle glaucoma or ocular hypertension
naphazoline hydrochloride	Clear Eyes; Vasoclear	0.012%, 0.02%, 0.03%, 0.1% solution	1-2 drops q3-4h (up to four times daily)	Used as a topical vasoconstrictor; therapy should not exceed 3 days
Oxymetazoline hydrochloride	Visine LR	0.025% solution	1-2 drops q6h	Used as a topical vasoconstrictor for minor eye irritation
phenylephrine	Altafrin, Neofrin, Mydfrin	0.12%, 2.5%, 10% solution	1-2 drops two or three times daily	0.12% used as a decongestant for minor eye irritation; 2.5% and 10% solutions used for pupil dilation in uveitis, open-angle glaucoma, and diagnostic procedures
tetrahydrozoline hydrochloride	Visine, Opti-Clear	0.05% solution	1-2 drops two to four times daily	Used as a topical vasoconstrictor

IOP, intraocular pressure.

reduce the brightness. Caution the patient to temporarily avoid tasks that require visual acuity, such as driving or operating power machinery.

Conjunctival irritation, lacrimation. These adverse effects are usually mild and tend to resolve with continued therapy. Encourage the patient not to discontinue therapy without first consulting the healthcare provider.

■ Serious Adverse Effects

Cardiovascular

Systemic adverse effects. Systemic effects from ophthalmic instillation are uncommon and minimal; however, systemic absorption may occur via the lacrimal drainage system into the nasopharyngeal passages. Systemic effects are manifested by palpitations, tachycardia, dysrhythmias, hypertension, faintness, trembling, and diaphoresis. These are indications of overdose or excessive administration. Report to the healthcare provider for treatment and dosage adjustment. Prevent systemic effects by carefully blocking the inner canthus for 3 to 5 minutes after instilling the medication to prevent absorption via the nasolacrimal duct. Monitor the pulse rate and blood pressure, and instruct the patient to continue to do this at home; report significant changes from the baseline data.

Diaphoresis, trembling. Touch the patient and bedding to assess for diaphoresis, particularly when these medications are used in surgery in which the patient is under sterile drapes, anesthetized, and unable to respond to verbal questioning.

■ Drug Interactions

Tricyclic Antidepressants. Tricyclic antidepressants (e.g., amitriptyline, imipramine, doxepin) may cause additive hypertensive effects. Monitor carefully for poor blood pressure control or a gradually increasing blood pressure.

DRUG CLASS: BETA-ADRENERGIC BLOCKING AGENTS

ACTIONS

Beta-adrenergic blocking agents are used in ophthalmology to reduce elevated IOP. Their exact mechanism of action is not known, but it is thought that they reduce the production of aqueous humor.

USES

Beta blockers are used to reduce IOP in patients with chronic open-angle glaucoma or ocular hypertension. Unlike anticholinergic agents, there is no blurred or dim vision or night blindness because IOP is reduced with little or no effect on pupil size or visual acuity.

THERAPEUTIC OUTCOME

The primary therapeutic outcome expected from adrenergic blocking agents is reduced IOP.

❖ NURSING IMPLICATIONS FOR BETA-ADRENERGIC BLOCKING AGENTS

■ Premedication Assessment

1. Obtain baseline vital signs, including pulse and blood pressure; hold the medication and contact the

Table 42-4   Beta-Adrenergic Blocking Agents

GENERIC NAME	BRAND NAME	AVAILABILITY	INITIAL DOSAGE	COMMENTS
betaxolol hydrochloride	Betoptic-S	0.25%, 0.5% solution in 5-, 10-, and 15-mL dropper bottles	1-2 drops twice daily	Beta-1 blocking agent; onset in 30 min, duration is 12 hr; several weeks of therapy may be required to determine optimal dosage
carteolol	—	1% solution in 5-, 10-, 15-mL dropper bottles	1 drop twice daily	Beta-1, beta-2 blocking agent; duration is up to 12 hr
levobunolol hydrochloride	Betagan	0.25%, 0.5% solution in 5-, 10-, 15-mL dropper bottles	1 drop once or twice daily	Beta-1, beta-2 blocking agent; onset within 60 min, duration is up to 24 hr
metipranolol	—	0.3% solution in 5-, 10-mL dropper bottles	1 drop twice daily in affected eye(s)	Beta-1, beta-2 blocking agent; onset within 30 min, duration is 12-24 hr
timolol maleate	Timoptic	Solution: 0.25%, 0.5% in 5-, 10-, 15-mL dropper bottles Gel: 0.25%, 0.5% solution, gel-forming	1 drop of 0.25% solution twice daily; 1 drop of gel solution once daily	Beta-1, beta-2 blocking agent; onset within 30 min, duration is up to 24 hr; gel may be used once daily

healthcare provider if bradycardia, hypertension, or respiratory disorders are present.

2. Record the premedication IOP readings and visual acuity data.

■ **Availability, Dosage, and Administration**
See Table 42-4.

■ **Common Adverse Effects**
Sensory
Conjunctival irritation, lacrimation. These adverse effects are usually mild and tend to resolve with continued therapy. Encourage the patient not to discontinue therapy without first consulting the healthcare provider.

■ **Serious Adverse Effects**
Cardiovascular
Bradycardia, hypotension. Systemic effects are uncommon, but may be manifested by bradycardia, dysrhythmias, hypotension, faintness, and bronchospasm. These adverse effects are more frequently observed in patients requiring higher dosages of beta-adrenergic blocking agents and in patients with hypertension, diabetes mellitus, heart disease, arteriosclerosis, or long-standing bronchial asthma. Report to the healthcare provider for treatment and dosage adjustment. Record the blood pressure and pulse rate at specific intervals.

■ **Drug Interactions**
Beta-Adrenergic Blocking Agents. Beta blockers (e.g., propranolol, atenolol, metoprolol) may enhance the systemic therapeutic and toxic effects of ophthalmic beta-adrenergic blocking medications. Monitor for an increase in severity of adverse effects such as fatigue, hypotension, bronchospasm, and bradycardia.

DRUG CLASS: PROSTAGLANDIN AGONISTS

ACTIONS

Prostaglandin agonists reduce IOP by increasing the outflow of aqueous humor.

USES

The prostaglandin agonists are used to reduce IOP in patients with chronic open-angle glaucoma or ocular hypertension who have not responded well to other IOP-lowering agents.

THERAPEUTIC OUTCOME

The primary therapeutic outcome expected from prostaglandin agonists is reduced IOP.

❖ NURSING IMPLICATIONS FOR PROSTAGLANDIN AGONISTS

■ **Premedication Assessment**
1. Obtain baseline vital signs.
2. Record the premedication IOP readings and visual acuity data.

■ **Availability, Dosage, and Administration**
See Table 42-5. If more than one drug is to be instilled in the same eye, administer the drugs at least 5 minutes apart.

[!] Medication Safety Alert

Do not administer prostaglandin agonists into the eyes when the patient is wearing contact lenses. Lenses may be reinserted 15 minutes following administration.

Table 42-5 Prostaglandin Agonists

GENERIC NAME	BRAND NAME	AVAILABILITY	DOSAGE	COMMENTS
bimatoprost	Lumigan	0.01% and 0.03% solution in 2.5-, 5-, 7.5-mL dropper bottles	1 drop in each affected eye in the evening	Do not exceed dosage because it may reduce IOP-lowering effect
latanoprost	Xalatan	0.005% solution in 2.5-mL dropper bottle	1 drop in each affected eye in the evening	Do not exceed dosage because it may reduce IOP-lowering effect
tafluprost	Zioptan	0.015 % solution in 0.3-mL pouches	1 drop in each affected eye in the evening	Do not exceed dosage because it may reduce IOP-lowering effect. If used with other ophthalmic agents, separate administration by at least 5 min
travoprost	Travatan Z	0.004% solution in 2.5- and 5-mL dropper bottles	1 drop in each affected eye in the evening	Do not exceed dosage because it may reduce IOP-lowering effect

IOP, Intraocular pressure.

■ Common and Serious Adverse Effects
Sensory

Conjunctival irritation, burning and stinging, lacrimation. These adverse effects are usually mild and tend to resolve with continued therapy. Encourage the patient not to discontinue therapy without first consulting the healthcare provider.

Eye pigment changes. The prostaglandin agonists may gradually cause changes to pigmented tissues, including change to eye color, increasing the amount of brown pigment in the iris. The change may take several months to years to develop and is thought to be permanent. Iris pigmentation changes may be more evident in patients with green-brown, blue- or gray-brown, or yellow-brown irises. The eyelids may also develop color changes. There may also be an increased growth of eyelashes.

■ Drug Interactions
Thimerosal. A precipitate occurs when eyedrops containing thimerosal (a commonly used preservative in ophthalmic solutions) are mixed with latanoprost. Administer eyedrops at least 5 minutes apart.

OTHER OPHTHALMIC AGENTS

DRUG CLASS: ANTICHOLINERGIC AGENTS

ACTIONS

Anticholinergic agents cause the smooth muscle of the ciliary body and iris to relax, producing mydriasis (extreme dilation of the pupil) and cycloplegia (paralysis of the ciliary muscle).

USES

Ophthalmologists use anticholinergic agents for their pharmacologic effects to examine the interior of the eye, measure the proper strength of lenses for eyeglasses (refraction), and rest the eye in inflammatory conditions of the uveal tract.

THERAPEUTIC OUTCOMES

The primary therapeutic outcomes expected from anticholinergic ophthalmic use are as follows:
1. Visualization of intraocular structures
2. Reduced uveal tract inflammation

❖ NURSING IMPLICATIONS FOR ANTICHOLINERGIC AGENTS

■ Premedication Assessment
1. Check for the diagnosis of increased IOP. If present, hold the medication and contact the healthcare provider for approval before instillation of the anticholinergic agent.
2. Take vital signs; if the patient has hypertension, contact the healthcare provider for approval before instilling the anticholinergic agent.

■ Availability, Dosage, and Administration
See Table 42-6.

> ### [!] Medication Safety Alert
>
> The pharmacologic effects of anticholinergic agents cause an increase in IOP. Use these agents with extreme caution in patients with narrow anterior chamber angle; in infants, children, and older adults; and in patients with hypertension, hyperthyroidism, and diabetes. Discontinue therapy if signs of increased IOP (i.e. blurred vision, halos around white lights, frontal headaches and eye pain) or systemic effects develop.

■ Common Adverse Effects
Sensory

Sensitivity to bright light. The mydriasis produced allows excessive light into the eyes, causing the patient to squint. Sunglasses will help reduce the brightness.

Table 42-6   Anticholinergic Agents

GENERIC NAME	BRAND NAME	AVAILABILITY	DOSAGE	COMMENTS
atropine sulphate	Isopto-Atropine	1% ointment; 1% solution	Uveitis: 1-2 drops up to three times daily	Onset of mydriasis and cycloplegia is 30-40 min, duration is 7-12 days; do not use in infants.
cyclopentolate hydrochloride	Cyclogyl	0.5%, 1%, 2% solutions	Refraction: 1 drop followed by another drop in 5-10 min	For mydriasis and cycloplegia necessary for diagnostic procedures; 1-2 drops of 1%-2% pilocarpine allows full recovery within 6-24 hr; CNS disturbances of hallucinations, loss of orientation, restlessness, and incoherent speech have been reported in children.
homatropine hydrobromide	Isopto-Homatropine	2%, 5% solutions	Uveitis: 1-2 drops q3-4h	Onset of mydriasis and cycloplegia is 40-60 min; duration is 1-3 days.
scopolamine hydrobromide	Isopto-Hyoscine	0.25% solution	Uveitis: 1-2 drops up to three times daily	Onset of mydriasis and cycloplegia is 20-30 min; duration is 3-7 days.
tropicamide	Mydriacyl	0.5%, 1% solutions	Refraction: 1-2 drops, repeated in 5 min	Onset of mydriasis and cycloplegia is 20-40 min; duration is 6 hr; CNS disturbances such as hallucinations, loss of orientation, restlessness, and incoherent speech have been reported in children.

CNS, Central nervous system.

Caution the patient to temporarily avoid tasks that require visual acuity, such as driving or operating power machinery.

Conjunctival irritation, lacrimation. These adverse effects are usually mild and tend to resolve with continued therapy. Encourage the patient not to discontinue therapy without first consulting the healthcare provider.

■ Serious Adverse Effects
Neurologic
Systemic adverse effects. Prolonged use may result in systemic effects manifested by flushing and dryness of the skin, dry mouth, blurred vision, tachycardia, dysrhythmias, urinary hesitancy and retention, vasodilation, and constipation. These are indications of overdose or excessive administration. Report to the healthcare provider for treatment and dosage adjustment. Prevent systemic effects by carefully blocking the inner canthus for 3 to 5 minutes after instilling the medication to prevent absorption via the nasolacrimal duct. Monitor the pulse rate and blood pressure, and instruct the patient to continue to do this at home; report significant changes from the baseline data. Children are particularly prone to developing systemic reactions.

■ Drug Interactions
No clinically significant drug interactions have been reported.

DRUG CLASS: ANTIFUNGAL AGENTS

natamycin (nă-tŭ-MĪ-sĭn)
Natacyn (NĂT-ă-sĭn)

ACTIONS
Natamycin acts by altering the cell wall of the fungus to prevent it from serving as a selective barrier, therefore causing loss of fluids and electrolytes.

USES
Natamycin is an antifungal agent that is effective against a variety of yeasts, including *Candida* species, *Aspergillus* species, and *Fusarium* species. It is effective in treating fungal blepharitis, conjunctivitis, and keratitis caused by susceptible organisms. If little or no improvement is noted after 7 to 10 days of treatment, resistance to the antifungal agent may have developed. Topical administration does not appear to result in systemic effects.

THERAPEUTIC OUTCOME
The primary therapeutic outcome expected from natamycin is eradication of fungal infection.

❖ NURSING IMPLICATIONS FOR NATAMYCIN
■ Premedication Assessment
1. Collect ordered cultures or smears before initiating drug therapy.

2. Record baseline data relating to symptoms accompanying the fungal infection and the degree of visual impairment.

■ Availability

Ophthalmic: 5% suspension.

■ Dosage and Administration

Fungal keratitis: One drop in the conjunctival sac at 1- or 2-hour intervals for the first 3 to 4 days. The dosage may then be reduced to one drop every 3 to 4 hours. Continue therapy for 14 to 21 days.

■ Common Adverse Effects

Sensory

Sensitivity to bright light. The slight mydriasis produced allows an excessive amount of light into the eyes, causing the patient to squint. Sunglasses will help reduce the brightness. Caution the patient to avoid tasks temporarily that require visual acuity, such as driving or operating power machinery.

Blurred vision, lacrimation, redness. Provide for patient safety during temporary visual impairment. Instruct the patient not to rub the eyes forcefully while tearing.

These adverse effects are usually mild and tend to resolve with continued therapy. Encourage the patient not to discontinue therapy without first consulting the healthcare provider.

■ Serious Adverse Effects

Sensory

Eye pain. If eye pain develops, discontinue use and consult an ophthalmologist immediately.

Therapeutic effect. If, after several days of therapy, the symptoms do not improve or if they gradually worsen, consult the prescriber treating the patient.

■ Drug Interactions

No significant drug interactions have been reported.

DRUG CLASS: ANTIVIRAL AGENTS

ACTIONS

The ophthalmic antiviral agents act by inhibiting viral replication.

USES

Trifluridine is used to treat keratitis caused by herpes simplex virus types 1 and 2. Ganciclovir is used to treat cytomegalovirus retinitis for patients with acquired immunodeficiency syndrome. These antiviral agents are not effective against infections caused by bacteria, fungi, or *Chlamydia* organisms.

THERAPEUTIC OUTCOME

The primary therapeutic outcome expected from antiviral agents is eradication of the viral infection.

❖ NURSING IMPLICATIONS FOR ANTIVIRAL AGENTS

■ Premedication Assessment

Record baseline data concerning the symptoms and the degree of visual impairment.

■ Availability, Dosage, and Administration

See Table 42-7.

Storage. Trifluridine should be stored in the refrigerator.

> **! Medication Safety Alert**
>
> If significant improvement has not occurred 7 to 14 days after initiating treatment with trifluridine, other therapy should be considered. Do not exceed 21 days of continuous therapy because of potential ocular toxicity.

■ Common Adverse Effects

Sensory

Visual haze, lacrimation, redness, burning. Patients may notice a mild, transient stinging, burning, and redness of the conjunctiva and sclera on instillation. Provide for patient safety during temporary visual impairment. Instruct the patient not to rub the eyes forcefully while tearing. These adverse effects are usually mild and tend to resolve with continued therapy. Encourage the patient not to discontinue therapy without first consulting the healthcare provider.

Sensitivity to bright light. The slight mydriasis produced allows excessive light into the eyes, causing the patient to squint. Sunglasses will help reduce the

Table 42-7 Antiviral Agents

GENERIC NAME	BRAND NAME	AVAILABILITY	DOSAGE
ganciclovir	Vitrasert	Implant: 4.5 mg	A device is surgically implanted to release drug over 5 to 8 mo for treatment of CMV retinitis in patients with AIDS
ganciclovir	Zirgan	0.15% gel	Initial dosage: 1 drop in affected eye five times daily (about q3h while awake) until the corneal ulcer heals Maintenance dose: 1 drop three times daily for 7 days
trifluridine	Viroptic	1% solution in 7.5 mL	Intraocular: Place 1 drop onto the cornea of the affected eye q2h during waking hours; do not exceed 9 drops daily Continue for 7 more days to prevent recurrence, using 1 drop q4h (5 drops daily).

CMV, Cytomegalovirus.

Drugs Used to Treat Cancer

Objectives

1. Cite the goals of chemotherapy.
2. Describe the role of targeted anticancer agents in treating cancer.
3. Identify how chemoprotective agents are used in treating cancer.
4. Discuss bone marrow stimulants and their effect and use.
5. Describe the nursing assessments and interventions needed to help alleviate the adverse effects of chemotherapy.

Key Terms

cancer (KĂN-sŭr) (p. 667)
metastases (mĕ-TĂS-tă-sēz) (p. 667)
neoplastic disease (nē-ō-PLĂS-tĭk dĭs-ĒZ) (p. 667)
malignant (mă-LĬG-nănt) (p. 667)
palliation (păl-ē-Ā-shŭn) (p. 668)

combination therapy (kŏm-bĭ-NĀ-shŭn THĀR-ŭ-pē) (p. 669)
targeted anticancer agents (TĂR-gĕt-ĕd ăn-tē-KĂN-sŭr) (p. 669)
chemoprotective agents (kē-mō-prō-TĔK-tĭv) (p. 670)

CANCER AND THE USE OF ANTINEOPLASTIC AGENTS

Cancer is a group of more than 100 different diseases that are characterized by uncontrolled cellular growth, local tissue invasion, and distant metastases (Chabner, 2010). It is a group of once-normal cells that have mutated to abnormal cells that generally multiply more rapidly than normal cells, lose the ability to perform specialized functions, invade surrounding tissues, and develop growths in other tissues distant to the site of original growth (metastases). Cancer is also referred to as a *neoplasm*, neoplastic disease, or *new growth*. The new growth may be subdivided into benign or malignant cells. Since benign cells do not metastasize, they are generally not as life threatening as the malignant cells. Malignant cells often metastasize to other organs of the body, making treatment and survival substantially less likely.

The American Cancer Society (2015) reports that the rate of cancer occurrences and deaths have decreased annually since the all-time high year of 1991. Declining rates are due to prevention; early detection; and better quality of treatment with chemotherapy, surgery, and radiation. Cancer was responsible for nearly one in four deaths in the United States in 2011, making it the second leading cause of death overall after cardiovascular disease. It is the leading cause of death among adults aged 40 to 79. In 2015, it is estimated that there will be almost 1.7 million new cancer cases and almost 600,000 deaths from cancer (Figure 43-1).

Cancers can occur anywhere in the body: within organs (e.g., liver, colon, lungs) and blood components (e.g., lymphatic system causing lymphoma) and bone marrow, causing leukemias. Treatment of cancer often requires a combination of surgery, radiation, chemotherapy, targeted drug therapy, and biologic therapy. Biologic therapies are made from a living organism or its byproducts and include antibodies, vaccines, growth factors, and cytokines. Surgery and radiation are considered to be local therapy, whereas chemotherapy, targeted drug therapy, and biologic therapies use the systemic circulation to treat the primary tumor and metastases. Recent advancements in understanding carcinogenesis, cellular and molecular biology, genetics, and tumor immunology have enhanced the role that antineoplastic agents may play in treatment. It is beyond the scope of this chapter to delve into the interrelationships of chemotherapy and neoplastic disease; however, a short discussion of the concepts of cancer chemotherapy will be presented. As a result of rapidly changing approaches to the treatment of specific malignancies and the changing nature of chemotherapeutic regimens, specific agents and dosages will not be discussed.

All cells, whether normal or malignant, pass through a similar series of phases during their lifetime, although duration of time spent in each phase differs with the type of cell (Figure 43-2). The cell cycle involves five stages: DNA replication (S phase), cell division (M phase), two resting phases (G_1 and G_2), and a resting (nondividing state [G_0]) phase. The cell cycle begins

Estimated New Cases*		Estimated Deaths	
Male	**Female**	**Male**	**Female**
Prostate 220,800 (26%)	Breast 231,840 (29%)	Lung & bronchus 86,380 (28%)	Lung & bronchus 71,660 (26%)
Lung & bronchus 115,610 (14%)	Lung & bronchus 105,590 (13%)	Prostate 27,540 (9%)	Breast 40,290 (15%)
Colon & rectum 69,090 (8%)	Colon & rectum 63,610 (8%)	Colon & rectum 26,100 (8%)	Colon & rectum 23,600 (9%)
Urinary bladder 56,320 (7%)	Uterine corpus 54,870 (7%)	Pancreas 20,710 (7%)	Pancreas 19,850 (7%)
Melanoma of the skin 42,670 (5%)	Thyroid 47,230 (6%)	Liver & intrahepatic bile duct 17,030 (5%)	Ovary 14,180 (5%)
Non-Hodgkin lymphoma 39,850 (5%)	Non-Hodgkin lymphoma 32,000 (4%)	Leukemia 14,210 (5%)	Leukemia 10,240 (4%)
Kidney & renal pelvis 38,270 (5%)	Melanoma of the skin 31,200 (4%)	Esophagus 12,600 (4%)	Uterine corpus 10,170 (4%)
Oral cavity & pharynx 32,670 (4%)	Pancreas 24,120 (3%)	Urinary bladder 11,510 (4%)	Non-Hodgkin lymphoma 8,310 (3%)
Leukemia 30,900 (4%)	Leukemia 23,370 (3%)	Non-Hodgkin lymphoma 11,480 (4%)	Liver & intrahepatic bile duct 7,520 (3%)
Liver & intrahepatic bile duct 25,510 (3%)	Kidney & renal pelvis 23,290 (3%)	Kidney & renal pelvis 9,070 (3%)	Brain & other nervous system 6,380 (2%)
All sites 848,200 (100%)	All sites 810,170 (100%)	All sites 312,150 (100%)	All sites 277,280 (100%)

*Excludes basal cell and squamous cell skin cancers and in situ carcinoma except urinary bladder.

FIGURE 43-1 Leading sites of new cancer cases and deaths—2015 estimates. (Data from American Cancer Society: *Cancer facts & figures 2015*, Atlanta, 2015, American Cancer Society. Retrieved from http://www.cancer.org/acs/groups/content/@editorial/documents/document/acspc-044552.pdf.)

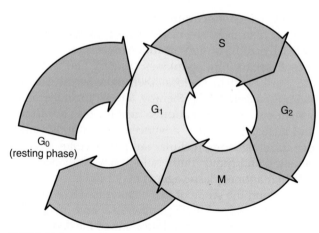

FIGURE 43-2 The cell cycle. G_0, Resting phase; G_1, gap 1 phase; G_2, gap 2 phase; *M*, mitosis; *S*, synthesis.

again when the cell is divided into two daughter cells. The daughter cells may advance again into the same cycle. The time required to complete one cycle is termed the *generation time*.

Many antineoplastic agents are cell cycle specific (i.e., the drug is selectively toxic when the cell is in a specific phase of growth, and therefore is schedule dependent). Malignancies most amenable to cell cycle–specific chemotherapy are those that proliferate or grow very rapidly. Cell cycle–nonspecific drugs are active throughout the cell cycle and may be more effective against slowly proliferating neoplastic tissue. These agents are not schedule dependent but are dose dependent. One implication of cell cycle specificity is the importance of correlating the dosage schedule of anticancer therapy with the known cellular kinetics of that type of neoplasm. Drugs are usually administered when the cell is most susceptible to the cytotoxic effects of the agent for a higher "kill rate" of neoplastic cells.

DRUG THERAPY FOR CANCER

The overall goal of cancer chemotherapy is to give a dose large enough to be lethal (cytotoxic) to the cancer cells but small enough to be tolerable for normal cells. It is hoped that a long-term survival or cure can be achieved by this means. A second goal may be control of the disease (arresting tumor growth). When a cancer is beyond control, the goal of treatment may be **palliation** (alleviation) of symptoms (e.g., administration of chemotherapy to reduce tumor size for easier breathing in a patient with lung cancer). Finally, in some types of cancer in which no tumor is

4. The nurse is administering epoetin alfa (Procrit) to a patient receiving chemotherapy. What is the best explanation to the patient why this medication is used?
   1. To stimulate WBC (white blood cell) production
   2. To stimulate RBC (red blood cell) production
   3. To prevent thrombocytopenia
   4. To protect the kidneys from toxic chemotherapy

5. The drugs that are used in conjunction with chemotherapy to reduce the toxic effects are called:
   1. chemoprotective agents.
   2. targeted anticancer agents.
   3. bone marrow stimulants.
   4. alkylating agents.

6. When teaching a patient about what to report to the healthcare provider, the nurse includes the following. *(Select all that apply.)*
   1. Any increase in pain
   2. Nasal stuffiness
   3. Bleeding
   4. Development of a fever
   5. Dry skin over heels

7. The nurse is discussing ways to counteract the effects of diarrhea caused by chemotherapy. The following suggestions should be included in the discussion. *(Select all that apply.)*
   1. Use products that protect the skin around the anus from excoriation (such as A&D Ointment).
   2. Drink more coffee or tea.
   3. Increase intake of potassium-containing foods depending upon other medications being taken.
   4. Obtain daily weights as an indicator of maintenance of hydration.
   5. Frequent walks should alleviate the symptoms.

Objectives

1. Describe the nursing assessment data needed to evaluate a patient with a skeletal muscle disorder.
2. Identify the therapeutic response and the common and serious adverse effects from skeletal muscle relaxant therapy.
3. Describe the effect of centrally acting skeletal muscle relaxants on the central nervous system

(CNS) and the safety precautions required during their use.
4. Describe the physiologic effects of neuromuscular blocking agents and assessments needed, as well as the equipment needed in the immediate patient care area when neuromuscular blocking agents are administered.

Key Terms

cerebral palsy (sĕ-RĒ-brăl PŎL-zē) (p. 678)
multiple sclerosis (MŬL-tĭ-pŭl sklĕ-RŌ-sĭs) (p. 678)
stroke syndrome (STRŌK SĬN-drōm) (p. 678)
hypercapnia (hī-pĕr-KĂP-nē-ă) (p. 679)

spasticity (spăs-TĬS-ĭ-tē) (p. 681)
muscle spasms (MŬ-sŭl SPĂ-zĭmz) (p. 681)
neuromuscular blocking agents (nyū-rō-MŬS-kyū-lăr BLŎK-ĭng Ā-jĕnts) (p. 684)

The muscular system involves all of the voluntary muscles that line the skeleton of the body and allow for movement. The most common musculoskeletal disorders are cerebral palsy and multiple sclerosis. **Cerebral palsy** is a condition in which movement of the extremities is marked by any combination of the following: exaggerated reflexes, abnormal posture, involuntary movements, and walking difficulties. Cerebral palsy can be caused by an injury or a birth defect.

Multiple sclerosis is an autoimmune disease that affects the brain and spinal cord. Symptoms may be mild, such as numbness in the limbs, or severe, such as paralysis or loss of vision. The progression, severity, and specific symptoms of multiple sclerosis are unpredictable and highly variable between persons. **Stroke syndrome** is a condition of sudden onset of vertigo, numbness, aphasia and dysarthria, marked by hemiplegia or hemiparesis due to vascular lesions of the brain, embolism, thrombosis or ruptured aneurysm.

MUSCLE RELAXANTS AND NEUROMUSCULAR BLOCKING AGENTS

❖ NURSING IMPLICATIONS FOR SKELETAL MUSCLE RELAXANTS AND NEUROMUSCULAR BLOCKING AGENTS

▪ Assessment

Assessment for Skeletal Muscle Disorders. Musculoskeletal disorders may produce varying degrees of pain and immobility, impairing the individual's ability

to perform the activities of daily living. The nursing assessments performed are individualized to the muscles affected and the underlying disease.

Current history
- What is the reason for seeking treatment now? Request a brief history of any symptoms present.
- What is the degree of impairment present (e.g., strength, gait, conservation effect, compensatory action)? What is the effect on usual daily activities (e.g., dressing, preparing meals, eating, performing basic hygiene, maintaining home)?
- Assess the pain level and extent, frequency of analgesic use, precipitating factors, and any measures the patient has identified that alleviate pain.
- Assess the extent of muscle spasticity and the muscle groups affected. Are there impairments that affect the patient's self-care, activities of daily living, or ability to fulfill work responsibilities?

History
- Ask the patient to describe disorders that cause musculoskeletal impairment (e.g., scoliosis, poliomyelitis, rickets, osteoarthritis, cerebral palsy, multiple sclerosis, muscular dystrophy, spinal cord injury, stroke).
- Have there been any injuries to, or surgeries on, the musculoskeletal system (e.g., dislocations, sprains, fractures, joint replacements)? If so, obtain details.
- Ask the patient if there is a family history of difficulties or abnormal responses to neuromuscular blocking agents during anesthesia.

Antimicrobial Agents

Objectives

1. Explain the major actions and effects of classes of drugs used to treat infectious diseases.
2. List the signs and symptoms of a secondary infection.
3. Describe the signs and symptoms of the common adverse effects of antimicrobial therapy.
4. Describe the nursing assessments and interventions for the common adverse effects associated with antimicrobial

agents: allergic reaction, nephrotoxicity, ototoxicity, and hepatotoxicity.
5. Cite the primary uses for antibiotic agents, antitubercular agents, antifungal agents, and antiviral agents.

Key Terms

pathogenic (păth-ō-JĔN-ĭk) (p. 687)
antibiotics (ăn-tĭ-bī-Ŏ-tĭks) (p. 687)
gram-negative microorganisms (GRĂM NĔG-ĭ-tĭv) (p. 687)
gram-positive microorganisms (GRĂM PŎ-zĭ-tĭv mī-krō-ŌR-găn-ĭz-ĕmz) (p. 687)
prophylactic antibiotics (prō-fĭ-LĂK-tĭk) (p. 688)

nephrotoxicity (nĕf-rō-tŏks-ĬS-ĭ-tē) (p. 689)
ototoxicity (ō-tō-tŏks-ĬS-ĭ-tē) (p. 690)
hypoprothrombinemia (hī-pō-prō-thrŏm-bĭn-Ē-mē-ă) (p. 695)
penicillinase-resistant penicillins (pĕn-ĭ-SĬL-ĭn-ās rē-ZĬS-tĕnt pĕn-ĭ-SĬL-ĭnz) (p. 702)

ANTIMICROBIAL AGENTS

Antimicrobial agents are chemicals that eliminate living microorganisms that are **pathogenic** (toxic) to the patient. Antimicrobial agents may be of chemical origin, such as the sulfonamides, or they may be derived from other living organisms. Those derived from other living microorganisms are called **antibiotics**; for example, penicillin was first derived from the mold *Penicillium notatum*. Most antibiotics used today are harvested from large colonies of microorganisms, which are then purified and chemically modified into semisynthetic antimicrobial agents. The chemical modification makes the antibiotic more effective against specific pathogenic organisms. Antimicrobial agents are often first classified according to the type of pathogen to be destroyed, such as bacteria (antibacterial agents), fungus (antifungal agents), or virus (antiviral agents). The antimicrobial agents are then subdivided by chemical families into drug classes such as the penicillins, tetracyclines, and aminoglycosides.

The selection of the antimicrobial agent must be based on the sensitivity of the pathogen and the possible toxicity to the patient. If at all possible, infecting organisms should first be isolated and identified. Culture and sensitivity tests should be completed to

identify the infective organism and determine the antibiotic to which the infecting organism is most sensitive. Bacteria are classified as **gram-negative microorganisms** (e.g., *Acinetobacter* spp., *Citrobacter* spp., *Enterobacter* spp., *Escherichia coli*, *Klebsiella* spp., *Providencia* spp., *Pseudomonas* spp., *Salmonella* spp., and *Shigella* spp.) or **gram-positive microorganisms** (e.g., *Staphylococcus aureus*, *S. epidermidis*, *Streptococcus pyogenes*, *S. pneumoniae*). However, if clinically indicated, a patient may be started on a broad-spectrum antibiotic regimen until the infecting organism is identified and its drug sensitivity is determined. The antimicrobial therapy is then started based on the sensitivity results and the clinical judgment of the healthcare provider. In the inpatient setting, however, it is routine to obtain specimens of the infecting organism from infected sites (e.g., blood, urine, wound) and then start therapy immediately with one or more antimicrobial agents that are most likely to stop the infection. This is known as *empirical treatment*. When the cultures identify the pathogen and the sensitivity tests indicate which antimicrobial agent will be most effective, that antimicrobial agent is started and all other antimicrobial agents are discontinued. Discontinuation of therapy of unneeded antimicrobial agents helps prevent the development of resistant organisms and reduce health care costs.

The use of **prophylactic antibiotics** is recommended for patients at risk for developing infective endocarditis before dental, gastric, and genitourinary surgery and other invasive procedures. The American Heart Association (Wilson et al, 2007) guidelines recommend prophylactic antibiotic treatment for patients with cardiac conditions that put them at highest risk for infection, such as prosthetic cardiac valve; previous infective endocarditis; congenital heart disease (CHD); unrepaired, cyanotic CHD, including palliative shunts and conduits; congenital heart defects completely repaired with prosthetic material or device—whether placed by surgery or by catheter intervention—during the first 6 months after the procedure; repaired congenital heart defects with residual defects at the site or adjacent to the site of prosthetic patch or prosthetic device; and cardiac transplantation.

❖ NURSING IMPLICATIONS FOR ANTIMICROBIAL THERAPY

Nurses must consider the entire patient when administering and monitoring antimicrobial therapy. It is essential that the nurse be knowledgeable about the drugs, including physiologic parameters for monitoring expected therapeutic activity and adverse effects. It is important to teach the individual with an infection the basic principles of self-care, which will enhance the recovery process, and measures to prevent the spread of infection. With communicable diseases, exposed individuals must be contacted for follow-up testing and appropriate treatment.

■ Assessment

History of Current Infection. What symptoms are described by the patient? Which of the symptoms described potentially relate to an infectious process? Extend questioning to help the patient focus—for example, when did the symptoms begin? Have they worsened? Is there fever, night sweats, malaise, chronic fatigue, weight loss, arthralgia, cough (type of secretions), diarrhea, painful urination, nausea, vomiting, lesions or skin rash, discharge, or drainage? Is there any swelling, pain, or heat in a particular area or discharge from a site? Has the patient been treated previously for a similar infection? Ask questions specific to the body systems affected by the infection (e.g., pain and burning with urination for a urinary tract infection [UTI]). Determine the patient's current living environment and review the institutional policy. Many patients residing in long-term care facilities are screened for methicillin-resistant *Staphylococcus aureus* (MRSA) and vancomycin-resistant *Enterococcus faecium* (VRE).

Health care-associated infections (HAIs) are common reasons for admission to hospitals, as well as reasons for extended stays. These infections occur when patients who are being treated for other conditions develop an additional infection while being cared for by healthcare workers. The common types of HAI are health care-associated pneumonia (HCAP) and UTIs.

When treating patients with sexually transmitted infections (STIs), ask about the number of sexual partners, sexual orientation, and use of precautions during intercourse. (See Chapter 40 for further details.)

Medication History
- Ask the patient to list all current prescribed and over-the-counter (OTC) medications or those taken in the past 6 months. Ask specifically about any medicines, such as corticosteroids, chemotherapy, or transplant suppressants, that may affect the immune status of the individual.
- Does the person take any type of allergy injections or medications?
- Is the person immunized against childhood diseases?
- Has the person been treated for an infection recently? If yes, what medications were taken, and were there any allergic responses? If so, ask for details of the symptoms of the allergic reaction.
- Has the patient taken this medication before? If so, what symptoms (e.g., nausea, vomiting, diarrhea, rash, itching, or hives) developed when taking it that led the patient to state that there was an allergy? Ask the patient to describe the appearance of a rash, where it started, and the course of recovery. How soon after starting the medication did the symptoms develop?
- Ask if the patient has ever developed a secondary infection (black hairy tongue, white patches [thrush] in mouth, or vaginal infection) when taking an antibiotic. For example, women taking antibiotics may develop a vaginal infection because of suppression of normal flora.

Physical Examination
- Perform a head-to-toe body or functional assessment, focusing on the areas pertinent to the admitting diagnosis.
- Assess for risk factors that may contribute to development of infection, such as extensive surgical procedures, obesity, underlying contributory conditions (e.g., chronic obstructive pulmonary disease, diabetes), immunotherapy drugs, malnutrition, and age extremes (infants or older adults).

Psychosocial. For an individual with a serious communicable disease, assess the response and adaptive processes used to cope with the disease and its treatments.

Assessments During Antimicrobial Therapy. Read each drug monograph for specific common and serious adverse effects, and individualize the assessments for the drugs prescribed. Nausea, vomiting, diarrhea, allergies, anaphylaxis, nephrotoxicity, hepatotoxicity, ototoxicity, hematologic dyscrasias, secondary infection, and photosensitivity are found with recurring frequency in the antimicrobial drug monographs.

- *Nausea, vomiting, and diarrhea:* These conditions are the "big three" adverse effects associated with antimicrobial drug therapy. When they occur, gather data such as the following:

  1. Did the patient have a history of nausea, vomiting, or diarrhea before starting the drug therapy?
  2. How soon after starting the medication did the symptoms start?
  3. Since starting the medication, has the diet or water source changed in any way?
  4. Was the patient taking other drugs, either prescription or OTC medications, before initiating antibiotic therapy?
  5. How much fluid is the patient consuming when taking medications? Inadequate fluid intake sometimes causes gastritis manifested by nausea.
  6. For diarrhea, what was the pattern of elimination before drug therapy? Report diarrhea and the character and frequency of stools, as well as any abdominal pain, promptly. Nausea, vomiting, and diarrhea are often dose related and result from changes in normal bacterial flora in the bowel, irritation, and secondary infection. Symptoms resolve within a few days, and discontinuation of therapy is rarely required.

When drug therapy causes nausea and vomiting, the healthcare provider may elect to give the antibiotic with food to decrease irritation, even though absorption may be slightly decreased, or may choose to switch to a parenteral dosage form. When reporting any incidence of nausea and vomiting, all significant data should be collected and reported. Administer prescribed antiemetics or antidiarrheal agents (see also Chapters 33 and 34).

- *Secondary infection:* Assess for symptoms of secondary infection such as oral infection. Observe for a black hairy tongue, white patches (thrush) in the oral cavity, cold sores, canker sores, and glossitis. There may be lesions and itching in the vaginal and anal areas. Secondary infection of the intestine, such as *Clostridium difficile,* can produce severe life-threatening diarrhea. Secondary infection may occur in patients receiving broad-spectrum antibiotic therapy, particularly in those who are immunosuppressed. Monitor for the development of symptoms of secondary infection, and notify the healthcare provider if this occurs. Instruct the patient to minimize exposure to people known to have an infection and to practice good personal hygiene measures.
- *Allergies and anaphylaxis:* The severity of allergic reaction ranges from a mild rash to fatal anaphylaxis. Allergic reactions may develop within 30 minutes of administration (e.g., anaphylaxis, laryngeal edema, shock, dyspnea, skin reactions) or may occur several days after discontinuing therapy (e.g., skin rashes, fever). All patients must be questioned for previous allergic reactions, and allergy-prone

patients must be observed closely. It is important that a patient not be labeled "allergic" to a particular medication without adequate documentation. Patients who report gastrointestinal (GI) symptoms of nausea, vomiting, and/or diarrhea with no other symptoms (e.g., skin rash, facial edema, dyspnea, hypotension) should not be labeled allergic to the medicine. The medication to which a patient claims an allergy may be a life-saving drug for that patient in the future.

Closely monitor all patients—particularly those with histories of allergies, asthma, or rhinitis and those who are taking multiple drug preparations—for an allergic response during antimicrobial therapy. All patients should be watched carefully for possible allergic reactions for at least 20 to 30 minutes after administration of a medication. However, some drug reactions may not occur for several days. Hold the prescribed antimicrobial medication if the person reports a possible allergy. In the event of suspected anaphylaxis, summon the healthcare provider and the emergency cart immediately.

Although a serious reaction may occur with the first administration of a drug, repeated exposures to a previously sensitized substance can be fatal. Respond immediately to any signs of reaction, including swelling, redness, or pain at the site of injection; hives; nasal congestion and discharge; wheezing progressing to dyspnea; pulmonary edema; stridor; and sternal retractions.

- *Nephrotoxicity:* Assess **nephrotoxicity** through an increasing blood urea nitrogen (BUN) and creatinine, decreasing urine output, decreasing urine specific gravity, casts or protein in the urine, frank blood or smoky-colored urine, or red blood cells (RBCs) in excess of 0 to 3 RBCs/high-power field (HPF) (see Table 41-1) on the urinalysis report.

Maintain an accurate intake and output record; report declining output or output below 30 mL/hr in the adult patient. Many antimicrobial agents are potentially nephrotoxic (e.g., aminoglycosides, tetracyclines, vancomycin). Concomitant therapy with diuretics enhances the likelihood of toxicity, particularly in the older or debilitated patient. When renal function is impaired, most drug dosages must be decreased or alternative drug therapy used.

- *Hepatotoxicity:* Assess for preexisting hepatic disease such as cirrhosis or hepatitis. Review laboratory studies (e.g., bilirubin, aspartate aminotransferase [AST], alanine aminotransferase [ALT], gamma-glutamyl transferase [GGT], alkaline phosphatase levels, prothrombin time [PT][international normalized ratio or INR]) and report abnormal findings to the healthcare provider. Several drugs to be studied in this chapter are potentially hepatotoxic (e.g., isoniazid, sulfonamides). The liver is active in the metabolism of many drugs, and drug-induced hepatitis may occur. The actual liver damage may occur shortly after exposure to the pharmacologic agent, or may not appear for several weeks after initial exposure. The symptoms of hepatotoxicity are anorexia, nausea, vomiting, jaundice, hepatomegaly, splenomegaly, and abnormal liver function test results (e.g., elevated bilirubin, AST, ALT, GGT, alkaline phosphatase levels, increased PT). Patients with preexisting hepatic disease such as cirrhosis or hepatitis will require lower dosages of drugs metabolized by the liver.

- *Ototoxicity:* Damage to the eighth cranial nerve, **ototoxicity,** can occur from drug therapy, particularly from aminoglycosides. This may initially be manifested by dizziness, tinnitus, and progressive hearing loss. Assess the patient for difficulty in walking unaided, and assess the level of hearing daily. Intentionally speak to patients softly; note if they are aware that you said anything. Take particular notice of the patient who repeatedly asks, "What did you say?" or who starts talking more loudly or progressively increases the volume on the television or radio. Report preexisting hearing impairment or symptoms of developing hearing deficits to the healthcare provider and initiate orders prescribed. Provide for patient safety if tinnitus or dizziness accompanies the symptoms of hearing impairment.

- *Blood dyscrasias*
  1. Ask specifically about any history of blood disorders diagnosed and treatments prescribed.
  2. Ask specifically about any types of anemia (e.g., aplastic, hemolytic, megaloblastic) or deficiencies of folic acid, vitamin B_{12}, or glucose-6-phosphate dehydrogenase.
  3. Ask whether the individual has received chemotherapy, radiation therapy, or transplant therapy, all of which may induce an immunocompromised state and changes in the blood.
  4. Has the patient received blood cell stimulator drugs such as Epogen or Neupogen?
  5. Does the patient have any bleeding disorders, such as hemophilia or thrombocytopenia?
  6. Observe for bleeding gums, prolonged bleeding at an injection site, petechiae, and epistaxis (nosebleeds).
  7. Review admission laboratory studies and report abnormalities (e.g., complete blood count [CBC] with differential, increased BUN or creatinine levels).
  8. Individualize care to the type of blood dyscrasia present. When hypoprothrombinemia is present, the usual treatment is administration of vitamin K. Serious and possibly fatal bone marrow suppression may occur after therapy is initiated with some antibiotics (e.g., chloramphenicol). Monitor for signs and symptoms such as sore throat, fatigue, elevated temperature, small petechial hemorrhages, and bruises on the skin, and if present, report these symptoms immediately.

- *Photosensitivity:* Assess for the development of dermatologic symptoms such as exaggerated sunburn, itching, rash, urticaria, pruritus, and scaling, particularly after exposure to sunlight. Photosensitivity is seldom evident during hospitalization. It is more commonly seen in ambulatory practice.

When the drug monograph lists this as a potential serious adverse effect, the nurse should provide health teaching to prevent its occurrence. Instruct the patient to avoid exposure to sunlight and ultraviolet light (e.g., sun lamps, suntanning beds); wear long-sleeved clothing, a hat, and sunglasses; and apply sunscreen to exposed skin when going out into the sunlight.

■ Implementation

- Routine monitoring of all individuals receiving antimicrobial therapy should include status of hydration, temperature, pulse, respirations, and blood pressure. Monitor at least every 4 hours and more frequently as the patient's clinical status warrants.
- Use the Centers for Disease Control and Prevention (CDC) recommended precautions for infection transmission—universal precautions and appropriate guidelines for isolation. Consult the CDC's website, as well as clinical policies and procedures, to prevent transmission of infection. Always remember the importance of adequate handwashing.
- Always monitor for phlebitis when antimicrobials are administered intravenously.
- Administer antimicrobials as prescribed on the time schedule established.
- In some cases, a second drug (e.g., probenecid) may be administered concurrently to inhibit the excretion of the antibiotic (e.g., penicillin, cephalosporin). When this is done, monitor closely for adverse effects.

Medication History

- Ask the patient to list all prescribed or OTC medications being taken. Ask specifically about the recent use of corticosteroids, chemotherapy, or transplant suppressants.
- Does the patient have any allergies? If so, obtain details of medications and actual symptoms that occur during an allergic reaction. What treatment was used for any past allergic responses? What antibiotics have been taken? Were there any problems during antibiotic therapy?

■ Patient Education

The following basic principles of patient care should not be overlooked when treating a patient with infections:

- Adequate rest with as little stress as possible. Rest decreases metabolic needs and enhances the physiologic repair process.
- Nutritional management, including attention to hydration, proteins, fats, carbohydrates, minerals, and vitamins, to support the body's needs during an inflammatory response. Adequate nutrients to meet the energy needs, especially during times of

fever, are essential so that the body will not break down its protein stores to meet energy requirements. The dietary teaching must be individualized to the patient's diagnosis and point of recovery. Unless contraindicated by coexisting disease, encourage adequate fluid intake of 2000 to 3000 mL/24 hr, and simultaneously monitor the patient for signs and symptoms of fluid volume deficit or fluid volume overload.

- Extensive teaching, individualized to the circumstances and mode of transmission of the disease, should be given to those with communicable infection. This should include contacting exposed individuals in accordance with institutional policies for disease screening, treatment, and follow-up counseling.
- Explain personal hygiene measures, such as handwashing techniques, management of excretions such as sputum, wound care, and the importance of not sharing personal hygiene items with others.
- Instruct the patient to refrain from sexual intercourse during therapy for STIs.

Medications

- Drug therapy specific for the type of microorganism causing the infection should be explained in detail so that the patient will realize the need for adherence with the prescribed regimen.
- Examine each drug monograph to identify suggestions to the patient on how to handle the common adverse effects associated with antimicrobial therapy. The patient also must be taught the signs and symptoms that must be reported to the healthcare provider. Stress to the patient the importance of not discontinuing the prescribed medication until the adverse effects have been discussed with the healthcare provider.
- Develop a medication schedule with the patient for at-home medications prescribed. Make sure that the patient understands why it is important to take antimicrobials for the entire course of drug therapy and not to discontinue them when feeling better. Completing treatment is critical to preventing microbial resistance to antibiotics. In addition, patients must know self-monitoring parameters for the prescribed drug therapy.
- Nursing mothers should remind their healthcare provider that they are breastfeeding so that antibiotics may be selected that will have no effect on the infant.
- After an allergic reaction, the patient and family should inform anyone treating the patient in the future of the allergy to a specific drug. Wearing an allergy bracelet or tag may be appropriate. A wallet card describing the type of allergy can be helpful to future healthcare providers.
- Follow recommendations for annual influenza vaccine and pneumococcal vaccine for high-risk individuals (e.g., children; patients with diabetes, asthma, or pulmonary disease; older adults; healthcare workers; people with chronic or debilitating diseases). Always check with the healthcare provider if in doubt about advisability of administering vaccine.

Fostering Health Maintenance

- Throughout the course of treatment, discuss medication information. Continue to emphasize those factors that the patient can control to alter the progression of the disease: maintenance of general health and nutritional needs, adequate rest and appropriate exercise, and taking the prescribed medication until the entire course of therapy has been completed.
- Discuss expectations of therapy so that the patient understands whether a satisfactory response to drug therapy is being achieved, such as the relief of symptoms for which treatment was sought (e.g., relief of burning with urination and frequency of urination, relief of cough, or end of drainage and healing of a wound).

Patient Self-Assessment. Enlist the patient's aid in developing and maintaining a written record of monitoring parameters (e.g., list presenting symptoms: cough with a large amount of phlegm, wound drainage, temperature, exercise tolerance). (See Patient Self-Assessment Form for Antibiotics on the Evolve website.) Complete the Premedication Data column for use as a baseline to track response to drug therapy. Ensure that the patient understands how to use the form, and instruct the patient to take the completed form to follow-up visits. During follow-up visits, focus on issues that will foster adherence to the therapeutic interventions prescribed.

DRUG THERAPY FOR INFECTIOUS DISEASE

DRUG CLASS: AMINOGLYCOSIDES

ACTIONS

Aminoglycoside antibiotics kill bacteria primarily by inhibiting protein synthesis. Other mechanisms of action have not yet been fully defined.

USES

The aminoglycosides are used primarily against gram-negative microorganisms that cause UTIs, meningitis, wound infections, and life-threatening septicemias. They are the mainstays in the treatment of health care–associated gram-negative infections (e.g., *Acinetobacter* spp., *Citrobacter* spp., *Enterobacter* spp., *E. coli*, *Klebsiella* spp., *Providencia* spp., *Pseudomonas* spp., *Salmonella* spp., and *Shigella* spp.). Kanamycin and neomycin may also be used before surgery to reduce the normal flora content of the intestinal tract.

THERAPEUTIC OUTCOME

The primary therapeutic outcome expected from aminoglycoside therapy is elimination of bacterial infection.

❖ NURSING IMPLICATIONS FOR AMINOGLYCOSIDES

■ Premedication Assessment

1. Obtain baseline assessments of the presenting symptoms.
2. Record temperature, pulse, respirations, blood pressure, and hydration status.
3. Assess for any allergies and symptoms of hearing loss or renal disease. If present, withhold drug and report findings to the healthcare provider.
4. If the patient has had anesthesia within the past 48 to 72 hours, check to see if skeletal muscle relaxants were administered. If used, withhold the drug and notify the healthcare provider.
5. Check for scheduled time of laboratory aminoglycoside serum-level testing. After levels have been determined, assess whether results are normal or toxic. Contact the healthcare provider as appropriate.
6. Obtain baseline laboratory studies ordered and review results (e.g., CBC with differential, BUN, creatinine, culture and sensitivity).

■ Availability, Dosage, and Administration

See Table 45-1.

Admixture Compatibilities. Do *not* mix other drugs in the same syringe or infuse together with other drugs. See Drug Interactions on this page for incompatibilities.

Rate of Infusion. Check with the hospital laboratory regarding timing of aminoglycoside blood-level tests. The rate of infusion is quite important for aminoglycoside antibiotics, especially if pre- and postinfusion serum levels are being measured. Consult with a pharmacist, or see the individual package literature for proper infusion rate. After levels have been determined, assess whether results are normal or toxic.

■ Serious Adverse Effects

Sensory

Ototoxicity. Damage to the eighth cranial nerve can occur as a result of aminoglycoside therapy. Continue to observe patients for ototoxicity after therapy has been discontinued. These adverse effects may appear several days later.

Genitourinary

Nephrotoxicity. Monitor urinalysis and kidney function tests for abnormal results. Report increasing BUN and creatinine levels, decreasing urine output or decreasing specific gravity (despite amount of fluid intake), casts or protein in the urine, frank blood or smoky-colored urine, or RBCs in excess of 0 to 3 RBCs/HPF (see Table 41-1) on the urinalysis report.

■ Drug Interactions

Nephrotoxic Potential. Cephalosporins, enflurane, vancomycin, and diuretics, when combined with aminoglycosides, may increase the nephrotoxic potential. Monitor the urinalysis and kidney function test findings for abnormal results.

Ototoxic Potential. Aminoglycosides, when combined with ethacrynic acid, torsemide, bumetanide, and furosemide, may increase ototoxicity. Therefore nursing assessments for tinnitus, dizziness, and decreased hearing should be done regularly every shift.

Table 45-1 Aminoglycosides

GENERIC NAME	BRAND NAME	AVAILABILITY	ADULT DOSAGE RANGE
amikacin ⇄ *Do not confuse amikacin with Anakinra.*	—	Injection: 500 mg/2 mL in 2-mL vial 1 g/4 mL in 4-mL vial	IM, IV: 15 mg/kg/24 hr (max 1.5 g/day)
gentamicin	—	Injection: 10, 40 mg/mL in 2- and 20-mL vials 60-, 80-, 90-, 100-, and 120-mg single-dose containers	IM, IV: 3-5 mg/kg/day in two or three doses or 5 mg/kg once daily
kanamycin	—	Injection: 333 mg/mL in 3-mL vial	IM, IV: Up to 15 mg/kg/24 hr in two divided doses, not to exceed 1.5 g/24 hr
neomycin	Neo-Fradin	Tablets: 500 mg Solution: 125 mg/5 mL in 480-mL bottle	PO: 4-12 g daily in four divided doses
streptomycin	—	Injection: 1-g vials	IM: 15 mg/kg/day once daily
tobramycin	—	Injection: 10 mg/mL in 2-mL vials; 40 mg/mL in 30-, 50-mL vials 80 mg/2 mL in 2-mL vials 1.2 g in 50-mL bulk vials 300-mg/5 mL nebulizer solution	IM, IV: 3-5 mg/kg/day in two or three doses or 5 mg/kg once daily

Neuromuscular Blockade. Taking aminoglycoside antibiotics in combination with skeletal muscle relaxants may produce respiratory depression.

Check the anesthesia records of postoperative patients to determine if skeletal muscle relaxants such as succinylcholine or pancuronium bromide were administered during surgery.

The nurse should monitor and assess the respiratory rate, depth of respirations, and chest movement and report apnea immediately. Because these effects may be seen for up to 48 hours after administration of skeletal muscle relaxants, continue monitoring respirations, pulse, and blood pressure beyond the usual postsurgical vital signs routine.

Compatibilities. Do not mix other drugs in the same syringe or infuse together with other drugs.

Heparin. The aminoglycoside gentamicin and heparin are physically incompatible. *Do not* mix together before infusion.

Beta-Lactam–Type Antibiotics (Penicillins, Cephalosporins). These drugs rapidly inactivate aminoglycoside antibiotics. *Do not* mix together or administer together at the same IV site.

DRUG CLASS: CARBAPENEMS

ACTIONS

The carbapenems are extremely potent broad-spectrum antibiotics resistant to beta-lactamase enzymes secreted by bacteria. They act by inhibiting bacterial cell wall synthesis.

USES

Imipenem-cilastatin (Primaxin) is a combination product containing a carbapenem antibiotic called imipenem and cilastatin, an inhibitor of the renal dipeptidase enzyme dehydropeptidase I. Cilastatin has no antimicrobial activity; it prevents the inactivation of imipenem by the renal enzyme. It is used for the treatment of lower respiratory tract and intraabdominal infections; infections of the urinary tract, bones, joints, and skin; gynecologic infections; endocarditis; and bacterial septicemia caused by gram-negative or gram-positive organisms. A primary therapeutic role of imipenem-cilastatin is in the treatment of severe infections caused by multiresistant organisms and in mixed anaerobic-aerobic infections, primarily those involving intraabdominal and pelvic sepsis in which *Bacteroides fragilis* is a common pathogen. It should be used in combination with antipseudomonal agents because of resistance of *Pseudomonas cepacia* and *P. aeruginosa* to imipenem.

Meropenem is a carbapenem antibiotic that has a chemical structure that protects it against dehydropeptidase I, so that cilastatin is not necessary. It has a broad spectrum of activity similar to that of imipenem, but it is more active against Enterobacteriaceae and less active against gram-positive bacteria. It is used alone by the IV route for the treatment of intraabdominal infections caused by *E. coli*, *Klebsiella pneumoniae*, *P. aeruginosa*, *B. fragilis*, and *Peptostreptococcus* spp. It is also used alone intravenously to treat bacterial meningitis caused by *S. pneumoniae*, *Haemophilus influenzae*, and *Neisseria meningitidis*.

Ertapenem is a carbapenem antibiotic that has a chemical structure that protects it against dehydropeptidase I, so that cilastatin is not necessary. It has a broad spectrum of activity and is approved to treat infections caused by aerobic and anaerobic gram-positive and gram-negative bacteria causing complicated intraabdominal infections, skin and skin structure infections, community-acquired pneumonia, UTIs (including pyelonephritis), and acute pelvic infections. It is effective against susceptible strains of *S. aureus*, *S. agalactiae*, *S. pneumoniae*, *S. pyogenes*, *E. coli*, *K. pneumoniae*, *Moraxella catarrhalis*, *H. influenzae*, *Bacteroides* spp., *Clostridium* spp., and *Peptostreptococcus* spp.

Doripenem is a single agent that has a gram-negative and gram-positive spectrum similar to imipenem and meropenem combined. It is used to treat complicated intraabdominal infections caused by *E. coli*, *K. pneumoniae*, *P. aeruginosa*, *Bacteroides caccae*, *B. fragilis*, *B. thetaiotaomicron*, *B. uniformis*, *B. vulgatus*, *S. intermedius*, *S. constellatus*, and *Peptostreptococcus micros*. It is also approved for use in complicated UTIs caused by *E. coli*, including cases with concurrent bacteremia, *K. pneumoniae*, *Proteus mirabilis*, *P. aeruginosa*, and *Acinetobacter baumannii*.

THERAPEUTIC OUTCOME

The primary therapeutic outcome expected from carbapenem therapy is elimination of bacterial infection.

❖ NURSING IMPLICATIONS FOR CARBAPENEMS

■ Premedication Assessment

1. Obtain baseline assessments of presenting symptoms.
2. Record temperature, pulse, respirations, blood pressure, and hydration status.
3. Assess for and record any gastric symptoms before initiating therapy.
4. Assess for any allergies. Ask specifically about penicillin and cephalosporin allergies.
5. Obtain baseline laboratory studies ordered and review results (e.g., CBC with differential, culture and sensitivity).
6. Perform a baseline assessment of the patient's degree of alertness and orientation to name, place, and time before beginning therapy.
7. Ask whether there is a history of seizure activity before initiating therapy.

■ Availability, Dosage, and Administration

See Table 45-2.

Hypersensitivity. Although these antibiotics are carbapenems rather than penicillins or cephalosporins,

Table 45-2   Carbapenems

GENERIC NAME	BRAND NAME	AVAILABILITY	DOSAGE RANGE
doripenem	Doribax	Injection: 250-, 500-mg vials	IV: 500 mg q8h over 1 hr.
ertapenem	Invanz ⇄ Do not confuse Invanz with Avinza.	Injection: 1-g vials	IM, IV: 1 g daily. Infuse IV solution over 30 min for up to 14 days. Limit IM injection to 7 days.
imipenem-cilastatin ⇄ Do not confuse imipenem with Omnipen.	Primaxin ⇄ Do not confuse Primaxin with Premarin.	Injection: IV: 250-, 500-mg vials	IV: 50 mg/kg/day up to 4 g/day in two to four doses. 125, 250, or 500 mg by IV infusion over 20-30 min. Infuse 750-mg or 1-g dose over 40-60 min. If nausea develops, slow the infusion rate. IM: 500-750 mg q12h, depending on severity of infection. Do not exceed 1500 mg/day.
meropenem	Merrem IV	Injection: 500-mg, 1-g vials	IV: 1 g IV q8h; infuse over 15-30 min or as a bolus over 3-5 min.

they also contain a beta-lactam nucleus. Cross-hypersensitivity may develop between these classes. Complete a history of hypersensitivity before starting therapy. If an allergic reaction to a carbapenem occurs, discontinue the infusion. Serious reactions may require epinephrine and other emergency measures.

Admixture Compatibilities. Do *not* mix other drugs in the same syringe or infuse together with other drugs. See "Drug Interactions" on this page for incompatibilities.

■ Common Adverse Effects

Gastrointestinal

Severe diarrhea. Severe diarrhea may develop from using carbapenems. Blood and mucus in the stool may also be present. This may be an indication of drug-induced pseudomembranous colitis and should be reported immediately. Withhold the next dose of antibiotic until the healthcare provider gives approval for administration.

Neurologic

Dizziness. Provide for patient safety during episodes of dizziness; report for further evaluation.

Confusion, seizures. Seizure activity—including myoclonic activity, focal tremors, confusional states, and other seizures—has been reported with the carbapenems. These episodes occur most commonly in patients with histories of previous seizure activity and renal impairment.

Perform a baseline assessment of the patient's degree of alertness and orientation to name, place, and time before initiating therapy. Make regularly scheduled subsequent mental status evaluations, and compare findings. Report alterations in consciousness.

Implement seizure precautions. Make sure that the patient continues with anticonvulsant therapy. If seizures develop, provide for patient safety and then record the exact time of seizure onset and duration of

each phase, a description of the specific body parts involved, and any progression in the affected parts. Describe automatic responses during the clonic phase: altered, jerky respirations or frothy salivation, dilated pupils and any eye movements, cyanosis, diaphoresis, or incontinence.

Vascular

Phlebitis. Carefully assess patients for thrombophlebitis. Inspect the IV area frequently when providing care; inspect visually during dressing changes and whenever the IV is changed to a new site. Report redness, warmth, tenderness to touch, and edema in the affected part; if the lower extremities are affected, dorsiflexion of the foot may cause pain in the calf area (Homans' sign). Compare the affected limb with the unaffected limb.

■ Drug Interactions

Probenecid. Probenecid inhibits the urinary excretion of carbapenems. Do not administer probenecid concurrently.

Valproic Acid. Carbapenem antibiotics may produce clinically significant reductions in valproic acid levels, which may lead to a loss of seizure control. If any carbapenem is administered with valproic acid, serum valproic acid levels should be monitored frequently.

Ganciclovir. Concurrent administration of ganciclovir and imipenem-cilastatin has resulted in an increased incidence of seizures. Avoid concurrent use if at all possible.

Admixture Compatibility. The carbapenems require special care regarding mixing and administration:
- Imipenem-cilastatin should not be mixed with or physically added to other antibiotics, but it may be administered concomitantly with other antibiotics, such as aminoglycosides.
- Meropenem should not be mixed with or physically added to solutions containing other medicines.

- Ertapenem for IV use should be reconstituted with bacteriostatic water, or 0.9% sodium chloride (normal saline) for injection. Do not reconstitute or dilute with dextrose solutions.
- Ertapenem for IM use should be reconstituted with 1% lidocaine injection (without epinephrine). Administer the injection within 1 hour of reconstitution.

DRUG CLASS: CEPHALOSPORINS

ACTIONS

The cephalosporins are chemically related to the penicillins and have a similar mechanism of activity. The cephalosporins act by inhibiting cell wall synthesis in bacteria. The cephalosporins may be divided into groups, or "generations," based primarily on antimicrobial activity. The first-generation cephalosporins have effective activity against gram-positive microorganisms (*S. aureus, S. epidermidis, S. pyogenes, S. pneumoniae*) and relatively mild activity against gram-negative microorganisms (*E. coli, K. pneumoniae, P. mirabilis*). Second-generation cephalosporins have somewhat increased activity against gram-negative bacteria but are much less active than the third-generation agents, which are generally less active than first-generation agents against gram-positive cocci, although they are much more active against penicillinase-producing bacteria. Some of the third-generation cephalosporins also are active against *P. aeruginosa*, a potent gram-negative microorganism. Fourth-generation cephalosporins are broad-spectrum agents, with both gram-negative and gram-positive coverage. Ceftaroline is a new fourth-generation cephalosporin that shows promise in treating methicillin resistant staphylococcus aureus (MRSA) and vancomycin-resistant *Staphylococcus aureus* (VRSA).

USES

Cephalosporins may be used with caution as alternatives when patients are allergic to the penicillins unless they are also allergic to the cephalosporins. The cephalosporins are used for certain urinary and respiratory tract infections, abdominal infections, bacteremia, meningitis, and osteomyelitis.

THERAPEUTIC OUTCOME

The primary therapeutic outcome expected from cephalosporin therapy is elimination of bacterial infection.

❖ NURSING IMPLICATIONS FOR CEPHALOSPORINS

▪ Premedication Assessment
1. Obtain baseline assessments of presenting symptoms.
2. Record temperature, pulse, respirations, blood pressure, and hydration status.
3. Assess for any allergies, symptoms of renal disease, or bleeding disorders. If present, withhold drug and report findings to the healthcare provider.
4. Obtain baseline laboratory studies ordered and review results (e.g., CBC with differential, culture and sensitivity).

▪ Availability, Dosage, and Administration
See Table 45-3.

▪ Common Adverse Effects
Gastrointestinal

Diarrhea. Cephalosporins cause diarrhea by altering the bacterial flora of the GI tract. The diarrhea is usually not severe enough to warrant discontinuing medication. Encourage the patient not to discontinue therapy without consulting the healthcare provider. When diarrhea persists, monitor the patient for signs of dehydration.

Immune System (Opportunistic Infections)

Secondary infections. Oral thrush, genital and anal pruritus, vaginitis, and vaginal discharge may occur with cephalosporin therapy. Report promptly because these infections are resistant to the original antibiotic used. Teach the importance of meticulous oral and perineal personal hygiene.

Gastrointestinal

Hepatotoxicity. Transient elevations of liver function test results (e.g., AST, ALT, alkaline phosphatase) have been reported. Monitor returning laboratory data and report abnormal findings to the healthcare provider.

Renal

Nephrotoxicity. Transient elevations of renal test results (e.g., BUN, serum creatinine) have been reported. Renal toxicity, as evidenced by proteinuria, hematuria, casts, decreased creatinine clearance, and decreased urine output, also has been reported. Monitor returning laboratory data and report abnormal findings to the healthcare provider.

Hematologic

Hypoprothrombinemia. Hypoprothrombinemia, a reduction in circulating prothrombin, with and without bleeding, has been reported. This rare occurrence is most frequent in older adult, debilitated, or otherwise compromised patients with borderline vitamin K deficiency. Treatment with broad-spectrum antibiotics eliminates enough GI flora to cause a further reduction in vitamin K synthesis.

Assess the patient for ecchymosis after minimal trauma; prolonged bleeding at an infusion site or from a surgical wound; or the development of petechiae, bleeding gums, or nosebleeds. Notify the healthcare provider of any of the signs of hypoprothrombinemia. The usual treatment is administration of vitamin K.

Electrolyte imbalance. If a patient develops hyperkalemia or hypernatremia, consider the electrolyte

Table 45-3 Cephalosporins

GENERIC NAME	BRAND NAME	GENERATION	AVAILABILITY	ADULT DOSAGE RANGE

cefaclor	Nu-Cefaclor ❦	2	Capsules: 250, 500 mg
			Extended-release tablets (12 hr):
			  500 mg
			Oral suspension: 125, 250 mg/5 ml
				PO: 250-500 mg q8h; do
				  not exceed 4 g/day

cefadroxil	—	1	Capsules: 500 mg Tablets: 1000 mg Suspension: 250, 500 mg/5 mL	PO: 1-2 g daily in one or two doses daily

cefazolin	—	1	Injection: 500-mg and 1-, 10-, 20-,
			  100-, 300-, 500-g vials
				IM, IV: 250 mg to 2 g
				  q6-8h

cefdinir	Omnicef
	⇄ Do not confuse
	  Omnicef with
	  Omnipen.
		3	Capsules: 300 mg
			Oral suspension: 125,
			  250 mg/5 mL
				PO: 300 q12h and
				  600 mg once daily

cefditoren	Spectracef	2	Tablets: 200, 400 mg	PO: 200-400 mg q12h
cefepime	Maxipime	4	Injection: 1-, 2-g vials	IM, IV: 0.5-2 g q8-12h

cefixime	Suprax
	⇄ Do not confuse
	  Suprax with
	  Surfak.
		3	Tablets: 400 mg
			Tablets, chewable: 100, 200 mg
			Capsules: 400 mg
			Suspension: 100, 200,
			  500 mg/5 mL
				PO: 200 mg q12h or
				  400 mg once daily

cefotaxime	Claforan	3	IV: 500-mg, 1-, 2-, 10-g vials	IV: 1-2 g q4-12h; do not exceed 12 g/day
cefotetan	—	3	Injection: 1-, 2-, 10-g vials	IM, IV: 1-3 g q12h; do not exceed 6 g/day

cefoxitin	—	2	Injection: 1-, 2-, 10-g vials	IM, IV: 1-2 g q4-6h or
				  2-3 g q6-8h; do not
				  exceed 12 g/day

cefpodoxime	Vantin	3	Tablets: 100, 200 mg Suspension: 50, 100 mg/5 mL	PO: 200 mg q12h for 7-14 days
cefprozil	Cefzil	2	Tablets: 250, 500 mg Suspension: 125, 250 mg/5 mL	PO: 250-500 mg q12h for 10 days
ceftaroline	Teflaro	4 MRSA active	IV: 400-, 600-mg vials	IV: 600 mg q12h for 5-14 days
ceftazidime	Fortaz, Tazicef	3	Injection: 500-mg, 1-, 2-, 6-, 10-g vials	IM, IV: 1-2 g q12h

ceftazidime/
avibactam
	Avycaz		Injection: 2 gm ceftazidime;
			  500 mg avibactam
				IV: 2.5 mg ceftazidime
				  q8hr

ceftibuten	Cedax	3	Capsules: 400 mg
			Suspension: 90, 180 mg/5 mL
				PO: 400 mg once daily
				  2 hr before or 1 hr after
				  meals for 10 days

ceftolozane/ tazobactam	Zerbaxa		Injection: 1 g ceftolozane; 500 mg tazobactam	IV: 1.5 g ceftolozane q8hr

ceftriaxone	Rocephin	3	Injection: 250-, 500-mg, 1-, 2-,
			  10-g vials
				IM, IV: 1-2 g once daily;
				  do not exceed 4 g daily

cefuroxime
⇄ Do not confuse
  cefuroxime with
  deferoxamine.
	Zinacef, Ceftin	2	Tablets: 250, 500 mg
			IV: 750-mg, 1.5-, 7.5-, 225-g vials
			Suspension: 125, 250 mg/5 mL
				PO: 250-500 mg q12h
				IV: 750 mg-1.5 g q8h

cephalexin	Keflex, Novolexin ❦	1	Tablets: 250, 500 mg Capsules: 250, 500, 750 mg Suspension: 125, 250 mg/5 mL	PO: 250-1000 mg q6h

❦ Available in Canada.

content of the antibiotics. Most cephalosporins have a high electrolyte content.

Vascular

Thrombophlebitis. Phlebitis and thrombophlebitis, or inflammation of the vein with a blood clot or thrombus, are recurrent problems associated with IV administration of cephalosporins. Use small IV needles in large veins and alternate infusion sites, if possible, to minimize irritation. Carefully assess patients receiving IV cephalosporins for the development of thrombophlebitis. Inspect the area frequently when providing care; inspect during dressing changes and when the IV is changed to a new site. Always investigate pain at the IV site. Report redness, warmth, tenderness to touch, or edema in the affected part. If in the lower extremities, dorsiflexion of the foot may cause pain in the calf area (Homans' sign). Compare findings in the affected limb with those in the unaffected limb.

■ **Drug Interactions**

Nephrotoxic Potential. Patients receiving cephalosporins, aminoglycosides, polymyxin B, vancomycin, and loop diuretics concurrently should be assessed for signs of nephrotoxicity. Monitor urinalysis and kidney function tests for abnormal results. Report increasing BUN and creatinine levels, decreasing urine output or decreasing specific gravity (despite amount of fluid intake), casts or protein in the urine, frank blood or smoky-colored urine, or RBCs in excess of 0 to 3 RBCs/HPF (see Table 41-1) on the urinalysis report.

Antacids. Antacids inhibit the absorption of cefaclor, cefdinir, and cefpodoxime. If antacids must be taken, the antibiotic should be taken 2 hours before or after the antacid.

Histamine-2 (H₂) Antagonists. H_2 antagonists (e.g., cimetidine, famotidine, nizatidine, ranitidine) inhibit the absorption of cefpodoxime and cefuroxime, decreasing the antibiotic effect. Because of the long duration of action of the H_2 antagonists, it is recommended that they not be administered when these cephalosporins are prescribed.

Iron Supplements. Iron supplements and food fortified with iron inhibit the absorption of cefdinir. If iron supplements must be taken, the antibiotic should be taken 2 hours before or after the iron supplement.

Probenecid. Patients receiving probenecid in combination with cephalosporins are more susceptible to toxicity because of the inhibition of excretion of the cephalosporins by probenecid. Monitor closely for adverse effects.

Alcohol. Instruct the patient to avoid alcohol consumption during cefmetazole, cefoperazone, cefotetan, and possibly ceftizoxime therapy. Patients ingesting alcohol during, and for 24 to 72 hours after, administration of these cephalosporins will become flushed, tremulous, dyspneic, tachycardic, and hypotensive.

Also, tell the patient not to use OTC preparations containing alcohol, such as mouthwash (e.g., Cēpacol, Listerine) or cough preparations.

Oral Contraceptives. Cephalosporins may interfere with the contraceptive activity of oral contraceptives. Oral contraceptives should not be discontinued, but counseling regarding use of additional methods of contraception (e.g., condoms and foam) should be planned.

DRUG CLASS: GLYCYLCYCLINES

tigecycline (tī-gĕ-SĪ-klēn)
Tygacil (TĪG-ă-sĭl)

ACTIONS

Tigecycline is the first of a new family of antimicrobial agents known as the glycylcyclines. Tigecycline is chemically related to the tetracyclines, but is not susceptible to the mechanisms that cause resistance to the tetracyclines. It acts by binding to the 30S ribosome, preventing protein synthesis. It is a bacteriostatic antibiotic effective against a broad spectrum of grampositive, gram-negative, and anaerobic microorganisms. It is not effective against viruses.

USES

Tigecycline is used to treat complicated skin and skin structure infections (cSSSIs) caused by *E. coli, Enterococcus faecalis, S. aureus* (methicillin-susceptible and methicillin-resistant isolates), *S. agalactiae,* and *Bacteroides fragilis.* It may also be used to treat complicated intraabdominal infections caused by *Citrobacter freundii, Enterobacter cloacae, E. coli, Klebsiella oxytoca, K. pneumoniae, E. faecalis, S. aureus* (methicillin-susceptible isolates only), *B. fragilis, B. vulgaris, C. perfringens,* and *Peptostreptococcus micros.* In an effort to slow the development of strains of bacteria resistant to tigecycline, it should be used only when the pathogen is resistant to other available antibiotics.

Tigecycline is not approved for use in people younger than 18 years. As with tetracyclines, tigecycline administered during the ages of tooth development (the last half of pregnancy through 8 years of age) may cause enamel hypoplasia and permanent yellow, gray, or brown staining of the teeth.

THERAPEUTIC OUTCOME

The primary therapeutic outcome expected from tigecycline therapy is elimination of bacterial infection.

❖ **NURSING IMPLICATIONS FOR TIGECYCLINE**

■ **Premedication Assessment**

1. Obtain baseline assessments of presenting symptoms.

2. Record temperature, pulse, respirations, blood pressure, and hydration status.
3. Assess for and record any gastric symptoms before initiating therapy.
4. Assess for any allergies.
5. Obtain baseline laboratory studies ordered and review results (e.g., CBC with differential, culture and sensitivity).

▪ Availability

IV: 50 mg in 5-mL vials.

▪ Dosage and Administration

IV: Initial: 100 mg followed by 50 mg every 12 hours. Administer by IV infusion over 30 to 60 minutes. Therapy is continued for 5 to 14 days, depending on the severity and site of the infection and the patient's clinical progress.

▪ Common Adverse Effects

Gastrointestinal

Gastric irritation. The most common adverse effects of tigecycline therapy are nausea and vomiting (30% and 20%, respectively). These adverse effects are usually mild to moderate in the first 1 to 2 days of therapy but tend to resolve with continued therapy.

Severe diarrhea. Rarely, severe diarrhea may develop from the use of tigecycline. Report diarrhea of five or more stools daily to the healthcare provider. This may be an indication of drug-induced pseudomembranous colitis. Blood or mucus in the stool also should be reported to the healthcare provider. **Warn patients not to treat diarrhea themselves when taking this drug.** The use of diphenoxylate, loperamide, or paregoric may prolong or worsen the condition.

Integumentary

Photosensitivity. Photosensitivity resulting in an exaggerated sunburn after short exposure has been reported. The patient should be cautioned to avoid exposure to sunlight and ultraviolet light. Suggest wearing long-sleeved clothing, a hat, and sunglasses when outdoors. Discourage the use of tanning lamps. Consult the healthcare provider about the advisability of discontinuing therapy.

▪ Drug Interactions

Warfarin. This medication may enhance the anticoagulant effects of warfarin. Observe for petechiae, ecchymoses, nosebleeds, bleeding gums, dark tarry stools, and bright red or coffee-ground emesis. Monitor the PT and INR, and reduce the dosage of warfarin if necessary.

Oral Contraceptives. Tigecycline may interfere with the activity of oral contraceptives. Oral contraceptives should not be discontinued, but counseling regarding use of additional methods of contraception (e.g., condoms and foam) should be planned.

DRUG CLASS: KETOLIDES

telithromycin (tĕl-ĭth-rō-MĪ-sĭn)
Ketek (KĒ-tĕk)

ACTIONS

Telithromycin is the first of a new family of antimicrobial agents known as the *ketolides*. They are chemically related to the macrolide antibiotics and have a similar mechanism of bactericidal action by preventing bacterial ribosomes from translating its mRNA, preventing the synthesis of new proteins.

USES

Telithromycin is used to treat acute lung (pneumonia) infections caused by susceptible strains of gram-positive bacteria such as *S. pneumoniae, H. influenzae, M. catarrhalis, S. aureus, Chlamydophila pneumoniae,* or *Mycoplasma pneumoniae.* It can be used cautiously as an alternative to a macrolide, oral cephalosporin, or fluoroquinolone antibiotic therapy. In an effort to slow the development of strains of bacteria resistant to telithromycin, it should be used only when the pathogen is resistant to other available antibiotics. Telithromycin is contraindicated in patients with myasthenia gravis. There have been reports of life-threatening and fatal respiratory failure in patients with myasthenia gravis associated with the use of telithromycin. It should also be used with extreme caution in patients with liver disease.

THERAPEUTIC OUTCOME

The primary therapeutic outcome expected from telithromycin therapy is the elimination of bacterial infection.

❖ NURSING IMPLICATIONS FOR TELITHROMYCIN

▪ Premedication Assessment

1. Obtain baseline assessments of presenting symptoms.
2. Record temperature, pulse, respirations, blood pressure, and hydration status.
3. Assess for and record any gastric symptoms before initiating therapy.
4. Assess for and record any visual acuity issues before initiating therapy.
5. Assess for any allergies.
6. Obtain baseline laboratory studies ordered and review results (e.g., CBC with differential, liver function tests, culture and sensitivity).

▪ Availability

PO: 300- and 400-mg tablets.

▪ Dosage and Administration

PO: 800 mg once daily for 5, 7, or 10 days, depending on the type of infection. In general, bacterial bronchitis and sinusitis are treated for 5 days, and pneumonia is treated for 7 to 10 days.

Common Adverse Effects

Gastrointestinal

Gastric irritation. The most common adverse effects of oral telithromycin therapy are diarrhea, nausea, and vomiting. These adverse effects are usually mild and tend to resolve with continued therapy. Encourage the patient not to discontinue therapy without first consulting the healthcare provider.

Serious Adverse Effects

Neurologic

Fainting. Fainting has been reported, especially when the patient is experiencing nausea, vomiting, and lightheadedness. If fainting occurs, patients should be advised to avoid driving a motor vehicle, operating heavy machinery, or engaging in otherwise hazardous activities. Any fainting episodes should be reported to the healthcare provider. The patient must obtain healthcare provider approval before taking another dose of telithromycin.

Sensory

Visual disturbances. Visual disturbances (e.g., blurred vision, difficulty focusing, double vision) may occur after the first or second dose and last for several hours. Visual disturbances may be particularly noted when quickly changing focus from distant objects to close objects. If visual difficulties occur, patients should be advised to avoid driving a motor vehicle, operating heavy machinery, or engaging in otherwise hazardous activities. Any visual disturbances should be reported to the healthcare provider. The patient must obtain healthcare provider approval before taking another dose of telithromycin.

Gastrointestinal

Hepatotoxicity. Potentially severe liver toxicity has occurred in patients during and immediately after completing telithromycin therapy. Signs of hepatotoxicity include increased tiredness, loss of appetite, right upper abdominal pain, cola-colored urine, yellowing of the skin or eyes, and itchy skin. Any of these signs and symptoms should be reported to the healthcare provider. The patient must obtain healthcare provider approval before taking another dose of telithromycin.

Drug Interactions

Toxicity Caused by Telithromycin. Telithromycin is a strong inhibitor of the cytochrome P450 3A4 (CYP3A4) enzyme system. It may inhibit the metabolism of several drugs, causing accumulation and potential toxicity. These drugs are benzodiazepines (e.g., midazolam, triazolam), cisapride, buspirone, carbamazepine, phenytoin, cyclosporine, digoxin, 3-hydroxy-3-methylglutaryl coenzyme A (HMG-CoA) reductase inhibitors (e.g., atorvastatin, lovastatin, simvastatin), azole-type antifungals (e.g., fluconazole, itraconazole), and metoprolol. Read individual drug monographs for monitoring parameters of toxicity from these agents.

Pimozide. Coadministration of telithromycin with pimozide is contraindicated.

Rifampin, Rifabutin, Carbamazepine, Phenobarbital. The coadministration of telithromycin with any of these medicines may cause a reduction in antimicrobial effect while increasing the frequency of GI adverse effects.

Oral Contraceptives. Telithromycin may interfere with the activity of oral contraceptives. Oral contraceptives should not be discontinued, but counseling regarding use of additional methods of contraception (e.g., condoms and foam) should be planned.

DRUG CLASS: MACROLIDES

ACTIONS

The macrolide antibiotics act by inhibiting protein synthesis in susceptible bacteria. They are bacteriostatic and bacteriocidal, depending on the organism and drug concentration present. Erythromycin is effective against gram-positive microorganisms and gram-negative cocci. Azithromycin is less active against gram-positive organisms than erythromycin, but has greater activity against gram-negative organisms that are resistant to erythromycin. Clarithromycin has a spectrum of activity similar to that of erythromycin, but has considerably greater potency.

USES

The macrolides are used for respiratory, GI tract, skin, and soft tissue infections and for STIs, especially when penicillins, cephalosporins, and tetracyclines cannot be used. Fidaxomicin is a new macrolide antibiotic used to treat *Clostridium difficile*–associated diarrhea. It should be used only for *C. difficile* infections.

THERAPEUTIC OUTCOME

The primary therapeutic outcome expected from macrolide therapy is elimination of bacterial infection.

❖ NURSING IMPLICATIONS FOR MACROLIDES

Premedication Assessment

1. Obtain baseline assessments of presenting symptoms.
2. Record temperature, pulse, respirations, blood pressure, and hydration status.
3. Assess for and record any gastric symptoms before initiating therapy.
4. Assess for any allergies.
5. Obtain baseline laboratory studies ordered and review results (e.g., CBC with differential, culture and sensitivity).

Availability, Dosage, and Administration

See Table 45-4.

PO: Azithromycin and erythromycin should be administered at least 1 hour before or 2 hours after meals. Clarithromycin may be taken without regard to meals.

Table 45-4 Macrolides

GENERIC NAME	BRAND NAME	AVAILABILITY	ADULT DOSAGE RANGE

azithromycin	Zithromax	Tablets: 250, 500, 600 mg
		Packets: 1 g
		Suspension: 100, 200 mg/5 mL;
		   2000 mg
		Injection: 500 mg in 10-mL vial
			PO: 500 mg as a single dose on day 1,
			   followed by 250 mg once daily on
			   days 2-5 for a total dose of 1.5 g
			IV: 500 mg daily. Dilute powder to a
			   concentration of 1-2 mg/mL; infuse
			   1-mg/mL concentration over 3 hr or
			   the 2-mg/mL concentration over 1 hr
			Do not administer as an IV bolus or IM

clarithromycin	Biaxin, Biaxin XL ⇄ *Do not confuse Biaxin with Bactrim.*	Tablets: 250, 500 mg Suspension: 125, 250 mg/5 mL Extended-release tablets (24 hr): 500, 1000 mg	PO: 250-500 mg q12h for 7-14 days

erythromycin	Erythrocin, Eryc, many
	others ♦
		Enteric-coated tablets: 250, 333,
		   500 mg
		Chewable tablets: 250, 500 mg
		Film-coated tablets: 250, 500 mg
		Enteric-coated pellets in
		   capsules: 333, 500 mg
		Suspension: 125, 200, 250,
		   400 mg/5 mL
		IV: 500-, 1000-mg vials for
		   reconstitution
			PO: 250 mg four times daily for 10-14
			   days
			IV: 15-20 mg/kg/24 hr; up to 4 g/24 hr

fidaxomicin	Dificid	Tablets: 200 mg	200 mg twice daily for 10 days

♦ Available in Canada.

IM: Because of pain on injection and the possibility of sterile abscess formation, IM administration of erythromycin is generally not recommended for multiple-dose therapy.

IV: Dilute the dosage of erythromycin in 100 to 250 mL of saline solution or 5% dextrose and administer over 20 to 60 minutes. Thrombophlebitis after IV infusion is a relatively common adverse effect.

- ■ **Common Adverse Effects**
  Gastrointestinal

Gastric irritation. The most common adverse effects of oral macrolide therapy are diarrhea, nausea and vomiting, and abnormal taste. These adverse effects are usually mild and tend to resolve with continued therapy. Encourage the patient not to discontinue therapy without first consulting his or her healthcare provider.

- ■ **Serious Adverse Effects**
  Gastrointestinal

Severe diarrhea. Severe diarrhea may develop from the use of erythromycin. Report diarrhea of five or more stools daily to the healthcare provider. This may be an indication of drug-induced pseudomembranous colitis. Blood or mucus in the stool should also be reported to the healthcare provider. **Warn patients not to treat diarrhea themselves when taking this drug.** The use of diphenoxylate, loperamide, or paregoric may prolong or worsen the condition.

Vascular

Thrombophlebitis. Carefully assess patients receiving IV erythromycin for thrombophlebitis. Inspect the IV area frequently when providing care; inspect during dressing changes and when the IV is changed to a new site. Always investigate pain at the IV site. Report redness and edema in the affected part. If the affected part is in the lower extremities, dorsiflexion of the foot may cause pain in the calf area (Homans' sign). Compare the affected limb with the unaffected limb.

- ■ **Drug Interactions**

Toxicity Caused by Macrolides. Macrolide antibiotics may inhibit the metabolism of several drugs, causing accumulation and potential toxicity. These drugs are alfentanil, benzodiazepines (e.g., alprazolam, diazepam, midazolam, triazolam), bromocriptine, cisapride, buspirone, carbamazepine, cyclosporine, digoxin, disopyramide, felodipine, HMG-CoA reductase inhibitors (e.g., atorvastatin, lovastatin, simvastatin), omeprazole, tacrolimus, theophyllines, vinblastine, warfarin, and other CYP3A-metabolized drugs. Read individual drug monographs for monitoring parameters of toxicity from these agents.

Pimozide. Coadministration of a macrolide antibiotic with pimozide is contraindicated. Death has resulted from this combination of drug therapy.

Rifampin, Rifabutin. The coadministration of a macrolide antibiotic with rifampin or rifabutin may cause a reduction in antimicrobial effect while increasing the frequency of GI adverse effects.

Oral Contraceptives. Macrolides may interfere with the activity of oral contraceptives. Oral contraceptives should not be discontinued, but counseling regarding use of additional methods of contraception (e.g., condoms and foam) should be planned.

DRUG CLASS: OXAZOLIDINONES

linezolid (lĭn-ā-ZŌ-lĭd)
Zyvox (ZĪ-vŏks)

⇄ *Do not confuse Zyvox with Zosyn or Zovirax.*

ACTIONS

Linezolid is the first of a new class of antimicrobial agents known as the *oxazolidinones.* It acts by inhibiting protein synthesis in bacterial cells. It is bactericidal in certain strains of bacteria and bacteriostatic in others. It is the only currently available agent in this class. It is also a reversible monoamine oxidase inhibitor, inhibiting the action of monoamine oxidase A, an enzyme responsible for metabolizing serotonin in the brain.

USES

Linezolid is used in the treatment of serious or life-threatening infections caused by gram-positive microorganisms. It is approved for use with VRE bacteria and uncomplicated and cSSSIs caused by methicillin-susceptible and methicillin-resistant *S. aureus, S. pyogenes,* or *S. agalactiae.* It may also be used to treat community-acquired pneumonia caused by penicillin-susceptible *S. pneumoniae.* It is not indicated for treatment of gram-negative infections. Other appropriate antibiotics to provide gram-negative coverage should be used concurrently. As a representative of a new class of antibiotics, linezolid should be reserved for those cases in which other antibiotics such as vancomycin are ineffective, so that resistant strains of bacteria do not rapidly develop.

THERAPEUTIC OUTCOME

The primary therapeutic outcome expected from linezolid therapy is elimination of bacterial infection.

❖ NURSING IMPLICATIONS FOR LINEZOLID

- **Premedication Assessment**
1. Obtain baseline assessments of presenting symptoms.
2. Record temperature, pulse, respirations, blood pressure, and hydration status.
3. Assess for and record any gastric and visual symptoms before initiating therapy.
4. Assess for any allergies.
5. Obtain baseline laboratory studies ordered and review results (e.g., CBC with differential, platelets, blood glucose, electrolytes, culture and sensitivity).

- **Availability**

PO: 600-mg tablets; 100-mg/5 mL oral suspension in 150 mL. *IV:* 400- and 600-mg prefilled containers at 2 mg/mL.

- **Dosage and Administration**
Adults

TYPE OF INFECTION	DOSE AND ROUTE OF ADMINISTRATION	DURATION (DAYS)
Skin (uncomplicated)	400 mg PO q12h	10-14
Skin (complicated)	600 mg PO or IV q12h	10-14
Community-acquired pneumonia		
HCAP		
Methicillin-resistant staphylococcal infections (MRSA)	600 mg PO or IV q12h	Determined clinically
VRE infections	600 mg PO or IV q12h	14-28
HCAP	600 mg PO or IV q12h	10-14

IV: Infuse the dose over 30 to 120 minutes. Do not administer concurrently with other medicines. If the same IV line is used for sequential infusion of other medicines, flush the line before and after infusion of linezolid with 5% dextrose, normal saline, or lactated Ringer's solution. Keep the linezolid infusion in its wrapper until ready for administration. Linezolid may exhibit a yellow color that may intensify over time but without a loss of potency.

No dosage adjustment is necessary when switching from IV to oral administration using the tablet or oral suspension dosage form.

- **Common Adverse Effects**
Gastrointestinal
Gastric irritation. The most common adverse effects of linezolid therapy are nausea and vomiting (9% and 11%, respectively). These adverse effects are usually mild and moderate in the first few days of therapy, but tend to resolve with continued therapy.
Neurologic
Headaches. Headache was reported in 1% to 11% of patients taking linezolid. Headaches were not severe enough to discontinue therapy and tended to resolve with continued therapy.

- **Serious Adverse Effects**
Gastrointestinal
Severe diarrhea. Rarely, severe diarrhea may develop from the use of linezolid. Report diarrhea of five or more stools daily to the healthcare provider. This may be an indication of drug-induced pseudomembranous colitis. Blood or mucus in the stool should also be reported to the healthcare provider. **Warn patients not to treat diarrhea themselves when taking this drug.** The use of diphenoxylate, loperamide, or paregoric may prolong or worsen the condition.

Hematologic

Bone marrow suppression. Serious and possibly fatal bone marrow suppression may occur after therapy is initiated with linezolid. Early signs include sore throat, fatigue, elevated temperature, and small petechial hemorrhages and bruises on the skin. If patients describe any of these symptoms, report them to the healthcare provider immediately. Routine laboratory studies (RBC, white blood cell [WBC] counts, differential counts, platelets) are scheduled for patients taking linezolid for 14 days or longer. Stress the importance of returning for this laboratory work. Monitor for the development of sore throat, fever, purpura, jaundice, or excessive or progressive weakness.

Immune System (Opportunistic Infections)

Secondary infections. Oral thrush, genital and anal pruritus, vaginitis, and vaginal discharge may occur. Report promptly because these infections are resistant to the original antibiotic used. Teach the importance of meticulous oral and perineal hygiene.

Metabolic

Lactic acidosis. Lactic acidosis has been reported in conjunction with linezolid therapy. Patients who develop recurrent nausea or vomiting, unexplained acidosis, or a low bicarbonate level should be reported to their healthcare provider as soon as possible.

Neurologic

Seizures. Seizures have been reported in patients receiving linezolid. Patients should be monitored for the development of seizures, particularly those with a history of seizure activity or whose clinical condition (e.g., hypoxia) may make the patient more susceptible to seizures.

Visual neuropathy. Changes in vision from blurred vision to loss of vision have been reported with linezolid, particularly with therapy longer than 28 days. Patients should be asked to report, and should be monitored for, changes in visual acuity, color vision, or visual field and blurred vision. These symptoms should be reported to the healthcare provider for further evaluation.

■ Drug Interactions

Monoamine Oxidase Inhibitors (e.g., Phenelzine, Isocarboxazid, Tranylcypromine, Meperidine, Selegiline, Rasagiline, Tramadol, Methadone). Linezolid is a monoamine oxidase A inhibitor and should not be used in patients taking other monoamine oxidase inhibitors or within 2 weeks of taking such products. Although not reported with linezolid, fatal drug interactions have been reported between monoamine oxidase inhibitors and these agents listed here.

Adrenergic Agents (e.g., Dopamine, Epinephrine, Norepinephrine, Ephedrine, Pseudoephedrine, Phenylpropanolamine). Linezolid is a monoamine oxidase inhibitor that will reduce the metabolism of adrenergic agents, potentially resulting in tachycardia and hypertension. Initial doses of the adrenergic agents should be reduced to see how the patient responds before using normal doses.

Serotonergic Agents (e.g., Fluoxetine, Paroxetine, Sertraline; Tricyclic Antidepressants, Buspirone, Triptans). As a monoamine oxidase A inhibitor, linezolid has the potential to interact with serotonergic agents to induce a serotonin syndrome. Patients developing signs and symptoms of serotonin syndrome, such as hyperreflexia (twitching) and incoordination, fever, excessive sweating, shivering or shaking, diarrhea, and confusion, should be reported to their healthcare provider for further evaluation.

DRUG CLASS: PENICILLINS

ACTIONS

Penicillins were the first true antibiotics to be grown and used against pathogenic bacteria in humans. They currently remain one of the most widely used classes of antibiotics.

The penicillins act by interfering with the synthesis of bacterial cell walls. The resulting cell wall is weakened because of defective structure, and the bacteria are subsequently destroyed by osmotic lysis. The penicillins are most effective against bacteria that multiply rapidly. They do not hinder growth of human cells because human cells have protective membranes but no cell wall.

Many bacteria that are initially sensitive to penicillins develop a protective mechanism and become resistant to penicillin therapy. These bacteria produce the enzyme penicillinase (beta-lactamase), which can destroy the antibacterial activity of most penicillins. Penicillinase inactivates the penicillin antibiotics by splitting open the beta-lactam ring of the penicillin molecule. Researchers have developed two mechanisms to prevent this inactivation. The first is to modify the penicillin molecule to "protect" the ring structure while retaining antimicrobial activity. This mechanism culminated in the development of the **penicillinase-resistant penicillins** (e.g., nafcillin, oxacillin, dicloxacillin). The second method is to add another chemical with a similar structure that will more readily bond to the penicillinase enzymes than the penicillin, leaving the free penicillin to inhibit cell wall synthesis. Potassium clavulanate is now added to amoxicillin (Augmentin) to bond to penicillinases that would normally destroy this antibiotic. Sulbactam has been added to ampicillin (Unasyn) and tazobactam to piperacillin (Zosyn) for similar reasons.

USES

Penicillins are used to treat middle ear infections (otitis media), pneumonia, meningitis, UTIs, syphilis, and gonorrhea, and as a prophylactic antibiotic before surgery or dental procedures for patients with histories of rheumatic fever.

THERAPEUTIC OUTCOME

The primary therapeutic outcome expected from penicillin therapy is elimination of bacterial infection.

❖ NURSING IMPLICATIONS FOR PENICILLINS

■ Premedication Assessment

1. Obtain baseline assessments of presenting symptoms.
2. Record temperature, pulse, respirations, blood pressure, and hydration status.
3. Assess for and record any allergies, symptoms of diarrhea, and abnormal liver or renal function test results. If present, withhold drug and report findings to the healthcare provider.
4. Obtain baseline laboratory studies ordered and review results (e.g., CBC with differential, culture and sensitivity).

■ Availability, Dosage, and Administration

See Table 45-5.

Admixture Compatibilities. Do not mix with other drugs in the same syringe or infuse with other drugs. See "Drug Interactions" section for incompatibilities.

■ Common Adverse Effects

Gastrointestinal

Diarrhea. Penicillins cause diarrhea by altering the bacterial flora of the GI tract. The diarrhea is usually not severe enough to warrant discontinuation. Encourage the patient not to discontinue therapy without first consulting the healthcare provider. If diarrhea persists, monitor the patient for signs of dehydration.

■ Severe Adverse Effects

Gastrointestinal

Hepatotoxicity. Transient elevations of liver function test results (e.g., AST, ALT, alkaline phosphatase levels) have been reported. Monitor returning laboratory data and report abnormal findings to the healthcare provider.

Renal

Nephrotoxicity. Transient elevations of renal test results (e.g., BUN, serum creatinine levels) have been reported. Renal toxicity, as evidenced by proteinuria, hematuria, casts, decreased creatinine clearance, and decreased urine output, also has been reported. Monitor returning laboratory data and report abnormal findings to the healthcare provider.

Table 45-5   Penicillins

GENERIC NAME	BRAND NAME	AVAILABILITY	ADULT DOSAGE RANGE
amoxicillin	—	Tablets: 500, 875 mg Extended-release tablets (24 hr): 775 mg Chewable tablets: 125, 250 mg Capsules: 250, 500 mg Suspension: 125, 200, 250, 400 mg/5 mL	PO: 250 to 875 mg q8-12h
ampicillin	—	Capsules: 250, 500 mg Suspension: 125, 250 mg/5 mL Injection: 0.25-, 0.5-, 1-, 2-, 10-g vials	IM, IV: 0.5-1 g q4-6h PO: 250-500 mg q6h
dicloxacillin ⇌ *Do not confuse dicloxacillin with doxycycline.*	—	Capsules: 250, 500 mg	PO: 250-500 mg q6h
nafcillin	—	IV: 1-, 2-, 10-g powder; 1-, 2-g premixed containers	IV: 500-1000 mg q4h
oxacillin	—	Injection: 1-, 2-, 10-g vials	IM, IV: 0.5-1 g q4-6h
penicillin G, potassium or sodium	Pfizerpen-G	Injection: Vials of 0.6, 1, 2, 3, 5, 20 million units	IM, IV: 600,000 to 30 million units daily
penicillin V potassium	—	Tablets: 250, 500 mg Suspension: 125, 250 mg/5 mL	PO: 125-500 mg q6h
Combination Products			
amoxicillin and potassium clavulanate (co-amoxiclav)	Augmentin, Clavulin ♣	Chewable tablets: 200, 400 mg Tablets: 250, 500, 875 mg Extended-release tablets (12 hr): 1000 mg Suspension: 250, 400, 600 mg/5 mL	PO: 250 q8h or 500-875 mg q12h Extended release: 2000 mg q12h Extra-strength suspension: 600 mg q12h
ampicillin and sulbactam sodium	Unasyn	Injection: 1.5-, 3-, 15-g bottles and vials	IM, IV: 1.5-3 g q6h
piperacillin and tazobactam	Zosyn	IV: 2.25-, 3.375-, 4.5-, 40.5-g vials	IV: 3.375 g q6h

♣ Available in Canada.

Hematologic

Electrolyte imbalance. The electrolyte content of the antibiotics may cause hyperkalemia or hypernatremia. Some of the penicillins (e.g., penicillin G IV, piperacillin, ticarcillin) have a high electrolyte content.

Vascular

Thrombophlebitis. Carefully assess patients receiving IV penicillins for the development of thrombophlebitis. Inspect the IV area frequently when providing care; inspect during dressing changes and when the IV is changed to a new site. Always investigate pain at the IV site. Report redness, warmth, tenderness to touch, and edema in the affected part. If in the lower extremities, dorsiflexion of the foot may cause pain in the calf area (Homans' sign). Compare the affected limb with the unaffected limb.

■ **Drug Interactions**

Probenecid. Patients receiving probenecid in combination with penicillins are more susceptible to toxicity because probenecid inhibits renal excretion of the penicillins. Monitor closely for adverse effects.

This combination may be used advantageously when treating gonorrhea and other infections in which high levels are indicated.

Ampicillin and Allopurinol. When used concurrently, these two agents are associated with a high incidence of rash. Do not label the patient as allergic to penicillins until further skin testing has verified that there is a true hypersensitivity to penicillins.

Antacids. Excessive use of antacids may diminish the absorption of oral penicillins.

Oral Contraceptives. Penicillins may interfere with the activity of oral contraceptives. Oral contraceptives should not be discontinued, but counseling regarding use of additional methods of contraception (e.g., condoms and foam) should be planned.

DRUG CLASS: QUINOLONES

ACTIONS

Quinolone antibiotics are an important class of therapeutic agents. The subclass known as the fluoroquinolones is effective against a wide range of gram-positive and gram-negative bacteria, including some anaerobes. The fluoroquinolones act by inhibiting the activity of DNA gyrase, an enzyme essential for the replication of bacterial DNA.

USES

- Ciprofloxacin was the first well-tolerated, broad-spectrum oral antibiotic in the quinolone series. It demonstrates rapid bactericidal activity against the pathogens that cause health care–associated and community-acquired UTIs, most of the strains that cause enteritis, gonococci, meningococci, *Legionella, Pasteurella, H. influenzae,* and methicillin-resistant staphylococci, and some gram-negative bacteria.

The activity of ciprofloxacin against gram-positive and gram-negative cocci is equal to or better than that of the penicillins, cephalosporins, and aminoglycosides, but most anaerobic organisms and most strains of *P. aeruginosa* are resistant.

- Gemifloxacin is similar in spectrum of activity and use to levofloxacin and moxifloxacin. It also has an advantage of once-daily oral dosing.

- Levofloxacin has broad-spectrum activity against gram-negative, gram-positive, and anaerobic bacteria. It is used to treat maxillary sinusitis, acute bacterial exacerbations of chronic bronchitis, community-acquired pneumonia, skin and soft tissue infections, chronic bacterial prostatitis, UTIs, acute pyelonephritis, and inhalational anthrax. It has an advantage of once-daily oral dosing. Levofloxacin should be used with caution in older patients who may be susceptible to prolongation of the QT interval and the development of potentially life-threatening dysrhythmias. Levofloxacin is contraindicated in patients with hypokalemia or those receiving quinidine, procainamide, amiodarone, or sotalol antiarrhythmic agents.

- Moxifloxacin is active against gram-positive microorganisms such as *S. pneumoniae* and *S. aureus,* gram-negative organisms such as *H. influenzae,* and atypical causes of pneumonia such as *C. pneumoniae* and *M. pneumoniae.* It is approved for use in patients with acute bacterial sinusitis, acute bacterial exacerbation of chronic bronchitis, and community-acquired pneumonia caused by susceptible organisms. Moxifloxacin should be used with caution in older patients who may be susceptible to prolongation of the QT interval and the development of potentially life-threatening dysrhythmias. Moxifloxacin is contraindicated in patients with hypokalemia or those receiving quinidine, procainamide, amiodarone, or sotalol antiarrhythmic agents.

- Ofloxacin has broad-spectrum activity against gram-negative, gram-positive, and anaerobic bacteria. It differs from ciprofloxacin in that it has greater activity against STIs such as *N. gonorrhoeae, C. trachomatis,* and genital ureaplasma. Ofloxacin is also less susceptible to drug interactions than are other fluoroquinolones. Ofloxacin is used to treat UTIs, prostatitis, skin infections (e.g., cellulitis and impetigo), lower respiratory pneumonia, and STIs other than syphilis.

THERAPEUTIC OUTCOME

The primary therapeutic outcome expected from quinolone therapy is elimination of bacterial infection.

❖ **NURSING IMPLICATIONS FOR QUINOLONES**

■ **Premedication Assessment**

1. Obtain baseline assessments of presenting symptoms.

Table 45-6   Quinolones

GENERIC NAME	BRAND NAME	AVAILABILITY	DOSAGE RANGE
ciprofloxacin ⇄ *Do not confuse ciprofloxacin with cephalexin.*	Cipro ⇄ *Do not confuse Cipro with Ceftin.*	Tablets: 100, 250, 500, 750 mg Tablets, extended-release (24 hr): 500, 1000 mg Suspension: 250, 500 mg/5 mL Injection: 200-, 400-mg vials; 1.2-g bulk package	PO: 0.2-1.5 g daily in two divided doses 2 hr after meals IV: 400-800 mg daily in two divided doses q12h
gemifloxacin	Factive	Tablets: 320 mg	PO: 320 mg once daily; may be taken with or without food
levofloxacin	Levaquin ⇄ *Do not confuse Levaquin with Lovenox, Tequin, or heparin.*	Tablets: 250, 500, 750 mg Suspension: 25 mg/mL Injection: 250-, 500-, 750-mg vials	PO: 250-500 mg once daily IV: 250-750 mg infused slowly over at least 60 min
moxifloxacin	Avelox ⇄ *Do not confuse Avelox with Avandia, Avapro, or Cerebyx.*	Tablets: 400 mg Injection: 400 mg/250 mL	IV, PO: 400 mg once daily; may be taken with or without food
ofloxacin	—	Tablets: 400 mg	PO: 400-800 mg daily in two divided doses q12h, 1 hr before or 2 hr after meals, with a large glass of fluid

2. Record temperature, pulse, respirations, blood pressure, and hydration status.
3. Assess for and record any gastric symptoms before initiation of therapy.
4. Assess for any allergies.
5. Obtain baseline laboratory studies ordered and review results (e.g., CBC with differential, culture and sensitivity).
6. Ensure that the patient is not pregnant.
7. Warn patients of possible phototoxicity to lomefloxacin (see "Serious Adverse Effects" section).

■ Availability, Dosage, and Administration

See Table 45-6.

Children and Adults Older Than 60 Years of Age. Fluoroquinolones should not be prescribed for patients younger than 18 years. Use in pediatric patients has resulted in an increased incidence of musculoskeletal disorders such as arthralgia, tendinopathy, and gait abnormality. This risk is further increased in older patients (usually older than 60 years of age), in patients taking corticosteroids (e.g., prednisone, dexamethasone), and in patients with organ transplants.

Pregnant Women. Quinolone therapy is not recommended during pregnancy unless the benefit of therapy outweighs the risk. No studies have been completed in human patients, but animal studies have demonstrated various teratogenic effects.

■ Common Adverse Effects

Gastrointestinal

Nausea, vomiting, diarrhea, abdominal discomfort. These adverse effects are usually mild and tend to resolve with continued therapy. Encourage the patient not to discontinue therapy without first consulting her or his healthcare provider. If the patient becomes debilitated, contact the healthcare provider.

Neurologic

Dizziness, lightheadedness. Although uncommon, ciprofloxacin may cause these disturbances. They tend to be self-limiting, and therapy should not be discontinued until the patient consults the healthcare provider. Caution the patient against driving or performing hazardous tasks until adjusted to the effects of the medication.

■ Serious Adverse Effects

Integumentary

Phototoxicity. Phototoxic reactions have been reported in patients treated with fluoroquinolones. Exposure to direct and indirect sunlight and the use of sun lamps should be avoided. These reactions have occurred with and without the use of sunblocks and sunscreens and with single doses of fluoroquinolones. The patient should not take additional doses and should contact the healthcare provider if a sensation of skin burning, redness, swelling, blisters, rash, itching, or dermatitis develops. Suggest wearing long-sleeved clothing, a hat, and sunglasses when exposed to sunlight.

Rash. Report a rash or pruritus immediately and withhold additional doses pending approval by the healthcare provider.

Gastrointestinal

Hepatotoxicity. Transient elevations of liver function test results (e.g., AST, ALT, alkaline phosphatase levels) have been reported. Monitor returning laboratory data and report abnormal findings to the healthcare provider.

Renal

Nephrotoxicity. Transient elevations of renal test results (e.g., BUN, serum creatinine levels) have been reported. Renal toxicity, as evidenced by proteinuria, hematuria, casts, decreased creatinine clearance, and decreased urine output, also has been reported. Monitor returning laboratory data and report abnormal findings to the healthcare provider.

Neurologic

Tinnitus, headache, dizziness, mental depression, drowsiness, confusion. Quinolone therapy may cause these disturbances. Consult with the healthcare provider when these effects occur. Caution the patient against driving or performing hazardous tasks until adjusted to the effects of the medication.

▪ Drug Interactions

Iron, Antacids, Sucralfate. Iron salts, zinc salts, sucralfate, and antacids containing magnesium hydroxide or aluminum hydroxide decrease the absorption of quinolones. Administer at least 4 hours before or 4 hours after ingestion of antacids, sucralfate, or iron-containing products.

Nonsteroidal Antiinflammatory Drugs. The concurrent administration of nonsteroidal antiinflammatory drugs (NSAIDs) with fluoroquinolones (e.g., levofloxacin, ofloxacin) may increase the risk of central nervous system (CNS) stimulation with seizures. Use with extreme caution. Consider the use of other analgesics or antiinflammatory agents.

Didanosine. Do not administer quinolone antibiotics within 4 hours of administration of didanosine tablets or pediatric powder for oral solution. The antacid present in these formulations inhibits the absorption of the quinolones.

Theophylline. The fluoroquinolones (e.g., ciprofloxacin, moxifloxacin, ofloxacin), when given with theophylline, may produce theophylline toxicity. Observe for vomiting, dizziness, restlessness, and cardiac dysrhythmias. Monitor theophylline serum levels. The dosage of theophylline may need to be reduced.

DRUG CLASS: STREPTOGRAMINS

quinupristin-dalfopristin (kwĭ-yū-PRĬS-tĭn dăl-fō-PRĬS-tĭn)
  Synercid (SĬN-ŭr-sĭd)

ACTIONS

Quinupristin-dalfopristin is the first of a new class of antimicrobial agents known as *streptogramins*. These two agents were developed from pristinamycin. When used in combination, they are synergistic and act by inhibiting protein synthesis in bacterial cells.

USES

Quinupristin-dalfopristin are agents that can be used in the treatment of serious or life-threatening infections that are associated with VRE bacteria and cSSSIs caused by methicillin-susceptible *S. aureus* or *S. pyogenes*. The use of quinupristin-dalfopristin, a representative of a new class of antibiotics, should be reserved for those cases in which other antibiotics such as vancomycin are ineffective, so that resistant strains of bacteria do not rapidly develop.

THERAPEUTIC OUTCOME

The primary therapeutic outcome expected from quinupristin-dalfopristin therapy is elimination of bacterial infection.

❖ NURSING IMPLICATIONS FOR STREPTOGRAMINS

▪ Premedication Assessment

1. Obtain baseline assessments of presenting symptoms.
2. Record temperature, pulse, respirations, blood pressure, and hydration status.
3. Assess for and record any gastric symptoms before initiating therapy.
4. Assess for any allergies.
5. Obtain baseline laboratory studies ordered and review results (e.g., CBC with differential, platelets, blood glucose, electrolytes, creatine kinase, liver function tests, culture and sensitivity).

▪ Availability

IV: 500 mg (150 mg quinupristin and 350 mg dalfopristin) in 10-mL vial. All dosage recommendations are based on total quinupristin and dalfopristin, in milligrams.

▪ Dosage and Administration

Adult: IV: 7.5 mg/kg every 8 hours for the treatment of vancomycin-resistant *E. faecium* bacteremia or every 12 hours for treatment of complicated skin infections. Infuse the dose over 60 minutes.

Admixture Compatibility. Reconstitute only with 5% dextrose or sterile water for injection and then dilute with 5% dextrose to a final concentration of 100 mg/mL. A precipitate will form if reconstituted with other standard diluents. If infused in IV tubing being used for other medicines, flush with 5% dextrose. Do not flush with heparin or sodium chloride.

▪ Serious Adverse Effects

Vascular

Pain, infusion site inflammation. The most frequent adverse venous events include pain at the administration site, edema, infusion site reaction, and thrombophlebitis.

Gastrointestinal

Nausea, vomiting, anorexia, abdominal cramps, diarrhea. These adverse effects are usually mild and tend to resolve with continued therapy.

Hepatotoxicity. The symptoms of hepatotoxicity are anorexia, nausea, vomiting, jaundice, hepatomegaly, splenomegaly, and abnormal liver function tests (e.g., elevated bilirubin, AST, ALT, GGT, alkaline phosphatase levels, increased PT).

Musculoskeletal

Arthralgia, myalgia. Arthralgias and myalgias may occur during therapy. Decreasing the frequency of administration to every 12 hours may minimize recurrence.

▪ Drug Interactions

Toxicity Induced by Quinupristin-Dalfopristin. Quinupristin-dalfopristin may decrease the metabolism of HMG-CoA reductase inhibitors (e.g., atorvastatin, lovastatin, pravastatin, fluvastatin, simvastatin), cyclosporine, delavirdine, nevirapine, indinavir, ritonavir, vincristine, paclitaxel, docetaxel, tamoxifen, diazepam, midazolam, cisapride, methylprednisolone, carbamazepine, nifedipine, verapamil, diltiazem, quinidine, lidocaine, disopyramide, and other potent CYP3A enzyme system inhibitors. Serum concentrations of these agents should be monitored closely if used concurrently with quinupristin-dalfopristin.

DRUG CLASS: SULFONAMIDES

ACTIONS

The sulfonamides are not true antibiotics because they are not synthesized by microorganisms. However, they are highly effective antibacterial agents. Sulfonamides act by inhibiting bacterial biosynthesis of folic acid, which eventually results in bacterial cell death. Human cells do not synthesize folic acid and therefore are not affected.

USES

Sulfonamides are used primarily to treat UTIs and otitis media. They may also be used to prevent streptococcal infection or rheumatic fever in those allergic to penicillin.

Because of an increasing incidence of organisms resistant to sulfonamide therapy and the unreliability of in vitro sulfonamide sensitivity tests, patients should be monitored closely for continued therapeutic response to treatment. This is particularly important for patients being treated for chronic and recurrent UTIs.

The sulfonamide most commonly used today is actually a combination of trimethoprim and sulfamethoxazole (e.g., co-trimoxazole, TMP-SMX). This combination blocks two steps in the pathway of folic acid production; therefore fewer resistant strains of microorganisms have developed. Co-trimoxazole is often used for treatment of UTIs, otitis media in children, traveler's diarrhea, acute exacerbations of chronic bronchitis in adults, and prophylaxis and treatment of *Pneumocystis jiroveci* (formerly *P. carinii*) pneumonia (PJP, formerly PCP) in immunocompromised patients.

THERAPEUTIC OUTCOME

The primary therapeutic outcome expected from sulfonamide therapy is elimination of bacterial infection.

❖ NURSING IMPLICATIONS FOR SULFONAMIDES

▪ Premedication Assessment

1. Obtain baseline assessments of presenting symptoms.
2. Record temperature, pulse, respirations, blood pressure, and hydration status.
3. Assess for and record any gastric symptoms before beginning therapy.
4. Assess for any allergies.
5. Obtain baseline laboratory studies ordered and review results (e.g., CBC with differential, culture and sensitivity).

▪ Availability, Dosage, and Administration

See Table 45-7.

 Medication Safety Alert

Patients should be encouraged to drink water several times daily while receiving sulfonamide therapy. In rare situations, crystals form in the urinary tract if the patient becomes too dehydrated.

▪ Common Adverse Effects

Gastrointestinal

Nausea, vomiting, anorexia, diarrhea. These adverse effects are usually mild and tend to resolve with continued therapy. Encourage the patient not to discontinue therapy without first consulting the healthcare provider. If the patient becomes debilitated, contact the healthcare provider.

Integumentary

Dermatologic reactions. Report a rash or pruritus immediately and withhold additional doses pending approval by the healthcare provider.

Photosensitivity. The patient should be cautioned to avoid exposure to sunlight and ultraviolet light. Suggest wearing long-sleeved clothing, a hat, and sunglasses when outdoors. Discourage the use of tanning lamps.

Hematologic

Hematologic reactions. Routine laboratory studies (e.g., CBC with differential) are scheduled for patients taking sulfonamides for 14 days or longer. Stress the importance of returning for this laboratory work. Monitor for the development of a sore throat, fever,

Table 45-7 Sulfonamides

GENERIC NAME	BRAND NAME	AVAILABILITY	ADULT DOSAGE RANGE
sulfadiazine	—	Tablets: 500 mg	PO: Initial dose: 2-4 g, then 2-4 g/day in three to six divided doses
sulfasalazine	Azulfidine	Tablets: 500 mg Delayed-release tablets: 500 mg	PO: Initial therapy: 3-4 g daily in three to four divided doses; maintenance dosage: 2 g daily
co-trimoxazole	Bactrim, Bactrim DS ⇄ *Do not confuse Bactrim with Biaxin.* Septra, Septra DS	Tablets, suspension, infusion	PO: 2-4 tablets daily, depending on strength, disease being treated IV: 8-10 mg/kg/day (based on trimethoprim) in two to four divided doses Pneumocystis pneumonia: 15-20 mg/kg/24 hr (based on trimethoprim) in three or four divided doses for up to 14 days

purpura, jaundice, or excessive and progressive weakness.

Neurologic

Neurologic effects. Report the development of tinnitus, headache, dizziness, mental depression, drowsiness, or confusion.

■ **Drug Interactions**

Oral Hypoglycemic Agents. Sulfonamides may displace sulfonylurea oral hypoglycemic agents (e.g., tolbutamide, tolazamide, chlorpropamide, glipizide, glyburide) and meglitinide oral hypoglycemic agents (repaglinide, nateglinide) from protein-binding sites, resulting in hypoglycemia. Monitor for hypoglycemia, headache, weakness, decreased coordination, general apprehension, diaphoresis, hunger, and blurred or double vision. The dosage of the hypoglycemic agent may need to be reduced. Notify the healthcare provider if any of these symptoms appear.

Warfarin. Sulfonamides may enhance the anticoagulant effects of warfarin. Observe for petechiae, ecchymoses, nosebleeds, bleeding gums, dark tarry stools, and bright red or coffee-ground emesis. Monitor PT and INR and reduce dosage of warfarin if necessary.

Methotrexate. Sulfonamides may produce methotrexate toxicity when given simultaneously. Monitor patients on concurrent therapy for oral stomatitis and for signs of nephrotoxicity (e.g., oliguria, hematuria, proteinuria, casts).

Phenytoin. Sulfisoxazole may displace phenytoin from protein-binding sites, resulting in phenytoin toxicity. Monitor patients on concurrent therapy for signs of phenytoin toxicity (e.g., nystagmus, sedation, lethargy); serum levels may be ordered. A reduced dosage of phenytoin may be required.

Angiotensin-Converting Enzyme Inhibitors. Concurrent use of sulfamethoxazole/trimethoprim and angiotensin-converting enzyme (ACE) inhibitors (e.g., lisinopril, captopril, ramipril) may act additively to suppress aldosterone, resulting in hyperkalemia that may lead to cardiac arrhythmias. Monitor serum potassium levels.

DRUG CLASS: TETRACYCLINES

ACTIONS

Tetracyclines are a class of antibiotics that are effective against gram-negative and gram-positive bacteria. They act by inhibiting protein synthesis by bacterial cells.

USES

The tetracyclines are often used in patients allergic to the penicillins for the treatment of certain venereal diseases, UTIs, upper respiratory tract infections, pneumonia, and meningitis. They are particularly effective against skin (acne), rickettsial, and mycoplasmic infections.

Tetracyclines administered during the ages of tooth development (last half of pregnancy through 8 years of age) may cause enamel hypoplasia and permanent yellow, gray, or brown staining of teeth. Tetracyclines are secreted in breast milk, so nursing mothers on tetracycline therapy are advised to feed their infants formula or cow's milk, as appropriate.

THERAPEUTIC OUTCOME

The primary therapeutic outcome expected from tetracycline therapy is elimination of bacterial infection.

❖ **NURSING IMPLICATIONS FOR TETRACYCLINES**

■ **Premedication Assessment**

1. Obtain baseline assessments of presenting symptoms.
2. Record temperature, pulse, respirations, blood pressure, and hydration status.
3. Assess for and record any gastric symptoms present before beginning therapy.
4. Assess for any allergies.

Table 45-8   Tetracyclines

GENERIC NAME	BRAND NAME	AVAILABILITY	ADULT DOSAGE RANGE
demeclocycline	Declomycin	Tablets: 150, 300 mg	PO: 150 mg four times daily or 300 mg twice daily
doxycycline ⇄ Do not confuse doxycycline with dicloxacillin or dicyclomine.	Vibramycin ⇄ Do not confuse Vibramycin with vancomycin. Adoxa, Doryx	Tablets: 20, 50, 75, 100, 150 mg Delayed-release tablets: 75, 100, 150 mg Capsules: 20, 40, 50, 100 mg Syrup: 25, 50 mg/5 mL IV: 100-mg vials	IV: 100 twice daily or 200 mg once daily PO: 100 mg twice daily
minocycline	Minocin	Capsules: 50, 75, 100 mg Tablets: 50, 75, 100 mg Tablets, extended release (24 hr): 45, 55, 65, 80, 90, 105, 115, 135 mg Extended-release powder in dental base: 1 mg IV: 100-mg vial	PO, IV: 200 mg, followed by 100 mg q12h
tetracycline		Capsules: 250, 500 mg	PO: 250-500 mg four times daily

5. Obtain baseline laboratory studies ordered and review results (e.g., CBC with differential, culture and sensitivity).

■ **Availability, Dosage, and Administration**
See Table 45-8. *PO:* Emphasize the importance of taking medication 1 hour before or 2 hours after ingesting antacids, milk, or other dairy products, or products containing calcium, aluminum, magnesium, or iron (e.g., vitamins). *Exception:* Food and milk do not interfere with the absorption of doxycycline.

■ **Common Adverse Effects**
Gastrointestinal
Nausea, vomiting, anorexia, abdominal cramps, diarrhea. These adverse effects are usually mild and tend to resolve with continued therapy. Encourage the patient not to discontinue therapy without first consulting the healthcare provider.
Integumentary
Photosensitivity. Photosensitivity resulting in an exaggerated sunburn after short exposure has been reported. The patient should be cautioned to avoid exposure to sunlight and ultraviolet light. Suggest wearing long-sleeved clothing, a hat, and sunglasses when outdoors. Discourage the use of tanning lamps. Consult the healthcare provider about the advisability of discontinuing therapy.

■ **Drug and Other Interactions**
Warfarin. This medication may enhance the anticoagulant effects of warfarin. Observe for petechiae, ecchymoses, nosebleeds, bleeding gums, dark tarry stools, and bright red or coffee-ground emesis. Monitor the PT and INR, and reduce the dosage of warfarin if necessary.
Impaired Absorption. Iron; calcium-containing foods (milk and dairy products); and calcium, aluminum, or magnesium preparations (antacids) decrease absorption of tetracyclines. Administer all tetracycline products 1 hour before or 2 hours after ingestion of these foods or products. *Exceptions:* Food and milk do not interfere with the absorption of doxycycline.

Phenytoin, Carbamazepine. These agents reduce the half-life of doxycycline. Monitor patients for lack of clinical improvement from the infection.
Tooth Development. Do not administer tetracyclines to pregnant patients or to children younger than 8 years. The infant's or child's tooth enamel may be permanently stained yellow, gray, or brown.
Lactation. Nursing mothers must switch their babies to formula while taking tetracyclines because tetracyclines are present in breast milk.
Oral Contraceptives. Tetracyclines may interfere with the activity of oral contraceptives. Oral contraceptives should not be discontinued, but counseling regarding use of additional methods of contraception (e.g., condoms and foam) should be planned.
Didanosine. Do not administer tetracycline antibiotics within 2 hours of taking didanosine tablets or pediatric powder for oral solution. The antacid present in these formulations inhibits the absorption of the tetracyclines.

DRUG CLASS: ANTITUBERCULAR AGENTS

ethambutol (ĕth-ĂM-byū-tŏl)

ACTIONS
Ethambutol inhibits tuberculosis bacterial growth by altering cellular RNA synthesis and phosphate metabolism.

USES
Ethambutol is an antitubercular agent. It must be used in combination with other antitubercular agents to prevent the development of resistant organisms.

THERAPEUTIC OUTCOME

The primary therapeutic outcome expected from ethambutol therapy is elimination of tuberculosis.

❖ NURSING IMPLICATIONS FOR ETHAMBUTOL

▪ Premedication Assessment

1. Obtain baseline assessments of presenting symptoms.
2. Record temperature, pulse, respirations, blood pressure, and hydration status.
3. Assess for and record any gastric symptoms before initiating therapy.
4. Assess for any allergies.
5. Perform baseline mental status assessment (e.g., orientation and alertness), assess for GI symptoms, and test color vision (e.g., red-green discrimination) before initiating therapy.
6. Review laboratory data of tuberculin testing and cultures in the patient's chart.

▪ Availability

PO: 100- and 400-mg tablets.

▪ Dosage and Administration

Adult: PO: Initial treatment: 15 mg/kg administered as a single dose every 24 hours. Retreatment: 25 mg/kg as a single daily dose. After 60 days, reduce the dosage to 15 mg/kg and administer as a single dose every 24 hours. Administer once daily with food or milk to minimize gastric irritation.

Counseling. The patient should be warned that omission or interrupted intake may result in drug resistance, reversal of clinical improvement, and increased susceptibility of family members and others to tuberculosis.

▪ Common Adverse Effects

Gastrointestinal

Nausea, vomiting, anorexia, abdominal cramps. These adverse effects are usually mild and tend to resolve with continued therapy. Encourage the patient not to discontinue therapy without first consulting his or her healthcare provider. Administer the daily dosage with food to minimize nausea and vomiting.

▪ Serious Adverse Effects

Neurologic

Confusion, hallucinations. Perform a baseline assessment of the patient's degree of alertness and orientation to name, place, and time before initiating therapy. Make regularly scheduled subsequent mental status evaluations, and compare findings. Report development of alterations. Provide for patient safety during episodes of altered behavior or periods of dizziness.

Sensory

Blurred vision, red-green vision changes. Before initiating therapy, check for any visual alterations using a color vision chart. Schedule subsequent evaluations on a regular basis. Report the development of visual disturbances for the healthcare provider's evaluation. These adverse effects disappear within a few weeks after therapy has been discontinued.

▪ Drug Interactions

Antacids. Aluminum salts may delay and reduce absorption of ethambutol. Separate administration by at least 2 hours.

---

isoniazid (ī-sō-NĪ-ă-zĭd)
INH

ACTIONS

Isoniazid has been a mainstay for many years in the prevention and treatment of tuberculosis. Despite this, its mechanism of action is still not fully known. It appears to disrupt the *Mycobacterium tuberculosis* cell wall and inhibit replication.

USES

Isoniazid is used for the prophylaxis and treatment of tuberculosis. It should be used in combination with other antitubercular agents for therapy of active disease.

THERAPEUTIC OUTCOMES

The primary therapeutic outcomes expected from isoniazid therapy are as follows:

- Prevention of tuberculosis in people with a positive skin test
- Elimination of tuberculosis in people with active disease

❖ NURSING IMPLICATIONS FOR ISONIAZID

▪ Premedication Assessment

1. Obtain baseline assessments of presenting symptoms.
2. Record temperature, pulse, respirations, blood pressure, and hydration status.
3. Assess for and record any gastric symptoms, abnormal liver function test results, or paresthesias present before initiation of therapy.
4. Assess for any allergies.
5. Check medication orders for concurrent administration of other antitubercular drugs and for an order for pyridoxine.

▪ Availability

PO: 100- and 300-mg tablets; 50-mg/5 mL syrup. *IM:* 100 mg/mL in 10-mL vials.

▪ Dosage and Administration

Adult: PO: Treatment of active tuberculosis is 5 mg/kg to a maximum of 300 mg daily or 15 mg/kg/day

(900 mg maximum per dose) two or three times per week. Isoniazid should be used in conjunction with other effective antitubercular agents. Prophylactic therapy: 300 mg daily in a single dose. Administer on an empty stomach for maximum effectiveness. Pyridoxine, 25 to 50 mg daily, is often given concurrently with isoniazid to diminish peripheral neuropathies, dizziness, and ataxia. *IM:* Same as for PO administration.

Pediatric: PO: 10 to 15 mg/kg/24 hr (maximum dose of 300 mg daily) in single dose or 20 to 40 mg/kg/day (900 mg maximum per dose) two or three times weekly. Infants and children tolerate larger dosages than adults.

■ Common and Serious Adverse Effects
Gastrointestinal

Nausea, vomiting. Nausea and vomiting are relatively common adverse effects of isoniazid and are dose related. Concurrent use of pyridoxine, 25 to 50 mg daily, will usually prevent these symptoms.

Hepatotoxicity. The incidence of hepatotoxicity increases with age and with the consumption of alcohol. This reaction usually occurs within the first 3 months of therapy and is thought to be an allergic reaction. The symptoms of hepatotoxicity are anorexia, nausea, vomiting, jaundice, hepatomegaly, splenomegaly, and abnormal liver function test results (e.g., elevated bilirubin, AST, ALT, GGT, alkaline phosphatase levels, increased PT).

Neurologic

Tingling, numbness. Tingling and numbness of the hands and feet are relatively common adverse effects of isoniazid and are dosage related. Concurrent use of pyridoxine, 25 to 50 mg daily, will usually prevent these symptoms. When paresthesias are present, the patient must be cautioned to inspect the extremities for any skin breakdown because of the diminished sensation. Caution patients not to immerse feet or hands in water without first testing the temperature. Monitor patients with paresthesias for adequate nutrition.

Dizziness, ataxia. Provide for patient safety and assistance in ambulation until either a dosage adjustment or addition of pyridoxine provides symptomatic relief.

■ Drug Interactions
Disulfiram. Patients may experience changes in physical coordination and mental affect and behavior. Provide for patient safety and monitor the patient's mental status before and during therapy. If possible, avoid concomitant therapy.

Carbamazepine. Isoniazid may inhibit the metabolism of carbamazepine. Monitor patients receiving concurrent therapy for signs of carbamazepine toxicity (e.g., ataxia, headache, vomiting, blurred vision, drowsiness, confusion).

Theophylline. Isoniazid may inhibit the metabolism of theophylline. Monitor patients receiving concurrent therapy for signs of theophylline toxicity (e.g., anxiety, tachycardia, nausea, headache, vomiting).

Phenytoin. Isoniazid may inhibit the metabolism of phenytoin. Monitor patients receiving concurrent therapy for signs of phenytoin toxicity (e.g., nystagmus, sedation, lethargy). Serum levels may be ordered and the dosage of phenytoin reduced.

---

rifampin (rĭf-ĂM-pĭn)
⇄ *Do not confuse rifampin with ramipril or rifabutin.*
Rifadin (RĬF-ă-dĭn)
⇄ *Do not confuse Rifadin with Rifater.*

ACTIONS
Rifampin prevents RNA synthesis in mycobacteria by inhibiting DNA-dependent RNA polymerase. This action blocks key metabolic pathways needed for mycobacterium cells to grow and replicate.

USES
Rifampin is used in combination with other agents for the treatment of tuberculosis. Rifampin is also used to eliminate meningococci from the nasopharynx of asymptomatic *N. meningitidis* carriers and to eliminate *H. influenzae* type b (Hib) from the nasopharynx of asymptomatic carriers.

THERAPEUTIC OUTCOMES
The primary therapeutic outcomes expected from rifampin therapy are as follows:
1. Elimination of tuberculosis
2. Eradication of meningococci or Hib from asymptomatic carriers of these diseases

❖ NURSING IMPLICATIONS FOR RIFAMPIN
■ Premedication Assessment
1. Obtain baseline assessments of presenting symptoms.
2. Record temperature, pulse, respirations, blood pressure, and hydration status.
3. Assess for and record any gastric symptoms present before beginning therapy.
4. Assess for any allergies.
5. Obtain baseline laboratory studies ordered (e.g., CBC with differential, tuberculin tests, chest radiography).

■ Availability
PO: 150- and 300-mg capsules. *IV:* 600-mg vials.

■ Dosage and Administration
Adult: PO: 10 mg/kg (maximum 600) mg once daily, either 1 hour before or 2 hours after a meal. *IV:* same as for PO.

Pediatric: PO: 10 to 20 mg/kg/24 hr, with a maximum daily dose of 600 mg. *IV:* same as for PO.

Medication Safety Alert

Patients should be warned that omission or interrupted intake of rifampin may result in drug resistance, reversal of clinical improvement, and increased susceptibility of family members to tuberculosis.

■ Common Adverse Effects

Excretory

Reddish orange secretions. Urine, feces, saliva, sputum, sweat, and tears may be tinged reddish orange. The effect is harmless and will disappear after discontinuing therapy. Rifampin may permanently discolor soft contact lenses.

■ Serious Adverse Effects

Gastrointestinal

Nausea, vomiting, anorexia, abdominal cramps. These adverse effects are usually mild and tend to resolve with continued therapy. Encourage the patient not to discontinue therapy without first consulting the healthcare provider. If these symptoms are accompanied by fever, chills, or muscle and bone pain, or if unusual bruising or a yellowish discoloration of the skin or eyes appears, contact the patient's healthcare provider.

■ Drug Interactions

Warfarin. This medication may diminish the anticoagulant effects of warfarin. Monitor the PT and INR and increase the dosage of warfarin if necessary.

Isoniazid. Concurrent therapy may rarely result in hepatotoxicity. Patients on combined therapy should have liver function tests monitored periodically.

Benzodiazepines (Diazepam, Midazolam, Triazolam), Quinidine, Amiodarone, Verapamil, Nifedipine, Mexiletine, Enalapril, Theophylline, Beta-Blocking Agents (Bisoprolol, Metoprolol, Propranolol), Disopyramide, Barbiturates, Fluoroquinolones, Ondansetron, Haloperidol, Losartan, Protease Inhibitors, Sulfonylureas, Many Other Drugs. Rifampin stimulates the metabolism of these agents. Long-term combined therapy may require an increase in dosages for therapeutic effect.

Ketoconazole. Administration of rifampin and ketoconazole decreases serum levels of both drugs. Avoid concurrent use if possible.

Oral Contraceptives. Rifampin interferes with the activity of oral contraceptives. Counseling regarding alternative methods of birth control should be planned.

DRUG CLASS: MISCELLANEOUS ANTIBIOTICS

aztreonam (ăz-TRĒ-ō-năm)
⇄ *Do not confuse aztreonam with azithromycin.*
Azactam (ăz-ĂK-tăm)

ACTIONS

Aztreonam is a monobactam antibiotic, acting by inhibition of cell wall synthesis.

USES

The monobactams have a high degree of activity against beta-lactamase–producing aerobic gram-negative bacteria, including *P. aeruginosa*. Aztreonam has essentially no activity against anaerobes or gram-positive microorganisms. It is used to treat urinary tract, lower respiratory tract, skin, intraabdominal, gynecologic, and bacteremic infections and meningitides caused by *P. aeruginosa*, *Salmonella*, *Shigella*, *N. gonorrhoeae*, and ampicillin-resistant *H. influenzae*. It is recommended that aztreonam be combined with a broad-spectrum antibiotic in the initial treatment of an infection of unknown cause to treat susceptible anaerobes or gram-positive organisms.

THERAPEUTIC OUTCOME

The primary therapeutic outcome expected from aztreonam therapy is elimination of bacterial infection.

❖ NURSING IMPLICATIONS FOR AZTREONAM

■ Premedication Assessment

1. Obtain baseline assessments of presenting symptoms.
2. Record temperature, pulse, respirations, blood pressure, and hydration status.
3. Assess for and record any gastric symptoms before initiating therapy.
4. Assess for any allergies.
5. Obtain baseline laboratory studies ordered and review results (e.g., CBC with differential, culture and sensitivity).

■ Availability

Injection: 1- and 2-g powders in 15-, 30-, and 100-mL bottles for reconstitution. *Inhalation:* 75 mg in 84-mL containers for reconstitution.

■ Dosage and Administration

Adult: IM or *IV:* Urinary tract infections: 0.5 to 1 g every 8 to 12 hours. Moderately severe systemic infections: 1 to 2 g every 8 to 12 hours. Life-threatening infections: 2 g every 6 to 8 hours.
IM: Reconstitute a 15-mL vial with at least 3 mL of diluent per gram of aztreonam. After adding diluent to container, shake immediately and vigorously. Inject deeply into the large muscle mass of the gluteus maximus. Discard unused portion of vial. *IV bolus:* Reconstitute a 15-mL vial with 6 to 10 mL of diluent. Immediately shake vigorously. Inject directly into a vein or into the tubing of a suitable IV set over 3 to 5 minutes. Discard any unused portion of the vial. *IV infusion:* Reconstitute the 100-mL bottle with at least

50 mL of diluent. Shake immediately and vigorously. Infuse over the next 30 to 60 minutes.

Inhalation: Usual dosage: 75 mg three times daily using an Altera Nebulizer system. Reconstitute the powder using the supplied diluent just prior to inhalation. Patients should use a short- or long-acting bronchodilator prior to administration of aztreonam.

■ **Common Adverse Effects**

Gastrointestinal

Nausea, vomiting, diarrhea. These adverse effects are usually mild and tend to resolve with continued therapy.

■ **Serious Adverse Effects**

Gastrointestinal

Severe diarrhea. Severe diarrhea may develop from the use of aztreonam. Report diarrhea of five or more stools daily to the healthcare provider. This may be an indication of drug-induced pseudomembranous colitis. Blood or mucus in the stool also should be reported to the healthcare provider. **Warn patients not to treat diarrhea themselves when taking this drug.** The use of diphenoxylate, loperamide, or paregoric may prolong or worsen the condition.

Vascular

Phlebitis. Avoid IV infusion in the lower extremities or in areas with varicosities. Use proper technique in starting the IV solution.

Carefully assess at regularly scheduled intervals for signs of developing phlebitis. Inspect for redness, warmth, tenderness to touch, edema, or pain. Always assess complaints of pain at the infusion site. If signs of inflammation accompany complaints, discontinue and restart elsewhere.

Immune System (Opportunistic Infections)

Secondary infections. Oral thrush, genital and anal pruritus, vaginitis, and vaginal discharge may occur. Report promptly because these infections are resistant to the original antibiotic used. Teach the importance of meticulous oral and perineal hygiene measures.

■ **Drug Interactions**

Beta-lactamase Antibiotics (e.g., Cefoxitin, Imipenem). These antibiotics induce the production of beta-lactamase in some gram-negative organisms, resulting in possible antagonism with a beta-lactam antibiotic such as aztreonam. It is recommended that beta-lactamase–stimulating antibiotics not be used concurrently with aztreonam.

---

chloramphenicol (klōr-ăm-FĔN-ĭ-kŏl)

ACTIONS

Chloramphenicol is an antibiotic that acts by inhibiting bacterial protein synthesis of a variety of gram-positive and gram-negative organisms.

USES

Chloramphenicol is particularly effective in treating rickettsial infections, meningitis, and typhoid fever. It must not be used in the treatment of trivial infections or when it is not indicated, such as in colds, influenza, or throat infections, or as a prophylactic agent to prevent bacterial infection.

THERAPEUTIC OUTCOME

The primary therapeutic outcome expected from chloramphenicol therapy is elimination of bacterial infection.

❖ NURSING IMPLICATIONS FOR CHLORAMPHENICOL

■ **Premedication Assessment**

1. Obtain baseline assessments of presenting symptoms.
2. Record temperature, pulse, respirations, blood pressure, and hydration status.
3. Assess for and record any gastric symptoms before initiating therapy.
4. Assess for any allergies.
5. Obtain baseline laboratory studies ordered and review results (e.g., CBC with differential, culture and sensitivity).

■ **Availability**

IV: 100 mg/mL in 1-g vials.

■ **Dosage and Administration**

Adult: IM: Not recommended because of poor absorption and clinical response. *IV:* 50 to 100 mg/kg every 6 hours. Reconstitute by adding 10 mL of sterile water for injection or 5% dextrose to 1 g of chloramphenicol to make a solution containing 100 mg/mL. Administer the calculated dose intravenously over 1 minute.

Pediatric: IM: Not recommended. *IV:* Neonates: 25 mg/kg/24 hr in four equally divided doses. Infants older than 2 weeks: 50 mg/kg/24 hr in four equally divided doses. Administer over 1 minute or by IVPB (intravenous piggyback) over 30 to 60 minutes. Use only chloramphenicol sodium succinate IV in children.

■ **Serious Adverse Effects**

Hematologic

Bone marrow suppression. Serious and possibly fatal bone marrow suppression may occur after therapy is initiated with chloramphenicol. Early signs include sore throat, fatigue, elevated temperature, and small petechial hemorrhages and bruises on the skin. If patients describe any of these symptoms, report them to the healthcare provider immediately. Routine laboratory studies (RBC, WBC, and differential counts) are scheduled for patients taking chloramphenicol for 14 days or longer. Stress the importance of returning for this laboratory work. Monitor for the development of sore throat, fever, purpura, jaundice, or excessive or progressive weakness.

Immune System (Opportunistic Infections)
Secondary infections. Oral thrush, genital and anal pruritus, vaginitis, and vaginal discharge may occur. Report promptly because these infections are resistant to the original antibiotic used. Teach the importance of meticulous oral and perineal hygiene.

■ **Drug Interactions**
Warfarin. Chloramphenicol may enhance the anticoagulant effects of warfarin. Observe for the development of petechiae, ecchymoses, nosebleeds, bleeding gums, dark tarry stools, and bright red or coffee-ground emesis. Monitor the PT and INR and reduce the dosage of warfarin if necessary.

Sulfonylureas. Monitor for hypoglycemia: headache, weakness, decreased coordination, general apprehension, diaphoresis, hunger, and blurred or double vision. The dosage of the hypoglycemic agent may need to be reduced. Notify the healthcare provider if any of these symptoms appear.

Phenytoin. Chloramphenicol inhibits the metabolism of phenytoin. Monitor patients with concurrent therapy for signs of phenytoin toxicity: nystagmus, sedation, and lethargy. Serum levels may be ordered and the dosage of phenytoin reduced.

---

clindamycin (klĭn-dă-MĬ-sĭn)
  Cleocin (klē-Ō-sĭn)

ACTIONS

Clindamycin is an antibiotic that acts by inhibiting protein synthesis.

USES

Clindamycin is useful against infections caused by gram-negative aerobic organisms and a variety of gram-positive and gram-negative anaerobes.

THERAPEUTIC OUTCOME

The primary therapeutic outcome expected from clindamycin therapy is elimination of bacterial infection.

❖ NURSING IMPLICATIONS FOR CLINDAMYCIN
■ **Premedication Assessment**
1. Obtain baseline assessments of presenting symptoms.
2. Record temperature, pulse, respirations, blood pressure, and hydration status.
3. Record pattern of bowel elimination before initiating drug therapy.
4. Assess for any allergies.
5. Obtain baseline laboratory studies ordered and review results (e.g., CBC with differential, culture and sensitivity).

■ **Availability**
PO: 75-, 150-, and 300-mg capsules; 75-mg/5 mL suspension. *IV:* 150 mg/mL in 2-, 4-, and 6-mL ampules.

■ **Dosage and Administration**
Adult: PO: 150 to 450 mg every 6 hours. *Do not* refrigerate the suspension. It is stable at room temperature for 14 days. *IM:* 600 to 2700 mg/24 hr. *Do not* exceed 600 mg per injection. Pain, induration, and sterile abscesses have been reported. Deep IM injection is recommended to help minimize this reaction. *IV:* 600 to 2700 mg/24 hr. Dilute to less than 6 mg/mL, and administer at a rate less than 30 mg/min. Administration by IV push is not recommended.
Pediatric: PO: suspension: 8 to 25 mg/kg/24 hr in three or four divided doses. Capsules: 8 to 20 mg/kg/24 hr in three or four divided doses. Capsules should be taken with a full glass of water to prevent esophageal irritation. *IM:* 15 to 40 mg/kg/24 hr in four divided doses. *IV:* same as for IM use. Dilute to less than 6 mg/mL, and administer at a rate less than 30 mg/min.

■ **Common Adverse Effects**
Gastrointestinal
Diarrhea. These adverse effects are usually mild and tend to resolve with continued therapy. Encourage the patient not to discontinue therapy without first consulting the healthcare provider.

■ **Serious Adverse Effects**
Gastrointestinal
Severe diarrhea. Severe diarrhea may develop from the use of clindamycin. Report diarrhea of five or more stools daily to the healthcare provider. This may be an indication of drug-induced pseudomembranous colitis. Blood or mucus in the stool should also be reported to the healthcare provider. **Warn patients not to treat diarrhea themselves when taking this drug.** The use of diphenoxylate, loperamide, or paregoric may prolong or worsen the condition.

■ **Drug Interactions**
Neuromuscular Blockade. Label charts of patients scheduled for surgery who are taking clindamycin. When combined with surgical muscle relaxants or aminoglycosides, neuromuscular blockade may result.

These combinations may potentiate respiratory depression. Check the anesthesia record of surgical patients. Monitor postoperative patients for respiratory depression for a prolonged period. This can occur 48 hours or more after the drug administration.

Erythromycin. Therapeutic antagonism has been reported between clindamycin and erythromycin. Do not administer concurrently.

---

daptomycin (dăp-tō-MĬ-sĭn)
  Cubicin (KYŪ-bĭ-sĭn)

ACTIONS

Daptomycin is in the class of antibiotics known as *cyclic lipopeptide antibiotics*. It has a unique mechanism of action among the antibiotics. It binds to bacterial membranes and causes a rapid depolarization of membrane potential leading to inhibition of protein, RNA, and DNA synthesis, leading to cell death. Because of its unique mechanism of action, daptomycin is effective against microorganisms that have developed resistance to other commonly used antibiotics.

USES

Daptomycin has been approved for the treatment of cSSSIs caused by *S. aureus*, *S. pyogenes*, *S. agalactiae*, and *E. faecalis*. It is particularly valuable in cases of gram-positive organisms becoming resistant to the beta-lactam (penicillins and cephalosporins) antibiotics and vancomycin. In an effort to slow the development of strains of bacteria resistant to daptomycin, it should be used only when the pathogen is resistant to other available antibiotics.

THERAPEUTIC OUTCOME

The primary therapeutic outcome expected from daptomycin therapy is elimination of bacterial infection.

❖ NURSING IMPLICATIONS FOR DAPTOMYCIN

■ Premedication Assessment

1. Obtain baseline assessments of presenting symptoms.
2. Record temperature, pulse, respirations, blood pressure, and hydration status.
3. Assess for any allergies.
4. Assess the bowel elimination patterns and record before initiating therapy.
5. Ensure that a baseline creatine phosphokinase (CPK, CK) has been drawn and sent to the laboratory before daptomycin is started. Also, inquire and record whether the patient has any particular muscle weakness or pains, particularly in the extremities.
6. Obtain other baseline laboratory studies ordered and review results (e.g., CBC with differential, culture and sensitivity).

■ Availability

IV: 500-mg vials.

■ Dosage and Administration

IV: 6 mg/kg infused over 30 minutes every 24 hours for 7 to 14 days. Patients who have reduced renal function with a creatinine clearance of less than 30 mL/min should have the same dose administered every 48 hours.

Admixture Compatibility. Daptomycin is not compatible with dextrose-containing diluents, and additives or other medications should not be added to daptomycin or infused simultaneously through the same IV line. If the same IV line is used for sequential infusion of several different drugs, the line should be flushed with a compatible infusion solution before and after infusions with daptomycin.

■ Common Adverse Effects

Gastrointestinal

Gastric irritation. The most common adverse effects of daptomycin therapy are diarrhea, constipation, nausea, and vomiting. These adverse effects are usually mild and tend to resolve with continued therapy.

■ Serious Adverse Effects

Gastrointestinal

Severe diarrhea. Severe diarrhea may develop from using daptomycin. Blood and mucus in the stool also may be present. This may be an indication of drug-induced pseudomembranous colitis and should be reported immediately. Withhold the next dose of antibiotic until the healthcare provider gives approval for administration.

Musculoskeletal

Skeletal muscle weakness and pain. Patients should be monitored for the development of muscle pain or weakness, particularly in the distal extremities. It is recommended that CPK concentrations be monitored weekly in patients treated with daptomycin, and more frequently in those who develop unexplained elevations of CPK levels during therapy.

■ Drug Interactions

HMG-CoA Reductase Inhibitors. The statins (e.g., atorvastatin, lovastatin, simvastatin, others) may infrequently cause skeletal muscle myopathy and potentially rhabdomyolysis. It is therefore suggested that statin therapy be discontinued in patients being treated with daptomycin. Statin therapy may be reinitiated after daptomycin therapy has been completed.

---

metronidazole (mĕt-rō-NĪ-dă-zŏl)
⇄ *Do not confuse metronidazole with metoclopramide, metoprolol, miconazole, or methazolamide.*
Flagyl (FLĂ-jĭl)

ACTIONS

Metronidazole is a nitroimidazole. It is a somewhat unusual medication in that it has bactericidal, trichomonacidal, and protozoacidal activity. Its mechanism of action is unknown.

USES

Metronidazole is used to treat trichomoniasis, giardiasis, amebic dysentery, amebic liver abscess, and anaerobic bacterial infections.

THERAPEUTIC OUTCOME

The primary therapeutic outcome expected from metronidazole therapy is elimination of infection.

❖ NURSING IMPLICATIONS FOR METRONIDAZOLE

▪ Premedication Assessment

1. Obtain baseline assessments of the presenting symptoms.
2. Record temperature, pulse, respirations, blood pressure, and hydration status.
3. Assess for and record any gastric symptoms, peripheral neuropathy, or seizure disorders before initiating therapy.
4. Assess for any allergies.
5. Perform a baseline assessment of the patient's degree of alertness and orientation to name, place, and time before initiating therapy.
6. Obtain baseline laboratory studies ordered and review results (e.g., CBC with differential, culture and sensitivity).

▪ Availability

PO: 250- and 500-mg tablets; 375-mg capsules; 750-mg extended-release tablets (24 hr). *Injection:* 500-mg powder/vial.

▪ Dosage and Administration

PO:

- Trichomoniasis: Men and women: 500 mg twice daily for 7 days (CDC) *or* 250 mg three times daily or 375 mg twice daily for 7 days (manufacturer). Sexual partners must be treated concurrently to prevent reinfection. Single doses of 2 g or two doses of 1 g each administered the same day appear to provide adequate treatment for trichomoniasis in men and women.
- Amebic dysentery: 750 mg three times daily for 5 to 10 days.
- Amebic liver abscess: 7.5 mg/kg every 6 hours for 7 to 10 days.
- Giardiasis: 250 mg three times daily for 5 to 7 days.
- Anaerobic bacterial infections: Start with parenteral therapy initially. The usual oral dosage is 7.5 mg/ kg every 6 hours. Do not exceed 4 g/24 hr. The usual duration is 7 to 10 days. Infections of the bone and joint, lower respiratory tract, and endocardium may require longer treatment.

IV:

- Anaerobic bacterial infections: Loading dose: 15 mg/kg infused over 1 hour. Maintenance dosage: 7.5 mg/kg infused over 1 hour every 6 hours. Do not exceed 4 g/24 hr. Convert to oral dosages when clinical condition is stable. Dosage reduction is necessary in patients with hepatic impairment but not renal impairment.

Pediatric: PO: Trichomoniasis: 15 mg/kg/24 hr in three divided doses for 7 days. Amebiasis: 35 to 50 mg/ kg/24 hr in three divided doses for 7 to 10 days. Giardiasis: 15 mg/kg/24 hr in three divided doses (maximum of 250 mg/dose) for 5 days.

▪ Common Adverse Effects

Gastrointestinal

Nausea, vomiting, diarrhea, metallic taste. These adverse effects are usually mild and tend to resolve with continued therapy.

▪ Serious Adverse Effects

Neurologic

Dizziness. Provide for patient safety during episodes of dizziness; report for further evaluation.

Confusion, seizures. Patients receiving high doses of metronidazole, those with histories of seizure activity, and those with significant hepatic impairment are at greater risk of confusion and seizures. Perform a baseline assessment of the patient's degree of alertness and orientation to name, place, and time before initiating therapy. Make regularly scheduled subsequent mental status evaluations and compare findings. Report the development of alterations. Implement seizure precautions (padded side rails, available oxygen, and suction sets). Make sure that the patient continues with anticonvulsant therapy. If seizures develop, provide for patient safety, and then record the exact time of seizure onset and duration of each phase, a description of the specific body parts involved, and any progression in the affected parts. Describe the automatic responses seen during the clonic phase—altered, jerky respirations; frothy salivation; dilated pupils and eye movements; cyanosis; diaphoresis; or incontinence.

Vascular

Phlebitis. Carefully assess patients for thrombophlebitis. Inspect the IV area frequently when providing care; visually inspect during dressing changes and whenever the IV is changed to a new site. Report redness, warmth, tenderness to touch, and edema in the affected part. If in the lower extremities, dorsiflexion of the foot may cause pain in the calf area (Homans' sign). Compare the affected limb with the unaffected limb.

▪ Drug Interactions

Alcohol. Use of alcohol and alcohol-containing preparations, such as OTC cough medications and mouthwashes (e.g., Listerine, Cēpacol), should be avoided during and up to 48 hours after discontinuation of metronidazole therapy. Metronidazole inhibits enzymes required to metabolize alcohol, resulting in mild symptoms of abdominal cramping, flushing, headache, nausea, vomiting, and sweating.

Warfarin. Metronidazole may enhance the anticoagulant effects of warfarin. Observe for the development of petechiae, ecchymoses, nosebleeds, bleeding gums, dark tarry stools, and bright red or coffee-ground emesis. Monitor the PT and INR, and reduce the dosage of warfarin if necessary.

Disulfiram. Combined use of disulfiram and metronidazole may result in mental confusion and psychoses. Concurrent therapy is not recommended.

Lithium. Patients receiving higher dosages of lithium are more susceptible to lithium toxicity and potential renal damage. Metronidazole should be initiated only if absolutely necessary. Frequently monitor serum lithium and creatinine concentrations when metronidazole and lithium are administered concurrently.

Phenytoin, Fosphenytoin. Metronidazole inhibits phenytoin metabolism. Monitor patients with concurrent therapy for signs of phenytoin toxicity: nystagmus, sedation, and lethargy. Serum levels may be ordered and the dosage of phenytoin reduced.

---

tinidazole (tĭn-Ĭ-dă-zōl)
Tindamax (TĬN-dă-măks)

ACTIONS

Tinidazole is a nitroimidazole similar to metronidazole. Its mechanism of action is unknown.

USES

Tinidazole is used to treat parasites such as trichomoniasis caused by *Trichomonas vaginalis* in female and male patients, giardiasis caused by *Giardia lamblia*, and intestinal amebiasis and amebic liver abscess caused by *Entamoeba histolytica*.

THERAPEUTIC OUTCOME

The primary therapeutic outcome expected from tinidazole therapy is elimination of parasitic infection.

❖ NURSING IMPLICATIONS FOR TINIDAZOLE

■ Premedication Assessment

1. Obtain baseline assessments of the presenting symptoms.
2. Record temperature, pulse, respirations, blood pressure, and hydration status.
3. Assess for and record any gastric symptoms, peripheral neuropathy, or seizure disorders before initiating therapy.
4. Assess for any allergies.
5. Perform a baseline assessment of the patient's degree of alertness and orientation to name, place, and time before initiating therapy.
6. Obtain baseline laboratory studies ordered and review results (e.g., CBC with differential, culture and sensitivity).

■ Availability

PO: 250- and 500-mg tablets.

■ Dosage and Administration

NOTE: Tinidazole should be administered with food to reduce the incidence of GI effects.
PO:
• Trichomoniasis: Men and women: 2 g once. Sexual partners must be treated concurrently to prevent reinfection.

• Amebic dysentery and amebic liver abscess: 2 g once daily for 3 days.
• Giardiasis: 2 g once.

■ Common Adverse Effects
Gastrointestinal
Nausea, vomiting, diarrhea. These adverse effects are usually mild and tend to resolve with continued therapy.

■ Serious Adverse Effects
Neurologic
Dizziness. Provide for patient safety during episodes of dizziness; report for further evaluation.

Confusion, seizures. Patients receiving high doses of tinidazole, those with histories of seizure activity, and those with significant hepatic impairment are at greater risk of confusion and seizures. Perform a baseline assessment of the patient's degree of alertness and orientation to name, place, and time before initiating therapy. Make regularly scheduled subsequent mental status evaluations and compare findings. Report the development of alterations. Implement seizure precautions. Make sure that the patient continues with anticonvulsant therapy. If seizures develop, provide for patient safety and then record the exact time of seizure onset and duration of each phase, a description of the specific body parts involved, and any progression in the affected parts. Describe the automatic responses seen during the clonic phase—altered, jerky respirations; frothy salivation; dilated pupils and eye movements; cyanosis; diaphoresis; or incontinence.

■ Drug Interactions
Alcohol. Use of alcohol and alcohol-containing preparations, such as OTC cough medications and mouthwashes (e.g., Listerine, Cēpacol), should be avoided during therapy and for 72 hours after discontinuation of tinidazole therapy. Tinidazole inhibits enzymes required to metabolize alcohol, resulting in mild symptoms of abdominal cramping, flushing, headache, nausea, vomiting, and sweating.

Warfarin. Tinidazole may enhance the anticoagulant effects of warfarin during and up to 8 days after taking tinidazole. Observe for the development of petechiae, ecchymoses, nosebleeds, bleeding gums, dark tarry stools, and bright red or coffee-ground emesis. Monitor the PT and INR and reduce the dosage of warfarin if necessary.

Lithium. Patients receiving higher dosages of lithium are more susceptible to lithium toxicity and potential renal damage. Tinidazole should be initiated only if absolutely necessary. Frequently monitor serum lithium and creatinine concentrations when tinidazole and lithium are administered concurrently.

Phenytoin, Fosphenytoin. Tinidazole inhibits phenytoin metabolism. Monitor patients with concurrent therapy for signs of phenytoin toxicity: nystagmus, sedation, and lethargy. Serum levels may be ordered and the dosage of phenytoin reduced.

---

vancomycin (văn-kō-MĪ-sĭn)
  ⇄ *Do not confuse vancomycin with vecuronium, Vibramycin, azithromycin, or gentamicin.*
  Vancocin (VĂN-kō-sĭn)

ACTIONS

Vancomycin is an antibiotic that prevents the synthesis of bacterial cell walls. This site of action is different from the sites sensitive to penicillin and other antibiotics interfering with cell wall synthesis.

USES

Vancomycin is effective against only gram-positive bacteria such as streptococci, staphylococci, *C. difficile, Listeria monocytogenes,* and *Corynebacterium* that may cause endocarditis, osteomyelitis, meningitis, pneumonia, or septicemia. It may be used orally against staphylococcal enterocolitis and antibiotic-associated pseudomembranous colitis produced by *C. difficile.* Because of potential adverse effects, vancomycin therapy is reserved for patients with potentially life-threatening infections who cannot be treated with less toxic agents such as penicillins or cephalosporins.

The most prominent and severe adverse effects associated with vancomycin are nephrotoxicity and ototoxicity. These occur with greater frequency and severity in patients with renal impairment or when large doses are administered. Hearing loss may be preceded by tinnitus and high-tone hearing loss and is often permanent. Older patients appear to be particularly susceptible to the ototoxic effects.

THERAPEUTIC OUTCOME

The primary therapeutic outcome expected from vancomycin therapy is elimination of bacterial infection.

❖ NURSING IMPLICATIONS FOR VANCOMYCIN

▪ Premedication Assessment
1. Obtain baseline assessments of presenting symptoms.
2. Record temperature, pulse, respirations, blood pressure, and hydration status.
3. Assess for normal renal function and hearing before initiating therapy.
4. Assess for any allergies.
5. Obtain baseline laboratory studies ordered and review results (e.g., CBC with differential, culture and sensitivity).

▪ Availability
PO: 125- and 250-mg capsules. *IV:* 0.5-, 1-, 5- and 10-g powder/vial.

▪ Dosage and Administration
Adult: PO: 500 mg to 2 g daily given in three to four divided does for 7 to 10 days. Pseudomembranous colitis produced by *C. difficile:* 125 to 500 mg every 6 hours for 10 to 14 days. *IM:* Not recommended because of poor absorption and clinical response. *IV:* 500 mg every 6 hours or 1 g every 12 hours (manufacturer); 15 to 20 mg/kg (based on actual body weight) every 8 to 12 hours in patients with normal renal function. Dosage must be adjusted for patients with impaired renal function. Check serum concentrations. *Pediatric: PO:* children: 40 mg/kg/day in three to four divided doses, not to exceed 2 g per day. *IM:* Not recommended because of poor absorption and clinical response. *IV:* Neonates: initial dose of 15 mg/kg followed by 10 mg/kg every 12 hours until 1 month of age, then every 8 hours thereafter; children: 40 mg/kg/day in divided doses every 6 hours.

Serum Levels. Serum trough levels of vancomycin should be routinely ordered to minimize adverse effects. Notify the healthcare provider of any abnormal serum levels reported so that dosage adjustments may be made. Consult laboratory reports for normal range.

⚠ Medication Safety Alert

Rapid IV administration of vancomycin may result in a severe hypotensive episode. Patients develop a red neck syndrome, or red man syndrome, characteristic of vancomycin. It is manifested by a sudden and profound hypotension, with or without a maculopapular rash over the face, neck, upper chest, and extremities. The rash generally resolves within a few hours after terminating the infusion. In rare cases, the administration of fluids, antihistamines, or corticosteroids may be necessary. Administer the solution diluted to less than 5 mg/mL over at least 60 minutes. Monitor blood pressure during infusion.

▪ Serious Adverse Effects
Sensory
Ototoxicity. This may initially be manifested by dizziness, tinnitus, and progressive hearing loss. Assess patients for difficulty in walking unaided, and assess the level of hearing daily. Intentionally speak to patients softly; note if they are aware that anything was said. Take particular notice of the patient who repeatedly asks, "What did you say?" or who starts talking more loudly or progressively increases the volume on the television or radio.
Urinary
Nephrotoxicity. Monitor urinalysis and kidney function tests for abnormal results. Report increasing BUN and creatinine levels, decreasing urine output or decreasing urine specific gravity (despite amount of fluid intake), casts or protein in the urine, frank blood or smoky-colored urine, or RBCs in excess of 0 to 3 RBCs/HPF (see Table 41-1) on the urinalysis report.
Immune System (Opportunistic Infections)
Secondary infections. Oral thrush, genital and anal pruritus, vaginitis, and vaginal discharge may occur.

Report promptly because these infections are resistant to the original antibiotic used. Teach the importance of meticulous oral and perineal personal hygiene.

■ Drug Interactions

Nephrotoxicity, Ototoxicity. Concurrent and sequential use of other ototoxic or nephrotoxic agents such as neomycin, streptomycin, kanamycin, gentamicin, paromomycin, polymyxin B, colistin, tobramycin, amikacin, cisplatin, furosemide, torsemide, and bumetanide requires careful monitoring.

Neuromuscular Blockade. Taking vancomycin in combination with skeletal muscle relaxants may produce respiratory depression.

Check the anesthesia record in postoperative patients to determine if skeletal muscle relaxants such as succinylcholine or pancuronium bromide were administered during surgery. The nurse should monitor and assess the respiratory rate, depth of respirations, and chest movement, and report apnea immediately. Because these effects may be seen for up to 48 hours after administration of skeletal muscle relaxants, continue monitoring respirations, pulse, and blood pressure beyond the usual postsurgical vital signs routine.

DRUG CLASS: TOPICAL ANTIFUNGAL AGENTS

ACTIONS

The exact mechanisms whereby antifungal agents act are unknown. However, it is known that cell membranes are altered, resulting in increased permeability, leakage of amino acids and electrolytes, and impaired uptake of essential nutrients needed for cell growth.

USES

The common topical fungal infections caused by several different dermatophytes are tinea pedis (athlete's foot), tinea cruris (jock itch), tinea corporis (ringworm), and tinea versicolor. *Candida albicans* is the most common cause of oral candidiasis (thrush), cutaneous candidiasis (e.g., diaper rash), and vaginal candidiasis (moniliasis [yeast infection]).

THERAPEUTIC OUTCOME

The primary therapeutic outcome expected from topical antifungal therapy is elimination of fungal infection.

❖ NURSING IMPLICATIONS FOR TOPICAL ANTIFUNGALS

■ Premedication Assessment

1. Obtain baseline assessments of presenting symptoms.
2. Assess for any allergies.

■ Availability, Dosage, and Administration

See Table 45-9.

Topical. Apply clean gloves. Wash hands thoroughly before and immediately after application. Cleanse skin with soap and water and dry thoroughly.

For athlete's foot, the powder is most effective in intertriginous areas and in patients for whom a dry environment may enhance the therapeutic response.

Table 45-9   Topical Antifungal Agents

GENERIC NAME	BRAND NAME	AVAILABILITY	ADULT DOSAGE RANGE
butenafine	Lotrimin Ultra, Mentax	Cream: 1%	For ringworm, jock itch, athlete's foot: Apply topically to affected area one or two times daily for 1-4 wk
butoconazole	Gynazole-1	Vaginal cream: 2%	For vaginal candidiasis: Gynazole-1: One applicatorful intravaginally at bedtime once.
ciclopirox	Loprox	Gel: 0.77% Shampoo: 1% Solution for nails: 8% Topical suspension: 0.77%	For ringworm, jock itch, athlete's foot, cutaneous candidiasis, and tinea versicolor: Massage product into affected skin twice daily for at least 4 wk; shampoo: twice weekly for 4 wk
clotrimazole	Gyne-Lotrimin-3 Desenex Lotrimin AF	Vaginal cream: 2% Cream: 1% Solution: 1% Oral lozenges: 10 mg (troches)	For vaginal candidiasis: Cream: one applicatorful at bedtime for 3-7 nights For ringworm, jock itch, athlete's foot: Apply topically to affected skin morning and evening; gently rub in For oral candidiasis: Allow one lozenge to dissolve slowly in mouth five times daily for 14 consecutive days
econazole	—	Cream: 1%	For ringworm, jock itch, athlete's foot, tinea versicolor: Apply over affected area once daily For cutaneous candidiasis: Apply twice daily (morning and evening)

Continued

Table 45-9 **Topical Antifungal Agents—cont'd**

GENERIC NAME	BRAND NAME	AVAILABILITY	ADULT DOSAGE RANGE
efinaconazole	Jublia	Solution: 10%	For fungal infections of the toes: Apply to affected toe nails one time daily for 48 wk.
ketoconazole	Nizoral	Cream: 2% Foam: 2% Gel: 2% Shampoo: 1%, 2%	For ringworm, jock itch, athlete's foot, cutaneous candidiasis, and tinea versicolor: Massage in cream to affected and surrounding tissue once daily; may require 2-4 wk of treatment For seborrheic dermatitis: Cream and foam: Massage in to affected area twice daily for 4 wk Gel: Massage in to affected area once daily for 2 wk For dandruff: Moisten hair and scalp with water; apply shampoo and lather gently for 1 min; rinse and reapply, leaving lather on scalp for 3 min; rinse thoroughly and dry hair; apply shampoo twice weekly for 4 wk with at least 3 days between shampooing
luliconazole	Luzu	Cream, external 1%	For jock itch or truncal lesions, apply once daily for 1 wk. For athlete's foot: apply once daily for 2 wk.
miconazole	Monistat 3 Monistat 7 Micatin	Vaginal suppositories: 200 mg Vaginal cream: 2% Vaginal suppositories: 100 mg Vaginal cream: 1% Cream: 2% Powder: 2% Spray: 2% Ointment: 2%	For vaginal candidiasis: Monistat 3: Insert one suppository intravaginally at bedtime for 3 days Monistat 7: Insert one applicatorful or one suppository at bedtime for 3-7 days For ringworm, jock itch, athlete's foot, cutaneous candidiasis, and tinea versicolor: Cover affected areas twice daily (morning and evening); treatment may require 2-4 wk
naftifine	Naftin	Cream: 1% Gel: 1%	For ringworm, jock itch, athlete's foot: Cream: massage into affected area once daily. Gel: massage into affected area twice daily
nystatin	—	Vaginal tablets: 100,000 units Oral suspension: 100,000 units/mL Oral tablets: 500,000 units Cream, ointment, powder	For vaginal candidiasis: One tablet intravaginally daily for 2 wk For oral candidiasis: 4-6 mL four times daily; retain in mouth as long as possible before swallowing 1 or 2 tablets four or five times daily; do not chew or swallow For cutaneous candidiasis: Apply to affected area two or three times daily
oxiconazole nitrate	Oxistat	Cream: 1% Lotion: 1%	For ringworm, jock itch, athlete's foot: Massage into affected areas once daily at bedtime
sertaconazole	Ertaczo	Cream: 2%	For athlete's foot: Apply twice daily for 4 wk
sulconazole	Exelderm	Cream: 1% Solution: 1%	For ringworm, jock itch, athlete's foot: Massage into affected area twice daily
terbinafine	Lamisil AT	Cream: 1% Spray: 1% Gel: 1% Solution: 1%	Massage into affected area twice daily; treatment may require 2-4 wk
terconazole	Terazol 7 Terazol 3	Vaginal cream: 0.4% Vaginal cream: 0.8% Vaginal suppository: 80 mg	For vaginal candidiasis: Insert one applicatorful intravaginally daily at bedtime for 3 (Terazol 3) or 7 (Terazol 7) consecutive days Insert one suppository intravaginally once daily at bedtime for 3 consecutive days
tioconazole	Vagistat-1 Monistat-1	Vaginal ointment: 6.5%	For vaginal candidiasis: Insert one applicatorful intravaginally at bedtime once
tolnaftate	Tinactin	Cream: 1% Solution: 1% Gel: 1% Spray: 1% Powder: 1%	For ringworm, jock itch, athlete's foot, cutaneous candidiasis, and tinea versicolor: Cover affected areas twice daily (morning and evening); treatment may require 2-4 wk

Instruct patients to wear cotton socks (avoid nylon) if possible, and change them two or three times daily. Treatments may be required for 6 weeks or longer with long-standing infections and in areas of thickened skin.

For jock itch or ringworm, wear well-fitting, non-constrictive, ventilated clothing.

For all fungal infections, instruct patients to avoid tight-fitting clothing and occlusive dressings unless otherwise instructed by the healthcare provider.

Eye Contact. Instruct patients to avoid contact with the eyes and to wash their eyes immediately if contact occurs.

Intravaginal. Give the patient the following instructions:
1. Wash the applicator in warm soapy water after each use so that it does not become a vehicle for reinfection.
2. Consider using a pad to protect clothing.
3. Use the number of doses prescribed even if symptoms disappear or menstruation begins.
4. Refrain from sexual intercourse during therapy (or the male should wear a condom to avoid reinfection).
5. When being treated with vaginal ointment (e.g., Vagistat), use contraception other than a diaphragm or condom. Prolonged contact with petrolatum-based products may cause the diaphragm and condom to deteriorate.

■ **Common and Serious Adverse Effects**
Integumentary

Irritation. Some patients experience vulvar or vaginal burning, vulvar itching, discharge, soreness, or swelling from the intravaginal products. These adverse effects are usually mild and tend to resolve with continued therapy. Encourage the patient not to discontinue therapy without first consulting the healthcare provider.

Redness, swelling, blistering, oozing. These signs may be an indication of hypersensitivity. Inform the healthcare provider.

■ **Drug Interactions**
No clinically significant drug interactions have been reported.

DRUG CLASS: SYSTEMIC ANTIFUNGAL AGENTS

amphotericin B (ăm-fō-TĒR-ĭ-sĭn), **amphotericin B sodium desoxycholate ("conventional")**
   amphotericin B cholesteryl sulfate complex
   Amphotec
   amphotericin B lipid complex
   Abelcet
   amphotericin B liposome
   AmBisome

ACTIONS
Amphotericin B is a fungistatic agent that disrupts the cell membrane of fungal cells, resulting in a loss of cellular contents.

USES
Amphotericin B is used primarily in treating systemic life-threatening fungal infections. It should not be used to treat noninvasive fungal infections such as oral thrush, vaginal candidiasis, and esophageal candidiasis in immunocompetent patients with normal neutrophil counts. There are four dosage forms of amphotericin B, each with different brand names and somewhat different approval for use. Each has different requirements for reconstitution, dilution, filtration, and administration rate. Work closely with the pharmacy department to ensure that the correct dosage form is being reconstituted and diluted properly, and that proper administration technique, including the use of appropriate inline filters and rate of infusion, is being used.

THERAPEUTIC OUTCOME
The primary therapeutic outcome expected from amphotericin B therapy is elimination of fungal infection.

❖ **NURSING IMPLICATIONS FOR AMPHOTERICIN B**
■ **Premedication Assessment**
1. Obtain baseline assessments of presenting symptoms.
2. Record temperature, pulse, respirations, blood pressure, and hydration status.
3. Assess for normal renal function and normal electrolytes before initiating therapy.
4. Assess for any allergies.
5. Gather baseline data about the patient's mental status (e.g., alertness, orientation, confusion), muscle strength, presence of muscle cramps, tremors, nausea, and general appearance (e.g., drowsy, anxious, lethargic).
6. Obtain baseline laboratory studies ordered and review results (e.g., CBC with differential, culture and sensitivity).

■ **Availability**
IV:
• Amphotericin B sodium desoxycholate ("conventional" amphotericin B): 50 mg/vial
• Amphotericin B cholesteryl sulfate complex (Amphotec): 50 and 100 mg/vial
• Amphotericin B lipid complex (Abelcet): 5 mg/mL in 100-mg concentrate
• Amphotericin B liposome (AmBisome): 50 mg/vial

■ **Dosage and Administration**
Dosage varies depending on the dosage form and the organism for which the medicine is being used. Consult

the healthcare provider, laboratory results, and the pharmacist to provide checks on the appropriate dose and administration of the antifungal agent.

■ Common and Serious Adverse Effects

General

Malaise, fever, chills, headache, nausea, vomiting. These adverse effects tend to be dose related and may be minimized by slow infusion, reduction of dosage, and alternate-day administration. Check PRN and standing orders for drugs (e.g., antihistamines, aspirin, antiemetics) that may alleviate these symptoms.

Urinary

Nephrotoxicity. Nephrotoxicity may be manifested by increases in excretion of uric acid, potassium, and magnesium; oliguria; granular casts in the urine; proteinuria; and increased BUN and serum creatinine levels.

Monitor urinalysis and kidney function tests for abnormal results. Report increasing BUN and creatinine levels, decreasing urine output or decreasing urine specific gravity (despite amount of fluid intake), casts or protein in the urine, frank blood or smoky-colored urine, or RBCs in excess of 0 to 3 RBCs/HPF (see Table 41-1) on the urinalysis report. Report input and output, as well as a progressive decrease in daily urine volume or changes in visual characteristics.

Hematologic

Electrolyte imbalance. The electrolytes most commonly altered are potassium (K^+) and magnesium (Mg^{2+}). Hypokalemia is most likely to occur. Many symptoms associated with altered fluid and electrolyte balance are subtle and resemble general symptoms of drug toxicity or the disease process itself. Gather data about changes in the patient's mental status (e.g., alertness, orientation, confusion), muscle strength, muscle cramps, tremors, nausea, and general appearance (e.g., drowsy, anxious, lethargic). Always check the electrolyte reports for early indications of electrolyte imbalance. Keep accurate records of input and output, daily weights, and vital signs.

Vascular

Thrombophlebitis. Carefully assess patients receiving IV amphotericin B for the development of thrombophlebitis. Inspect the IV area often when providing care; inspect during dressing changes and whenever the IV is changed to a new site. Always investigate pain at the IV site. Report redness, warmth, tenderness to touch, and edema in the affected part. If in the lower extremities, dorsiflexion of the foot may cause pain in the calf (Homans' sign). Compare the affected limb with the unaffected one.

■ Drug Interactions

Corticosteroids (e.g., Prednisone). The concurrent use of amphotericin B and corticosteroids may enhance the loss of potassium. Check potassium levels and monitor more closely for hypokalemia.

Nephrotoxic Potential. Combining amphotericin B with other nephrotoxic agents such as aminoglycosides, diuretics, or cisplatin should be done with extreme caution. Monitor closely for signs of nephrotoxicity.

Digoxin. Because amphotericin B may induce hypokalemia, use cautiously in patients receiving digoxin. Hypokalemia may induce digoxin toxicity. Monitor patients for dysrhythmias, nausea, and bradycardia.

Diuretics. Thiazide and loop diuretics may induce hypokalemia. Monitor patients receiving amphotericin B and diuretic therapy very closely for hypokalemia.

---

fluconazole (flū-KŎN-ă-zōl)
  Diflucan (DĪ-flū-kăn)
  ⇄ *Do not confuse Diflucan with Dilantin or Diprivan.*

ACTIONS

Fluconazole is an antifungal agent chemically related to ketoconazole and itraconazole. It acts by inhibiting certain metabolic pathways in fungi, thus interfering with cell wall synthesis.

USES

Fluconazole is used for oral and IV treatment of cryptococcal meningitis and oropharyngeal, esophageal, vulvovaginal, or systemic candidiasis. Fluconazole therapy is usually reserved for patients in whom other antifungal therapy was not tolerated or was ineffective. Fluconazole is also used prophylactically to prevent candidiasis in bone marrow transplant patients who are receiving radiation or chemotherapy treatment and in patients with human immunodeficiency virus (HIV) infection. Fluconazole is also approved as a single-dose treatment of vaginal candidiasis in immunocompetent patients.

THERAPEUTIC OUTCOMES

The primary therapeutic outcomes expected from fluconazole therapy are as follows:
1. Prevention of systemic fungal infections
2. Elimination of fungal infection

❖ NURSING IMPLICATIONS FOR FLUCONAZOLE

■ Premedication Assessment

1. Obtain baseline assessments of presenting symptoms.
2. Record temperature, pulse, respirations, blood pressure, and hydration status.
3. Assess for and record any gastric symptoms and abnormal liver and renal function before initiating therapy.
4. Assess for any allergies.
5. Obtain baseline laboratory studies ordered and review results (e.g., CBC with differential, culture and sensitivity).

■ **Availability**

PO: 50-, 100-, 150-, and 200-mg tablets; 10 and 40 mg/mL in 35-mL bottle. *IV:* 100-, 200- and 400-mg vials.

■ **Dosage and Administration**

PO: 100 to 400 mg daily; dosage must be individualized to type of infection being treated. *IV:* same as for PO.

■ **Common Adverse Effects**

Gastrointestinal

Nausea, vomiting, diarrhea. These adverse effects are usually mild and tend to resolve with continued therapy. Encourage the patient not to discontinue therapy without first consulting his or her healthcare provider.

■ **Serious Adverse Effects**

Integumentary

Rash. Report symptoms for further evaluation by the healthcare provider. Do not administer any further doses until so ordered by the healthcare provider.

Gastrointestinal

Hepatotoxicity. The symptoms of hepatotoxicity are anorexia, nausea, vomiting, jaundice, hepatomegaly, splenomegaly, and abnormal liver function test results (e.g., elevated bilirubin, AST, ALT, GGT, alkaline phosphatase levels, increased PT).

■ **Drug Interactions**

Cimetidine. Cimetidine inhibits the absorption of fluconazole. Concurrent use is not recommended.

Diuretics. Diuretics inhibit the excretion of fluconazole. Monitor patients for an increase in frequency of adverse effects. The dosage of fluconazole may need to be decreased if concurrent therapy with diuretics is required.

Toxicity Induced by Fluconazole. Fluconazole can increase serum concentrations of alfentanil, benzodiazepines, buspirone, cyclosporine, losartan, phenytoin, vincristine, zidovudine, zolpidem, tricyclic antidepressants (TCAs), HMG-CoA reductase inhibitors (e.g., simvastatin, atorvastatin), protease inhibitors (e.g., ritonavir, indinavir), and oral sulfonylurea hypoglycemic agents (e.g., tolbutamide, glipizide, and glyburide). Fluconazole can also potentiate the anticoagulant effects of warfarin. Read individual drug monographs for monitoring parameters of toxicity from these agents.

flucytosine (flū-SĪ-tō-sēn)
  ⇄ *Do not confuse flucytosine with fluorouracil.*
  Ancobon (ĂN-kō-bŏn)

ACTIONS

Flucytosine is an antifungal agent. Its mechanism of action is thought to be inhibition of RNA and protein synthesis.

USES

Flucytosine is effective against susceptible candidal septicemia, endocarditis, UTIs, cryptococcal meningitis, and pulmonary infections.

THERAPEUTIC OUTCOME

The primary therapeutic outcome expected from flucytosine therapy is elimination of fungal infection.

❖ **NURSING IMPLICATIONS FOR FLUCYTOSINE**

■ **Premedication Assessment**

1. Obtain baseline assessments of presenting symptoms.
2. Record temperature, pulse, respirations, blood pressure, and hydration status.
3. Assess for and record any gastric symptoms or abnormal liver or renal function before initiating therapy.
4. Assess for any allergies.
5. Record baseline mental status assessment data.
6. Obtain baseline laboratory studies ordered and review results (e.g., CBC with differential, culture and sensitivity).

■ **Availability**

PO: 250- and 500-mg capsules.

■ **Dosage and Administration**

Adult: PO: 50 to 150 mg/kg/day divided into doses every 6 hours. Nausea may be reduced if the capsules are given a few at a time over 20 to 30 minutes.

■ **Common Adverse Effects**

Gastrointestinal

Nausea, vomiting, diarrhea. These adverse effects are usually mild and tend to resolve with continued therapy. Encourage the patient not to discontinue therapy without first consulting the healthcare provider. Adverse effects may be reduced by administering a few capsules at a time over 30 minutes.

■ **Serious Adverse Effects**

Hypersensitivity. Monitor the patient for sore throat, fever, purpura, jaundice, or excessive and progressive weakness.

Renal

Nephrotoxicity. Monitor the patient's urinalysis and kidney function tests for abnormal results. Report an increasing BUN and creatinine, decreasing urine output or decreasing urine specific gravity (despite amount of fluid intake), casts or protein in the urine, frank blood or smoky-colored urine, or RBCs in excess of 0 to 3 RBCs/HPF (see Table 41-1) on the urinalysis report.

Gastrointestinal

Hepatotoxicity. The symptoms of hepatotoxicity are anorexia, nausea, vomiting, jaundice, hepatomegaly, splenomegaly, and abnormal liver function test results (e.g., elevated bilirubin, AST, ALT, GGT, alkaline phosphatase levels, increased PT).

▪ Drug Interactions

Amphotericin B. Flucytosine and amphotericin B display enhanced activity when used concurrently.

---

griseofulvin microsize (grĭz-ē-ō-FŬL-vĭn)
   Grifulvin V (grĭ-FŬL-vĭn)
   griseofulvin ultramicrosize
   Gris-PEG

ACTIONS

Griseofulvin is a fungistatic agent that acts by stopping cell division and new cell growth.

USES

Griseofulvin is used to treat ringworm of the scalp, body, nails, and feet. After griseofulvin is absorbed, it is incorporated into the keratin of the nails, skin, and hair in therapeutic amounts. The infecting fungus is not killed, but its growth into new cells is prevented. Once the cells are shed or removed, they are replaced by new cells that are free from the infection. Because of slow nail growth, treatment is often required for several months.

THERAPEUTIC OUTCOME

The primary therapeutic outcome expected from griseofulvin therapy is elimination of fungal infection.

❖ NURSING IMPLICATIONS FOR GRISEOFULVIN

▪ Premedication Assessment

1. Obtain baseline assessments of presenting symptoms.
2. Record temperature, pulse, respirations, blood pressure, and hydration status.
3. Assess for and record any gastric symptoms or abnormal hematologic, liver, or renal function tests before initiating therapy.
4. Assess for any allergies.
5. Obtain baseline laboratory studies ordered (e.g., CBC with differential, culture and sensitivity, liver and renal function tests).
6. Record results of baseline mental status examination.

▪ Availability

PO: Microsize (Grifulvin V) 500-mg tablets; 125-mg/5 mL oral suspension.
Ultramicrosize (Gris-PEG) 125- and 250-mg tablets.

▪ Dosage and Administration

Adult: PO: Microsize: depending on the specific organism and the location of the infection, 500 mg to 1 g in single or divided doses daily. Absorption from the GI tract may be increased by administering griseofulvin with a high-fat meal.
Adult: PO: Ultramicrosize: depending on the specific organism and the location of the infection, 350 to 750 mg daily in divided doses. Absorption from the GI tract may be increased by administering griseofulvin with a high-fat meal.

▪ Common Adverse Effects

Gastrointestinal

Nausea, vomiting, anorexia, abdominal cramps. These adverse effects are usually mild and tend to resolve with continued therapy. Encourage the patient not to discontinue therapy without first consulting the healthcare provider.

▪ Serious Adverse Effects

Integumentary, Hypersensitivity

Urticaria, rash, pruritus. Hypersensitivity reactions, manifested by itching, urticaria, and rash, are relatively common. Report symptoms for further evaluation by the healthcare provider. Pruritus may be relieved by adding baking soda to the bath water.

Photosensitivity. The patient should be cautioned to avoid exposure to sunlight and ultraviolet light. Suggest wearing long-sleeved clothing, hat, and sunglasses when outdoors. Discourage the use of tanning lamps. Notify the healthcare provider for the advisability of continuing therapy.

Neurologic

Confusion. Perform a baseline assessment of the patient's degree of alertness and orientation to name, place, and time before initiating therapy. Make regularly scheduled subsequent mental status evaluations, and compare findings. Report the development of alterations.

Dizziness. Provide for patient safety during episodes of dizziness; report for further evaluation.

Immune System (Opportunistic Infections)

Secondary infections. With griseofulvin, oral thrush, genital and anal pruritus, vaginitis, and vaginal discharge may occur. Report promptly because these infections are resistant to the original antimicrobial agent. Teach the importance of meticulous oral and perineal personal hygiene.

Hematologic. Routine laboratory studies (e.g., RBC, WBC, differential counts) are scheduled for patients taking griseofulvin for 30 days or longer. Stress the importance of returning for this laboratory work. Monitor for sore throat, fever, purpura, jaundice, or excessive and progressive weakness.

Renal

Nephrotoxicity. Monitor urinalysis and kidney function tests for abnormal results. Report increasing BUN and creatinine levels, decreasing urine output or decreasing urine specific gravity (despite amount of fluid intake), casts or protein in the urine, frank blood status, edema, dyspnea, crackles and rhonchi, tachycardia, and bounding pulses. Dehydration may be noted by loss of skin turgor, sticky oral mucous membranes, a shrunken or deeply furrowed tongue, crusted lips, weight loss, deteriorating vital signs, soft or sunken eyeballs, weak pedal pulses, delayed capillary refill, excessive thirst, and mental confusion.

Electrolyte imbalances. Check for indications of electrolyte imbalance (e.g., mental status [alertness, orientation, confusion], muscle strength, muscle cramps, tremors, nausea, decline in general appearance). Check laboratory values and report abnormal values to healthcare provider.

Vitamin deficiencies. Fat-soluble vitamins (A, D, E, K):
- *Vitamin A:* Diarrhea; dry, scaly, rough, cracked skin; alterations in adaptation to light and dark
- *Vitamin D:* Involuntary spasms and twitching, decreased calcium and phosphorus, demineralization of bones
- *Vitamin E:* Hemolysis of red blood cells; in older children, neurologic syndrome of vitamin E deficiency
- *Vitamin K:* Symptoms of bleeding and/or delayed clotting

Deficiencies of water-soluble vitamins (cyanocobalamin, folic acid, niacin, pyridoxine, riboflavin, thiamine, and vitamin C):
- *Cyanocobalamin:* Anorexia, ataxia, diarrhea, constipation, irritability, paresthesia, delirium, hallucinations
- *Folic acid:* Diarrhea, glossitis, macrocytic anemia, low serum levels

- *Niacin:* Glossitis, diarrhea, rashes, weakness, anorexia, indigestion; as deficiency progresses, central nervous system involvement is manifested by confusion, disorientation, neuritis
- *Pyridoxine:* Anemia, dyspnea, cheilosis, glossitis, convulsions
- *Riboflavin:* Cheilosis, glossitis, seborrheic dermatitis, photophobia, poor wound healing
- *Thiamine:* Anorexia, constipation, indigestion, confusion, edema, muscle weakness, cardiomegaly, heart failure
- *Vitamin C:* Anemia, petechiae, depression, delayed wound healing

Gastrointestinal

Hepatotoxicity. Fatty liver may develop. Check liver function tests (elevated bilirubin, aspartate aminotransferase [AST], alanine aminotransferase [ALT], gamma-glutamyltransferase [GGT], alkaline phosphatase levels, increased prothrombin time) and report abnormal laboratory values to the healthcare provider.

Hypersensitivity, Immune System

Rash, chills, fever, respiratory difficulty. These signs are an indication of allergy to formula. Provide emergency care, as needed. Immediately discontinue feedings and await further healthcare provider's orders.

■ Drug Interactions

No other drugs should be administered concurrently with TPN. Consult a pharmacist for parenteral nutrition solutions and compatibility with specific medicines.

Get Ready for the NCLEX® Examination!

Key Points

- Energy sources required for balanced metabolism are the macronutrients—fats, carbohydrates, and proteins. Other essential nutrients include vitamins, minerals, fiber, and water. Nutritional requirements vary based not only on the age of the individual, but also on the gender and level of activity.
- No one food source can meet all of the basic nutritional requirements. Healthful diets provide a balance of carbohydrates, fiber, fat, protein, and essential nutrients to reduce the risks of chronic diseases and support a full and productive lifestyle. Healthful nutrition must be accompanied by regular mild-to-moderate physical activity to help maintain muscle tone and agility.
- Nutrition plays a vital role in helping a patient recover from illness. Adequate intake of nutrients is critical to restoring normal homeostasis and rebuilding damaged tissue. If nutritional needs are not adequately addressed, malnutrition results. Malnutrition is a major source of morbidity and mortality in patients who are suffering from disease because they are much more susceptible to infections and organ failure than are healthy individuals.

- During illness, patients may require partial or full supplementation of their nutritional needs. One of two forms of supplementation is often used. Enteral nutrition is administered orally, either by the patient drinking the liquid or by administration into the GI tract by a feeding tube. Administration of nutrients directly into veins is known as *parenteral nutrition*.
- Nurses need to understand the importance of cultural beliefs whenever special diets are prescribed. Because the nurse may not have knowledge of the cultural aspects of dietary adaptations, it is essential to involve a nutritionist in the dietary planning process.

Additional Learning Resources

SG Go to your Study Guide for additional Review Questions for the NCLEX® Examination, Critical Thinking Clinical Situations, and other learning activities to help you master this chapter content.

evolve Go to your Evolve website (http://evolve.elsevier.com/Clayton) for additional online resources.

Review Questions for the NCLEX® Examination

1. The nurse asked the patient to pick out good food sources of dietary fiber from the menu. Which selection indicates adequate patient understanding?
   1. Lettuce salad with dressing
   2. Potatoes, pasta, and white bread
   3. Cereal brans, sweet potatoes, vegetables, and fruits
   4. Beef, chicken, fish, and tofu

2. After discussing sources of dietary fats that have health benefits with the patient, the nurse expects that the patient will identify these sources. *(Select all that apply.)*
   1. Whole milk
   2. Olive oil
   3. Coconut oil
   4. Ice cream
   5. Avocados

3. A patient who has a diet high in fruits and vegetables is getting plenty of:
   1. vitamin E.
   2. vitamin A.
   3. vitamin C.
   4. vitamin B.

4. A patient who had been instructed by the physician to increase the amount of calcium in her diet asked the nurse what would be recommended. The nurse responded with:
   1. "Cook with ginger and cloves, and eat more whole grains."
   2. "Be sure to eat more chicken, beans, and green leafy vegetables."
   3. "I think that you can have more oysters and liver, as well as oatmeal."
   4. "Milk, cheese, and vegetables should be part of your diet."

5. The nurse was assessing the patient's nutritional status and became concerned about these findings that point to possible malnutrition. *(Select all that apply.)*
   1. Reports of increased physical activity
   2. Dry, dull hair that falls out easily
   3. Generalized weakness and lethargy
   4. Recent intended weight loss
   5. Laboratory tests that indicate hypoalbuminemia

6. This assessment finding that the nurse discovered during a gastrostomy feeding requires the prescriber to be notified:
   1. a gastric residual of 120 mL after the tube feeding was held for 1 hour.
   2. the tube-feeding formula was kept at room temperature in a cabinet.
   3. the patient's abdomen was soft and nausea was absent.
   4. the feeding tube was kinked and only half of the formula was administered during that hour.

7. The nurse reviewing an order for PPN notifies the healthcare provider after checking the formula and finding the dextrose amount to be:
   1. 10%.
   2. 15%.
   3. 7%.
   4. 5%.

Herbal and Dietary Supplement Therapy

Objectives

1. Summarize the primary actions and potential uses of the herbal and dietary supplement products cited.

2. Describe the interactions between commonly used herbal and dietary supplement products and prescription medications.

Key Terms

dietary supplements (DĪ-ĕ-tār-ē SŬP-lĕ-mĕnts) (p. 755)
herbal medicines (ĔR-băl MĔD-ĭ-sĭnz) (p. 757)
botanicals (bō-TĂN-ĭ-kălz) (p. 758)

phytomedicine (fĭ-tō-MĔD-ĭ-sĭn) (p. 758)
phytotherapy (fĭ-tō-THĔR-ă-pē) (p. 758)

HERBAL MEDICINES, DIETARY SUPPLEMENTS, AND RATIONAL THERAPY

Over the past two decades, there has been a tremendous resurgence in the popularity of self-care and alternative therapies, including acupuncture, aromatherapy, homeopathy, vitamin and other supplement therapy, and herbal medicine. When herbal preparations are labeled "all natural," these products become attractive to the general public because the general perception is that "all natural" is synonymous with "better" and not harmful.

There also has been a greater emphasis on health, wellness, and disease prevention, which contributes to the perception that herbal preparations are harmless. Some of the more than 250 herbal medicines and hundreds of combinations of other supplements may be beneficial, but unfortunately the whole field of complementary medicine is fraught with false claims, lack of standardization, and adulteration and misbranding of products.

REGULATORY LEGISLATION

In the early 1990s, the U.S. Food and Drug Administration (FDA) threatened to ban from the U.S. market herbal medicines and other types of supplements that were being touted as good for health until appropriate scientific studies were completed to prove that these products were safe and effective. Such an uproar was created by this threat that Congress passed the Dietary Supplement Health and Education Act of 1994. Under this act, almost all herbal medicines, vitamins, minerals, amino acids, and other supplemental chemicals used for health were reclassified legally as dietary supplements, a food category. The legislation also allows manufacturers to include information on the label and through advertisements about how these products affect the human body. These labels and advertisements also must contain a statement that the product has not yet been evaluated by the FDA for treating, curing, or preventing any disease. The law does not prevent other people (e.g., nutritionists, health food store clerks, herbalists, strength coaches, or other unlicensed individuals) from making claims (founded or unfounded) about the therapeutic effects of supplement ingredients.

The result of the new law is that dietary supplements are not required to be safe and effective, and unfounded claims of therapeutic benefit abound. Hundreds of herbal medicines and other dietary supplements are marketed in the United States as single- and multiple-ingredient products for an extremely wide variety of uses, all implying that they will improve one's health.

INDEPENDENT PRODUCT TESTING

The vast majority of the popular claims made for herbal medicines and dietary supplements are unproven. The FDA issued good manufacturing practices, which became mandatory for the dietary supplement industry as of June 2010 (www.fda.gov/Drugs/DevelopmentApprovalProcess/Manufacturing/ucm090016.htm).

Since 1999, ConsumerLab.com has been testing dietary supplements, and the U.S. Pharmacopeia (USP) launched the Dietary Supplement Verification Program

A   B   C

FIGURE 47-1 The certification marks signify that the dietary supplements to which their mark is affixed contain ingredients as listed on the label and that they were manufactured using good manufacturing practices, but they do not certify whether the products are safe and effective for the labeled use. (**A,** Used with permission from ConsumerLab.com; **B,** used with permission from NSF International; **C,** used with permission from the USP.)

in 2001 and began testing products that year. U.S. Pharmacopeia is a scientific nonprofit organization that establishes federally recognized standards for the quality of drugs and dietary supplements. It is the only such organization that also offers voluntary verification services to help ensure dietary supplement quality, purity, and potency. U.S. Pharmacopeia is the only nonprofit standards-setting organization recognized in U.S. federal law that also offers verification services. Its standards for prescription drugs and over-the-counter (OTC) medicines are FDA enforceable per the Federal Food, Drug, and Cosmetic Act. In 2003 the National Sanitation Foundation International began testing dietary supplements. Products that pass testing are eligible to bear the mark of approval from the testing agency (Figure 47-1).

It is important to remember that the products are tested for labeled potency, good manufacturing practices, and lack of contamination, but they are not tested for safety and efficacy or for manufacturer's claims on the label. Dietary supplement therapy, under current legal standards, creates an ethical dilemma for nurses and other healthcare professionals. Licensed healthcare professionals have a moral and ethical responsibility to recommend only medicines that are proven to be safe and effective. They should be aware of a medicine's legal use versus its popular use, its potential for toxicity, and its potential for interactions with other medicines. Box 47-1 lists the factors to consider when discussing dietary supplements.

Studies have shown that 40% to 78% of patients fail to disclose the use of complementary and herbal therapy to their healthcare provider, resulting in a lack of guidance for these products (Chong, 2006).

It is important for the nurse to inquire about the use of these products when obtaining a history from the patient. The nurse can direct the patient and family toward reliable web resources, such as the National Institutes of Health website, which provide sound scientific data on supplements.

❖ NURSING IMPLICATIONS FOR HERBAL AND DIETARY SUPPLEMENT THERAPY

▪ Assessment

- Discuss specific dietary supplement products and the patient's reasons for using these products.
- Obtain a list of the specific symptoms that the patient is treating with the supplement products and details of whether the symptoms have improved (or worsened) since beginning therapy. Ask whether the patient has informed his or her healthcare provider of this use of supplement products.
- Did anyone in particular recommend herbal products? If yes, what was the basis of the recommendations?
- Obtain a detailed list of all prescribed, OTC, and supplemental products in use. Have any prescribed medications been discontinued in lieu of initiating supplements?
- What cultural or ethnic beliefs does the individual espouse?

History of Symptoms. Examine data to determine the individual's understanding of the symptoms or the disease process for which the individual began taking supplements.

Medication History

- Check the history and physical assessment by the healthcare provider to determine whether any supplement products are listed.
- Research supplements being taken and identify drug interactions, actions, and adverse effects that may occur.
- Check the hospital policy regarding the administration and recording of the products. Because they are not medications, but rather are classified legally

Box **47-1**	Factors to Consider When Recommending Herbal Medicines and Other Dietary Supplements

1. Dietary supplements are not miraculous cure-alls. Most of those intended for therapeutic use are technically unapproved drugs. They may have been used for centuries, but substantial data on safety and efficacy of long-term use are often lacking.
2. Prospective consumers may be seriously misinformed about the value of certain dietary supplements as a result of false advertising and unsubstantiated claims made by advocacy literature.
3. Dietary supplements are generally mild medications and should not be endorsed for the treatment of HIV infection, cancer, self-diagnosed heart disease, or other serious conditions.
4. Quality control of dietary supplements is often deficient in the United States. Purchase them only from the most reliable producers. Purchase standardized products when possible.
5. Do not recommend dietary supplement use for pregnant women, lactating mothers, infants, or young children without approval from the patient's healthcare provider.
6. Advise patients to cease taking a dietary supplement immediately if adverse effects (e.g., allergy, stomach upset, skin rashes, headache) occur.
7. Products containing many different ingredients, such as herbs, should be carefully examined to determine whether the ingredients are present in therapeutic amounts. Some contain only a few milligrams of each ingredient in quantities insufficient for any beneficial effect.
8. Be cautious in recommending any product that does not indicate, or permit calculation of, the quantity of individual ingredients contained in it.
9. The labels of dietary supplement products should also show the scientific name of the ingredients, the name and address of the actual manufacturer, a batch or lot number, the date of manufacture, and the expiration date.
10. Do not confuse herbal medicine, which uses therapeutic doses of drugs of botanical origin, with homeopathy, which uses products containing few or no active ingredients.

Adapted from Tyler VE: What pharmacists should know about herbal remedies, *J Am Pharm Assoc* NS36(1):29, 1996.

as dietary supplements, a food category, how are the orders for their use handled? Are they self-administered? If so, how often and in what quantity?

Cultural and Ethnic Beliefs. If cultural issues are involved in the use of the supplement products, research the belief system and ways that the nurse can appropriately be involved in supporting the individual.

■ **Implementation**

• Perform detailed nursing assessments of the symptoms for which the products are being taken, including any adverse effects.
• Record data in the nursing notes regarding the use, response, or lack of response to the products.
• Label the front of the chart with a listing of supplement products being used in case the healthcare provider does not have knowledge of their use.
• Discuss cultural and ethnic beliefs with the individual patient, and consult other members of the healthcare team regarding appropriate approaches for patient care and education.

■ **Patient Education**

Expectations of Therapy. Discuss the expectations of therapy with the patient and why self-treatment needs to be discussed with other members of the healthcare team. Emphasize to the patient that supplement products can and do interact with other medications.

Fostering Health Maintenance

• Discuss medication information and how it will benefit the course of treatment to produce an optimal response. Have the healthcare provider or pharmacist discuss implications of medications and products being used.
• Seek cooperation and understanding of the following points so that medication compliance is increased: name of medication; dosage, route, and times of administration; and common and serious adverse effects. The patient must understand not only prescribed medication data, but that of the supplement products as well. The individual must believe in the prescribed regimen in order for compliance to be enhanced.

Patient Self-Assessment. Enlist the patient's aid in developing and maintaining a written record of monitoring parameters (e.g., blood pressure, pulse, daily weight, degree of pain relief). (See Appendix B: Template for Developing a Written Record for Patients to Monitor Their Own Therapy.) Complete the Premedication Data column for use as a baseline to track response to drug therapy. Ensure that the patient understands how to use the form, and instruct the patient to take the completed form to follow-up visits. During follow-up visits, focus on issues that will foster adherence with the therapeutic interventions prescribed. The healthcare team members must understand that simply telling the patient not to take supplements may result in the patient's hiding the use of these products, creating additional problems.

HERBAL THERAPY

Herbal medicine is perhaps as old as the human race. For thousands of years, civilizations have depended on substances found in nature to treat illnesses. **Herbal**

medicines are defined as natural substances of botanical or plant origin. Other names for herbal medicines are *botanicals*, *phytomedicine*, and *phytotherapy*.

> **Common name: aloe** (ĂL-ō)
> Other names: Aloe vera, salvia, burn plant
> Botanical source: *Aloe barbadensis*
> Parts used: Aloe gel: clear, jellylike secretion obtained from the thin-walled, sticky cells of the inner portion of the leaf; aloe latex: cells just below the outer skin of the aloe plant

ACTIONS

Two products derived from aloe plant leaves are aloe gel and aloe latex. Aloe gel (commonly known as *aloe vera*) is a gelatinous extract from the sticky cells lining the inner portion of the leaf. Aloe gel is composed of polysaccharides and lignin, salicylic acid, saponin, sterols, triterpenoids, and a variety of enzymes. Aloe gel may possibly inhibit bradykinin and histamine, reducing pain and itching. Aloe latex (resin), also known as an *aloin*, contains pharmacologically active anthraquinone derivatives that, when taken orally, act as a laxative by irritating the intestinal lining, increasing peristalsis and fluid and electrolyte secretions.

USES

Aloe has been used as a medicinal agent for more than 5000 years for a vast array of internal and external illnesses, including arthritis, colitis, the common cold, ulcers, hemorrhoids, seizures, and glaucoma. Aloe gel is the form most commonly used in the cosmetic and health food industries. Most recently, aloe gel has been marketed for topical use to treat pain, inflammation, and itching and as a healing agent for sunburn, skin ulcers, psoriasis, and frostbite. The FDA has reviewed clinical studies of aloe gel and has not found adequate scientific evidence to support these claims. Therefore aloe gel is not classified as a drug but is allowed to remain on the market as a cosmetic for topical use. It is frequently used as a co-ingredient in skin care products; however, the product labeling should not make therapeutic claims of the aloe gel because none have been substantiated through scientific studies.

Aloe latex contains anthraquinone derivatives that, when taken orally, act as a laxative. There is a concern, however, about carcinogenicity, so aloe latex has been removed from the pharmaceutical market because it is not proven to be safe and effective. Historically, aloe has been known as a fragrant wood used as incense, unrelated to aloe vera.

❖ NURSING IMPLICATIONS FOR ALOE

■ Availability

Aloe gel: Moisturizing lotion, shampoo, hair conditioner, gels, toothpaste, aloe juice for topical application. Capsules and tinctures are also available for oral use. There are no proven therapeutic effects from these products.
Aloe latex: Aloe juice drinks for catharsis; whole-leaf aloe vera: juice.

■ Adverse Effects

When applied to the skin, no adverse effects have been reported. When taken orally, aloe products may cause diarrhea due to anthraquinone content.

■ Drug Interactions

Diabetic Therapy. Monitor blood glucose levels closely because of claims that when taken orally, aloe may have hypoglycemic effects.

> **Common name: black cohosh** (KŌ-hŏsh)
> Other names: Squawroot, black snakeroot, bugbane, bugwort
> Botanical source: *Cimicifuga racemosa*
> Parts used: Fresh and dried root

ACTIONS

The active ingredients in black cohosh are complex triterpenes and flavonoids. It is thought that these agents have estrogenlike effects by suppressing release of luteinizing hormone and by binding to estrogen receptors in peripheral tissue.

USES

Black cohosh is used to reduce symptoms of premenstrual syndrome, dysmenorrhea, and menopause. Therapy is not recommended for longer than 6 months. Black cohosh should not be used in the first two trimesters of pregnancy because of its uterine-relaxing effects.

Avoid use in the following situations:
- Hypotension: may cause low blood pressure; avoid concurrent use with antihypertensive agents.
- People with a history of hormone-sensitive conditions, for example, breast cancer, uterine cancer, or endometriosis.
- People with known seizure disorders, liver disease, or a history of stroke or blood clots.

❖ NURSING IMPLICATIONS FOR BLACK COHOSH

■ Availability

PO: Elixirs, tablets, capsules.

■ Adverse Effect

Upset stomach is rare.

■ Comments

Do not confuse black cohosh with blue cohosh. Blue cohosh is used as an antispasmodic and uterine stimulant to promote menstruation or labor, but it is different and potentially more toxic than black cohosh.

Beware of commercial products that contain both black and blue cohosh when only black cohosh is sought.

 Herbal Interactions

Black Cohosh

HORMONE REPLACEMENT THERAPY

Women already receiving hormone replacement therapy (usually estrogen and progestin) to treat symptoms associated with menopause and to prevent osteoporosis should be cautious about receiving additional estrogenic effects from concurrent use of black cohosh.

ANTIHYPERTENSIVE THERAPY

Black cohosh may cause added antihypertensive effects when taken with other antihypertensive agents. If black cohosh is being taken, monitor the blood pressure response to the cumulative effects. Take blood pressures in the supine and erect positions.

Common name: chamomile (KĂM-ō-mē-ŭl)

Other names: German or Hungarian chamomile: pinheads, chamomilla, genuine chamomile; Roman or English chamomile: ground apple, whig plant, common chamomile

Botanical source: *Matricaria recutita* (German or Hungarian chamomile); *Chamaemelum nobile* (Roman or English chamomile)

Parts used: Predominantly flower heads, but other above-ground parts also contain the volatile oils

---

ACTIONS

Two herbs are known as chamomile: German chamomile and Roman chamomile. The therapeutic effects of chamomile derive from a complex mixture of different compounds. The antiinflammatory and antispasmodic effects come from a volatile oil containing matricin, bisabolol, bisabolol oxides A and B, and flavonoids such as apigenin and luteolin. Coumarins, herniarin, and umbelliferone exhibit antispasmodic properties. Chamazulene has also been shown to possess antiinflammatory and antibacterial properties.

USES

Both chamomiles are used in herbalism and medicine; however, German chamomile is the species most commonly used in the United States and Europe, whereas Roman chamomile is favored in Great Britain. Chamomile is used as a digestive aid for bloating, an antispasmodic and antiinflammatory in the gastrointestinal (GI) tract, an antispasmodic for menstrual cramps, an antiinflammatory for skin irritation, and a mouthwash for minor mouth irritation or gum infections. Plant extracts are used in cosmetic and hygiene products in the form of ointments, lotions, and vapor baths for topical application. For internal use, chamomile is taken in the form of a strong tea.

❖ NURSING IMPLICATIONS FOR CHAMOMILE

▪ Availability

German chamomile is available as ointment and gel in strengths of 3% to 10%. As a bath additive, 50 g is added to 1 L of water. For internal use as a tea, pour 150 mL of boiling water over 3 g of chamomile (1 teaspoon = 1 g of chamomile), cover for 5 to 10 minutes, and then strain.

▪ Adverse Effects

Rare hypersensitivity reactions may occur in patients who are allergic to ragweed, asters, chrysanthemums, or daisies.

▪ Drug Interactions

No clinically significant drug interactions have been reported with chamomile.

Common name: echinacea (ĕk-ĭn-Ā-shĕ)

Other names: Purple coneflower, coneflower, black sampson

Botanical source: *Echinacea angustifolia*, *E. purpurea*, and other related species

Parts used: Roots, rhizomes, above-ground parts

ACTIONS

Echinacea is a nonspecific stimulator of the innate (nonspecific) immune system. It stimulates phagocytosis and effector cell activity. There is an increased release of tumor necrosis factors and interferons from macrophages and T lymphocytes, which increases the body's resistance to bacterial and viral infection. It may have antiinflammatory effects by inhibiting hyaluronidase, a potent inflammatory agent. Echinacea has no direct bactericidal or bacteriostatic effects.

USES

As a nonspecific immunostimulant, echinacea may prevent or treat viral respiratory tract infections such as the common cold or flu. Well-designed clinical studies have shown equivocal results. Symptoms of the common cold may be reduced if echinacea is taken during the early, acute phase. Echinacea has also been used to treat urinary tract infections and may be applied externally to difficult-to-heal superficial wounds. Because of its immunomodulating effects, it is recommended that it not be used for more than 8 weeks at a time.

Avoid use in the following situations:

- People with heart disease. Echinacea may cause abnormal or irregular heartbeat.
- People taking anticoagulants or who are at increased risk of bleeding.

- People with skin disorders; echinacea may cause burning sensations, hives, itching, rashes, and skin redness.
- People who are taking agents that may be toxic to the liver, including anabolic steroids, amiodarone, methotrexate, and ketoconazole. Echinacea may cause hepatotoxicity.

❖ NURSING IMPLICATIONS FOR ECHINACEA

▪ Availability

PO: Echinacea is available as dried roots, teas, tinctures, and dry powder extracts.

▪ Adverse Effects

Rare hypersensitivity reactions may occur in patients who are allergic to ragweed, asters, chrysanthemums, or daisies.

▪ Comments

Because echinacea appears to be an immunomodulator, it is not recommended for patients with autoimmune diseases, such as multiple sclerosis or lupus erythematosus, or diseases affecting the immune system, such as acquired immunodeficiency syndrome (AIDS).

 Herbal Interactions

Echinacea

Echinacea may interfere with immunosuppressive therapy. Concurrent use with immunosuppressants (e.g., azathioprine, cyclosporine) is not recommended.

Common name: ephedra (ē-FĔD-ră)
  Other names: Ma-huang, desert herb, ephedrine
  Botanical source: *Ephedra sinica*
  Parts used: Stems, rhizomes with roots

ACTION

The active ingredient in ephedra is the alkaloid ephedrine.

USES

Ephedra was perhaps the first Chinese herbal medicine to be used in Western medicine. It is used as a bronchodilator for asthma, as a nasal decongestant, and as a central nervous system (CNS) stimulant. It is contraindicated in patients with heart conditions, hypertension, diabetes, and thyroid disease. The FDA first banned the sale of all dietary supplements containing ephedra in April 2004 based on a lack of evidence to support efficacy claims and more than 16,000 reported cases of adverse reactions. The ban was later overturned by a federal judge in April 2005 for products containing ephedra 10 mg or less. However, in May 2007, the ban was upheld by the U.S. Supreme Court based on a final FDA regulation declaring dietary supplements containing adulterated ephedrine

alkaloids as presenting an unreasonable risk of illness or injury.

❖ NURSING IMPLICATIONS FOR EPHEDRA

▪ Adverse Effects

Ephedra elevates systolic and diastolic blood pressures and heart rate, causing palpitations. It also causes nervousness, headache, insomnia, and dizziness.

▪ Comments

- In recent years, popular culture has touted ephedra as a weight loss product, an energy booster, an aphrodisiac, and a mental stimulant. There is no substantial evidence that supports these claims. It is commonly found in OTC weight loss products. Deaths have been reported from its overuse and in those patients who may have underlying cardiovascular disease.
- Because ephedrine can serve as a precursor to the synthesis of illegal methamphetamine (speed), several states have passed laws regulating the sale of products containing ephedrine.
- Ephedrine is a medicine approved as safe and effective by the FDA and is readily available commercially. There are several other medicines that are safer, with fewer adverse effects (e.g., pseudoephedrine). There is really no need to use herbal ephedra for rational medical therapy.

 Herbal Interactions

Ephedra

DRUGS THAT ENHANCE TOXIC EFFECTS
Beta-adrenergic stimulants (e.g., pseudoephedrine, phenylpropanolamine) and monoamine oxidase inhibitors (MAOIs) (e.g., isocarboxazid, tranylcypromine, phenelzine):
- Excessive use may result in significant hypertension.
- Patients already receiving antihypertensive therapy should not use decongestants such as ephedrine because they raise blood pressure.

METHYLDOPA, RESERPINE
Frequent use of decongestants inhibits the antihypertensive activity of these agents. Concurrent therapy is not recommended.

Common name: feverfew (FĒ-vĕr-fyū)
  Other names: Featherfoil, flirtwort, bachelor's buttons
    Botanical source: *Tanacetum parthenium*
    Parts used: Leaves

ACTIONS

There is significant controversy as to which ingredients in feverfew are therapeutic. Several sesquiterpene lactones are smooth muscle relaxants in the walls of the cerebral blood vessels and may be the source of antimigraine activity. Feverfew has also been shown to inhibit the release of arachidonic acid, which serves as a substrate for production of prostaglandins and leukotrienes. It also inhibits release of serotonin and histamine from platelets and white cells, which helps prevent or control migraine headaches. Parthenolide, long thought to be the primary active ingredient, has been shown by one well-controlled study to be of minimal therapeutic effect. Perhaps additional compounds work synergistically with parthenolide to prevent migraine headaches.

USES

Feverfew is used to reduce the frequency and severity of migraine headaches. Its antiinflammatory effects have also been used to treat rheumatoid arthritis. Feverfew is contraindicated in women who are pregnant. It may cause uterine contractions, increasing the risk of miscarriage or premature delivery.

❖ NURSING IMPLICATIONS FOR FEVERFEW

■ Availability
PO: Leaf powder for making tea; tablets.

■ Adverse Effects
Fresh feverfew leaves appear to be most effective in reducing the frequency and pain associated with migraine headaches. Ulcerations of the oral mucosa and swelling of the lips and tongue have been reported by 7% to 12% of patients. Feverfew therapy should be discontinued if these lesions develop. Rare hypersensitivity reactions may occur in patients who are allergic to ragweed, asters, chrysanthemums, or daisies.

■ Comments
- The sesquiterpene lactone content is higher in the flowering tops than in the leaves, stalks, and roots. This diminishes with time and with exposure to light. Because the active ingredients are not known, there are no standards established for purity. Many products sold in the United States have been found to have low, variable quantities of sesquiterpene lactones.
- People who take feverfew for a long time and then stop taking it may have difficulty sleeping, headaches, joint pain, nervousness, and stiff muscles.

 Herbal Interactions

Feverfew

NONSTEROIDAL ANTIINFLAMMATORY DRUGS
Even though feverfew has antiinflammatory properties, concurrent use with nonsteroidal antiinflammatory drugs (NSAIDs) may reduce the effectiveness of feverfew.

ANTICOAGULANTS
Because feverfew reduces platelet aggregation, it should be used with extreme caution in patients who are also receiving platelet inhibitors (e.g., aspirin, ticlopidine, dipyridamole, clopidogrel), anticoagulants (e.g., warfarin), and herbal medicines (e.g., ginkgo, garlic, ginger, ginseng). Monitor patients for signs of bleeding.

> **Common name: garlic** (GĂR-lĭk)
> Other names: None
> Botanical source: *Allium sativum*
> Parts used: Bulb

ACTIONS

Garlic contains a large variety of chemicals, making it difficult to determine which ingredients are responsible for its biologic effects. Alliin is a major component of garlic that, when crushed, is acted on by the enzyme allinase to produce allicin. Allicin is thought to have the greatest pharmacologic activity, but is also responsible for garlic's characteristic odor. A metabolite of allicin, ajoene (Ō-hō-wĕn) is also thought to have biologic activity.

USES

Garlic has been one of the most widely used herbal medicines for centuries. At various times, claims have been made for it curing almost all diseases, as well as being an excellent aphrodisiac. It also has been widely used in folklore to ward off vampires, demons, and witches. Its most frequent use supported by scientific literature is in reducing cholesterol and triglyceride levels. Garlic has been shown to lower levels of serum cholesterol by 9% to 12% and triglycerides by as much as 17%. It also demonstrates antiplatelet activity similar to aspirin, and may also modestly lower high blood pressure.

❖ NURSING IMPLICATIONS FOR GARLIC

■ Availability
PO: Cloves, oil, enteric-coated tablets, capsules, elixirs.

■ Adverse Effects
The most common adverse effect of garlic is its characteristic taste and odor, frequently resulting in halitosis. Enteric-coated oral preparations minimize this problem. There are rare reports of patients developing nausea and vomiting and burning of the mouth and stomach after ingesting various commercial preparations.

■ Comments
Fresh garlic is the most potent from a biologic standpoint, releasing the active ingredients in the mouth when chewed. The enzyme allinase, necessary for conversion of alliin to the active principles of allicin and ajoene, is inactivated in stomach acid. The active ingredients of garlic are easily destroyed by freeze drying or heat drying, and commercial products are of variable potency. Dried garlic preparations are most effective if they are enteric coated, allowing them to pass into the intestine before dissolution. These products tend to have less of the characteristic odor associated with garlic because the allicin is released in the intestine. One fresh clove daily or a daily dose of 8 mg of

alliin from a product standardized for alliin content is the current dosage recommendation to treat hypercholesterolemia. Diet and exercise will aid the garlic in reducing high blood pressure and cholesterol levels.

 Herbal Interactions

Garlic

ANTICOAGULANTS

Because garlic reduces platelet aggregation, it should be used with extreme caution in patients who are also receiving platelet inhibitors (e.g., aspirin, ticlopidine, dipyridamole, clopidogrel), anticoagulants (e.g., warfarin), and herbal medicines (e.g., ginkgo, ginger, feverfew, ginseng). Monitor patients for signs of bleeding.

Common name: ginger (JĬN-jĕr)
   Other names: African ginger, Jamaica ginger, race ginger
   Botanical source: *Zingiber officinale*
   Parts used: Roots and rhizomes

ACTIONS

The active ingredients in ginger roots and rhizomes are known as *gingerols*. They increase the rate of GI motility, act as serotonin antagonists, and inhibit cyclooxygenase pathways.

USES

Ginger has been used for centuries to alleviate nausea and vomiting from a variety of causes. It is thought to act as an antiemetic by increasing gastroduodenal motility and by blocking serotonin receptors that, when stimulated, may trigger nausea and vomiting. Ginger is possibly safe when used in pregnancy, and a few controlled studies indicate that it may reduce the frequency of morning sickness. The use of ginger in pregnancy is controversial, however, because it has never been studied thoroughly for safety in this patient population.

Ginger has also been shown to be modestly effective in reducing inflammation and pain in patients with rheumatoid arthritis, osteoarthritis, and muscle discomfort because it is a cyclooxygenase-2 (COX-2) inhibitor.

The rhizome is used as the source for the dried powder used in food preparation.

❖ NURSING IMPLICATIONS FOR GINGER

▪ Availability

PO: Powdered ginger root; ginger tea made from ginger root; tinctures. The dosages are quite variable, but it is recommended that the dosage not exceed 4 g daily.

▪ Adverse Effects

Generally, ginger is well tolerated. There have been reports of heartburn, diarrhea, and irritation to the mouth and throat.

▪ Comments

Ginger is generally recognized as safe when used in food preparation. The dosages used for nausea, vomiting, and analgesia are substantially higher and have not been proven to be safe or effective.

 Herbal Interactions

Ginger

ANTICOAGULANTS

Because ginger reduces platelet aggregation, it should be used with extreme caution in patients who are also receiving platelet inhibitors (e.g., aspirin, ticlopidine, dipyridamole, clopidogrel), anticoagulants (e.g., warfarin), and herbal medicines (e.g., garlic, ginkgo, ginseng, feverfew). Monitor for signs of bleeding.

Common name: ginkgo (GĬNK-ō)
   Other names: Maidenhair tree
   Botanical source: *Ginkgo biloba*
   Parts used: Green-picked leaves

ACTIONS

The active ingredients in ginkgo leaves are flavonoids and terpenes. Because higher concentrations of these chemicals are necessary for biologic activity, the green-picked leaves are processed to form a concentrated ginkgo biloba extract (GBE). Ginkgo biloba extract is standardized to a potency of 24% flavonoids (primarily flavonoid glycosides and quercetin) and 6% terpenes (primarily composed of ginkgolides A, B, C, and J and bilobalide). Ginkgo biloba extract is a smooth muscle relaxant and vasodilator that improves blood flow in arteries and capillaries. It may also be a free radical scavenger, preventing endothelial cell damage. Ginkgolides inhibit platelet-activating factor, inhibiting platelet aggregation.

USES

Ginkgo biloba extract is used primarily for increasing cerebral blood flow, particularly in geriatric patients. Conditions treated are short-term memory loss, headache, dizziness, tinnitus, and emotional instability with anxiety. Patients with Alzheimer's disease may show modest improvement in cognitive performance and social functioning. Other uses include improved walking distance in patients with intermittent claudication, improvement in erectile dysfunction secondary to antidepressant therapy, improved peripheral blood flow in patients with diabetes mellitus, and improved hearing in patients whose hearing is impaired secondary to poor circulation to the ears. Therapy must be continued for up to 6 months to assess optimal response.

❖ NURSING IMPLICATIONS FOR GINKGO

■ Availability

PO: 40 mg GBE in liquid, tablets, and capsules. Dosages range from 120 to 240 mg of GBE twice daily.

■ Adverse Effects

Large doses of GBE may cause mild restlessness, diarrhea, nausea, vomiting, and dizziness. Adverse effects may be minimized by slowly titrating the dose upward as tolerated.

 Herbal Interactions

Ginkgo

ANTICOAGULANTS

Because ginkgo reduces platelet aggregation, it should be used with extreme caution in patients who are also receiving platelet inhibitors (e.g., aspirin, ticlopidine, dipyridamole, clopidogrel), anticoagulants (e.g., warfarin), and herbal medicines (e.g., ginger, garlic, feverfew, ginseng). Monitor patients for signs of bleeding.

> **Common name: ginseng** (JĬN-sĭng)
>   Other names: Aralia cinquefoil, five fingers, tartar root, red berry
>   Botanical source: *Panax ginseng* (Chinese or Korean ginseng)
>   Parts used: Root

ACTIONS

Ginseng contains a large variety of chemicals, making it difficult to determine which components are responsible for its biologic effects. The ingredients believed to be responsible are triterpenoid saponins, classified into panaxosides, ginsenosides, and chikusetsusaponins. Unfortunately, the literature is extremely difficult to interpret because of differences in composition between Asian and American ginseng species, different scientific terms for active ingredients, and the lack of well-controlled scientific studies.

USES

Ginseng is not used to cure a disease, but is an "adaptogen" in maintaining health. Current claims for ginseng are that it increases the body's resistance to stress, overcomes disease by building up defenses, and strengthens general vitality. It has also been used for centuries as an aphrodisiac. There is no scientific basis for its claims as an aphrodisiac and little scientific evidence as an adaptogen.

❖ NURSING IMPLICATIONS FOR GINSENG

■ Availability

PO: Teas, powders, capsules, tablets, liquids. There are no standardized methods of purity. Commercial ginseng extract products range from 100 to 600 mg standardized to a percentage of ginsenosides.

■ Adverse Effects

Many adverse effects have been reported with the use of ginseng, but most are single case reports, and may be the pharmacologic effect of adulterants added to ginseng. Adverse effects most commonly attributed to ginseng are insomnia, diarrhea, and skin eruptions.

■ Comments

Even though thousands of articles have been written lauding its praises, ginseng has not undergone much scientific study. Most of the literature is based on superstition and anecdotal reports. Many of the reports have been written by governments and companies making claims for financial gain. Ginseng is an herbal medicine that is commonly adulterated, so it is difficult to know whether the results of studies are because of the ginseng content or the added ingredients.

Siberian ginseng (*Eleutherococcus senticosus;* also known as *eleuthero*) is different from American or Asian ginseng and should not be substituted. It has been marketed as a cheaper form of ginseng but is known to have many adulterants, and there are no scientific studies to support its claims as an immune system stimulant and enhancer of endurance.

 Herbal Interactions

Ginseng

ANTICOAGULANTS

Ginseng may affect platelet aggregation and blood coagulation. It should be used with extreme caution in patients who are also receiving platelet inhibitors (e.g., aspirin, ticlopidine, dipyridamole, clopidogrel), anticoagulants (e.g., warfarin), and herbal medicines (e.g., garlic, feverfew, ginger, ginkgo). Monitor for signs of bleeding.

INSULIN

Ginseng has been shown to raise insulin levels in laboratory animals. It may have the potential to induce hypoglycemia. Blood glucose levels of patients with type 1 or type 2 diabetes mellitus should be monitored closely if the patient insists on taking ginseng.

> **Common name: goldenseal** (GŌL-dĕn-sē-ăl)
>   Other names: Yellow root, Indian dye, Indian paint, jaundice root
>   Botanical source: *Hydrastis canadensis*
>   Parts used: Rhizomes with root fibers

ACTIONS

The active ingredients in goldenseal are contained in a group of plant alkaloids, the most active of which are hydrastine and berberine. Berberine gives the herb its characteristic golden color.

USES

Goldenseal is popular in herbal medicine as an antiseptic and astringent, reducing inflammation of mucous membranes. It is used topically as a tea for treatment of canker sores, sore mouth, and cracked and bleeding lips. Goldenseal may have weak antibacterial properties and may stimulate the immune system to help fight viral upper respiratory infections such as a cold or flu. Goldenseal is sometimes marketed in combination with echinacea to ward off bouts of the common cold. No controlled studies have been completed to validate this combined therapy. In high doses, goldenseal may have uterine stimulant effects and should not be taken during pregnancy. In recent years, there has been a common myth that goldenseal, when taken as tea, or put into urine, will mask assays for street drugs (see "Comments").

❖ NURSING IMPLICATIONS FOR GOLDENSEAL

▪ Availability

PO: Powder for tea, tincture, fluid extract, freeze-dried root.

▪ Adverse Effects

The alkaloids in goldenseal are not absorbed to any extent when swallowed, producing no systemic effects. High doses may cause nausea, vomiting, diarrhea, and CNS stimulation.

▪ Comments

One of the more recent popular uses for goldenseal is to mask the presence of illicit drugs in urine samples. Contrary to popular belief, goldenseal does not prevent detection of drugs by urine tests, nor does it flush illicit drugs from the body. When goldenseal is present, the urine takes on a distinctive dark amber or brown color.

> **Common name: green tea**
>   Other names: Chinese tea, teagreen
>   Botanical source: *Camellia sinensis*, evergreen shrub
>   Parts used: Leaf, leaf bud, and stem

ACTIONS

When steamed, green tea leaves and stems yield high concentrations of polyphenols such as gallic acid, and catechins and caffeine, which are thought to be the active ingredients of green tea. Mechanisms of action are unknown. Green tea also contains B vitamins and ascorbic acid.

USES

Green tea has been used as a very common beverage in Asian cultures for centuries. The caffeine produces CNS stimulation and is thought to improve cognitive performance. It raises blood pressure, heart rate, and contractility and acts as a diuretic. Green tea has been shown to lower cholesterol, triglyceride, and low-density lipoprotein (LDL) levels and raise high-density lipoprotein (HDL) level. There is some evidence that green tea might reduce the risk of bladder, esophageal, and pancreatic cancers and reduce or prevent the onset of parkinsonism. Green tea is also used to treat diarrhea.

❖ NURSING IMPLICATIONS FOR GREEN TEA

▪ Availability

PO: Green tea is readily available in premade tea bags and in bulk form for brewing. Moderate consumption of one to four cups daily appears to provide therapeutic benefits. Consumption of five or more cups daily has significantly more adverse effects that are associated with excessive caffeine.

▪ Adverse Effects

Many of the adverse effects of green tea are an extension of the pharmacologic effects of caffeine: anxiety, nervousness, headache, diuresis, insomnia, tremor, irritability, palpitations, and dysrhythmias. The chronic use and consumption of high quantities can produce tolerance, habituation, and psychological dependence. The abrupt discontinuation may cause withdrawal headaches, irritation, and nervousness.

 Herbal Interactions

Green Tea

INCREASED THERAPEUTIC AND TOXIC EFFECTS

The following drugs, when used concurrently with green tea, may significantly increase the stimulant effects and the adverse effects of the caffeine in green tea by inhibiting its metabolism: ephedrine, cimetidine, disulfiram, grapefruit juice, MAOIs (e.g., tranylcypromine, phenelzine, isocarboxazid), mexiletine, oral contraceptives, quinolones (e.g., ciprofloxacin, enoxacin, norfloxacin, sparfloxacin), theophylline, and verapamil.

BETA-ADRENERGIC AGENTS (ALBUTEROL, METAPROTERENOL, TERBUTALINE)

Concurrent consumption of green tea (caffeine) with beta agonists can increase the heart rate and the potential for dysrhythmias. Use with caution. Discontinue green tea consumption if palpitations develop.

EPHEDRA

Concurrent consumption of ephedra and the caffeine in green tea results in significantly more stimulant effects with greater possibility of adverse effects.

WARFARIN

Concurrent consumption of large quantities of green tea with warfarin may antagonize the anticoagulant effects of warfarin. Monitor the patient's international normalized ratio (INR) for therapeutic effect of warfarin.

Common name: St. John's wort (SĂNT JŎNZ WŌRT)

Other names: Klamath weed, hardhay, amber
Botanical source: *Hypericum perforatum*
Parts used: Fresh buds and flowers

ACTIONS

The active ingredients of St. John's wort are unknown. Studies indicate that it behaves as a reuptake inhibitor, prolonging the effect of serotonin, dopamine, and norepinephrine.

USES

St. John's wort is used orally to treat mild depression and to heal wounds.

❖ NURSING IMPLICATIONS FOR ST. JOHN'S WORT

▪ Availability

St. John's wort is available as powder, tablets, capsules, and liquid. It is also found in semisolid preparations for topical use. It is commonly standardized to hypericin content, but it has been shown that hypericin content is not related to antidepressant effect, so this standard is of little value. Therapeutic effects are variable between various products and different batches of the same product. Because the therapeutic ingredients are unknown, there is no effective standardization for St. John's wort products. The average daily dosage for internal use is 2 to 4 g of herb or 0.2 to 1 mg of total hypericin.

▪ Adverse Effects

St. John's wort may cause photosensitivity. Patients should discontinue the herbal medicine and report excessive sunburn, pruritus, and edema immediately.

There is concern about St. John's wort contributing to the development of serotonin syndrome. The seriousness of this adverse effect warrants that patients be informed of this complication of therapy. Serotonin syndrome may result from taking two or more drugs that affect serotonin levels. Symptoms associated with the syndrome are confusion, agitation, shivering, fever, diaphoresis, nausea, diarrhea, muscle spasms, and tremor. These symptoms have a sudden onset, somewhat like a panic attack, and may progress to a coma. The syndrome is life threatening. When switching between serotonergic agents and St. John's wort, a 5- to 7-day washout period is recommended (see Chapter 16).

▪ Comments

- Folklore tells us that St. John's wort received its name because its golden flower is particularly abundant on June 24, the day celebrated as the birthday of John the Baptist.
- St. John's wort products are light and heat sensitive. Exposure to light and excessive heat for 2 weeks will alter the content of the chemical constituents.

- Depression is a serious, potentially fatal illness. It is important that patients discuss their symptoms and the use of St. John's wort before starting self-treatment.

🔖 Herbal Interactions

St. John's Wort

SEROTONIN STIMULANTS

Selective serotonin reuptake inhibitors (SSRIs) (e.g., paroxetine, sertraline, fluoxetine), tricyclic antidepressants (e.g., amitriptyline, imipramine, doxepin), MAOIs (e.g., isocarboxazid, phenelzine, tranylcypromine), and dopamine agonists (e.g., bromocriptine) may induce a serotonin syndrome when taken concurrently with St. John's wort. Patients should contact their healthcare provider immediately if they start noticing symptoms of this syndrome (see "Adverse Effects").

Common name: valerian (văl-ĀR-ē-ăn)

Other names: Amantilla, setwall, heliotrope, vandal root
Botanical source: *Valeriana officinalis*
Parts used: Dried roots and rhizomes

ACTIONS

The chemical constituents that are responsible for the therapeutic effects of valerian have not been fully identified.

USES

Valerian has been used for more than 1000 years as a mild tranquilizer. It is used for restlessness and may promote sleep.

❖ NURSING IMPLICATIONS FOR VALERIAN

▪ Availability

PO: Valerian may be administered in the form of a tea, tincture, extract, tablets, or capsules. Some preparations are standardized for valepotriate content, but it is not known whether these compounds are the active ingredients.

▪ Adverse Effects

Adverse effects are rare; chronic users may experience excitability, uneasiness, and headache.

▪ Comments

Because of similarity in names, valerian and Valium have sometimes been confused. Valerian is a mild tranquilizer, whereas Valium is the brand name of a much more potent tranquilizer (generic name, diazepam). Diazepam is a member of the benzodiazepines (see Chapter 15, p. 222).

▪ Drug Interactions

No clinically significant drug interactions have been reported, but concurrent use of other medicines with sedative properties, such as antihistamines, benzodiazepines, alcohol, and barbiturates, should be avoided.

OTHER DIETARY SUPPLEMENTS

Common name: coenzyme Q10 (kō-ĔN-zīm)
  Other names: CoQ10, ubiquinone
  Sources: Commercial sources—fermentation of cane sugar and beets using special strains of yeast; natural sources—beef, soy oil, sardines, peanuts

DESCRIPTION AND ACTIONS

Coenzyme Q10 is a provitamin found in every living cell and is essential for energy production in the mitochondria. Organs with high energy requirements contain the highest levels of CoQ10; these organs are the heart muscle, liver, kidney, and pancreas. Human cells synthesize CoQ10 from the amino acid tyrosine in a series of chemical reactions that also require folic acid, niacin, riboflavin, and pyridoxine. A deficiency of any of these vitamins may result in a deficiency in CoQ10. Deficiency of CoQ10 also results from diminished dietary intake, impairment of biosynthesis, and increased usage of CoQ10 by the body.

USES

CoQ10 has been used to treat a variety of disorders. Its primary use is as an adjunctive therapy for chronic heart failure. It has also been tested with varying degrees of success in other cardiovascular diseases (e.g., ischemic heart disease [angina], hypertension, dysrhythmias, toxin-induced cardiomyopathy, surgery for heart valve replacement), cancer (breast, lung, prostate, pancreatic, colon), muscular dystrophy, periodontal disease, and AIDS. Additional studies are required to determine the degree of therapeutic benefit for these diseases.

❖ NURSING IMPLICATIONS FOR COQ10

▪ Availability

PO: Powder-filled capsules, tablets, liquid-filled gel capsules, chewable wafers, intraoral spray.

▪ Dosage

- Prevention of deficiency: 30 to 60 mg daily.
- Treatment of deficiency: 100 to 200 mg daily.
- Administer with meals that contain some fat to enhance absorption.
- Doses of more than 100 mg daily should be divided into two or three dosages.
- The safety of CoQ10 in pregnancy and lactation has not been established, and its use is not recommended.

▪ Adverse Effects

No serious adverse effects have been reported. Less than 1% of patients describe symptoms of nausea, upset stomach, diarrhea, and appetite suppression. Doses of 100 mg or more taken at bedtime may cause mild insomnia. Patients taking 300 mg daily for extended periods demonstrate mild elevations of liver enzyme levels, but no cases of hepatotoxicity have been reported.

 Herbal Interactions

Coenzyme Q10

HMG-COA (3-HYDROXY-3-METHYLGLUTARYL COENZYME A) REDUCTASE INHIBITORS ("STATINS"), GEMFIBROZIL
These antilipemic agents appear to reduce total body levels of CoQ10 by inhibiting its synthesis by the body. The clinical significance of this interaction is not known at this time.

BETA-ADRENERGIC BLOCKING AGENTS
Beta-adrenergic blocking agents appear to reduce total body levels of CoQ10 by inhibiting its synthesis. The clinical significance of this interaction is not known at this time.

INSULIN, ORAL HYPOGLYCEMIC AGENTS
CoQ10 supplementation has been reported to reduce insulin requirements in diabetes mellitus. Oral hypoglycemic agents (e.g., tolazamide, glyburide) have also been reported to reduce total body levels of CoQ10; therefore patients with diabetes who are taking CoQ10 require close monitoring of blood glucose levels with adjustment in dosages of antidiabetic medicines as needed.

WARFARIN
The chemical structure of CoQ10 and vitamin K are similar. There are reports that administration of CoQ10 to patients receiving warfarin causes a decrease in the INR. Monitor the INR closely for therapeutic effect.

Common name: creatine (KRĒ-ă-tēn)
  Other names: Creatine monohydrate
  Sources: Natural sources: meat and fish (muscle)

DESCRIPTION AND ACTIONS

Creatine is a naturally occurring, energy-producing substance in the human body synthesized from amino acids. It plays a key role in providing energy to muscles for short-duration, high-intensity exercise. About 95% of the body's creatine is in skeletal muscle, of which 60% is in the form of creatine phosphate. Muscle adenosine triphosphate (ATP) provides immediate energy for muscle contraction, after which it is replenished by creatine phosphate. The rapidity with which creatine phosphate is replenished depends on the amount of free creatine available.

USES

Creatine is used as a performance-enhancing substance. Creatine supplementation is thought to enhance muscle performance for short bouts of repeated, intense exercise such as sprinting, jumping, and power lifting. Increasing creatine phosphate stores enhances rapid replenishment of ATP, and increased supplies of free creatine shorten muscle recovery time by rebuilding depleted creatine phosphate stores faster. Many small studies have attempted to document the benefits of creatine supplementation, but with mixed results. At best, some studies indicate a 1% to 3% improvement in performance for brief periods.

Small clinical studies also indicate that patients with heart failure and muscular dystrophy might benefit from creatine supplementation by preserving energy stores in the myocardium and skeletal muscle, respectively. Additional studies are needed to assess long-term benefits of creatine therapy in these and other conditions.

❖ NURSING IMPLICATIONS FOR CREATINE

▪ Availability
PO: Powder, candy, gum, and liquid. It is often combined with other supplements for energy.

▪ Dosage
A loading dose of 5 to 6 g four times daily for 5 to 7 days, followed by doses of 2 g daily to maintain elevated creatine concentrations in the muscle, or 3 g per day for 28 days.

▪ Adverse Effects
No serious adverse effects have been reported, but long-term studies have not been completed that might document adverse effects. Creatine causes weight gain of 3 to 6 pounds because of water retention. Other adverse effects of creatine may include muscle cramping, dehydration, and GI bloating and diarrhea.

▪ Comments
- It is recommended that at least eight 8-ounce glasses of water be consumed daily while taking creatine supplements.
- Creatine supplementation should be avoided by people who have impaired renal function or are taking potentially nephrotoxic medicines.
- The safety of creatine in pregnancy and lactation has not been established, and its use is not recommended.

Common name: gamma-hydroxybutyrate (GHB)
(GĂ-mă hī-drŏk-sē-BYŪ-tĭr-āt)
   Other names: Georgia home boy (GHB), liquid ecstasy, salty water, many others

---

DESCRIPTION AND ACTIONS

Gamma-hydroxybutyrate occurs naturally in the brain, kidneys, heart, and skeletal muscle. It is a metabolite of gamma-aminobutyric acid, an inhibitory neurotransmitter. A wide variety of physiologic responses occur when GHB receptors are stimulated, including dopamine release, growth hormone release, and induction of sleep.

USES

In the late 1980s GHB was marketed and sold in the health food industry as a growth hormone stimulator to help bodybuilders promote muscle mass and maintain weight, and as an OTC sedative. The drug was banned by the FDA in 1990 after several reports of adverse reactions in individuals using nutritional and weight loss supplements containing GHB. Despite the FDA ban, GHB continues to be marketed as a dietary supplement. Home manufacturing kits can be purchased, and recipes are readily available on the Internet.

Gamma-hydroxybutyrate is usually abused for its intoxicating, sedative, and euphoric properties. It is an increasingly popular drug of abuse, particularly at rave parties where it is used as a euphoriant, and as a date rape drug that is added to alcoholic drinks. Like alcohol, GHB's intoxicating effects begin 10 to 20 minutes after ingestion. The effects typically last up to 4 hours, depending on the dose. In progressively higher doses, the sedative effects may progress from sleep to coma to death. As with other commonly abused substances, repeated exposure leads to reinforcement, tolerance, and dependence. Dependence may be manifested by withdrawal symptoms, such as the need to continue to take the drug, anxiety, insomnia, and abnormal thinking.

❖ NURSING IMPLICATIONS FOR GHB

▪ Availability
Gamma-hydroxybutyrate is available as a prescription product (sodium oxybate, Xyrem) for treating a small population of patients with narcolepsy who experience episodes of cataplexy, a condition characterized by weak or paralyzed muscles. Because of safety concerns associated with the use of the drug, sodium oxybate is a Schedule III controlled substance, and the distribution of Xyrem is tightly restricted. The medicine is to be used only at bedtime because it induces sleep very quickly.

▪ Adverse Effects
Adverse effects related to GHB ingestion are highly variable among individuals, possibly relating to contaminating chemicals from home manufacturing kits. A wide range of effects have been reported, including impairment of judgment, aggression, and hallucinations, but those that are potentially life threatening are vomiting (with aspiration into the lungs), respiratory depression, bradycardia, and hypotension.

 Herbal Interactions

Gamma-Hydroxybutyrate

DRUGS THAT INCREASE TOXIC EFFECTS
Alcohol, antihistamines, analgesics, anesthetics, tranquilizers, antidepressants, valproic acid, phenytoin, and sleep aids will increase the sedative-hypnotic effects of GHB.

Common name: lycopene (LĪ-kō-pēn)
Sources: Natural: tomatoes, watermelon, pink grapefruit

DESCRIPTION AND ACTIONS

Lycopene is a carotenoid, a family of more than 50 nutrients from yellow, red, and orange plant pigments that act as antioxidants to protect the body against free radicals (unstable molecules released when the body uses oxygen).

USES

There is some evidence to suggest that diets high in lycopene may reduce the risk of prostate cancer and possibly lung, colon, and breast cancer. Small studies also indicate that the antioxidant properties have a lowering effect on LDL cholesterol and can protect against heart attack and stroke. Lycopene may also help prevent ophthalmic conditions such as macular degeneration and cataracts.

❖ NURSING IMPLICATIONS FOR LYCOPENE

▪ Availability

Research indicates that lycopene in tomatoes can be absorbed more efficiently by the body if processed into tomato juice, sauce, paste, and ketchup. Most products are sold as carotenoid complex containing natural tomato powder and tomato extract.

▪ Dosage

Optimal dosages of lycopene have not been established. Analysis of major studies indicates that 5 to 10 servings per week of tomato-based sauces and other products (juices, extracts) may have a protective effect against developing prostate cancer. A common dosage is 1- to 15-mg tablets two or three times daily with meals.

▪ Adverse Effects

No serious adverse effects have been reported.

Common name: melatonin (mĕl-ă-TŌ-nĭn)
Other names: Sleep hormone, MEL, MLT

DESCRIPTION AND ACTIONS

Melatonin is a human hormone synthesized from serotonin and secreted by the pineal gland. Its secretion is increased by dark and suppressed by light through the retina.

USES

Melatonin is best known as a sleep aid and treatment for jet lag. It may also be helpful in patients withdrawing from benzodiazepine therapy. Melatonin has also been recommended as an antiaging medicine, but good clinical studies do not support this claim.

❖ NURSING IMPLICATIONS FOR MELATONIN

▪ Availability

PO: 1-, 1.3-, 2-, 3-, 5-, 10-mg tablets and capsules; 1 mg/mL liquid.

▪ Dosage

Insomnia: 1 to 3 mg about 30 minutes before going to bed. Drowsiness develops within 30 to 40 minutes and lasts about 4 hours.

Jet lag prevention: 1 to 3 mg at bedtime on the day before travel, and 1 to 3 mg for the first 2 to 3 days after arrival. Stay awake during the daytime hours after arrival to help adjust to changes in time zones.

▪ Comments

The safety of melatonin in children and during pregnancy and lactation has not been established, and its use is not recommended.

▪ Adverse Effects

Neurologic

Drowsiness, sedation, lethargy. Because melatonin causes drowsiness, people who work around machinery, drive a car, administer medicines, or perform other duties in which they must remain mentally alert should not take melatonin while working.

Paradoxical response. Occasionally, melatonin causes a paradoxical reaction such as agitation and insomnia. Provide supportive care and safety during these responses. Assess the level of excitement and deal calmly with the individual. During periods of excitement, protect the patient from harm and provide for physical channeling of energy (e.g., walking). Seek a change in the medication order.

 Herbal Interactions

Melatonin

CENTRAL NERVOUS SYSTEM DEPRESSANTS
Melatonin may add to CNS depression caused by alcohol, benzodiazepines, sleep aids, and other sedative-hypnotics. Do not administer melatonin to patients already receiving any of these medications without healthcare provider approval.

Common name: policosanol (pŏl-ē-KŌ-săn-ŏl)
Other names: Polycosanol, *N*-octacosanol, octacosyl alcohol, octacosanol, wheat germ oil

DESCRIPTION AND ACTIONS

Policosanol is a plant sterol that contains a mixture of waxy-type alcohols derived from plant sources, including sugarcane and wheat germ oil. The alcohols that comprise policosanol are primarily octacosanol, tetracosanol, hexacosanol, heptacosanol, nonacosanol, triacosanol, dotriacontanol, and tetratriacontanol. Policosanol appears to lower cholesterol levels by inhibiting hepatic cholesterol synthesis and by increasing the degradation of LDL cholesterol. Policosanol also reduces platelet aggregation but does not seem to significantly affect coagulation time.

USES

Plant sterols are included in the National Cholesterol Education Program guidelines as part of the Therapeutic Lifestyle Changes program. Orally, policosanol is used to treat dyslipidemia, lowering LDL cholesterol 17% to 27% and increasing HDL 7% to 10%. It has no effect on triglyceride levels. Clinical studies indicate that policosanol has similar efficacy in treating dyslipidemias as do lower doses of the statins. As a platelet inhibitor, policosanol is used to treat intermittent claudication in patients with peripheral artery disease and myocardial ischemia in patients with coronary heart disease.

❖ NURSING IMPLICATIONS FOR POLICOSANOL

▪ Availability

PO: 10- and 20-mg tablets.

▪ Dosage

The dosage of 5-10 mg twice daily in a product containing at least 60% octacosanol. Two months of therapy may be required to see significant changes in cholesterol levels. Doses of 40 mg daily do not appear to have added benefit.

▪ Adverse Effects

No serious adverse effects have been reported. Only mild adverse effects such as nervousness, headache, diarrhea, and insomnia have been reported. In long-term studies of 2 to 4 years, adverse effects occurred in less than 1% of patients. Weight loss, excessive urination, and insomnia were reported.

▪ Drug Interactions

Aspirin, Warfarin, Heparin, Clopidogrel, Ticlopidine, Pentoxifylline. The blood-thinning properties of policosanol may enhance the anticoagulant effects of these agents. Use with extreme caution and monitor closely for bruising and bleeding.

Garlic, Ginkgo, High-Dose Vitamin E. The blood-thinning properties of policosanol may enhance the blood-thinning effects of these agents. Use with extreme caution and monitor the patient closely for bruising and bleeding.

Common name: omega-3 fatty acids (ō-MĔG-ă)
Other names: Fish oils, omega-3 polyunsaturated fatty acids (ω-3 PUFAs)

DESCRIPTION AND ACTIONS

Omega-3 polyunsaturated fatty acids (ω-3 fatty acids) are found in a variety of plant (flaxseed, soybean, walnut, canola) and fish (tuna, salmon, herring, mackerel, sardine) oils. However, it is now recognized that the cardioprotective benefits of ω-3 fatty acids are primarily caused by the eicosapentaenoic acid (EPA) and docosahexaenoic acid (DHA), which are found primarily in fish oils. Alpha-linolenic acid, an ω-3 polyunsaturated fatty acid derived from plant sources, does not demonstrate as much reduction in heart attacks and stroke as do EPA and DHA and is much less studied. Although the exact mechanisms whereby ω-3 fatty acids reduce the incidence of myocardial infarction are unknown, they are thought to prevent dysrhythmias, lower triglycerides, stabilize plaque formation, reduce the risk of blood clot formation, and modestly lower blood pressure.

USES

Omega-3 fatty acids are used for the prevention of myocardial infarction.

❖ NURSING IMPLICATIONS FOR OMEGA-3 FATTY ACIDS

▪ Availability

Omega-3 fatty acid content is highly variable in OTC supplements, ranging from 300 to 2700 mg of EPA-DHA per teaspoonful or capsule. It is also available as a prescription-only product (Lovaza capsules) containing 840 mg of EPA-DHA, which is a highly purified product with a low incidence of adverse effects.

▪ Dosage

The American Heart Association recommends a daily intake of omega-3 fatty acids (Table 47-1).

▪ Adverse Effects

Dyspepsia and eructation (burping or belching) with a fishy aftertaste are the most common problems reported. These adverse effects can be minimized by using a more purified product (more EPA-DHA per serving), taking smaller doses with meals throughout the day, gradually building up the dosage over several weeks, taking enteric-coated tablets, and freezing non–enteric-coated tablets prior to administration.

▪ Comments

Factors to consider in product selection are purity, strength, calories, cholesterol count, and other ingredients, such as vitamins. Different products may need to be tried for optimal benefit to the consumer. More purified products generally have fewer adverse effects, such as a fishy aftertaste, but are usually more expensive. Some products are available with an enteric coating that reduces aftertaste.

Table 47-1	American Heart Association Recommended Daily Intake of Omega-3 Fatty Acids*
PATIENT POPULATION	**RECOMMENDATIONS**
No CHD	Consume a variety of preferably oily fish at least twice weekly.*
CHD present	1 g EPA-DHA daily, preferably from fatty fish (tuna, salmon, herring, mackerel, sardines); use supplements under physician supervision.
Elevated triglyceride levels	2 to 4 g EPA-DHA daily from a supplement under physician supervision.

Data from Kris-Etherton PM, Harris WS, Appel LJ; American Heart Association, Nutrition Committee: Fish consumption, fish oil, omega-3 fatty acids and cardiovascular disease, *Circulation* 106:2747-2757, 2002.
CHD, coronary heart disease; *DHA*, docosahexaenoic acid; *EPA*, eicosapentaenoic acid.
*Pregnant and nursing women and young children should avoid swordfish, shark, king mackerel, and tilefish and limit their consumption of other fish to 12 ounces per week (recommendation of the U.S. Food and Drug Administration).

Labels of supplement products should be read carefully because it is routine to report fish oil content per serving as much higher (e.g., 1000 mg) than it actually is because of including other fish oils (impurities), whereas the actual content of EPA-DHA is only 300 mg (EPA, 180 mg, plus DHA, 120 mg). Carbohydrates are often added as sweetening agents, making the product more palatable, but some products, when used in therapeutic doses, may be a hidden source of over 100 calories daily. Some products also contain cholesterol (an impurity) that can be significant for patients on a reduced cholesterol diet. Vitamin content (sometimes an impurity) can also be a potential for toxicity if the product is being taken in higher doses to treat hypertriglyceridemia.

Common name: S-adenosylmethionine (SAM-e)
 Other names: Sammy, SAM

DESCRIPTION AND ACTIONS

SAM-e is a naturally occurring substance found in all cells of the human body, particularly in the brain and liver. It is produced from ATP, an energy-producing compound, and methionine, an amino acid. SAM-e is involved in a wide range of essential biochemical reactions, including synthesis, activation, and metabolism of hormones, neurotransmitters, proteins, and phospholipids, and deactivation of toxic substances.

USES

As a supplement, SAM-e has been proposed for treating depression, osteoarthritis, and fibromyalgia. It is thought that SAM-e may have a dopaminergic effect in treating depression, but study results have been highly variable and inconclusive. In small studies for the treatment of osteoarthritis, SAM-e has been compared with NSAIDs (e.g., ibuprofen, naproxen, indomethacin) and placebo, and produced mild symptomatic improvement after 2 weeks. Other small studies suggest a possible benefit in relieving symptoms associated with liver disease (e.g., chronic fatigue) and fibromyalgia (e.g., pain, depression, morning stiffness). SAM-e is relatively expensive, so other, more conventional treatments for osteoarthritis and depression are warranted for several weeks before considering courses of SAM-e treatment.

❖ NURSING IMPLICATIONS FOR S-ADENOSYLMETHIONINE

■ Availability

A variety of tablet and capsule dosage forms are available, but it is recommended that the enteric forms that dissolve in the intestines (not the stomach) are more effective. There are two forms of SAM-e: the preferred form is S-adenosylmethionine 1,4-butanedisulfonate (sulfate form) rather than the toluene sulfonate (tosylate) form. There are cases of misleading labeling; for example, 400 mg SAM-e tosylate-disulfate actually contains only 200 mg or less of the preferred sulfate form.

■ Dosage

PO: 400 mg three or four times daily is recommended. Patients should start with lower dosages and gradually increase to a higher dosage to avoid mild stomach distress.

■ Comments

- Do not administer to patients diagnosed with manic depression. SAM-e has been reported to trigger manic episodes in patients with bipolar disease.
- The safety of SAM-e in pregnancy and lactation and in children has not been established, and its use is not recommended.

■ Adverse Effects

No serious adverse effects have been reported. Mild stomach distress has been reported at starting doses of 400 mg three or four times daily.

 Herbal Interactions

S-Adenosylmethionine

ANTIDEPRESSANTS (TRICYCLIC ANTIDEPRESSANTS, SSRIs, MAOIs)
SAM-e may interfere with the actions of these antidepressants or magnify their adverse effects. Combined use of antidepressants and SAM-e should be recommended only by a healthcare provider.

LEVODOPA
It is reported that SAM-e may reduce some of the adverse effects of levodopa used to treat parkinsonism, but it is also thought that SAM-e may reduce the beneficial effects of levodopa in the treatment of parkinsonism over time.

Get Ready for the NCLEX® Examination!

Key Points

- Herbal therapies are as old as the human race. Herbal medicines are defined as those natural substances derived from botanic or plant origin.
- Over the past two decades, there has been a tremendous resurgence in the popularity of self-care and alternative therapies, including acupuncture, aromatherapy, homeopathy, vitamin therapy, and herbal therapy. Some of the more than 250 herbal medicines may be beneficial, but unfortunately the whole field of herbal therapy is fraught with false claims, lack of standardization, and adulteration and misbranding of products.
- Dietary supplement therapy under the current legal standards creates an ethical dilemma for nurses and other healthcare professionals. Licensed healthcare professionals have a moral and ethical responsibility to recommend only medicines that are proven to be safe and effective. Regarding dietary supplements, including herbal medicines, the healthcare professional should be aware of their legal uses versus their popular uses, their potential for toxicity, and their potential for interaction with other medicines.

Additional Learning Resources

SG Go to your Study Guide for additional Review Questions for the NCLEX® Examination, Critical Thinking Clinical Situations, and other learning activities to help you master this chapter content.

evolve Go to your Evolve website (http://evolve .elsevier.com/Clayton) for additional online resources.

Review Questions for the NCLEX® Examination

1. After reviewing the medication history with the patient, the nurse noted that the herbal therapy St. John's wort was on the list. The nurse then made the following correct statement:
   1. "I see you are taking St. John's wort. Please tell me if you think it is working for you."
   2. "I see you are taking St. John's wort. I would advise you to stop immediately, as it is not safe to take."
   3. "I take St. John's wort, too. It works great for me. Tell me, how do you like it?"
   4. "I believe this St. John's wort is available in premade tea bags and also in bulk form."

2. Coenzyme Q10 is used primarily as an adjunctive therapy for which of the following disorders.
   1. Chronic heart failure
   2. Insomnia
   3. Depression
   4. Migraine headaches

3. A patient was discussing with the nurse the dietary supplement melatonin, and stated that he intended to take it to help his recent insomnia. Which statement by the nurse would be appropriate?
   1. "I would recommend that you take it if you wake up after falling asleep, as it will help you get back to sleep."
   2. "It should be okay to take it with other sleeping pills."
   3. "I believe it can be used for treatment of jet lag, as it can help you adjust to changes in time zones."
   4. "I don't believe these dietary supplements work."

4. A pregnant patient came into the clinic and was discussing with the nurse some options for her persistent nausea. She asked the nurse which herbal supplement might help. The nurse responded with:
   1. ginger.
   2. garlic.
   3. feverfew.
   4. ephedra.

5. While teaching a patient about home-going medications, the nurse asked a patient about the use of any dietary supplements or herbal medications. The nurse knows that further education is needed after the patient made this statement:
   1. "I do not take any supplements or over-the-counter medications anymore."
   2. "I heard that there is a new law requiring herbal medicines and supplements to be standardized."
   3. "From what I understand, the herbal medications and dietary supplements have been unproven to work."
   4. "Herbal therapy has been around a long time and involves the use of plant leaves and such to make teas and salves."

Objectives

1. Identify the differences between mild, moderate, and severe substance abuse disorder.
2. Differentiate between the screening instruments for substance use disorders.
3. Cite the responsibilities of professionals who suspect substance abuse by a colleague.
4. Explain the primary long-term goals in the treatment of substance abuse.
5. Identify the withdrawal symptoms for major substances that are commonly abused.

Key Terms

substance use disorder (SŬB-stăns ăb-YŪS) (p. 772)
impairment (ĭm-PĂR-mĕnt) (p. 772)
dependence (dē-PĔN-dĕns) (p. 773)

illicit substance (ĭl-LĬS-ĭt) (p. 773)
intoxication (ĭn-tŏks-ĭ-KĀ-shŭn) (p. 780)

CLASSIFICATION OF SUBSTANCE ABUSE

The new *Diagnostic and Statistical Manual of Mental Disorders,* 5th edition, (*DSM-5*) redefines substance abuse under a new category termed *Substance Use Disorders*, with the specific substance used defining the specific disorder (e.g., alcohol use disorder, cannabis use disorder, inhalant use disorder), each with its own diagnostic criteria. The *DSM-5* groups substances of abuse into 12 categories (Box 48-1). Many other medications taken for therapeutic purposes can induce substance-related disorders as an adverse effect, especially when large doses of the medications are taken (Box 48-2) for longer periods. Symptoms usually disappear when the dosage is lowered or the medication is stopped.

SUBSTANCE USE DISORDERS

The diagnosis of a substance use disorder is based on a pathological pattern of behaviors related to the use of the substance. Over time, an important characteristic of substance use disorders is an underlying change in brain chemistry. The criteria for diagnosis can be subdivided into groupings of impaired control, social impairment, risky use, and pharmacologic criteria (Table 48-1). Substance use disorders occur in a broad range of severity, from mild to severe, based on the number of symptom criteria present. As a general rule, a *mild* substance use disorder has the presence of two or three symptoms, *moderate* four to five symptoms, and *severe* six or more symptoms. Severity can fluctuate over time based on changes in frequency and/or dose of substance use.

A term no longer used in the *DSM-5* diagnostic criteria for substance use disorder is *addiction*, although it is often used in medical and common terminology. There is no true definition of the term addiction, and its use often has negative connotations. The more neutral term *substance use disorder* is used to describe the wide range of the disorder, from a mild form to a severe state of chronically relapsing, compulsive drug taking.

Substance abuse is the periodic, purposeful use of a substance that leads to clinically significant impairment. The impairment results in failure to fulfill major obligations at work, school, or home (e.g., absenteeism, poor work performance, neglect of responsibilities); places the person in physically hazardous situations (e.g., operating a vehicle or machinery when impaired); and creates legal problems (e.g., arrests for intoxication, disorderly conduct) or social problems that are aggravated by the substance (e.g., physical fights, spousal arguments). If the substance use disorder is not stopped, substance abuse may lead to more serious medical conditions known as *tolerance* and *withdrawal*, which are normal physiologic responses to long-term use of substances (see Table 48-1). Symptoms of severe abuse include overwhelming compulsive use, tolerance of higher amounts of the substance, and withdrawal symptoms on discontinuation. A phrase that characterizes chemical dependency is "using a substance to live and living to use." The amount of drug exposure and the frequency of use necessary to develop **dependence** are unknown and highly individual, based on the pharmacology of the drug, emotional condition, heredity, and environmental factors. A term frequently associated with substance abuse is *illicit substance*—any chemical or mixture of chemicals that alters biologic function and is not required to maintain health. The term applies primarily to illegal substances. Any chemical that can produce a pleasurable state of mind has potential for abuse. Commonly abused substances, their pharmacologic effects, their street names, and their potential long-term consequences are listed in Table 48-2.

Substance abuse is a societal issue that plagues many cultures and all races throughout the world. In the United States, as many as one in four individuals meet the criteria for a substance use disorder at some time in their lives. According to the National Survey on Drug Use and Health, an estimated 17.3 million individuals (6.6% of the U.S. population) age 12 and older were classified in 2013 with dependence on, or abused alcohol. The percentage of alcohol dependence

---

Box 48-1	**Substances of Abuse**

- Alcohol (ethanol)
- Caffeine
- Cannabis (marijuana)
- Hallucinogens
- Inhalants
- Opioids
- Phencyclidine (PCP) or similarly acting arylcyclohexylamines
- Sedatives, hypnotics, and anxiolytics
- Stimulants (including amphetamines, cocaine)
- Tobacco
- Other (or unknown) substance-related disorders
- Nonsubstance-related disorder: gambling disorder

Data from the National Institute of Drug Abuse: Commonly Abused Prescription Drugs Chart, 2015, Washington, D.C. Retrieved from www.drugabuse.gov/drugs-abuse/commonly-abused-drugs-charts-0. *American Psychiatric Association: Diagnostic and statistical manual of mental disorders*, ed 5, Washington DC, 2013, American Psychiatric Publishing.

Box 48-2	**Medications Whose Adverse Effects May Induce Substance Abuse**

- Analgesics
- Anesthetics
- Anticholinergic agents
- Anticonvulsants
- Antidepressants
- Antihistamines
- Antihypertensive and cardiovascular medications
- Antimicrobial medications
- Antiparkinsonian medications
- Chemotherapeutic agents
- Corticosteroids
- Gastrointestinal medications
- Muscle relaxants
- Nonsteroidal antiinflammatory drugs

Data from the National Institute of Drug Abuse: Commonly Abused Prescription Drugs Chart, 2015, Washington, D.C. Retrieved from www.drugabuse.gov/drugs-abuse/commonly-abused-drugs-charts-0.

Table 48-1	**Measures of Substance Use Disorders**

GROUPING	DESCRIPTION
Impaired Control	Intake of substance in larger quantities or over a longer time period than originally planned or prescribed. The desire to cut down substance use may exist along with multiple unsuccessful attempts to reduce or discontinue use. Substantial time spent in obtaining, using or recovering from the effects of the substance. Craving exhibited by a powerful urge for the substance; more common in circumstances in which the substance was used before.
Social Impairment	Failure to meet responsibilities at work, school, or home because of recurrent substance use. Substance use continues despite repeated social or interpersonal problems caused by the effects of the substance. Reduction or cessation of important social, occupational or recreational pursuits because of substance use. Withdrawal from family activities and hobbies to use the substance.
Risky Use	Repeated substance use even when in settings or circumstances where doing so may be physically risky. Continued substance use regardless of known recurrent physical or psychological problems caused by or worsened by the substance. (Failure to abstain despite the problems it is causing.)
Pharmacologic	Development of tolerance manifested by the necessity to consume larger quantities to reach the desired effect, or a reduced effect achieved when the usual dose is consumed. Development of withdrawal symptoms occurs when blood levels decline. Symptoms vary widely across the classes of substances.

Data from American Psychiatric Association: *Diagnostic and statistical manual of mental disorders*, ed 5, Washington DC, 2013, American Psychiatric Publishing, pp 483-484.

Table 48-2 — Substances of Abuse: Psychoactive Drugs Identification Chart

DRUGS	MEDICAL USES	MEDICAL NAMES	SLANG NAMES	FORMS	USUAL METHOD OF ADMINISTRATION
Stimulants					
Nicotine	None	Nicotine	Butt, chew, smoke, cig	Pipe, tobacco, cigarettes, snuff	Sniff, chew, smoke
Caffeine	Hyperkinesis, stimulant	Caffeine	Java, cup of joe, morning thunder	Chocolates, tea, soft drinks, coffee	Swallow
Amphetamines	Hyperkinesis, narcolepsy, weight control, mental disorders	Dexedrine, Benzedrine	Speed, bennies, dexies, pep pills; crank, crystal, Meth	Capsules, liquid, tablets, powder	Inject, swallow; inhale
Cocaine	Local anesthetic	Cocaine	Coke, rock, crack, blow, tool, white, blast, snow, flake	Powder, rock	Inject, smoke, inhale
Depressants					
Alcohol	None	Ethyl alcohol	Booze	Liquid	Swallow
Sedatives	Anesthetic, sedative-hypnotic, anticonvulsant	Secobarbital, phenobarbital, Seconal	Barbs, reds, downers, spoors	Capsules, tablets, powder	Inject, swallow
Tranquilizers	Antianxiety, sedative-hypnotic	Valium, Librium, Meprobamate	Downers	Capsules, tablets	Swallow
Narcotics					
Opium	Analgesic, antidiarrheal	Paregoric	Midnight oil, tar, hop	Powder	Smoke, swallow
Morphine	Analgesic, antitussive	Morphine	None	Powder, tablet, liquid	Inject, smoke, swallow
Heroin	Research	Diacetylmorphine	China white, smack, junk, H, horse	Powder	Inject, swallow
Codeine	Analgesic, antitussive	Codeine, Empirin compound with codeine, Robitussin AC	None	Capsules, tablets, liquid	Inject, swallow
Cannabis					
THC	Research, cancer chemotherapy antinauseant	Tetrahydrocannabinol	THC	Tablets, liquid	Swallow
Hashish	None	Tetrahydrocannabinol	Hash	Solid resin	Smoke
Marijuana	Research	Tetrahydrocannabinol	Pot, grass, doobie, ganja, dope, gold, herb, weed, reefer	Plant particles	Smoke, swallow

EFFECTS SOUGHT	POSSIBLE EFFECTS	OVERDOSAGE	LONG-TERM EFFECTS
Relaxation	Respiratory difficulties, fatigue, high blood pressure	None	Dependency, lung cancer, heart attacks, respiratory ailments
Alertness	Increased alertness, pulse rate, blood pressure; excitation, insomnia, loss of appetite	Irritability	Dependency may aggravate organic actions
Alertness, activeness	Increased alertness, pulse rate, and blood pressure; excitation, insomnia, loss of appetite	Agitation, increase in body temperature, hallucinations, convulsions, possible death	Severe withdrawal, possible convulsions, toxic psychosis; periodontitis, advanced tooth decay; dermatitis
Excitation, euphoria	Increased alertness, pulse rate, and blood pressure; excitation, insomnia, loss of appetite	Agitation, increase in body temperature, hallucinations, convulsions, possible death	Dependency, depression, paranoia, convulsions
Sense alteration, anxiety reduction	Loss of coordination, sluggishness, slurred speech, disorientation, depression	Total loss of coordination, nausea, unconsciousness, possible death	Dependency, toxic psychosis, neurologic damage
Anxiety reduction, euphoria, sleep	Loss of coordination, sluggishness, slurred speech, disorientation, depression	Cold clammy skin, dilated pupils, shallow respiration, weak and rapid pulse, coma, possible death	Dependency, severe withdrawal, possible convulsions, toxic psychosis
Anxiety reduction, euphoria, sleep	Loss of coordination, sluggishness, slurred speech, disorientation, depression	Cold clammy skin, dilated pupils, shallow respiration, weak and rapid pulse, coma, possible death	Dependency, severe withdrawal, possible convulsions, toxic psychosis
Euphoria, prevent withdrawal, sleep	Euphoria, drowsiness, respiratory depression, constricted pupils, sleep, nausea	Clammy skin, slow and shallow breathing, convulsions, coma, possible death	Dependency, constipation, loss of appetite, severe withdrawal
Euphoria, prevent withdrawal, sleep	Euphoria, drowsiness, respiratory depression, constricted pupils, sleep, nausea	Clammy skin, slow and shallow breathing, convulsions, coma, possible death	Dependency, constipation, loss of appetite, severe withdrawal
Euphoria, prevent withdrawal, sleep	Euphoria, drowsiness, respiratory depression, constricted pupils, sleep, nausea	Clammy skin, slow and shallow breathing, convulsions, coma, possible death	Dependency, constipation, loss of appetite, severe withdrawal
Euphoria, prevent withdrawal, sleep	Euphoria, drowsiness, respiratory depression, constricted pupils, sleep, nausea	Clammy skin, slow and shallow breathing, convulsions, coma, possible death	Dependency, constipation, loss of appetite, severe withdrawal
Relaxation, euphoria, increased perception	Relaxed inhibitions, euphoria, increased appetite, distorted perceptions, disoriented behavior	Fatigue, paranoia, possible psychosis	Amotivational syndrome, respiratory difficulties, lung cancer, interference with physical and emotional development
Relaxation, euphoria, increased perception	Relaxed inhibitions, euphoria, increased appetite, distorted perceptions, disoriented behavior	Fatigue, paranoia, possible psychosis	Amotivational syndrome, respiratory difficulties, lung cancer, interference with physical and emotional development
Relaxation, euphoria, increased perception	Relaxed inhibitions, euphoria, increased appetite, distorted perceptions, disoriented behavior	Fatigue, paranoia, possible psychosis	Amotivational syndrome, respiratory difficulties, lung cancer, interference with physical and emotional development

Continued

Table 48-2	Substances of Abuse—cont'd				
DRUGS	**MEDICAL USES**	**MEDICAL NAMES**	**SLANG NAMES**	**FORMS**	**USUAL METHOD OF ADMINISTRATION**
Hallucinogens					
PCP	None	Phencyclidine	Angel dust, zoot, peace pill, hog	Tablets, powder	Smoke, swallow
LSD	Research	Lysergic acid diethylamide	Acid, sugar	Capsules, tablets, liquid	Swallow
Organics	None	Mescaline, psilocybin	Mesc, mushroom	Crude preparations, tablets, powder	Swallow
Inhalants					
Aerosols and solvents	None	None	Glue, benzene, toluene, Freon	Solvents, aerosols	Inhale

For more information, contact the Florida Alcohol and Drug Abuse Association Resource Center, 1030 E. Lafayette St., Suite 100, Tallahassee, FL, 32301.
From the Center for Substance Abuse Prevention: *Curriculum modules on alcohol and other drug problems for schools of social work,* Rockville, MD, 1995, Center for Substance Abuse Prevention.

or abuse decreased from 7.5% in 2009 to 6.6% in 2013. This decrease was found for adolescents aged 12-17 and your adults aged 18-25 but not for those in older age groups. During this same time period, 2.6 million persons (2.6% of the U.S. population) age 12 or older were dependent on or abused illicit drugs. This percentage has not changed significantly since 2009. (SAMSHA, 2014).

SIGNS OF IMPAIRMENT

When signs of impairment start showing, it is usually not one sign alone, but a cluster that raises questions of an impairment problem. The disease is usually first manifested in family life (e.g., domestic violence, separation, financial problems, problem behavior in children) and then in social life (e.g., overt public intoxication; isolation from friends, peers, church). Physical and mental changes may be manifested by excessive tiredness, multiple illnesses, frequent injuries or accidents, and emotional crises. Deterioration in physical status is an important sign, but occurs late in the disease. Flagrant evidence of impairment at the worksite is relatively rare and usually occurs after the disease is advanced. In many cases, the workplace is the source of the drug of choice, so the impaired person will strive to protect the source with appropriate behavior.

SCREENING FOR ALCOHOL AND SUBSTANCE ABUSE

Because of the large number of health problems associated with alcohol and substance abuse, *Healthy People 2020*, the U.S. Preventive Services Task Force, the American Medical Association, and the American Nurses Association support and encourage screening patients for alcohol and other substance abuse. Screening instruments for substance abuse can be divided into the following four categories: (1) comprehensive drug abuse screening and assessment; (2) brief drug abuse screening; (3) alcohol abuse screening; and (4) drug and alcohol abuse screening for use with adolescents (Table 48-3). All the screening instruments listed have been validated for accuracy for specific purposes (e.g., differentiating between early detection of excessive drinking versus alcoholism; the potential for a substance use disorder). Another example of assessment for specific purposes is the Drug Abuse Screening Test, which can be used to differentiate among alcohol problems only, drug problems only, and both drug and alcohol problems. Some instruments are designed to be administered through an interview by a trained health professional, whereas others are designed for self-assessment by the patient using pencil and paper or computer entry. It is crucial that the proper assessment instrument be selected for use with a specific patient to attain meaningful results for an appropriate diagnosis. A disadvantage of some of the comprehensive screening instruments is the length of time required to administer the assessment and the availability of a qualified data interpreter. Many of the comprehensive instruments have been modified to be used as quick-screening instruments. A four-question assessment for alcohol abuse commonly used in the primary care setting because of its ease of administration is the CAGE questionnaire. CAGE (*c*ut down, *a*nnoyed, *g*uilty, and *e*ye opener) is an acronym that provides the interviewer with a quick reminder of questions to be asked about the patient's feelings

EFFECTS SOUGHT	POSSIBLE EFFECTS	OVERDOSAGE	LONG-TERM EFFECTS
Distortion of sense, insight, exhilaration	Illusions and hallucinations, distorted perception of time and distance	Longer and more intense "trips" or episodes, psychosis, convulsions, possible death	May intensify existing psychosis, flashbacks, panic reactions
Distortion of sense, insight, exhilaration	Illusions and hallucinations, distorted perception of time and distance	Longer and more intense "trips" or episodes, psychosis, convulsions, possible death	May intensify existing psychosis, flashbacks, panic reactions
Distortion of sense, insight, exhilaration	Illusions and hallucinations, distorted perception of time and distance	Longer and more intense "trips" or episodes, psychosis, convulsions, possible death	May intensify existing psychosis, flashbacks, panic reactions
Intoxication	Exhilaration, confusion, poor concentration	Heart failure, unconsciousness, asphyxiation, possible death	Impaired perception, coordination, and judgment; neurologic damage

Table 48-3 Screening Instruments for Substance Abuse

NAME OF INSTRUMENT	ACRONYM	NAME OF INSTRUMENT	ACRONYM
Comprehensive Drug Abuse Screening and Assessment Instruments		**Alcohol Abuse Screening Instruments**	
		CAGE	CAGE
Addiction Severity Index	ASI	Michigan Alcohol Screening Test	MAST
Alcohol, Smoking and Substance Involvement Screening Test	ASSIST	Millon Clinical Multiaxial Inventory	MCMI
		Millon Clinical Multiaxial Inventory Alcohol Dependence Scale	MCMI-III
Alcohol Use Disorders Identification Test	AUDIT		
Composite International Diagnostic Interview Substance Abuse Module	CIDI-SAM	Short Michigan Alcohol Screening Test	SMAST
		Drug and Alcohol Screening Instruments for Adolescents	
Drug Abuse Screening Test	DAST	Adolescent Alcohol Involvement Scale	AAIS
Drug Use Screening Inventory	DUSI	Adolescent Drug Abuse Diagnosis	ADAD
Individual Assessment Profile	IAP	Adolescent Drinking Inventory	ADI
MacAndrew Scale	MAC	Adolescent Drug Involvement Scale	ADIS
Millon Clinical Multiaxial Inventory	MCMI	Comprehensive Adolescent Severity Inventory	CASI
Minnesota Multiphasic Personality Inventory	MMPI		
Minnesota Multiphasic Personality Inventory-2	MMPI-2	Drug and Alcohol Quick Screen	DAP
Brief Drug Abuse Screening Instruments		Home, Education/Employment, Activities, Drugs, Sexuality, Suicide/Depression	HEADSS
CAGE–Adapted to Include Drugs	CAGE-AID		
Millon Clinical Multiaxial Inventory	MCMI	Home, Education, Abuse, Drugs, Safety, Friends, Image, Recreation, Sexuality, and Threats	HEADS FIRST
Millon Clinical Multiaxial Inventory Drug Dependence Scale	MCMI-III		
Minnesota Multiphasic Personality Inventory–2	MMPI-2	Problem-Oriented Screening Instrument for Teenagers	POSIT
Addiction Potential Scale	API		
Addiction Acknowledgment Scale	AAS		
Screening Instrument of Substance Abuse Potential	SISAP		
Short Michigan Alcohol Screening Test—Adapted to Include Drugs	SMAST-AID		

Modified from McPherson TL, Hersch PK: Brief substance use screening instruments for primary care settings: A review, *J Subst Abuse Treat* 18:193-202, 2000.

toward his or her intake of substances (Ewing, 1984). A disadvantage of many of the instruments is that they were developed using adult male patients and have not been validated in special populations (e.g., women, older adults, and adolescents).

HEALTH PROFESSIONALS AND SUBSTANCE ABUSE

Although the prevalence of substance abuse among physicians, nurses, pharmacists, and other health professionals is not precisely known, it is probably similar to that of the general population. There is thought to be more prescription drug use and less street drug use because of easier access to prescription drugs. It is a misperception that education somehow protects healthcare professions from substance use disorders because "they know better." An individual's inability to manage stress brought on by intense patient care practice, managing more patients with the same resources, zero tolerance for making a mistake in association with the expectation of 100% perfection, and financial debt are thought to be major contributing factors to substance abuse among healthcare professionals.

Healthcare professionals are responsible for maintaining a code of ethics and standards of care, and the inappropriate use of substances puts these principles in jeopardy. Signs that raise suspicion of substance abuse include behavioral changes (e.g., wearing long-sleeved garments all the time, diminished alertness, lack of attention to hygiene, mood swings) and performance deterioration (e.g., requests for frequent schedule changes, errors in clinical judgment, excessive absenteeism, frank odor of alcohol on the breath and attempts to camouflage it with breath fresheners, frequent or long breaks, or deterioration in professional practice and patient care).

If a healthcare professional suspects that a colleague is impaired, a confidential report should be made to an appropriate supervisor familiar with institutional policy. An investigation should be initiated; observation and documentation are crucial to building a record of repeat instances over time to support the suspicion of impairment. Because of faulty memory on the part of the impaired individual, examples of inappropriate actions need to be well documented over time. An accurate record can also be useful in helping the impaired individual recognize the problem and submit voluntarily to treatment.

When considering whether to report a colleague for suspected drug abuse, remember the following:
- Clinical practice is a privilege, not a right.
- Good-faith reporting should not be considered unfair or disloyal to a colleague; protecting patients and the profession from harm should be paramount.
- It is very unlikely that an individual making a confidential report to a supervisor will be sued if a reasonable effort is made to establish that the concerns are legitimate and it is clear that patient safety is the primary concern.
- An unreported colleague is more likely than a reported one to die as a result of the impairment (from suicide, accidental overdose, other accident, disease, or violence).
- Colleagues who are reported to licensing authorities (especially those who self-report) have a very good chance of retaining their license and salvaging their careers.
- If a healthcare professional has knowledge of suspected impairment of another healthcare professional but fails to report it, that healthcare professional may potentially be named in a civil lawsuit or be named as a contributor in a malpractice suit against the impaired healthcare provider.
- In some states, if impairment of a colleague is suspected, filing a report with the licensing authority is mandatory. Failure to do so may result in a reprimand or probation from the licensing authority.

LEGAL CONSIDERATIONS OF SUBSTANCE ABUSE AND DEPENDENCE

All states have laws pertaining to the reporting of impairment of healthcare workers. Some require that suspected impairment be reported to the healthcare professional's licensure or disciplinary board. Other states allow referral to a professional society's impairment committee, which then contracts with the impaired individual to participate in a recovery program. As long as the healthcare professional continues to participate, the committee can refrain from notifying the licensure board.

The healthcare professional who makes a conscious effort to be treated for a substance use disorder has a variety of legal protections that can be helpful to reestablishing a career. The Americans with Disabilities Act (ADA) (1992) defines a disabled person as one "with a physical or mental impairment seriously limiting one or more major life activities." People dependent on drugs, but who are no longer using drugs illegally and are receiving treatment for chemical dependence or who have been rehabilitated successfully, are protected by the ADA from discrimination on the basis of past drug addiction. However, a substance abuser whose current use of chemicals impairs job performance or conduct may be disciplined, discharged, or denied employment to the extent that this person is not a "qualified individual with a disability." An individual who is currently engaging in the illegal use of drugs is not an "individual with a disability" under the ADA. State and federal handicap laws also mandate that every employer, including healthcare institutions, ensure that each recovering chemically impaired individual who applies for employment or reinstatement be afforded the same protection received by anyone with a handicap.

Once a chemically dependent person has been through treatment, an ongoing monitoring program is routinely established to help ensure that the person is free of the abused substance. Urinalysis for drugs is the most common form of drug testing. The Drug-Free Workplace Act of 1988 encourages (but does not require) drug screening in an effort to provide drug-free workplaces. The Drug-Free Schools and Communities Act Amendments of 1989 extend this act to all educational institutions.

The Supreme Court has ruled that drug screening does not violate one's constitutional right to privacy or represent unreasonable search. Drug screening may be required for employment and can be requested for cause (e.g., suspicious behavior, arrest, after an accident), or a random test can be requested as a part of a return-to-work agreement for people in recovery. A positive drug test means that the reported drug is present in the specimen. It does not establish that the person is dependent on the drug, and it does not, by itself, prove the drug was the cause of an impaired performance.

EDUCATING HEALTHCARE PROFESSIONALS ABOUT SUBSTANCE ABUSE

The curricula of healthcare profession educational programs should ensure that all students have multiple opportunities during their development of professional attitudes and behaviors to consider and formulate values about self-medication and substance abuse consistent with professional and legal standards. Employers should make available drug abuse resources, such as information about employee assistance programs and policies, professional recovery assistance (e.g., recovery networks), and educational opportunities. Prevention of drug misuse, whether it is illegal or inappropriate use or drug abuse, is an important priority in the practice of every healthcare profession.

PRINCIPLES OF TREATMENT FOR SUBSTANCE ABUSE

It is important to recognize that substance-related disorders as described in *DSM-5* cover 10 separate classes of drugs and are considered treatable disorders. This focus is essential to successful treatment. The American Psychiatric Association lists long-term goals in treating substance abuse as follows:

- Reduction or abstinence in the use and effects of substances
- Reduction in the frequency and severity of relapse
- Improvement in psychological and social functioning

By the time a person seeks treatment for substance abuse or is ordered into a treatment program by the courts, the illness has become very complex, affecting almost every aspect of the person's life. Treatment requires lifelong effort, with a combination of psychosocial support and sometimes pharmacologic treatment. Key factors associated with long-term recovery are negative consequences of substance use (e.g., deteriorating health, divorce, loss of job, problems with family and friends) and social and community support, particularly with participation by self-help organizations whose goals include total abstinence of substances being abused (e.g., Alcoholics Anonymous, Narcotics Anonymous, Women for Sobriety, Rational Recovery). The types of social support given by the 12-step programs (e.g., Alcoholics Anonymous, Narcotics Anonymous), such as 24-hour availability when cravings arise, networking, role modeling, and advice on abstinence based on direct personal experiences, appear to be primary characteristics for success in maintaining recovery (Box 48-3).

Diagnostic criteria for assessment of substance use disorders are defined in the *DSM-5*. A combination of interviews, screening tools (see Table 48-3), information from colleagues, and laboratory tests will determine whether there is a single diagnosis of abuse of

---

Box 48-3   The 12 Steps of Alcoholics Anonymous

1. We admitted we were powerless over alcohol—that our lives had become unmanageable.
2. Came to believe that a Power greater than ourselves could restore us to sanity.
3. Made a decision to turn our will and our lives over to the care of God as we understood Him.
4. Made a searching and fearless moral inventory of ourselves.
5. Admitted to God, to ourselves, and to another human being the exact nature of our wrongs.
6. Were entirely ready to have God remove all these defects of character.
7. Humbly asked Him to remove our shortcomings.
8. Made a list of all people we had harmed, and became willing to make amends to them all.
9. Made direct amends to such people wherever possible, except when to do so would injure them or others.
10. Continued to take personal inventory and when we were wrong promptly admitted it.
11. Sought through prayer and meditation to improve our conscious contact with God as we understood Him, praying only for knowledge of His will for us and the power to carry that out.
12. Having had a spiritual awakening as the result of these steps, we tried to carry this message to alcoholics and to practice these principles in all our affairs.

From Alcoholics Anonymous World Services, Inc. The Twelve Steps are reprinted with permission of Alcoholics Anonymous World Services, Inc. (AAWS). Permission to reprint the Twelve Steps does not mean that AAWS has reviewed or approved the contents of this publication, or that AAWS necessarily agrees with the views expressed herein. AA is a program of recovery from alcoholism only; use of the Twelve Steps in connection with programs and activities patterned after AA but which address other problems or in any other non-AA context, does not imply otherwise.

one or more substances or if there are multiple diagnoses. Other psychiatric conditions (e.g., depression, psychosis, delirium, dementia) and medical conditions (e.g., anemia, cirrhosis, hepatic encephalopathy, nutrition deficiencies, cardiomyopathy) may be induced by substance abuse. Based on the findings, priorities must be assigned. Immediate medical needs must be addressed first (e.g., thiamine deficiency, withdrawal and detoxification, safety). Detoxification programs are an important first step in substance abuse treatment. Detoxification initiates abstinence, reduces the severity of withdrawal symptoms, and retains the person in treatment to forestall relapse. During detoxification, behavioral interventions (e.g., contingency management, motivational enhancement, and cognitive therapies) can also be started.

ALCOHOL

In the United States, the Behavior Risk Factor Surveillance System sponsored by the Centers for Disease Control and Prevention (CDC) (2010) reports that binge drinking, defined as five or more drinks on one or more occasions in the past month, is reported to have occurred in approximately 15% of the survey population from 1990 to 2010. Recent studies indicate that the frequency of binge drinking appears to be rising on college campuses. Chronic drinking—defined as two or more drinks per day or more than 60 drinks per month—is rising. The median in 1990 was 3.2% of the survey population, grew to 5.9% in 2002, and was reported as 5.0% in 2010. It has climbed to 6.7% (15.1 million individuals) in 2013. (SAMSHA, 2014). A common characteristic of alcohol abusers is denial of a problem. Individuals who abuse alcohol may continue to consume alcohol despite the knowledge that continued consumption poses a significant social and health hazard to themselves.

Research over the past 25 years indicates that with *acute* ingestion of alcohol, the central nervous system (CNS) depressant effects of alcohol come from release of the major inhibitory neurotransmitter gamma-aminobutyric acid (GABA) and suppression of the major excitatory neurotransmitter, glutamate, a byproduct of the *N*-methyl-d-aspartate (NMDA) receptors. With long-term *chronic* ingestion, the reverse occurs: tolerance to alcohol leads to reduced GABAergic activity and higher levels of NMDA activity. There are also inconsistent effects on the serotonin, dopamine, and opioid receptors of the CNS that may account for some of the acute and chronic effects of alcohol ingestion. Stimulation of opioid and dopamine receptors appears to be related to the alcohol "high," or the rewarding aspects of drinking alcohol.

Intoxication

Alcohol abuse, or more appropriately ethanol abuse, is commonly called *alcohol intoxication*. **Intoxication** is defined as the ingestion of ethanol to the point of clinically significant maladaptive behavioral or psycho-logical changes (e.g., inappropriate sexual or aggressive behavior, mood lability, impaired judgment, impaired social or occupational functioning). These changes are accompanied by evidence of slurred speech, incoordination, unsteady gait, nystagmus, impairment in attention or memory, or stupor or coma (*DSM-5*, 2013).

Withdrawal

When alcohol is ingested in quantities leading to intoxication, symptoms of overindulgence (e.g., "hangover," queasy stomach, headache) are common over the next several hours because of direct toxic effects on body cells. If a person frequently drinks to intoxication over long periods (i.e., months to years), a physical dependence develops and a decrease in the blood alcohol level over 4 to 12 hours may cause symptoms of alcohol withdrawal. Development of withdrawal symptoms and craving often induces the person to continue to abuse alcohol (see Figure 48-1 for symptoms and a time sequence of alcohol withdrawal). The person may no longer get much effect from the alcohol other than its ability to prevent withdrawal.

Alcohol withdrawal symptoms can begin within a few hours of discontinuation of drinking and may continue for 3 to 10 days. Withdrawal can progress to more severe symptoms, including visual and auditory hallucinations and seizures (usually of the tonic-clonic type). Less than 10% of patients develop delirium tremens (the DTs), the worst of the withdrawal symptoms. This syndrome is manifested by hyperactivity, delirium, and severe hyperthermia. The mortality rate of patients who progress to DTs is 20%, most commonly as a result of stroke or cardiovascular collapse. Because it is difficult to predict who may have severe withdrawal, anyone experiencing alcohol withdrawal should be observed closely and treated if necessary.

Treatment

Patients who appear to be developing withdrawal symptoms should be quickly assessed for hydration and electrolyte and nutritional status. Excessive loss of fluids and electrolytes may occur through vomiting, sweating, and hyperthermia. Dehydration also may be caused by inadequate fluid intake and diuresis during prolonged and heavy alcohol consumption. Thiamine and multiple vitamins should be administered routinely to patients in alcohol withdrawal. Intravenous (IV) fluid therapy for rehydration may be necessary, but thiamine must be administered before glucose infusion to prevent Wernicke's encephalopathy.

If a person with an alcohol-related disorder seeks treatment for withdrawal symptoms, benzodiazepines (e.g., diazepam, chlordiazepoxide, clorazepate, oxazepam, lorazepam) are commonly used for detoxification because they enhance GABA activity that has been suppressed by chronic alcohol ingestion. The benzodiazepines are effective in sedating and controlling autonomic hyperactivity and reducing seizure risk in

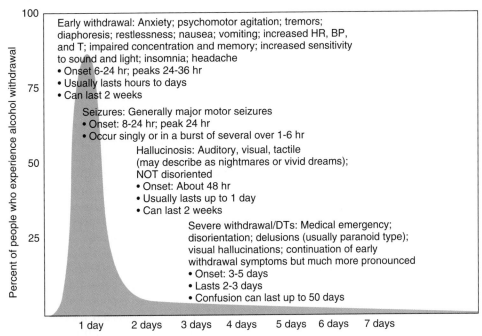

FIGURE 48-1 Alcohol withdrawal syndrome. (From Stuart GW: Principles and practice of psychiatric nursing, ed 10, St. Louis, 2013, Mosby.)

patients experiencing alcohol withdrawal. They are not effective in treating or controlling delirium.

There are two approaches for benzodiazepine dosing in treating withdrawal symptoms. The fixed-dose schedule uses a set dose of benzodiazepine administered at specific intervals. Usually, at about the second day, smaller tapering doses of benzodiazepines are administered on a fixed schedule. The symptom-triggered schedule depends on the use of a rating scale such as the Clinical Institute Withdrawal Assessment–Alcohol, Revised (CIWA-AR). The CIWA-AR protocol calls for administration of a benzodiazepine when the patient shows certain symptoms (symptom-triggered regimen) rather than a fixed-schedule regimen. It is hypothesized that the symptom-triggered medication regimen significantly reduces the amount of medication given and may shorten the length of treatment necessary.

The longer-acting benzodiazepines (e.g., chlordiazepoxide, diazepam, clorazepate) offer advantages of less fluctuation in blood levels and appear to be associated with fewer rebound effects and fewer withdrawal seizures on discontinuation. Because of the longer half-lives and active metabolites, patients taper themselves off just by discontinuing the dosage. The short-acting benzodiazepines (e.g., oxazepam, lorazepam) have the advantage of having no active metabolites that may produce additional adverse effects in older adults or those with concurrent liver disease. They do, however, have to be administered more often, and tapering may be required. Carbamazepine is also effective in decreasing seizure frequency and some of the psychiatric symptoms associated with withdrawal (e.g., anxiety, agitation). Beta blockers (e.g., atenolol, propranolol)

and an alpha agonist such as clonidine may reduce craving and decrease the severity of withdrawal symptoms.

Relapse Prevention

Lifelong effort with a combination of psychosocial support and sometimes pharmacologic treatment is necessary to prevent relapse. Key factors associated with long-term recovery are social and community support through participation with self-help organizations and negative consequences of substance use (e.g., job loss, divorce, loss of child custody). Current treatments are effective for about 50% of patients and significantly reduce the cost of health care, morbidity, and mortality associated with alcoholism.

Three medicines have been approved for use in helping to promote abstinence. Disulfiram (Antabuse) (later in this chapter) helps reduce the desire for alcohol by inducing nausea and vomiting (disulfiram reaction) if alcohol is ingested while disulfiram is being taken. Reactions can be severe, so it is essential that the patient understand the consequences of drinking alcohol while taking the medicine. It also means that the patient must avoid alcohol taken in the form of medicines (e.g., cough and cold elixirs, nighttime sedatives, mouthwashes), soups and sauces containing cooking sherry, and aftershave lotions or perfumes that contain alcohol that can be absorbed through the skin. Success with disulfiram very much depends on adherence to the medication regimen, and many alcoholics become lax in taking their medication as prescribed.

Naltrexone (ReVia) (see Chapter 19) is an opioid antagonist prescribed to block the pharmacologic effects of the high associated with opioids and alcohol. Studies report less alcohol craving and fewer drinking days, especially when naltrexone is combined with psychosocial treatment. Success is somewhat limited with naltrexone, because although it blocks the high from drinking, it provides no relief or promise of reward against the emotions that trigger the desire to drink in the first place.

Acamprosate (Campral) (later in this chapter) is the newest agent available to help individuals maintain abstinence from alcohol. It enhances abstinence and reduces drinking rates in alcohol-dependent patients who are abstinent at the beginning of treatment. It is neither a sedative nor an anxiolytic, and it is not habit forming. Unlike naltrexone, it does not reduce the rewarding effects of alcohol, and unlike disulfiram, it does not cause nausea and vomiting when alcohol is consumed. Studies indicate similar rates of success with naltrexone and acamprosate and a slightly higher success rate when used together.

OPIOIDS

Commonly abused opiates (i.e., derived from opium) are heroin, morphine, hydromorphone (Dilaudid), codeine, oxycodone, and hydrocodone, as well as the synthetic opiatelike (opioid) substances such as methadone, meperidine, fentanyl, pentazocine, buprenorphine, and butorphanol. Heroin is a street drug derived from opium; there are no approved medicinal uses for heroin. Heroin use has been growing in recent years because it is now available in a purer form. Improved purity means a heroin user can get high from smoking or sniffing heroin and can avoid injecting it. There is also a misconception that inhaling heroin does not lead to dependence. As many as 40% of individuals who initially sniff heroin become IV users of it. The other opiates and opioids are made by legitimate manufacturers in specific concentrations for prescription use as anesthetics, analgesics, antidiarrheal agents, and cough suppressants, but have been diverted from medicinal use into the illicit drug market for pleasure and profit. Obtaining prescriptions from one or more healthcare providers simultaneously for fake or exaggerated medical conditions (e.g., "severe" pain, back injury) is another mechanism of acquisition for illicit use by abusers. Healthcare providers who abuse opioids may write prescriptions for self-use or steal medicines intended for other patients or from pharmacy or floor stock. The National Center for Health Statistics show drug overdose deaths increased for the eleventh consecutive year in 2010 (CDC, 2012). Opioids (75.2%), benzodiazepines (29.4%), antidepressants (17.6%), and antiepileptic and antiparkinson drugs (7.8%) were the pharmaceuticals (prescription medicines used for nonmedical uses) that accounted for over 38,000 deaths in 2010. More people are dying annually now from prescription drug overdoses than from illicit street drug abuse (heroin, cocaine, amphetamines).

Intoxication

Indications of opioid intoxication are the presence of inappropriate behaviors after administration, such as initial euphoria (high) followed by apathy, dysphoria, agitation, impaired judgment, and/or impaired social and occupational functioning. Additional signs are pupillary constriction (miosis) and one or more of the following: drowsiness, slurred speech, and impairment of attention and memory. Intoxicated people also may show an indifference to placing themselves in potentially hazardous situations. The extent to which an intoxicated person shows these signs and symptoms depends on the dosage taken, route of administration, frequency of use, and acquired tolerance. Intoxication will usually last for several hours but depends on the half-life of the drug taken and the frequency of readministration of the opioid. Overdosage, especially with street drugs in which the concentration of drug is not known, can lead to severe intoxication manifested by coma, respiratory depression, pupillary dilation (mydriasis), and death.

Withdrawal

All opioids produce similar signs and symptoms of withdrawal. Onset of withdrawal symptoms in opioid-dependent people is somewhat predictable based on the half-life of the drug being abused; the symptoms begin two or three half-lives after the last dose has been taken. Onset of withdrawal symptoms from heroin or morphine is usually within 6 to 12 hours after the last dose, whereas it may take 2 to 4 days following discontinuation of longer-acting drugs such as methadone. Onset of withdrawal for people who abuse a variety of drugs and alcohol is extremely variable. Physical signs and symptoms associated with withdrawal are anxiety and restlessness, increased blood pressure and pulse, pupillary dilation, rhinorrhea, sweating, nausea, vomiting, and diarrhea. In severe cases, piloerection and fever may be present. Subjectively, the person may complain of an achy feeling, often located in the back and legs, an increased sensitivity to pain, and drug-seeking behavior (craving). Acute withdrawal symptoms from short-acting opiates (e.g., heroin) usually peak in 1 to 3 days and dissipate over the next 5 to 7 days. Chronic withdrawal symptoms (e.g., insomnia, anxiety, drug craving, apathy toward the pleasures in life [anhedonia]) may require weeks to months to dissipate.

Treatment

Withdrawal from opioids is uncomfortable but usually not life threatening unless there are coexisting medical conditions. Treatment is focused on relieving the acute symptoms. Clonidine (see Chapter 22 Alpha-1 Adrenergic Blocking Agents) is useful for decreasing tremors, sweating, and agitation; cyclobenzaprine (see Table 44-1, p. 682) reduces skeletal muscle spasms; and dicyclomine (see Table 12-5, p. 184 and Table 32-4, p. 505) reduces gastrointestinal cramping and diarrhea. A protocol such as the Clinical Institute Narcotic Assessment rating scale is helpful for assessing and monitoring a patient undergoing opioid withdrawal.

Another approach to treatment of opioid dependence is the substitution of another opioid, usually long-acting methadone, to reduce the severity of withdrawal symptoms. Once the person has been detoxified from the abused opiate substance, the methadone can be tapered gradually to allow the person to be drug free. The long half-life of the methadone requires that the taper be prolonged over several weeks.

Another treatment alternative is an opioid maintenance program. The patient is started on methadone to minimize withdrawal symptoms. Instead of being tapered off the methadone, however, the person is maintained on a daily dose to prevent the development of withdrawal symptoms. The benefits to this approach are that the person can be maintained on a stable dosage without tolerance and substantial craving developing and can function more normally in the work and home environment, although still addicted to an opiate. Opioid maintenance programs have been shown to reduce opioid use, criminal activity, and the transmission of human immunodeficiency virus (HIV) and hepatitis in opioid-dependent people.

Relapse Prevention

As with alcoholism, a lifelong effort with a combination of psychosocial support and sometimes pharmacologic treatment is necessary to prevent relapse. Key factors associated with long-term recovery are social and community support through participation with self-help organizations (e.g., Narcotics Anonymous) and the negative consequences of substance use. Current treatments are effective for maintaining abstinence for some patients and significantly reduce the cost of health care, morbidity, and mortality associated with opioid addiction.

Naltrexone (ReVia; see Chapter 19) is an opioid antagonist prescribed to block the pharmacologic effects of the high associated with opioids and alcohol. Studies report less drug craving and a reduced use of illicit drugs, especially when naltrexone is combined with psychosocial treatment. Success is somewhat limited with naltrexone, however, because although it blocks the high from opioid use, it provides no relief or promise of reward against the emotions that triggered the desire to get high in the first place.

Another approach to reducing the abuse of opioids is the methadone long-term maintenance program described as a treatment option. A disadvantage of this program is that the drug is available only through specially registered clinics, and patients often have to travel long distances to the clinics, sometimes as often as six times per week. The Drug Addiction Treatment Act of 2000 opened up the possibility of physician office–based management of addicted patients who meet certain criteria by legalizing the prescribing of Schedule III, IV, and V medications for the treatment of opioid dependence. A drug that has been well studied in office practice is buprenorphine (see Chapter 19), a partial opioid agonist. Because it has opioid agonist and antagonist properties, it has a ceiling effect on analgesia and respiratory depression, giving it a much greater safety profile. Two dosage forms of buprenorphine have been approved for maintenance opioid programs: buprenorphine only (Subutex), a sublingual tablet; and buprenorphine-naloxone (Suboxone), a sublingual film. The naloxone in the Suboxone product is to prevent abuse of the buprenorphine as a narcotic antagonist. Specifically trained prescribers administer the buprenorphine-only sublingual tablets directly to the patient in their offices, usually for 2 days. After dosage adjustment, the patient is switched to Suboxone for maintenance therapy.

AMPHETAMINE-TYPE STIMULANTS

Amphetamine-type stimulants (ATSs) are a group of chemically related compounds that are manufactured synthetically as CNS stimulants. Amphetamine, levoamphetamine, dextroamphetamine, and methamphetamine are all members of the ATS class. The amphetamines have been used medically over the years to treat schizophrenia, depression, opiate and nicotine addiction, and radiation sickness and have been used as bronchodilators in treating asthma. Dextroamphetamine and amphetamine are combined in the product Adderall, which is approved for the treatment of attention deficit hyperactivity disorder. The amphetamines have been commonly used for those in occupations that require mental stimulation during long hours of monotony, such as interstate truck drivers and assembly line workers.

The amphetamines have a high potential for abuse and dependence with prolonged use. Methamphetamine is most commonly used for nontherapeutic purposes. The World Health Organization (WHO) estimates that methamphetamine is the second most widely abused illicit drug after marijuana. It is more frequently used than heroin and cocaine combined. Worldwide, WHO reports that about 34 million individuals abuse methamphetamine, compared with 15 million people who regularly abuse cocaine (United Nations, 2008).

The amphetamines became popular in the 1960s because of the perception of enhanced performance and communication, embodying a modern and fashionable lifestyle. Recreational use was not thought to be harmful and was perceived as easily controlled compared with cocaine or heroin. Methamphetamine ("meth" or "crystal meth"), in particular, is cheaper than cocaine and has a longer half-life (10 to 12 hours) than cocaine (1.5 to 2 hours) for longer duration of effect. Although it is most commonly smoked for its quick onset (euphoric rush), methamphetamine can also be taken orally, rectally, injected, or snorted through the nostrils. In some social circles, it is perceived as being acceptable to take methamphetamine orally rather than by injection or smoking, which carries negative connotations.

From a manufacturing standpoint, methamphetamine is not dependent on climate or geographic location like heroin (poppy plants) and cocaine (coca trees). Manufacture does not require advanced knowledge of chemistry, and recipes are readily available on the Internet. Some recipes use ephedrine or pseudoephedrine, easily purchased over the counter (OTC) in some states as nasal decongestants. (Most states now require that these products be kept behind the prescription counter and sold only by a pharmacist in limited quantities.) Other ingredients are available for legitimate purposes in hardware and convenience stores. Although most methamphetamine is smuggled into the United States, "meth labs" are very easily assembled in the trunk of a car, the back of a van, or a rural farmhouse. A "cooker" can set up a lab, cook a batch, and then move on to another location. There is also a high margin of profit when the product is sold.

Intoxication

The intensity of physiologic response to methamphetamine intake depends on how it is ingested. If smoked, snorted, or injected, it produces a rapid, pleasurable "rush" within a few minutes because of the release of dopamine, norepinephrine, and serotonin neurotransmitters in the CNS. If taken orally, onset starts in about 20 minutes and peaks in 2 to 3 hours. Low doses tend to produce a sense of heightened alertness, attentiveness, self-confidence, powerfulness, and energy, whereas high doses produce a sense of well-being, euphoria, and enhanced self-esteem. Hypomania and grandiosity are more common with prolonged use. There is an increased libido and enhanced sense of sexual pleasure that is often associated with high-risk sexual behavior during a high. A methamphetamine high may last for 12 hours, but a user "on a run" taking additional doses may stay awake for 7 to 10 days, often with little food or water intake. As the drug starts to wear off, users may experience anxiety, depression, mental confusion, fatigue, and headaches. Prolonged sleep often follows.

Tolerance can occur with repeated use, requiring that larger and more frequent doses are needed to get high. The most common adverse effects are weight loss, insomnia, paranoia, hallucinations, and psychosis with violent behavior. Poor oral hygiene, in combination with the effects of methamphetamine use, such as dry mouth, teeth grinding, and jaw clenching, can lead to periodontitis and advanced tooth decay known as *meth mouth*. Other physiologic effects of methamphetamine are hypertension and tachycardia. Overdoses may induce myocardial infarction, stroke, and seizures.

Withdrawal

Abrupt discontinuation of methamphetamine after long-term use may result in withdrawal symptoms of severe depression, fatigue, lack of energy, loss of memory, and inability to manipulate information. These symptoms are frequently accompanied by drug craving. Because of its longer half-life and affinity for lipid tissues, methamphetamine withdrawal is substantially more prolonged than that of cocaine, and patients should be monitored closely for suicidal ideation.

Treatment

There are no antidotes to reverse methamphetamine intoxication, so treatment is largely supportive. If methamphetamine has been taken orally, activated charcoal may be administered. Rehydration is often necessary. Patients should be placed in a quiet area to reduce environmental stimuli. Patients demonstrating severe agitation may be sedated with a benzodiazepine such as diazepam. Antipsychotic agents such as haloperidol, a dopamine antagonist, may be necessary, but haloperidol may lower the seizure threshold in patients already at higher risk for seizures.

After withdrawal symptoms have subsided, the patient should be encouraged to undergo a psychiatric evaluation because methamphetamine is a neurotoxin that damages dopaminergic and serotonergic neurons in the brain. Damage to the dopaminergic centers may result in symptoms of parkinsonism, and serotonergic damage may result in depression, anxiety, and impulsive behavior that may be treatable with appropriate medication. Ongoing outpatient behavioral therapies such as cognitive behavioral therapy, contingency management programs, and support groups or 12-step drug treatment programs may also be beneficial.

COCAINE

Cocaine is obtained from the leaves of trees indigenous to Bolivia, Colombia, Peru, Indonesia, and other parts of the world. For centuries, workers who traveled in mountainous South American countries have chewed coca leaves to improve stamina and suppress hunger. It has been used in Western medicine as a topically applied local anesthetic, particularly in ophthalmic, nasal, oral, and laryngeal procedures, for more than 100 years. Pharmacologically, cocaine blocks the transmission of nerve impulses when applied to tissues in these areas. When injected intravenously, inhaled as smoke, or sniffed onto the mucous membranes of the nose (snorted using a straw), it blocks the reuptake of catecholamines in the brain, causing sudden CNS stimulation with euphoria (the rush).

Popular as a recreational drug for its euphoric efforts, cocaine use soared in the United States through the 1970s and 1980s. When treated with hydrochloric acid, cocaine becomes cocaine hydrochloride, which can be dried to a powder for sniffing or dissolved in water for IV injection for an immediate rush. Another method of extraction of cocaine led to the creation of the more potent "free-base" and "crack" cocaine. Free-base is formed when cocaine hydrochloride is mixed with ammonia to form a base, which then is dissolved in ether. The ether evaporates, leaving a powder residue. The powder is then smoked for the rush, but ether vapors remaining are extremely flammable and can ignite, causing a small explosion, with severe burns to the face and airways if inhaled. Crack cocaine is formed when the cocaine hydrochloride is mixed with baking soda and then heated. The resulting mass that forms is left to harden into slabs of cocaine. Chunks of the slab are sold as "rocks" of cocaine. This form of cocaine is the cheapest and most potent. When smoked, it makes a crackling sound, hence its name. Other drugs (e.g., nicotine, alcohol, heroin) are frequently used at the same time to enhance and prolong the euphoria. Cocaine smoking and IV use tend to be particularly associated with a rapid progression from use to abuse to dependence, often occurring over weeks to months. Intranasal use is associated with a more gradual progression, usually occurring over months to years. With continued use, tolerance and dependence develop, leading to increases in dosage and a reduction in the pleasurable effects of the euphoria.

Intoxication

Acute cocaine intoxication usually begins with a euphoric feeling and can then lead to a variety of other behaviors, including enhanced vigor, hyperactivity, restlessness, hypervigilance, talkativeness, anxiety, tension, alertness, grandiosity, anger, and impaired judgment. Signs and symptoms that develop are tachycardia or bradycardia, pupillary dilation, hyper- or hypotension, sweating or chills, and nausea and vomiting. With chronic use, fatigue, sadness, social withdrawal, respiratory depression, chest pain, cardiac dysrhythmias, and confusion may manifest. Severe intoxication can lead to hyperpyrexia, seizures (primarily tonic-clonic), respiratory depression, coma, and death.

Withdrawal

Because cocaine has a short half-life, withdrawal symptoms (a "crash") may begin within a few hours of a reduction in dosage, frequency of administration, or discontinuation. Acute withdrawal symptoms are more likely to be seen after periods of repetitive high-dose use ("runs" or "binges"). People often complain of fatigue, vivid and unpleasant dreams, extreme depression, insomnia or hypersomnia, and increased appetite. There is often an intense craving and drug-seeking behavior. These symptoms cause significant distress and social withdrawal, with the inability to continue work. Several days of rest and recuperation are required for symptoms to resolve. Depression with suicidal ideation is generally the most serious problem associated with cocaine withdrawal.

Treatment

There are no medicines approved to treat cocaine dependence. Many classes of drugs (e.g., dopamine agonists, antidepressants, anticonvulsants, calcium channel blockers, serotonin reuptake inhibitors) have been tested in controlled studies, with minimal effect. Studies are ongoing with GABA, the inhibitory neurotransmitter. Two additional areas of investigation are vaccines and maintenance drugs. Animal studies have shown that vaccines trigger the formation of antibodies that might increase the metabolism of cocaine. Long-acting maintenance medicines similar to methadone or buprenorphine for opioid addiction are also under investigation. Unfortunately, the rate of relapse for patients who develop a cocaine dependency is very high.

❖ NURSING IMPLICATIONS FOR SUBSTANCE ABUSE

▪ Assessment

Despite early detection of an overdose of a substance, the adverse effects of the ingested substance on multiple body systems may result in death. Assess the ABCs—*a*irway, *b*reathing, and *c*irculation—immediately on admission. A thorough physical and neurologic examination must be taken to detect life-threatening symptoms. Care must be prioritized, based on the individual patient's care needs.

Refer to Table 48-2 for a listing of substances abused and symptoms associated with each substance. Table 48-3 can serve as a reference for screening instruments for substance abuse, and the CAGE questionnaire (http://psychology-tools.com/cage-alcohol-questionnaire/) can be used as an index for individuals suspected of alcoholism. Screening instruments will have to be administered in a manner appropriate to circumstances and the overall condition of the patient.

History of the Event, Accident, or Behavior. For the person who appears to be intoxicated, ask simple, direct questions about whether the person has been drinking or using drugs. "Do you drink alcohol?" If yes, ask, "When was your last drink (time)?" "How much have you had to drink?" "Approximately how much alcohol have you consumed over the past week or month?" This would be an appropriate time to administer the CAGE questionnaire if other, more urgent care is not needed. If the answer to the question regarding drug and alcohol use is "no," ask whether the individual has a history of drinking alcohol or treatment for alcohol abuse, or has lost a driver's license, been fined, or ordered to a treatment program as a result of alcohol or drug abuse. Ask specific questions regarding the use of any "street drugs" or prescription drugs. Be direct and name examples, such as cocaine, marijuana, amphetamines, crack cocaine, barbiturates, tranquilizers, narcotics, phencyclidine (PCP), and lysergic acid diethylamide (LSD). It is essential to try to identify the abused substance so that reversal agents may be used to minimize respiratory depression.

People with symptoms of bizarre or inappropriate behavior and who are combative, violent, and possibly hallucinating should be screened not only for substance abuse, but also for possible psychiatric disorders that may be the primary cause of the presenting symptoms, a result of substance abuse, or a combination of both (see also Chapters 15, 16, and 17 for further information). Know how to summon security personnel or have them present to provide for patient and personnel safety. It is important to include past medical history in the nursing assessment. For example, a history of stroke may include slurred speech as a residual deficit that will not improve with an overdose treatment regimen.

If the patient has been injured, follow emergency department policies regarding forms and legal documents that need to be completed (e.g. screening toxicology, rape kit procedures) to meet the medicolegal requirements.

Vital Signs. Persistent abnormal vital signs during routine testing should raise suspicion of substance abuse. Vital signs should be taken as often as necessary to monitor the patient's status.

- *Blood pressure:* Blood pressure may be elevated from the use of stimulants and other coexisting conditions. Blood pressure should be determined at least twice daily and more often if indicated by the patient's symptoms or the healthcare provider's orders. Use the proper-sized blood pressure cuff and position the patient's arm at heart level.
- Record the blood pressure in both arms. A systolic pressure variance of 5 to 10 mm Hg is normal; readings reflecting a variance of more than 10 mm Hg should be reported for further evaluation. **Always report a narrowing pulse pressure** (difference between systolic and diastolic readings).
- *Pulse:* Assess bilaterally the rhythm, quality, equality, and strength of the pulses (i.e., carotid, brachial, radial, femoral, popliteal, posterior tibial, dorsalis pedis). If any pulse is diminished or absent, record the level at which initial changes are noted. The usual words to describe the pulse are *absent, diminished,* or *average; full and brisk;* or *full bounding, frequently visible.* **Report irregular rate, rhythm, and palpitations.** Check for delayed capillary refill.
- *Respirations:* Table 48-2 notes that respirations are affected by narcotics and depressants; however, because the patient may have coexisting medical conditions, respiratory rate cannot be relied on as a definitive observation for substance abuse. Lungs also may have substantial damage from smoking

or prolonged inhalations of drugs, aerosols, and solvents, making the patient susceptible to respiratory abnormalities. Observe and chart the rate and depth of respirations. Check breath sounds at least every shift, making specific notations regarding the presence of abnormal breath sounds (e.g., crackles, wheezes). Observe the degree of dyspnea that occurs and whether it happens with or without exertion.

- *Temperature:* Record the temperature at least every shift.

Basic Mental Status. Be particularly alert for fluctuating levels of consciousness; lack of awareness or attention; paranoid thoughts; visual, auditory, or tactile hallucinations; and confusion about the immediate surroundings.

Identify the person's level of consciousness and clarity of thought; both are indicators of cerebral perfusion. Terms frequently used to chart levels of consciousness include the following: *alert* (mentally functioning), *confused* (poor mental coordination), *obtunded* (sleepy, can respond appropriately when aroused or stimulated), *stuporous* (difficult to arouse, responds only to vigorous stimulation), *light coma* (grimaces and withdraws to painful stimulation), and *deep coma* (no observable response to painful stimulation). Assess regularly for improvement or deterioration. **Always report declining mental status to the healthcare provider.**

Appearance. Describe the individual's gait, coordination, and physical appearance.

Neurologic Assessment. Determine the Glasgow Coma Score if appropriate (Table 48-4).

Heart Assessment. Heart palpitations and irregularity may occur during withdrawal. Cocaine is associated with causing cardiotoxicity that can be fatal to a first-time user or to an individual who has cardiovascular disease. (See Chapters 22, 23, 24, 25, 26, and 27 for further details relating to heart assessments.)

Table 48-4	Determination of Glasgow Coma Score*		
EYE OPENING (E)	**VERBAL RESPONSE (V)**	**MOTOR RESPONSE (M)**
4 = Spontaneous	5 = Normal conversation	6 = Normal
3 = To voice	4 = Disoriented conversation	5 = Localizes to pain
2 = To pain	3 = Words, but not coherent	4 = Withdraws to pain
1 = None	2 = No words, only sounds	3 = Decorticate posture
	1 = None	2 = Decerebrate posture
		1 = None

*Total = E + V + M.

Auscultation and Percussion. Nurses with advanced skills can perform auscultation and percussion to note changes in heart size and heart and lung sounds. (See a medical-surgical nursing text for details of performing these advanced skills.) As appropriate to nursing skill level, note changes in cardiac rate and rhythm, heart sounds, and murmurs.

Eyes. Check pupil size, equality, light reaction, and accommodation (normal—equal, round, react to light, and react to accommodation). Note ptosis, nystagmus, or other abnormal eye movements. Abnormal pupil changes include either enlarged dilated pupils (mydriasis); very small, pinpoint pupils (miosis); or nonreactive pupils (do not respond to light).

Dry eyes may be a problem in a person with alcoholism. Blurred vision is common with alcoholism, and the condition may resolve after approximately 3 to 4 months of sobriety, but if the condition persists or increases, an eye examination should be scheduled.

Ears, Oral Cavity, Nose, and Throat. The range of symptoms associated with substance abuse is extensive in these tissues. Ringing, buzzing, and roaring in the ears are most common among benzodiazepine users.

The oral cavity, which is often ignored by people who abuse drugs, may have bleeding gums, canker sores, cold sores, dental caries, and infections. During withdrawal, the mouth may be very dry. The long-term use of alcohol, especially when combined with smoking, increases the risk of oral cancer, so a thorough examination of the mouth and throat should be completed.

Snorting of cocaine and heroin can seriously damage tissues in the nose, showing evidence of inflammation, ulceration, and perforation of the nasal septum. Nosebleeds are common.

Skin Assessment. Check skin color (jaundice may indicate hepatitis, which is common in drug abusers who share needles and in alcoholics with advanced disease) and for rashes, abscesses, and evidence of "tracking" along veins on the forearm, wrist, dorsum of hand, antecubital area, ankle, scrotal area, between the toes, and under the tongue. Is the skin dry, moist or clammy? Sweating may be observed during withdrawal.

Musculoskeletal Assessment. Alcohol depletes calcium from the bones, making them more susceptible to fractures. Osteoporosis also may be prevalent in alcoholics. Muscle pains (myalgia) and weakness in the muscles may be associated with withdrawal. Fine hand tremors may be observed with alcohol withdrawal.

Medication History. Ask specific questions relating to the use of prescription, OTC, and street or illicit drugs. Does the individual also use any herbal products?

Coexisting Diseases and Disorders. Is the individual currently under treatment for other diseases? Is there a history of any cardiac, respiratory, renal, endocrine, or neurologic disorders? Is there a history of head trauma or seizures?

Sexually Transmitted Infections. The individual will need examination and testing for the entire scope of sexually transmitted infections. Sexual activity is common during drug and alcohol intoxication. Prostitution is commonly used to support a substance abuse habit.

Pregnancy. Ask female patients if they are pregnant. Use of drugs and alcohol while pregnant has a strong likelihood of harming not only the mother, but also the baby before and after birth. Alcohol and drug use during pregnancy may cause preterm birth, low birth weight, birth defects, fatal bleeding disorders, and behavioral problems later in life. IV drug abusers who share needles may expose the fetus to hepatitis B, HIV, or acquired immunodeficiency syndrome (AIDS). Sexually transmitted infections also place both the mother and fetus at risk. Infants of drug addicts must be monitored closely for symptoms of withdrawal after delivery.

Laboratory Tests. Urine and/or blood toxicology screening; complete blood cell count; electrolyte studies; renal and liver function tests; thyroid levels; serologic tests for hepatitis B virus, venereal disease, and HIV; chest x-ray; tuberculosis skin test; and electrocardiography constitute a routine panel for most individuals suspected of substance abuse.

The sensitivity of the blood and urine testing for drugs depends on the amount, frequency of use, and time of last use. The presence of any drug depends on the drug's half-life and metabolites. Hallucinogens may be detected in urine for up to 28 days after last use in regular users, whereas opiates and narcotics may be detectable for only 12 to 36 hours after the last use.

Emergency Treatment. The nurse should be aware of the policy for calling codes, location of the emergency cart, and procedures used to check the emergency cart supplies and understand the procedure for defibrillation and cardioversion. The nurse should also be familiar with the medicolegal components of providing care to injured or impaired patients.

Safety. Provide for patient safety during and following detoxification until the individual is able to assume self-responsibility.

Medications. Order medications prescribed, and administer and document these on the medication administration record or in the electronic medical record. (See "Principles of Treatment for Substance Abuse" earlier in this chapter.)

Basic Mental Status. Schedule basic neurologic checks at least once per shift.

Physical and Psychological Status. Perform physical and psychological assessments at least once per shift or as indicated by the patient's condition and/or healthcare provider's orders.

Goal Setting for the Patient. Establish goals and outcomes for the immediate needs of an individual who has had an injury or has inflicted injury on others.

Plan for the patient's immediate care needs and arrange for follow-up in an inpatient or outpatient detoxification and rehabilitation program designed to help the individual reach the goal of long-term abstinence. Involve the patient in goal setting as the ability to assume responsibility for his or her own actions evolves.

In a rehabilitation program, the individual will be given factual information regarding the harmful use of drugs and/or alcohol. The individual will often not acknowledge that he or she has a problem (denial); when the problem is recognized, the person does not have insight into how to overcome the problem. Throughout the program, the patient will need to explore positive and negative aspects of his or her behavior to develop new behaviors that do not include the use of drugs and alcohol. The person will evolve through the following five stages of change: precontemplation, contemplation, preparation, action, and maintenance (Prochaska and DiClemente, 1986) as he or she advances through the rehabilitation program (Fig. 48-2).

Family and Support Involvement. Integrate family and others within the patient's support network into the interdisciplinary team for long-term planning for treatment and support. Encourage them to become involved in the rehabilitation program. Family members and friends need guidance in appropriate ways to be involved in the recovery of an individual who exhibits symptoms of a dysfunctional family relationship. Enrollment in community groups (e.g., Al-Anon, Nar-Anon) designed to provide support for family and friends will assist them in understanding the addiction problem and provide guidance in coping with potential problems.

Laboratory Tests. Obtain stat and subsequent laboratory studies.

■ **Implementation**

- In an emergency department setting, the immediate care needs of the individual must be met to stabilize the person and provide for patient safety. Deliver physical care and provide psychological support of the individual and significant others. Orient the patient to date, time, place, person, and situation. Once stabilized, the patient may be admitted to an intensive care, acute care, psychiatric, or rehabilitation facility designed to provide treatment of the presenting problems.

- The nurse needs to be familiar with the protocol and healthcare provider orders used during detoxification. Refer to the earlier section, "Principles of Treatment for Substance Abuse," and to other textbooks with more extensive coverage of substance abuse for details regarding detoxification for specific agents being abused.

- During withdrawal, patients need a quiet, safe care environment with staff experienced in detoxification methods.

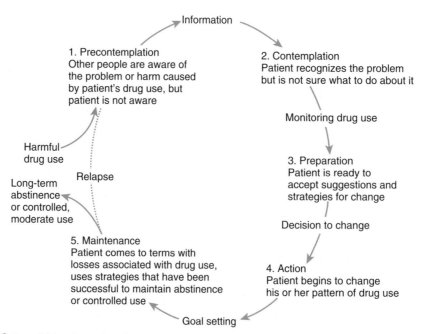

FIGURE 48-2 A model for change in substance use disorders. (Modified from Prochaska J, DiClemente C: Towards a comprehensive model of change. In Miller W, Heather N, editors: *Treating addictive behaviors: a process of change,* New York, 1986, Plenum Press.)

- Provide for patient and staff safety. Have emergency equipment available at all times, and be particularly vigilant for seizure activity.
- Perform physical assessments of the patient in accordance with clinical policies (e.g., every 2, 4, or 8 hours, or as indicated by the patient's status).
- Have medications listed in the protocol or healthcare provider's orders readily available for administration (e.g., benzodiazepines, clonidine, beta blockers for treatment of withdrawal; carbamazepine for seizures; cyclobenzaprine for muscle spasms; naltrexone to reduce craving).
- Implement measures to reduce anxiety, including administering prescribed medications that can best alleviate the patient's symptoms and provide maximum level of comfort. Support the patient in a calm manner, even if the patient responds in a hostile or confrontational way. React appropriately to the patient's expressions of resistance (e.g., arguing, denying, ignoring).
- As the patient progresses, encourage the patient to make choices and take responsibility for those decisions. See discussion earlier in the chapter for intoxication, withdrawal, treatment, and relapse prevention.

■ **Patient Education**

Design an individualized approach to help the patient modify factors that are in the patient's control.

Ongoing Health Care

- The patient must place himself or herself under the care of a healthcare provider who is trained to treat substance use disorders and who can guide the patient through the challenges of withdrawal and recovery. The rehabilitation center or abuse counselor may have a list of healthcare providers, or the patient can contact the American Society of Addiction Medicine (301-656-3920; email@asam.org) for a list of healthcare providers experienced in treating people with addictions.
- The patient should inform all healthcare providers (e.g., physician, dentist, psychiatrist, podiatrist) of the history of addictive behavior so that a comprehensive plan can be implemented for medication when necessary.
- If planning to get pregnant, the patient should consult with a healthcare provider about planning for a pregnancy that can be safe for the recovering addict and the baby.

Nutrition Status

- Encourage a well-balanced diet. Consultation with a dietitian may be necessary. The B vitamins, especially thiamine, are vital to the repair of the nervous system; calcium may be needed for weakened bones; and excessive vitamins A and D may be harmful.
- If the patient is anemic, an iron preparation may also be prescribed. Consult with the healthcare provider or a pharmacist about an appropriate vitamin supplement.
- Have the patient drink eight to ten 8-ounce glasses of water daily, unless coexisting medical problems prohibit it.
- Sugars may affect the mood of some individuals. If mood swings are a problem, it may be wise to limit the patient's sugar intake.

Stress Management

- Identify stress-producing situations in the patient's life and seek means to reduce these factors significantly. In some cases, referral for training in stress management, relaxation techniques, mediation, or biofeedback may be necessary. If stress is produced in the work setting, it may be appropriate to involve the nurse at the patient's place of employment.

Financial Status

- What is the financial status of the individual? Has the individual borrowed money from everyone? Are legal charges pending for theft or for writing bad checks? As part of the rehabilitation process, a social worker or counselor should assist the individual in creating a plan for assuming responsibility for social and financial debts.

Job or Employment

- The person may need assistance to establish a plan for how to integrate back into the work environment. Many fears are associated with the work environment (e.g., fear of being fired, fear of being tempted to use again because of stress at work, fear of not being able to perform the job duties satisfactorily).
- The person may need to contact the employer to see if returning to the job that she or he had before admission is acceptable. Often, the person may have displayed poor work habits while using alcohol or drugs and may have been terminated. The employer may also have an assistance program that can provide support to the employee in recovery.
- Drug testing may be a requirement of a court order, rehabilitation program, or returning to employment. The individual needs to understand the policies in place.
- If it is necessary to find a new job, the individual may need guidance in how to go about finding job leads, how to apply for a new position, and how to interview.

Career Changes. Depending on the circumstances, the individual may need to make a career change to a less demanding work environment or to one that is better suited to his or her abilities.

Licenses and Insurance. If a driver's license has been revoked, the state licensing agency should be contacted for guidance in steps to be taken for reinstatement. Once the license is reinstated, the person must also hold insurance to license and drive a car. Contact the auto insurance company for a list of companies that may sell automobile insurance to at-risk individuals. Understand that even with a valid driver's license, the cost of insurance is usually rated based on the previous driving violations.

If the patient holds a license to practice a profession, and if employment requires licensure, contact the state agency that issued the license to determine eligibility for continued licensure and potential employment in the field. Licensing boards usually require participation in a recovery program, with urine testing as well as periodic reports to the licensing agency, to maintain a license and practice a profession.

Fostering Health Maintenance. Seek the patient's cooperation and understanding of the following points so that medication adherence is increased: name of medication; dosage, route, and times of administration; and common and serious adverse effects. The person who has an alcohol or drug abuse problem needs to reveal his or her history to all healthcare providers so that the prescriber can take this into account when selecting agents for use. At the supermarket, pharmacy, or nutrition center, the patient should always read labels thoroughly to avoid food and medicinal products that contain alcohol.

Patient Self-Assessment. Enlist the patient's aid in developing and maintaining a written record of monitoring parameters for coexisting medical problems (e.g., pulse rate, blood pressure, degree of dyspnea and what precipitates it, chest pain, edema) (see Appendix B: Template for Developing a Written Record for Patients to Monitor Their Own Therapy). Complete the Premedication Data column for use as a baseline to track response to drug therapy. Ensure that the patient understands how to use the form, and instruct the patient to take the completed form to follow-up visits. During follow-up visits, focus on issues that will foster adherence with the therapeutic interventions prescribed.

DRUGS USED TO TREAT ALCOHOLISM

> **acamprosate** (ā-KĂM-prō-sāt)
> **Campral** (KĂM-prăl)

ACTIONS

Acamprosate is classified as a weak NMDA receptor antagonist. It is a synthetic compound structurally related to GABA. A variety of mechanisms have been proposed, but none have been well proven.

USES

Acamprosate is used in alcohol rehabilitation programs for chronic alcoholic patients who want to maintain sobriety. It should be used only in conjunction with other rehabilitative therapy. It enhances abstinence and reduces drinking rates in alcohol-dependent patients who are abstinent at the beginning of treatment. It is neither a sedative nor an anxiolytic, and it is not habit forming. It does not reduce the rewarding effects of alcohol as does naltrexone, and it does not cause nausea and vomiting when alcohol is consumed, as does disulfiram. Studies indicate similar rates of success with naltrexone and acamprosate and a slightly higher success rate when used together. Acamprosate may also be used in cases when naltrexone is contraindicated, such as for patients with liver disease or those receiving concurrent opioid therapy or methadone maintenance therapy. Acamprosate does not treat withdrawal symptoms.

THERAPEUTIC OUTCOME

The primary therapeutic outcome expected from acamprosate is improved adherence with an alcohol treatment program by abstinence from alcohol.

❖ NURSING IMPLICATIONS FOR ACAMPROSATE

▪ Premedication Assessment

1. Perform baseline neurologic assessment (e.g., orientation to date, time, and place; mental alertness; bilateral hand grip; motor functioning).
2. Take vital signs (temperature, blood pressure, pulse, respirations).
3. Check laboratory values for urine screen for alcohol use and blood urea nitrogen and serum creatinine levels for renal function.
4. Monitor for gastrointestinal symptoms before and during therapy.

▪ Availability

PO: 333-mg delayed-release tablets.

▪ Dosage and Administration

Adult: PO: Two 333-mg tablets (666 mg) three times daily. Tablets may be taken without regard to meals. Acamprosate should be started as soon as possible after the period of alcohol withdrawal, when the patient has become abstinent.

Patients with moderate renal function as indicated by a creatinine clearance of 30 to 50 mL/min should take one 333-mg tablet three times daily.

Behavior Modification. Acamprosate therapy in combination with behavioral therapy has been shown to be more effective than acamprosate or behavioral therapy alone in prolonging alcohol cessation in patients who were formerly physically dependent on alcohol.

⚠ **Medication Safety Alert**

Acamprosate is contraindicated in patients with severe renal failure as indicated by a creatinine clearance lower than 30 mL/min.

■ **Common Adverse Effects**

Gastrointestinal

Diarrhea. Diarrhea may occur in 10% to 20% of patients taking acamprosate, but rarely is it a cause for discontinuing therapy. Symptoms are usually mild and tend to resolve with continued therapy. Encourage the patient not to discontinue therapy without first consulting with the healthcare provider and treatment program.

■ **Serious Adverse Effects**

Psychological

Suicidal actions. In clinical studies with acamprosate, suicidal ideation, suicide attempts, and completed suicides were infrequent but were more common in acamprosate-treated patients than in patients treated with placebo (2.4% vs. 0.8%). The interrelationship of alcohol dependence, depression, and suicide is well recognized and complex. Monitor alcohol-dependent patients, including those patients being treated with acamprosate, for symptoms of negative thoughts, feelings, behaviors, depression, or suicidal thinking. Alert families and caregivers of patients being treated with acamprosate of the need to monitor patients for the emergence of these symptoms, and ask them to report such symptoms to the patient's healthcare provider.

■ **Drug Interactions**

No clinically significant drug interactions have been reported.

---

disulfiram (dī-SŬL-fĭr-ăm)
Antabuse (ĂN-tĕ-byūs)

ACTIONS

Disulfiram is an agent that, when ingested before any form of alcohol is consumed, produces a very unpleasant reaction to the alcohol. Disulfiram blocks the metabolism of acetaldehyde, a metabolite of alcohol. Elevated levels of acetaldehyde produce the disulfiram-alcohol reaction, which is manifested by nausea, severe vomiting, sweating, throbbing headache, dizziness, blurred vision, and confusion. The intensity of the reaction depends somewhat on the sensitivity of the individual and the amount of alcohol consumed. The duration of the reaction depends on the presence of alcohol in the blood. Mild reactions may last from 30 to 60 minutes, whereas more severe reactions may last for several hours. Prolonged administration of disulfiram does not produce tolerance; indeed, the longer a patient remains on therapy, the more exquisitely sensitive the person becomes to alcohol.

USES

Disulfiram is used in alcohol rehabilitation programs for chronic alcoholic patients who want to maintain sobriety. It should be used only in conjunction with other rehabilitative therapy. Patients must be fully informed of the consequences of drinking alcohol while receiving disulfiram therapy. As little as 10 to 15 mL of alcohol may produce a reaction. Patients must not drink or apply alcohol in any form, including OTC products such as sleep aids, cough and cold products, aftershave lotions, mouthwashes, and rubbing alcohol. Dietary sources, such as sauces and vinegars containing alcohol, are prohibited. A disulfiram-alcohol reaction may occur with the ingestion of any alcohol for 1 to 2 weeks after discontinuing disulfiram therapy. Disulfiram must never be administered to a patient who is intoxicated. Because of the consequence of a disulfiram-alcohol reaction on other disease states, disulfiram therapy must be used very cautiously in patients with diabetes mellitus, hypothyroidism, epilepsy, cerebral damage, chronic or acute nephritis, hepatic cirrhosis, or hepatic failure.

THERAPEUTIC OUTCOME

The primary therapeutic outcome expected from disulfiram is improved adherence to an alcohol treatment program by abstinence from alcohol.

❖ NURSING IMPLICATIONS FOR DISULFIRAM

■ **Premedication Assessment**

1. Perform baseline neurologic assessment (e.g., orientation to date, time, and place; mental alertness; bilateral hand grip; motor functioning).
2. Take vital signs (i.e., temperature, blood pressure, pulse, respirations).
3. Check laboratory values for hepatotoxicity; screen urine for alcohol use.
4. Monitor for gastrointestinal symptoms before and during therapy.
5. The manufacturer recommends that baseline determinations of liver function should be performed in all patients before initiation of therapy and repeated in 10 to 14 days. A baseline complete blood cell count and serum chemistries are recommended and should also be repeated every 6 months, along with the liver function tests.

■ **Availability**

PO: 250- and 500-mg tablets.

■ **Dosage and Administration**

Adult: PO: Initially a maximum of 500 mg once daily for 1 to 2 weeks. The maintenance dosage is usually 250 mg daily (range 125 to 500 mg). Do not exceed 500 mg daily. Administer at bedtime to avoid the complications of sedative effects.

Behavior Modification. Disulfiram therapy, in combination with behavioral therapy, has been shown to be more effective than disulfiram or behavioral therapy alone in prolonging alcohol cessation in patients who were formerly physically dependent on alcohol.

- Disulfiram must never be administered to patients when they are in a state of intoxication or when they are unaware that they are receiving therapy. Family members should be told about the treatment so that they can provide motivation and support and help the patient avoid accidental disulfiram-alcohol reactions.
- Do not administer disulfiram until the patient has abstained from alcohol for a period of at least 12 hours.
- It is recommended that all patients who are receiving disulfiram carry a patient identification card stating the use of disulfiram and describing the symptoms that are most likely to occur as a result of the disulfiram-alcohol reaction. This card also should indicate the healthcare provider or institution that should be contacted in an emergency.

■ Common Adverse Effects

These adverse effects are usually mild and tend to resolve with continued therapy. Encourage the patient not to discontinue therapy without first consulting with the healthcare provider and treatment program.

Neurologic. Drowsiness, fatigue, headache.

Reproductive. Impotence.

Gastrointestinal. Metallic taste.

■ Serious Adverse Effects

Gastrointestinal

Hepatotoxicity. The symptoms of hepatotoxicity are jaundice, nausea, vomiting, anorexia, hepatomegaly, splenomegaly, and abnormal liver function tests (e.g., elevated bilirubin, aspartate aminotransferase [AST], alanine aminotransferase [ALT], alkaline phosphatase levels, and increased prothrombin time). Because many of these patients do not develop clinical symptoms but do develop abnormal liver function test results, strongly encourage patients to report for blood tests as scheduled. Report abnormal values to the appropriate healthcare provider.

Hypersensitivity, Immune System

Hives, pruritus, rash. Report symptoms of hives, pruritus, or rash for further evaluation by the healthcare provider. Pruritus may be relieved by taking antihistamines and adding baking soda to the bath water.

■ Drug Interactions

Warfarin. Disulfiram may enhance the anticoagulant effects of warfarin. Observe for the development of petechiae, ecchymoses, nosebleeds, bleeding gums, dark tarry stools, and bright red or coffee-ground emesis. Monitor the prothrombin time (international normalized ratio) and reduce the dosage of warfarin if necessary.

Phenytoin. Disulfiram inhibits the metabolism of phenytoin. Monitor patients with concurrent use for signs of phenytoin toxicity (i.e., nystagmus, sedation, lethargy). Serum levels may be monitored and the dosage of phenytoin may need to be reduced.

Isoniazid. Disulfiram alters the metabolism of isoniazid. Perform a baseline assessment of the patient's degree of alertness (e.g., orientation to name, place, time) and coordination before initiating therapy. Make regularly scheduled subsequent mental status evaluations and compare findings. Report to the healthcare provider any development of alterations in mental status.

Metronidazole. Concurrent administration of disulfiram and metronidazole may result in psychotic episodes and confusional states. Concurrent therapy is not recommended.

Benzodiazepines. Disulfiram inhibits the metabolism of specific benzodiazepines (e.g., chlordiazepoxide, diazepam, clorazepate, halazepam, flurazepam, quazepam, estazolam). When benzodiazepine therapy is indicated, use oxazepam, alprazolam, temazepam, or lorazepam because of a different metabolic pathway not inhibited by disulfiram.

Caffeine. The cardiovascular and CNS stimulant effects of caffeine may be increased by disulfiram. If tachycardia or nervousness is noted, cut back on the consumption of caffeine-containing products such as coffee.

Get Ready for the NCLEX® Examination!

Key Points

- Substance abuse is defined as the periodic, purposeful use of a substance that leads to clinically significant impairment.
- Table 48-3 summarizes several screening instruments used for substance abuse.
- Frequency of substance abuse among healthcare providers is probably similar to that of the general population.
- Healthcare professionals suspecting a colleague of substance abuse need to observe, document, and

report relevant data to the supervisor and to the licensing agency or disciplinary board in states in which mandatory reporting is required. Many states have licensee assistance programs and procedures for reporting or seeking counseling from this resource.

- The *DSM-5* has redefined substance use disorders and recognizes they are treatable disorders. Treatment needs to be individualized to the person's needs.
- Professionals providing health care to people with a substance abuse problem need to be vigilant for coexisting medical or psychiatric problems.

- People with a substance use disorder must be encouraged to assume responsibility for their own actions and to focus not only on the need for a change in behavior, but also on strategies for managing their lives and approaches to coping more effectively with life situations.
- Group support for the individual and for family and significant others needs to be established. Many rehabilitation programs involve family as part of the treatment regimen. Others suggest community resources such as Alcoholics Anonymous or Narcotics Anonymous for the person in recovery and Al-Anon for family members.

Additional Learning Resources

SG Go to your Study Guide for additional Review Questions for the NCLEX® Examination, Critical Thinking Clinical Situations, and other learning activities to help you master this chapter content.

evolve Go to your Evolve website (http://evolve.elsevier.com/Clayton) for additional online resources.

Review Questions for the NCLEX® Examination

1. A patient reported to the clinic in a state of intoxication. The nurse questioned the patient about alcohol use and determined that the patient may be considered under the classification of moderate alcohol use disorder with the finding of:
   1. two symptoms.
   2. four symptoms.
   3. six symptoms.
   4. eight symptoms.

2. The screening instrument used commonly in acute care settings to determine alcohol abuse is referred to by the acronym:
   1. DAST.
   2. HEADSS.
   3. CAGE.
   4. MMPI-2.

3. These signs and symptoms raise the suspicion of substance use disorder by a healthcare professional. *(Select all that apply.)*
   1. Wearing long-sleeved garments all the time
   2. Diminished alertness
   3. Requests for frequent schedule changes
   4. Rarely being absent from work
   5. Infrequent breaks

4. The nurse recognizes that the amphetamine-type stimulants can have the following effects. *(Select all that apply.)*
   1. They are used in the treatment of attention deficit hyperactivity disorder (ADHD).
   2. They have a shorter half-life compared with cocaine.
   3. They produce hypotension and bradycardia.
   4. They may produce parkinsonism symptoms as a result of long-term use.
   5. They cause prolonged withdrawal due to their affinity for lipid tissues.

5. These symptoms are associated with alcohol withdrawal. *(Select all that apply.)*
   1. Nausea
   2. Vomiting
   3. Psychomotor agitation
   4. Diaphoresis
   5. Hypotension

6. The nurse realizes that the patient who is being treated for cocaine dependence has insight about cocaine use after stating the following:
   1. "When getting clean, I sometimes have thoughts of ending it all."
   2. "Cocaine withdrawal is relatively easy."
   3. "The only form of cocaine that is dangerous is free-base."
   4. "There are several approved treatment medications for cocaine dependence."

7. The nurse was instructing a patient taking disulfiram (Antabuse) on the following precautions while on the medication: *(Select all that apply.)*
   1. Review all drug labels for ingredients, particularly alcohol.
   2. Avoid all alcoholic beverages.
   3. Avoid foods high in tyramine.
   4. Avoid topical products and lotions with alcohol.
   5. Avoid foods high in purines.

Objectives

1. Summarize the primary actions and potential uses of the miscellaneous agents cited.

2. Describe patient education needed when miscellaneous agents are used.

MISCELLANEOUS AGENTS

colchicine (KŌL-chĭ-sēn)

ACTIONS

The exact mechanism of action is not known, but colchicine interrupts the cycle of urate crystal deposition in the tissues that results in an acute attack of gout. It does not affect the amount of uric acid in the blood or urine; therefore it is not a uricosuric agent.

USES

Colchicine is an alkaloid that has been used for hundreds of years to prevent or relieve acute attacks of gout. Joint pain and swelling begin to subside within 12 hours and are usually gone within 48 to 72 hours after initiating therapy.

THERAPEUTIC OUTCOME

The primary therapeutic outcome expected from colchicine therapy is elimination of joint pain secondary to acute gout attack.

❖ NURSING IMPLICATIONS FOR COLCHICINE

■ Premedication Assessment

1. Assess for and record any gastrointestinal complaints present before initiation of drug therapy.
2. Assess for a history of allergy to colchicine. If present, withhold the drug and consult with the healthcare provider.
3. Obtain baseline complete blood count and differential, uric acid level, blood urea nitrogen (BUN), creatinine, aspartate aminotransferase (AST), alanine aminotransferase (ALT), and other values as requested by healthcare provider for future comparison and for monitoring for development of blood dyscrasias, renal dysfunction, and liver impairment, as well as tracking progress in control of uric acid level.

4. Assess the patient's level and location of pain using the pain rating scale (0 to 10); assess affected area for signs of inflammation—erythema, edema, and mobility.

■ Availability
PO: 0.6-mg tablets.

■ Dosage and Administration
Adult: PO: Acute gout: 1.2 mg PO at first sign of gout flare followed by 0.6 mg PO 1 hour later; do not exceed 1.8 mg PO over 1 hour. After the acute attack, 0.6 mg should be administered one to two times daily to prevent relapse. Do not repeat high-dose therapy for at least 3 days.

> **[!] Medication Safety Alert**
>
> Use with extreme caution in older adults or debilitated patients and in patients with impaired renal, cardiac, or gastrointestinal function.

Fluid Intake. Monitor intake and output during therapy. Maintain fluid intake at eight to twelve 8-ounce glasses daily.

■ Common Adverse Effects
Gastrointestinal

Nausea, vomiting, diarrhea. These are common adverse effects of colchicine therapy. Discontinue therapy when gastrointestinal symptoms develop. Always report bright red blood in vomitus, coffee-ground vomitus, or dark tarry stools.

■ Serious Adverse Effects
Hematologic

Blood dyscrasias. Serious, potentially fatal, blood dyscrasias, including anemia, agranulocytosis, and thrombocytopenia, have been associated with colchicine therapy. Although the development of blood dyscrasias is rare, periodic differential blood counts are recommended if the patient requires prolonged treatment. Routine laboratory studies (e.g., red blood cell [RBC], white blood cell [WBC], differential counts) should be scheduled. Stress to the patient the importance of returning for this laboratory work. Monitor for the development of sore throat, fever, purpura, jaundice, or excessive and progressive weakness, and report any such development immediately to the healthcare provider.

■ **Drug Interactions**

No clinically significant drug interactions have been reported.

---

donepezil (dŏn-ĔP-ĭ-zĭl)
   Aricept (ĀR-ĭ-sĕpt)

ACTIONS

Donepezil is an acetylcholinesterase inhibitor that allows acetylcholine to accumulate at cholinergic synapses, causing a prolonged and exaggerated cholinergic effect.

USES

Although the causes are unknown, Alzheimer's disease is characterized by a loss of cholinergic neurons in the central nervous system (CNS), resulting in memory loss and cognitive deficits (dementia). Donepezil is used in patients with mild-to-moderate dementia to enhance cholinergic function. Its function diminishes with ongoing loss of cholinergic neurons. Donepezil does not prevent or slow the neurodegeneration caused by Alzheimer's disease.

THERAPEUTIC OUTCOME

The primary therapeutic outcome expected from donepezil therapy is improved cognitive skills (e.g., word recall, object naming, language, word finding, task performance).

❖ **NURSING IMPLICATIONS FOR DONEPEZIL**

■ **Premedication Assessment**

1. Obtain baseline assessments of presenting symptoms.
2. Record baseline pulse, respirations, and blood pressure.
3. Assess for and record any gastric symptoms present before initiation of therapy.

■ **Availability**

PO: 5-, 10-, and 23-mg tablets; 5- and 10-mg orally disintegrating tablets.

■ **Dosage and Administration**

Adult: PO: Initial dosage: 5 mg daily at bedtime. After 4 to 6 weeks of therapy, dosage may be increased to 10 mg daily to assess therapeutic benefit. After 3 months, dose may be increased to 23 mg in moderate-to-severe Alzheimer's disease. Donepezil may be taken with or without food. The orally disintegrating tablets may be helpful for patients who have difficulty swallowing. Allow tablets to dissolve on the tongue, and follow with a glass of water.

■ **Common Adverse Effects**

Gastrointestinal

Nausea, vomiting, dyspepsia, diarrhea. These are natural extensions of the pharmacologic effects of cholinergic agents. The dosage may need to be reduced if the patient has difficulty with these adverse effects. Symptoms are less common with lower doses and tend to subside after 2 to 3 weeks of therapy. Gradually increasing the dose may help avoid these complications.

■ **Serious Adverse Effects**

Cardiovascular

Bradycardia. Cholinergic agents cause a slowing of the heart. Notify the healthcare provider if the heart rate is regularly less than 60 beats/min.

■ **Drug Interactions**

Drugs That Enhance Therapeutic and Toxic Effects. Ketoconazole and quinidine may inhibit the metabolism of donepezil. Monitor closely for enhancement of adverse effects.

Drugs That Reduce Therapeutic Effects. Carbamazepine, dexamethasone, phenobarbital, phenytoin, and rifampin increase the metabolism of donepezil, reducing its therapeutic effects. The dose of donepezil may need to be increased or the patient switched to another medicine to treat Alzheimer's disease.

Anticholinergic Agents. As a cholinergic agent, donepezil has the potential to reduce the activity of anticholinergic agents (e.g., benztropine, diphenhydramine, orphenadrine, procyclidine, trihexyphenidyl).

Succinylcholine-Type Muscle Relaxants, Cholinergic Agents. As a cholinesterase inhibitor, donepezil is likely to exaggerate the actions of the depolarizing muscle relaxant (succinylcholine) during anesthesia and enhance the pharmacologic activity of cholinergic agents such as bethanechol.

---

memantine (MĔM-ăn-tēn)
   Namenda (năm-ĔN-dă)

ACTIONS

Memantine is an *N*-methyl-d-aspartate (NMDA) receptor inhibitor. It is a synthetic compound structurally related to gamma-aminobutyric acid (GABA).

USES

Although the causes are unknown, one of the neurochemical characteristics of Alzheimer's disease is persistent activation of NMDA receptors in the CNS. Memantine blocks these receptors and is used alone or in combination with an acetylcholinesterase inhibitor for the treatment of moderate-to-severe Alzheimer's-associated dementia. Patients taking memantine show improvement in cognitive function and behavioral symptoms and a slower decline in activities of daily living, but memantine does not prevent or slow the neurodegeneration of Alzheimer's disease.

THERAPEUTIC OUTCOME

The primary therapeutic outcome expected from memantine therapy is improved cognitive skills (e.g., word recall, object naming, language, word finding, task performance).

❖ NURSING IMPLICATIONS FOR MEMANTINE

▪ Premedication Assessment

1. Obtain baseline assessments of presenting symptoms.
2. Record baseline pulse, respirations, and blood pressure.

▪ Availability

PO: 5- and 10-mg tablets; capsules, extended release (24 hr): 7, 14, 21, and 28 mg. Oral solution: 2 mg/mL in 360 mL.

▪ Dosage and Administration

Adult: PO: 5 mg once daily. The dose should be increased in 5-mg increments to 10, 15, and 20 mg daily. The minimal interval between dose increases is 1 week. Memantine can be taken with or without food.

Conversion: Patients taking 10-mg immediate-release tablets twice daily may switch to a 28-mg extended-release capsule once daily the day following the last dose of a 10-mg immediate-release tablet.

Reduction in dose for renal impairment: A target dose of 14 mg/day is recommended in patients with severe renal impairment (creatinine clearance of 5 to 29 mL/min, based on the Cockcroft-Gault equation).

▪ Common and Serious Adverse Effects
Neurologic

Headache, dizziness, akathisia, insomnia, restlessness, increased motor activity, excitement, agitation. Many of these symptoms decline with continued therapy and can be reduced with a longer dosage titration. Dosage may need to be reduced if the patient has difficulty with these adverse effects.

▪ Drug Interactions
Acetazolamide, Sodium Bicarbonate. Medicines that alkalinize the pH of the urine will reduce excretion of memantine. Severe medical conditions such as renal tubular acidosis and severe urinary tract infections also may cause alkalization of the urine, with potential toxicity of memantine.

probenecid (prō-BĚN-ě-sĭd)

ACTIONS

Uricosuric agents act on the tubules of the kidneys to enhance the excretion of uric acid. Probenecid promotes renal excretion of a number of substances, including uric acid. It inhibits the reabsorption of urate in the kidney, which results in reduction of uric acid in the blood.

USES

Probenecid is used to treat hyperuricemia and chronic gouty arthritis. It is not effective for acute attacks of gout and is not an analgesic.

THERAPEUTIC OUTCOME

The primary therapeutic outcome expected with probenecid therapy is prevention of acute attacks of gouty arthritis.

❖ NURSING IMPLICATIONS FOR PROBENECID

▪ Premedication Assessment

1. Inquire about the time of onset of the last gout attack; do not administer medication during or within 2 to 3 weeks of an acute attack.
2. Assess for and record any gastrointestinal complaints before initiating drug therapy.
3. Ask about any history of blood dyscrasias or kidney stones; if present, withhold drug and contact a healthcare provider.
4. Obtain baseline blood studies as requested (e.g., uric acid and serum creatinine levels) to assess appropriateness and to monitor response to therapy.

> **[!] Medication Safety Alert**
>
> - Do NOT start probenecid therapy during an acute attack of gout; wait 2 to 3 weeks.
> - Do NOT administer to patients with histories of blood dyscrasias or uric acid kidney stones.
> - Do NOT administer to patients with a creatinine clearance lower than 40 mL/min or a BUN level higher than 40 mg/100 mL.

▪ Availability
PO: 500-mg tablets.

▪ Dosage and Administration
Adult: PO: Initially 250 mg twice daily for 1 week, then 500 mg twice daily. The dosage may be increased by 500 mg every few weeks to a maximum of 2 g daily. Administer with food or milk to diminish gastric irritation. Maintain fluid intake at 2 to 3 L daily.

▪ Common Adverse Effects
Metabolic

Acute gout attacks. Patients should be told that the incidence of gout attacks may increase for the first few months of therapy and that they should continue therapy without changing the dosage during the attacks.

■ Serious Adverse Effects

Gastrointestinal

Nausea, anorexia, vomiting. Use with caution in patients with a history of peptic ulcer disease. Individuals who experience symptoms of ulcers and are still undiagnosed should be encouraged to report gastrointestinal symptoms if they increase in intensity or frequency. Always report bright red blood in vomitus, coffee-ground vomitus, or dark tarry stools.

Hypersensitivity/Immune System

Hives, pruritus, rash. These are signs of hypersensitivity. Notify the healthcare provider. Therapy may have to be discontinued.

■ Drug Interactions

Oral Hypoglycemic Agents. Monitor for hypoglycemia (e.g., headache, weakness, decreased coordination, general apprehension, diaphoresis, hunger, blurred or double vision). The dosage of the hypoglycemic agent may need to be reduced. Notify the healthcare provider if any of these symptoms appear.

Acyclovir, Famciclovir, Valacyclovir, Zidovudine, Dapsone, Indomethacin, Sulfinpyrazone, Rifampin, Sulfonamides, Naproxen, Penicillins, Cephalosporins, Methotrexate, Clofibrate. Probenecid blocks the renal excretion of these agents. See individual drug monographs of the drugs listed for serious adverse effects that may indicate development of toxicity.

Salicylates. Although occasional use of aspirin will not interfere with the effectiveness of probenecid, regular use of aspirin or aspirin-containing products should be discouraged. If analgesia is required, suggest acetaminophen.

Antineoplastic Agents. Because of the potential development of renal uric acid stones, probenecid is not recommended for increased uric acid levels caused by antineoplastic therapy.

DRUG CLASS: XANTHINE OXIDASE INHIBITORS

ACTIONS

Xanthine oxidase inhibitors block the terminal pathways in uric acid formation by inhibiting the enzyme xanthine oxidase. The two drugs currently available are allopurinol and febuxostat.

USES

Allopurinol is used to treat primary hyperuricemia in patients with gout or gout secondary to antineoplastic therapy. It is not effective for treating acute attacks of gouty arthritis. Allopurinol has an advantage over uricosuric agents (probenecid) in that gouty nephropathy and the formation of urate stones are less likely because

the drug inhibits the production of uric acid. It may also be used in patients with renal failure. Uricosuric agents should not be used in this case.

Febuxostat is approved for the chronic management of hyperuricemia in patients with gout. Febuxostat is not approved for use in asymptomatic hyperuricemia.

THERAPEUTIC OUTCOME

The primary therapeutic outcome associated with xanthine oxidase inhibitor therapy is reduced serum uric acid levels with a lower frequency of acute gout attacks.

❖ NURSING IMPLICATIONS FOR XANTHINE OXIDASE INHIBITORS

■ Premedication Assessment

1. Inquire about the time of onset of gout attack; do not start the medication during an acute attack.
2. Assess for and record any gastrointestinal complaints before initiating drug therapy.
3. Obtain baseline blood studies, blood counts, and renal and liver function studies as requested.

■ Availability, Dosage, and Administration

See Table 49-1.

Allopurinol. **Adult:** *IV:* Infuse at a concentration no greater than 6 mg/mL. When possible, allopurinol therapy should be started 24 to 48 hours before chemotherapy known to cause tumor lysis. Dosage must be reduced in patients with a creatinine clearance of 20 mL/min or lower.

Febuxostat. Dosage must be reduced in patients with a creatinine clearance of 30 mL/min or lower.

Fluid Intake. Maintain fluid intake at eight to twelve 8-ounce glasses daily.

■ Common Adverse Effects

Metabolic

Acute gout attacks. Patients should be told that the frequency of gout attacks may increase for the first few months of therapy with xanthine oxidase inhibitors. The patient should continue therapy without changing the dosage during the attacks. Patients may be treated with nonsteroidal antiinflammatory agents or colchicine to prevent acute gout flare-ups.

Gastrointestinal

Gastric irritation. If gastric irritation occurs, administer with food or milk. If symptoms persist or increase in severity, report for healthcare provider evaluation.

Nausea, vomiting, diarrhea. These adverse effects are usually mild and tend to resolve with continued therapy. Encourage the patient not to discontinue therapy without first consulting with the healthcare provider.

Neurologic

Dizziness, headache. These adverse effects are usually mild and tend to resolve with continued therapy. Encourage the patient not to discontinue therapy

Table 49-1 **Xanthine Oxidase Inhibitors**

GENERIC NAME	BRAND NAME	AVAILABILITY	DAILY DOSAGE	MAXIMUM DAILY DOSAGE
allopurinol	Zyloprim	PO: 100-, 300-mg tablets	PO: 300 mg	800 mg
febuxostat	Uloric	PO: 40-, 80-mg tablets	PO: Initially, 40 mg *Dosage adjustment:* If serum uric acid level is not <6 mg/dL after 2 wk therapy, raise the dosage to 80 mg	Unspecified

without first consulting with his or her healthcare provider.

■ Serious Adverse Effects

Gastrointestinal

Hepatotoxicity. The symptoms of hepatotoxicity are anorexia, nausea, vomiting, jaundice, hepatomegaly, splenomegaly, and abnormal liver function test results (elevated bilirubin, AST, ALT, gamma-glutamyl transpeptidase [GGT], alkaline phosphatase levels, increased prothrombin time). Periodic measurement of liver function tests is appropriate when initiating therapy and in patients with hepatic impairment.

Hematologic

Bone marrow suppression. Routine laboratory studies (RBC, WBC, differential counts) should be scheduled. Stress the importance of the patient returning for this laboratory work. Monitor for sore throat, fever, purpura, jaundice, or excessive and progressive weakness.

Hypersensitivity

Fever, pruritus, rash. Report symptoms for further evaluation by the healthcare provider. Pruritus may be relieved by adding baking soda to the bathwater.

■ Drug Interactions

Theophylline Derivatives. Xanthine oxidase inhibitors, when given with theophylline derivatives, may cause theophylline toxicity. Observe for vomiting, dizziness, restlessness, and cardiac arrhythmias. The dosage of theophylline may need to be reduced.

Azathioprine, Mercaptopurine. Xanthine oxidase inhibitors inhibit the metabolism of these agents. When initiating therapy with azathioprine or mercaptopurine, start at one fourth to one third of the normal dosage and adjust subsequent dosages according to the patient's response.

Chlorpropamide. Allopurinol may reduce the metabolism of chlorpropamide. Monitor for hypoglycemia (headache, weakness, decreased coordination, general apprehension, diaphoresis, hunger, and blurred or double vision). The dosage of the hypoglycemic agent may need to be reduced. Notify the healthcare provider if any of these symptoms appear.

Ampicillin, Amoxicillin. There is a high incidence of rash when patients are taking both allopurinol and ampicillin or amoxicillin. Do not consider the patient allergic to either drug until sensitivity tests identify a hypersensitivity reaction.

Cyclophosphamide. There is a greater incidence of bone marrow depression in patients receiving allopurinol and cyclophosphamide concurrently. Monitor for sore throat, fever, purpura, jaundice, or excessive and progressive weakness.

Didanosine. Febuxostat increases serum levels of didanosine when used concurrently. Use of these agents concurrently is contraindicated.

Get Ready for the NCLEX® Examination!

Key Points

- Colchicine, probenecid, and the xanthine oxidase inhibitors are used to treat gout.
- Donepezil (Aricept) and memantine (Namenda) are used to treat dementia in Alzheimer's disease.

Additional Learning Resources

SG Go to your Study Guide for additional Review Questions for the NCLEX® Examination, Critical Thinking Clinical Situations, and other learning activities to help you master this chapter content.

evolve Go to your Evolve website (http://evolve .elsevier.com/Clayton) for additional online resources.

Review Questions for the NCLEX® Examination

1. The nurse is preparing to administer the medication allopurinol (Zyloprim) to an elderly patient and understands that this is used to treat:
   1. Alzheimer's disease.
   2. alcohol abuse.
   3. gout secondary to antineoplastic therapy.
   4. acute attacks of gouty arthritis.

2. The nurse is educating the family of an elderly patient on the mechanism of action for donepezil (Aricept). Which statement by the family indicated further teaching is needed?
   1. "As I understand it, this drug will improve the cognitive skills of my dad."
   2. "So you are saying that this drug is used in patients with mild-to-moderate dementia caused by Alzheimer's."
   3. "Are you saying that the enzyme that normally breaks down acetylcholine is inhibited by this medication?"
   4. "As I understand it, this medication will slow the progress of the neurodegeneration caused by Alzheimer's."

3. The nurse is teaching a patient about proper administration for probenecid. What information does the nurse include in the teaching plan? *(Select all that apply.)*
   1. "You will need to wait 2 to 3 weeks after an acute attack before starting the medicine."
   2. "The incidence of acute gout attacks will start to decrease in the first few months of therapy."
   3. "Before you start taking this, we need to get a blood sample for a baseline creatinine and BUN to monitor kidney function."
   4. "You will need to drink 2 to 3 quarts of fluid every day while taking this medicine."
   5. "If you are taking a hypoglycemic agent, be sure to monitor your glucose levels closely, as this may increase your blood sugar."

4. Because of the risk for hepatotoxicity, initial measurement and periodic monitoring of these liver function tests is appropriate for patients taking xanthine oxidase inhibitors. *(Select all that apply.)*
   1. BUN
   2. AST
   3. WBC
   4. ALT
   5. Platelets

5. When monitoring for adverse effects, the nurse will recognize which of the following as reportable symptoms related to colchicine? *(Select all that apply.)*
   1. Nausea, vomiting, diarrhea
   2. Dark tarry stools
   3. Nasal congestion
   4. Reduction in joint swelling
   5. Sore throat, fever, and progressive weakness

Nomogram for Calculating the Body Surface Area of Adults, Children, and Infants

evolve

http://evolve.elsevier.com/Clayton

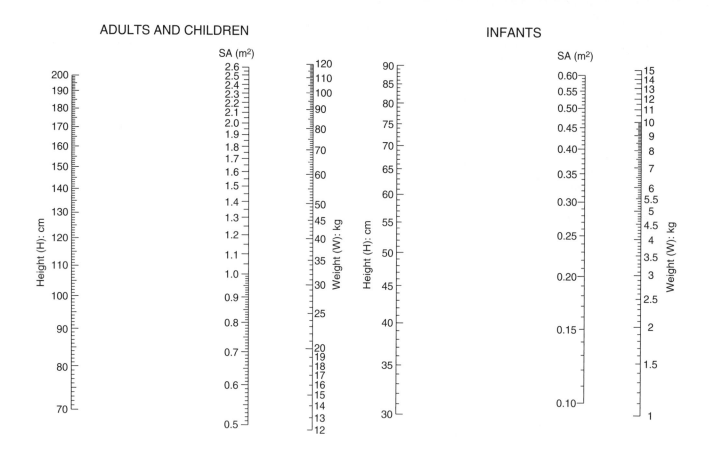

ADULTS AND CHILDREN

INFANTS

Template for Developing a Written Record for Patients to Monitor Their Own Therapy

PATIENT SELF-ASSESSMENT FORM **Self-Monitoring Drug Therapy Record**

MEDICATIONS	COLOR	TO BE TAKEN

Patient _____

Health Care Provider _____

Health Care Provider's phone _____

Next appt.* _____

What I Should Monitor	Premedication Data	Date	Date	Date	Date	Date	Date	Comments

Complete the premedication data column for use as a baseline to track response to drug therapy.
Instruct patient to bring this record to the next appointment.
Use the back of this sheet for additional information.

Bibliography

ONLINE RESOURCES

cpmcnet.columbia.edu/dept/partnership/publications.html Columbia University: *Partnership for Gender-Specific Medicine*, New York, 2009, Columbia University.

http://consumer.healthday.com/encyclopedia/pain-manage-ment-30/pain-health-news-520/pain-care-bill-of-rights-646163.html Pain Care Bill of Rights, American Pain Foundation.

http://health.gov/dietaryguidelines/2015-scientific-report/pdfs/scientific-report-of-the-2015-dietary-guidelines-advi-sory-committee.pdf

http://ibogaine.desk.nl/graphics/3639b1c_23.pdf: Beck depression inventory.

http://iom.nationalacademies.org/Reports.aspx?Series ={508F5CFF-EE88-4FF6-92BF-8D6CAB46F52E}&page=1 (1970-2014)

http://naturaldatabase.therapeuticresearch.com. Therapeutic Research Faculty.

http://www.nlm.nih.gov/medlineplus/ency/article/004024. htm Drugs that my cause impotence, 10/22/2012

rarediseases.info.nih.gov/Resources.aspx?PageID=1 National Institutes of Health, Office of Rare Diseases Research: *Rare diseases information*, 2015.

www.acc.org/qualityandscience/clinical/guidelines/failure/update/index.pdf American College of Cardiology; Hunt SA, et al: ACC/AHA 2005 Guideline Update for the Diagnosis and Management of Chronic Heart Failure in the Adult: A Report of the American College of Cardiology/American Heart Association Task Force on Practice Guidelines (Writing Committee to Update the 2001 Guidelines for the Evaluation and Management of Heart Failure), 2005, American College of Cardiology Foundation and the American Heart Association.

www.cancer.org/research/cancerfactsstatistics/cancerfactsfig-ures2015/index American Cancer Society: *Cancer facts and figures, 2015*, Atlanta, 2015, American Cancer Society.

www.cdc.gov/brfss Centers for Disease Control and Prevention: *National Center for Chronic Disease Prevention and Health Promotion: Behavioral risk factor surveillance system: Survey data and downloads*, Atlanta, 2015, U.S. Department of Health and Human Services.

www.cdc.gov/diabetes/pubs/pdf/ndfs_2015.pdf Centers for Disease Control and Prevention: *National diabetes fact sheet: General information and national estimates on diabetes in the U.S.*, Atlanta, 2015, U.S. Department of Health and Human Services.

www.cdc.gov/obesity/data/trends.html 2011-13 www.cdc.gov/nchs/fastats/deaths.htm Centers for Disease Control and Prevention; National Center for Health Statistics: *Deaths and mortality*, Atlanta, 2013, U.S. Department of Health and Human Services.

www.cordem.org/wellness.htm Council of Emergency Medicine Residency Directors; McNamara RM, Bouzoukis JK, Perina DG: Chemical dependency issues in emergency medicine residency programs. Lansing, MI, Council of Emergency Medicine Residency Directors.

www.drugabuse.gov/publications/drugfacts/methamphetamine –2014

www.fda.gov/consumer/updates/ucm101653 U.S. Food and Drug Administration: *How to dispose of unused medicines*, Rockville, MD, 2013, U.S. Food and Drug Administration.

www.fda.gov/downloads/Drugs/DrugSafety/UCM353335. pdf Magnesium Sulfate Drug Safety Communication—Recommendation against prolonged use in pre-term labor; U.S. Food and Drug Administration

www.fda.gov/drugs/scienceresearch/researchareas/pharma-cogenetics/ucm083378 Center for Drug Evaluation and Research: *Table of valid genomic biomarkers in the context of approved drug labels*, Rockville, MD, 2012, U.S. Food and Drug Administration.

www.ginasthma.org Global Initiative for Asthma (GINA): *Global strategy for asthma management and prevention* Revised 2014.

www.ginasthma.org Global Strategy for Asthma Management and Prevention, Global Initiative for Asthma (GINA) 2015.

www.goldcopd.org/guidelines-global-strategy-for-diagnosis-management.html 2014

www.health.gov/dietaryguidelines. *Dietary guidelines for Americans*, Washington, D.C., 2010, Department of Health and Human Services and Department of Agriculture.

www.idf.org/. The IDF consensus worldwide definition of the metabolic syndrome, Metabolic Syndrome 2014, Brussels, Belgium. International Diabetes Federation.

www.ins1.org Infusion Nurses Society: Infusion nursing. The Infusion Nurses Society promotes excellence in infusion nursing through standards, education, advocacy, and outcomes research.

www.iom.edu/activities/Nutrition/SummaryDRIs/DRI-Tables.aspx Institute of Medicine: Dietary Reference Intakes Tables and Application.

www.ismp.org/Tools/highalertmedications.pdf Institute for Safe Medication Practices: *ISMP's list of high-alert medications*, Horsham, PA, 2014, Institute for Safe Medication Practices.

www.isomerdesign.com/Cdsa/index.php Isomer Design: *Canadian Controlled Drugs and Substances Act.* 2008.

www.jointcommission.org/SentinelEvents/SentinelEventAl-ert/sea_35.htm The Joint Commission: Sentinel event alert: *Using medication reconciliation to prevent errors*, Oakbrook Terrace, IL, 2006, The Joint Commission.

www.nanda.org/nanda-international-publications.html NANDA International Nursing: Definitions and classification, 2015-17

www.nap.edu/openbook.php?isbn=0309085373 Food and Nutrition Board; Institute of Medicine of the National Academies: *Dietary reference intakes for energy, carbohydrate, fiber, fat, fatty acids, cholesterol, protein, and amino acids*, Washington DC, 2005, National Academies Press.

www.nccn.org/professionals/physician_gls/PDF/antiemesis. pdf *NCCN Guidelines Version 2. 2014.* Antiemesis; National Comprehensive Cancer Network, 2015.

www.nhlbi.nih.gov/about/factbook/chapter4.htm#4_7.

www.nhlbi.nih.gov/guidelines/asthma/asthgdln.htm National Heart Lung and Blood Institute: Expert Panel Report 3 (EPR3): *Guidelines for the diagnosis and management of asthma*, Bethesda, MD, 2007, National Institutes of Health, U.S. Department of Health and Human Services.

www.nhlbi.nih.gov/guidelines/asthma/index.htm National Asthma Education and Prevention Program: *Executive summary of the NAEPP expert panel report: Guidelines for the diagnosis and management of asthma*, Bethesda, MD, 2007, U.S. Department of Health and Human Services, Public Health

Service, National Institutes of Health, National Heart, Lung, and Blood Institute.

www.nhlbi.nih.gov/health/public/heart/obesity/phy_active.pdf U.S. Department of Health and Human Services; National Institutes of Health; National Heart, Lung, and Blood Institute: *Your guide to physical activity and your heart. NIH Publication No. 06–5714*, Bethesda, MD, 2006, U.S. Department of Health and Human Services.

www.oldwayspt.org *Food issues think tank. Oldways*, 2015.

www.painfoundation.org. Pain care bill of rights, Baltimore, MD, American Pain Foundation.

www.samhsa.gov/data/NSDUH/2012SummNatFindDetTables/Index.aspx: Substance Abuse and Mental Health Services Administration, *Results from the 2012 National Survey on Drug Use and Health: Mental Health Findings, NSDUH Series H-47, HHS Publication No. (SMA) 13-4805.* Rockville, MD: Substance Abuse and Mental Health Services Administration, 2013.

www.surgeongeneral.gov/library/mentalhealth/home.html. U.S. Department of Health and Human Services: *Mental health: A report of the Surgeon General*, Rockville, MD, 1999, U.S. Department of Health and Human Services.

www.unodc.org/documents/scientific/ATS/Global-ATS-Assessment-Exec-summary.pdf United Nations Office on Drugs and Crime: *Executive summary: Amphetamines and ecstasy. Global ATS Assessment*, 2011.

www.unodc.org/documents/scientific/ATS/Global-ATS-Assessment-Exec-summary.pdf *United Nations Office of Drug Control and Crime Prevention: Methamphetamine*, 2008.

PUBLICATIONS

Aboa-Eboule C, et al: Job strain and risk of acute recurrent coronary heart disease events, *JAMA* 298:1652, 2007.

Abramowicz M: *Treatment guidelines, Medical letter*, New Rochelle, NY, 2015, The Medical Letter.

Abrams P, et al: The standardisation of terminology of lower urinary tract function: Report from the Standardisation Subcommittee of the International Continence Society, *Neurourol Urodynam* 21:167, 2002.

Alberti KG, et al: Harmonizing the metabolic syndrome: a joint interim statement of the International Diabetes Federation Task Force on Epidemiology and Prevention; National Heart, Lung, and Blood Institute; American Heart Association; World Heart Federation; International Atherosclerosis Society; and International Association for the Study of Obesity, *Circulation* 120(16):1640–1645, 2009.

Alden K, Lowdermilk DL, et al: *Maternity and women's health care*, ed 10, St Louis, 2011, Mosby.

American Association of Clinical Endocrinologists: Medical guideline for Clinical Practice for Developing a Diabetes Mellitus Comprehensive Care Plan. 2011, *Endocr Pract* 17(Suppl 2):2011.

American College of Gastroenterology Chronic Constipation Task Force: An evidence-based approach to the management of chronic constipation in North America, *Am J Gastroenterology* 100(Suppl 1):S1, 2005.

American Diabetes Association: Standards of Medical Care in Diabetes, *Diabetes Care* 38(Suppl 1):S4, 2015.

American Pain Society: *Principles of analgesic use in the treatment of acute pain and cancer pain*, ed 6, Chicago, IL, 2008, American Pain Society.

American Psychiatric Association: *Diagnostic and statistical manual of mental disorders*, ed 5, Washington DC, 2013, American PsychiatricPublishing.

Baldwin JN, Thibault ED: Substance abuse by pharmacists: stopping the insanity, *J Am Pharm Assoc* 41:373, 2001.

Beck AT, Steer RA, Brown GK: *Beck depression inventory II (BDI-II) manual*, ed 2, Indianapolis, 1996, Pearson Education.

Beers H: Explicit criteria for determining potentially inappropriate medication use by the elderly: an update, *Arch Intern Med* 157:1531, 1997.

Bickley LS: *Bates' guide to physical examination and history taking*, ed 10, Philadelphia, 2009, Wolters Kluwer Health/Lippincott Williams & Wilkins.

Billups NF, Billups SM, editors: *American Drug Index 2014*, ed 58, Philadelphia, 2014, Lippincott, Williams & Wilkins.

Brown LM, Isetts BJ: Patient assessment and consultation. In *Handbook of non-prescription drugs*, ed 17, Washington, DC, 2012, American Pharmacists Association, p 27.

Brunton L, et al: *Goodman and Gilman's* the Pharmacological Basis of Therapeutics, ed 12, New York, 2010, McGraw-Hill.

Canadian Pharmacists Association, editor: *Compendium of pharmaceuticals and specialties 2014*, Ottawa, Canada, 2014, Canadian Pharmacists Association.

Canadian Pharmacists Association, editor: *Compendium of self-care products 2010*, Ottawa, Canada, 2010, Canadian Pharmacists Association.

Carpenito LJ: *Nursing diagnosis: application to clinical practice*, ed 14, Philadelphia, 2013, Wolters Kluwer Health/Lippincott Williams & Wilkins.

Centers for Disease Control and Prevention: *National Diabetes Statistics Report: Estimates of Diabetes and Its Burden in the United States, 2014*, Atlanta, GA, 2014, U.S. Department of Health and Human Services.

Centers for Disease Control and Prevention: Sexually transmitted diseases treatment guidelines. 2010, *MMWR Recomm Rep* 59(RR12):1–110, 2010.

Chabner BA: Clinical Strategies for Cancer Treatment. The role of drugs. In Chabner BA, Longo DL, editors: *Cancer Chemotherapy and Biotherapy: Principles and Practice*, ed 5, Philadelphia, 2010, Lippincott Williams & Wilkins.

Chandola T, Brunner E, Marmot M: Chronic stress at work and the metabolic syndrome: prospective study, *BMJ* 332:521, 2006.

Chen JJ, Swope DM: Parkinson's Disease. In DiPiro JT, et al, editors: *Pharmacotherapy, a pathophysiologic approach*, ed 9, New York, 2014, McGraw-Hill, pp 911–924.

Chong OT: An integrative approach to addressing clinical issues in complementary and alternative medicine in an outpatient oncology center, *Clin J Oncol Nurs* 10:83, 2006.

Clayton BD, Brown BK: Nausea and vomiting. In Helms RA, et al, editors: *Textbook of therapeutics, drug and disease management*, ed 8, Philadelphia, 2006, Lippincott Williams & Wilkins.

Cohen H: What are high-alert drugs and what role do they play in medication errors?, *Nursing Made Incredibly Easy* 7:7, 2008.

Criteria Committee of the New York Heart Association: *Nomenclature and criteria for diagnosis of diseases of the heart and great vessels*, ed 9, Boston, 1994, Little, Brown.

DiPiro JT, et al: *Pharmacotherapy, a pathophysiologic approach*, ed 9, New York, 2014, McGraw-Hill.

Dopheide JA, Stimmel GL: Sleep disorders. In Koda-Kimble MA, Young LY, editors: *Applied therapeutics*, ed 9, Philadelphia, 2009, Lippincott Williams & Wilkins.

Eckel RH, et al: 2013 AHA/ACC Guidelines on Lifestyle Management to Reduce Cardiovascular Risk: A Report of the American College of Cardiology/American Heart Association Task Force on Practice Guidelines, *Circulation* 2013. doi: 10.1161/01.cir.0000437740.48606.d1.

Ewing JA: Detecting alcoholism: The CAGE questionnaire, *JAMA* 252:1905, 1984.

Expert Panel on Detection, Evaluation, and Treatment of High Blood Cholesterol in Adults: *Third report of the National Cholesterol Education Program (NCEP), NIH Publication No. 025215*, Bethesda, MD, 2002, National Heart, Lung, and Blood Institute, National Institutes of Health.

Facts and Comparisons: *Drug facts and comparisons, 2015*, St Louis, 2015, Wolters Kluwer.

Fick D, et al: Updating the Beers Criteria for potentially inappropriate medication use in older adults: Results of a U.S. consensus panel of experts, *Arch Intern Med* 163:2716, 2003.

French JA, Pedley TA: Clinical practice. Initial management of epilepsy, *N Engl J Med* 359:166, 2008.

Garber AJ, et al: AACE Comprehensive Diabetes Management Algorithm 2013, *Endocr Pract* 19:327, 2013.

Gilbert DN, et al: *The Sanford Guide to Antimicrobial Therapy 2014*, ed 44, Sperryville, Va, 2014, Antimicrobial Therapy, Inc.

Go AS, Mazaffarian D, Roger JD, et al: Heart Disease and Stroke Statistics 2014 Update; A report from the American Heart Association, *Circulation* 129:e28–e292, 2013.

Goldman L, et al, editors: *Cecil textbook of medicine*, ed 24, Philadelphia, 2012, Saunders.

Guyton AC, Hall J: *Textbook of medical physiology*, ed 12, Philadelphia, 2011, Saunders.

Haas DM, Caldwell DM, Kirkpatrick P, et al: Tocolytic therapy for preterm delivery: systematic review and network meta-analysis, *BMJ* 345:e6226, doi: 10.1136/bmj.e6226. (published Oct. 9, 2012).

Hatcher RA, et al: *Contraceptive technology*, ed 20, New York, 2008, Ardent Media.

Helms RA, editor: *Textbook of therapeutics, drug and disease management*, ed 8, Philadelphia, 2006, Lippincott Williams & Wilkins.

Henderson ML: Self-care and nonprescription pharmacotherapy. In Krinsky DL, et al, editors: *Handbook of non-prescription drugs*, ed 17, Washington, DC, 2012, American Pharmacists Association.

Hines LE, et al: Critical issues associated with drug-drug interactions: highlights of a multistakeholder conference, *Am J Health-System Pharmacy* 68(10):941–946, 2011.

Hockenberry M, Wilson D: *Wong's nursing care of infants and children*, ed 9, St Louis, 2011, Mosby.

Ignatavicius DD, Workman ML: *Medical-surgical nursing: patient-centered collaborative care*, ed 7, Philadelphia, 2013, Saunders.

Infusion Nurses Society: *Infusion nursing standards of practice (2011)*, Store.untreedreads.com Institute of Medicine, Food and Nutrition Board: Dietary reference intakes: a risk assessment model for establishing upper intake levels for nutrients, Washington, DC, 1998, National Academy Press.

International Association for the Study of Pain, Subcommittee on Taxonomy: Classification of chronic pain. Descriptions of chronic pain syndromes and definitions of pain terms, *Pain Suppl* 3:S1, 1986.

James PA, et al: 2014 Evidence-based Guideline for the Management of High Blood Pressure in Adults; Report From the panel Members Appointed to the Eighth Joint National Committee (JNC 8), *JAMA* 2014. doi: 10.1001/jama.2013.284427.

Jarvis C: *Physical examination and health assessment*, ed 6, St Louis, 2011, Saunders.

Joint National Committee on Detection, Evaluation and Treatment of High Blood Pressure: *The seventh report of the National Committee on Detection, Evaluation and Treatment of High Blood Pressure (JNC 7)*, NIH Publication 03–5233, Bethesda, MD, 2003, National Institutes of Health.

Jones CM, Mack KA, Paulozzi LJ: Pharmaceutical Overdose Deaths, United States, 2010, *JAMA* 309(7):657–659, 2013.

Kaskutas LA, Bond J, Humphreys K: Social networks as mediators of the effects of Alcoholics Anonymous, *Addiction* 97:891, 2002.

Keltner NL, Steele D: *Psychiatric nursing*, ed 7, St Louis, 2014, Mosby.

Koda-Kimble MA, Young LY, editors: *Applied therapeutics*, ed 10, Philadelphia, 2012, Wolters Kluwer/Lippincott, Williams and Wilkins.

Kotecki JE: *Physical activity and health: an interactive approach*, ed 4, Boston, 2013, Jones & Bartlett Learning, Inc.

Lasser KE, et al: Timing of new black box warnings and withdrawal for prescription medications, *JAMA* 287:2215, 2002.

Laudet AB, Savage R, Mahmood D: Pathways to long-term recovery: a preliminary investigation, *J Psychoactive Drugs* 34:305, 2002.

Lazarou J, Pomeranz B, Corey P: Incidence of adverse drug reactions in hospitalized patients: a meta-analysis of prospective studies, *JAMA* 279:1200, 1998.

Leininger M: *Transcultural nursing:concepts, theories, and practices*, ed 3, New York, 2002, McGraw-Hill.

LeMone P, Burke K: *Medical-surgical nursing: critical thinking in client care*, ed 5, Upper Saddle River, NJ, 2010, Pearson.

Lewis S, et al: *Medical-surgical nursing: assessment and management of clinical problems*, St Louis, 2014, Mosby.

Lindenfeld J, et al: Executive summary: HFSA 2010 comprehensive heart failure practice guideline, *J Card Fail* 16:475–539, 2010.

Lindholm LH, Carlberg B, Samuelsson O: Should beta blockers remain first choice in the treatment of primary hypertension? A meta-analysis, *Lancet* 366:1545, 2005.

Lineberry TW, Bostwick JM: Methamphetamine abuse: A perfect storm of complications, *Mayo Clin Proc* 81:77, 2006.

McCance KL, Huether SE: *Pathophysiology: the biologic basis for disease in adults and children*, ed 7, St Louis, 2013, Mosby.

McEvoy G, editor: *AHFS drug information 2015*, Bethesda, MD, 2015, American Society of Health-System Pharmacists.

McPherson TL, Hersch RK: Brief substance use screening instruments for primary care settings: a review, *J Substance Abuse Treat* 18:193, 2000.

McVary KT: Clinical practice. Erectile dysfunction, *N Engl J Med* 357:2472, 2007.

Meiner S, Lueckenotte AG: *Gerontologic nursing*, ed 4, St Louis, 2011, Mosby.

Melzack R: The McGill pain questionnaire: major properties and scoring methods, *Pain* 1:277, 1975.

Moore N, et al: Frequency and cost of serious adverse drug reactions in a department of general medicine, *Br J Clin Pharmacol* 45:301, 1998.

Mulhall A: Nursing, research, and the evidence, *Evid Based Nurs* 1:4, 1998.

National High Blood Pressure Education Program Coordinating Committee: Seventh report of the Joint National Committee on Prevention, Detection, Evaluation, and Treatment of High Blood Pressure, *Hypertension* 42:1206, 2003.

National Research Council: *To err is human: building a safer health system*, Washington, DC, 2000, The National Academies Press.

Niebyl JR: Nausea and vomiting in pregnancy, *N Engl J Med* 363:1544–1550, 2010.

Nix S: *Williams' basic nutrition and diet therapy*, ed 14, St Louis, 2012, Mosby.

O'Gara PT, Kushner FG, Aschei DD, et al: 2013 ACCF/AHA Guideline for the Management of ST-Elevation Myocardial Infarction, *Circulation* 127:e362–e425, 2013. doi: 10.1161/CIR. Ob013e3182742cf6.

Pagana KD, Pagana TJ: *Mosby's manual of diagnostic and laboratory tests*, ed 5, St Louis, 2013, Mosby.

Parker RB, Nappi JM, Cavallari LH: Chronic heart failure. In DiPiro JP, et al, editors: *Pharmacotherapy: a pathophysiologic approach*, ed 9, New York, 2014, McGraw-Hill, pp 85–122.

Physicians' desk reference, ed 69, Montvale, NJ, 2015, PDR Network, LLC.

Potter PA, Perry AG: *Fundamentals of nursing*, ed 8, St Louis, 2012, Mosby.

Prochaska J, DiClemente C, Towards a comprehensive model of change: Miller W, Heather N, editors: *Treating addictive behaviors: a process of change*, New York, 1986, Plenum Press.

Reid WH: Recognizing and dealing with impaired clinicians, part I: recognition and reporting, *J Med Pract Manage* 17:97, 2001.

Reid WH: Recognizing and dealing with impaired clinicians, part II: treatment options, *J Med Pract Manage* 17:145, 2001.

Repchinsky C, editor: *Patient self-care: helping patients make therapeutic choices*, ed 2, Ottawa, Canada, 2010, Canadian Pharmacists Association.

Roger VL, et al: Heart Disease and Stroke Statistics—2011 Update: A Report From the American Heart Association, *Circulation* 123:e18–e209, 2011. originally pubished online Dec 15, 2010.